Microcirculation in Cancer Metastasis

Editors

F. William Orr, M.D.
Professor
Department of Pathology
McMaster University
Hamilton, Ontario, Canada

Michael R. Buchanan, Ph.D.
Associate Professor
Department of Pathology
McMaster University
Hamilton, Ontario, Canada

Leonard Weiss, M.D., Ph.D.
Chief Cancer Research Clinician and Director
Department of Experimental Pathology
Roswell Park Cancer Institute
Buffalo, New York

CRC Press
Taylor & Francis Group
Boca Raton London New York

CRC Press is an imprint of the
Taylor & Francis Group, an **informa** business

CRC Press
Taylor & Francis Group
6000 Broken Sound Parkway NW, Suite 300
Boca Raton, FL 33487-2742

ISBN 13: 978-0-8493-6154-8 (hbk)

Visit the Taylor & Francis Web site at
http://www.taylorandfrancis.com

and the CRC Press Web site at
http://www.crcpress.com

Library of Congress Cataloging-in-Publication Data

Microcirculation in cancer metastasis / editors, F. William Orr,
Michael R. Buchanan, Leonard Weiss.
p. cm
Includes bibliographical references.
Includes index.
ISBN 0-8493-6154-0
1. Metastasis. 2. Microcirculation. 3. Cancer invasiveness.
4. Lymphatic metastasis. I. Orr, F. William. II. Buchanan,
Michael R., Ph.D. III. Weiss, Leonard.
[DNLM: 1. Microcirculation--physiopathology. 2. Neoplasm
Metastasis. QZ 202 M6263]
RC269.5.M53 1991
616.99'4071--dc20
DNLM/DLC
for Library of Congress 91-195
Library of Congress Number 91-195 CIP

PREFACE

Metastasis is the major clinical complication of most types of cancer and is a major consideration in its staging and treatment.

Cancer cells from primary lesions enter various disseminative routes, particularly the veins, lymphatics, and body cavities. Usually, but not always, this involves an invasive process characterized by degradation of basement membranes, which separate the primary cancer from the adjacent "normal" tissues, surround the vessels, and inhibit the intravasation and extravasation of the cancer cells.

The most frequent disseminative routes are via the lymphatic system and the bloodstream. Metastasis via the lymphatic system usually results in lymph node involvement, which provides a useful, though limited, index of the extent of the disease and, consequently, an indication for treatment and prognosis. Although some cancer cells within the lymphatic system may also enter the bloodstream via the thoracic duct and other common connections, entry of cancer cells from the extravascular tissue directly into the bloodstream is probably the more common route for metastastic dissemination to many, if not most, of the target organs. Blood-borne cancer cells interact with the host leukocytes, platelets, plasma proteins of the coagulation system, and additionly, the vascular endothelium, a necessary step for their extravasation. Most cancer cells arrested in the microvasculature are killed by a variety of rapid and slow processes involving mechanical trauma, inflammation, and immune responses. The efficiency of these processes in terms of cancer cell survival is a major determinant in regulating the subsequent rate and pattern of hematogenous metastasis.

The trapping of cancer cells in the microvasculature involves an initial arrest process followed by an adhesion process. Cancer cell arrest is determined predominantly by mechanical factors such as the types of vessels through which cancer cell emboli traverse and by the topographical relationship between the primary cancer and the vascular network. Multicellular emboli become trapped in small veins and arterioles, whereas single cancer cells become trapped in the capillary network. For example, in colon cancer, most cancer cells entering the portal vein or its tributaries arrest in the liver sinusoids, and a very small proportion of the cancer cells is shunted via the inferior vena cava into the pulmonary arteries and the lungs. In contrast, the majority of cancer cells entering systemic veins arrest in the lung, and only a small proportion of them passes through the lungs into the pulmonary veins to be delivered to other end organs. Those cancer cells that do leave the lungs disseminate ultimately via an arterial route. While most arrested cancer cells do not survive the host's defense mechanisms, those cancer cells that do survive arrest-related events must extravasate in order to become clinically significant. The expression of adhesion molecules facilitates cancer cell attachment to the endothelium or its underlying basement membrane. Extravasation is then accomplished by a "bursting-out" process due to the forces generated by expansile, intravascular growth coupled with the degradation of specific components of the vessel wall. The enzymes that contribute to this latter process appear to be released not only from the cancer cells, but also from the vascular endothelium and from the blood cells responsible for the inflammatory response. In some cases, particularly with lymphoreticular cancer, extravasation may be accomplished predominantly by the cancer cells that actively migrate through the vessel walls.

The extent of both intravascular and extravascular growth is limited by diffusion of nutrients from the host vasculature and by host responses. Early growth culminates in *micrometastases* with diameters of 0.1 to 0.2 cm, which are not detectable by presently available, noninvasive clinical procedures. The subsequent development of clinically detectable metastasis is dependent upon acquisition of a neovasculature by the process of angiogenesis. This removes the diffusion-limited restraints on growth into larger metastases. Although neovascularization is a major factor in the growth of metastases, it is only one parameter of a set of complex host responses, which either promote or inhibit tumor growth and other metastasis-related processes.

The final step in the metastatic cycle is the metastasis of metastases, which poses a threat to the long-term survival of patients who have had their primary lesions resected.

In summary, the interactions of cancer cells with the microvasculature appear to play a pivotal role in hematogenous metastasis. The purpose of this publication is to provide an in-depth review that focuses on these and related interactions from a multidisciplinary viewpoint. The sequence of chapters in this volume is presented as far as possible in the same order as the events of the metastatic cascade outlined above.

In Chapter 1, Varani and Chakrabarty describe the regulation and synthesis of extracellular matrix molecules by cancer cells with an emphasis on the relationship to cancer cell transformation and differentiation. Terranova (Chapter 2) outlines the structure of basement membranes and extracellular matrices and describes how these components modulate the metastatic properties of cancer cells. Subsequent interactions between the cancer cells and the vessel wall must take into account the basic biology of endothelial cells (reviewed by Buchanan and Bertomeu in Chapter 3). Specific aspects of intravasation are then discussed by De Bruyn and Hellmann with respect to destructive and nondestructive entry. De Bruyn (Chapter 4) notes apparent similarities between leukemic cells and lymphocytes, while Hellmann (Chapter 5) explores the importance of tumor neovasculature to intravasation and reviews the possibilities for pharmacologic control. Interactions between circulating cancer cells and host leukocytes are reviewed by Glaves (Chapter 6). She discusses evidence that leukocytes may act in a dual capacity by (1) contributing to intravascular tumor cell death and (2) promoting cancer cell attachment and metastasis. Honn et al. (Chapter 7) review the mechanisms and effects of interactions between cancer cells and platelets. Chelladurai (Chapter 8) describes pathways by which cancer cells initiate the generation of active thrombin and summarizes evidence that blood coagulation promotes metastasis. Biophysical aspects of arrest, together with an account of the rapid deformation-associated trauma to which intravascular cancer cells are exposed, are discussed by Weiss (Chapter 9). The role of adhesive macromolecules that play an important part in adhesion of cancer cells to the endothelium and basement membrane is reviewed by Kramer et al. (Chapter 10). Organ-specific arrest in relation to metastatic pattern is reviewed by Auerbach (Chapter 11). Intraorgan-specific localization of metastasis is then discussed in the context of the liver, which is a common target organ for hematogenous metastasis; Barberá-Guillem and Vidal-Vanaclocha (Chapter 12) address the question of where in the liver sinusoid arrest occurs. The morphology of cancer cell arrest in the microvasculature is discussed by Crissman et al. (Chapter 13), and the events leading to extravasation also are described. The effects of fatty acid metabolism on cancer cell-endothelial cell interactions are described by Buchanan et al. in Chapter 14, and the related effects of eicosanoids are described by Honn et al. in Chapter 7. Orr surveys the effects of microvascular injury and inflammatory reactions on metastasis, which emphasize the influence of drugs and environmental factors and similarities between the processes of metastasis and inflammation (Chapter 15). Vascularization not only plays a central role in tumor biology, but also profoundly affects response to local therapy and provides access points for the intravasation of cancer cells. The key processes of angiogenesis and neovascularization are reviewed by Moses in Chapter 16. The related complexities of the tumor microcirculation are reviewed by Peterson in Chapter 17.

F. William Orr
Michael R. Buchanan
Leonard Weiss

THE EDITORS

Frederick William Orr, M.D., is a Professor in the Department of Pathology at McMaster University, Hamilton, Ontario. Dr. Orr graduated from the Faculty of Medicine at the University of Alberta, Edmonton, Canada, and subsequently trained in Pathology at the College of Physicians and Surgeons, Columbia University, New York City.

Dr. Orr is a Fellow of the Royal College of Physicians and Surgeons of Canada and a member of the Canadian Association of Pathologists, the American Association for Cancer Research, the American Association of Pathologists, the Canadian Society for Clinical Investigation, and the Metastases Research Society.

Among other awards, he has been a Fellow of the R. Samuel McLaughlin Foundation and a Research Scholar and Clinical Research Associate of the National Cancer Institute of Canada. Dr. Orr is the author of more than 75 papers. His current research interests relate to interactions between cancer cells and the blood vessel wall and to studies on the metastasis of cancer to bone.

Michael R. Buchanan, Ph.D., is an Associate Professor in the Department of Pathology, Experimental Thromboembolism Program, McMaster University, Hamilton, Ontario, a Senior Scientist at the Hamilton Civic Hospitals Research Centre, Henderson Hospital, Hamilton, Ontario, and the Director of Surgical Research, McMaster University and Hamilton Civic Hospitals, Hamilton General Hospital, Hamilton, Ontario.

Dr. Buchanan completed his undergraduate studies at the University of Toronto in 1970 and then obtained his M.Sc. and Ph.D. in Medical Sciences at McMaster University in 1974 and 1978. In 1980, he served both as a Research Fellow in the Department of Pathology at Harvard University, Boston, Massachusetts, and as a Research Associate at the Peter Bent Brigham Hospital, Boston, Massachusetts.

Dr. Buchanan is a member of the International Society of Thrombosis and Haemostasis, the American Heart Association, Council on Thrombosis, the Canadian Atherosclerosis Society, the International Society of Applied Cardiovascular Biology, the New York Academy of Sciences, and the Royal Society of Medicine.

Among other awards, Dr. Buchanan has received a number of Career Investigator awards from the Canadian Heart Foundation. In 1989, he was the recipient of the Third Sanofi Foundation for Thrombosis Research prize, awarded at the International Society of Thrombosis and Haemostasis meetings in Tokyo.

Dr. Buchanan has presented 101 invited lectures at various universities and institutes around the world and 106 presentations at international meetings. He also has published 145 research papers. His current research interests include both basic and applied studies, investigating (1) fatty acid metabolism as it relates to integrin expression by circulating blood and vessel wall cells and subsequent influences on thrombosis and metastasis and (2) the relative effects of anticoagulants on the inhibition of circulating vs. bound thrombin and subsequent benefit in venous and arterial thrombosis.

Leonard Weiss, M.D., Ph.D., is a Chief Cancer Research Clinician and the Director of the Department of Experimental Pathology, Roswell Park Cancer Institute, Buffalo, New York. He is also Research Professor of Biophysics and Interdisciplinary Sciences, State University of New York, Buffalo, New York.

Dr. Weiss is a graduate of the University of Cambridge: he received his B.A. in Natural Sciences in 1950, his M.B., B. Chir. in 1953, his M.D. in 1958, and his Ph.D. in 1963. He was awarded his Sc.D. in 1971.

Dr. Weiss is a Fellow of the Royal College of Pathologists, the College of American Pathologists, the Institute of Biology, and the American Association for the Advancement of Science.

Dr. Weiss has presented many invited lectures at international and national meetings and guest lectures at universities and institutes. He has published more than 250 research papers, in addition to writing three monographs and editing eight books. He has a long-standing interest in the pathobiology and biophysics of metastasis.

CONTRIBUTORS

Robert Auerbach, Ph.D.
Harold R. Wolfe Professor of Zoology
Center for Developmental Biology
University of Wisconsin
Madison, Wisconsin

Emilio Barberá-Guillem, M.D., Ph.D.
Professor and Head
Department of Cell Biology and Morphological Sciences
School of Medicine and Dentistry
University of the Basque Country
Leioa, Vizcaya
Spain

Maria C. Bertomeu, M.D.
Fellow
Department of Pathology
McMaster University
Hamilton, Ontario
Canada

Robert F. Cerra, Ph.D.
Department of Surgery
Henry Ford Hospital
Detroit, Michigan

Subhas Chakrabarty, Ph.D.
Assistant Professor
Department of Laboratory Medicine
M. D. Anderson Cancer Center
University of Texas
Houston, Texas

Mohan Chelladurai, Ph.D.
Assistant Professor
Department of Radiation Oncology
Wayne State University
Detroit, Michigan

Yao Fen Cheng, M.Sc.
Assistant Specialist
Department of Anatomy and Stomatology
University of California
San Francisco, California

Hemi Chopra, Ph.D.
Research Associate
Department of Radiation Oncology
Wayne State University
Gershenson Radiation Oncology Center
Harper Hospital
Detroit, Michigan

John D. Crissman, M.D.
Chief
Department of Pathology
Harper Hospital
Detroit, Michigan

Peter P. H. De Bruyn, M.D., Ph.D.
Professor Emeritus
Department of Organismal Biology and Anatomy
Committee on Immunology
University of Chicago
Chicago, Illinois

Judy Enenstein, Ph.D.
Postdoctoral Fellow
Department of Anatomy and Stomatology
University of California
San Francisco, California

Dorothy Glaves, Ph.D.
Cancer Research Scientist
Department of Experimental Pathology
Roswell Park Memorial Institute
Buffalo, New York

Irma M. Grossi, Ph.D.
Research Associate
Department of Radiation Oncology
Wayne State University
Gershenson Radiation Oncology Center
Harper Hospital
Detroit, Michigan

Thomas A. Haas, B.Sc.
Graduate Student
Department of Pathology
McMaster University
Hamilton, Ontario
Canada

Kurt Hellmann, D.M.
Honorary Professor
Department of Radiotherapy and Oncology
Westminster Hospital
London, England

Kenneth V. Honn, Ph.D.
Professor and Head
Cancer Biology Division
Department of Radiation Oncology
Wayne State University
Gershenson Radiation Oncology Center
Harper Hospital
Detroit, Michigan

Randall H. Kramer, Ph.D.
Associate Professor
Department of Anatomy and Stomatology
Cardiovascular Research Institute
University of California
San Francisco, California

David E. Maslow, Ph.D.
Scientific Review Administrator
Grants Review Branch
National Cancer Institute
National Institutes of Health
Bethesda, Maryland

Marsha A. Moses, Ph.D.
Instructor and Research Associate
Department of Surgical Research
Children's Hospital Medical Center
Harvard Medical School
Boston, Massachusetts

Hans-Inge Peterson, M.D., Ph.D.
Associate Professor
Laboratory of Biorheology
Department of Surgery I
Sahlgrenska University Hospital
Head, Department of Surgery
Lundby Hospital
Göteborg, Sweden

Daniel M. Ramos, D.D.S.
Postgraduate Research Dentist
Department of Anatomy and Stomatology
University of California
San Francisco, California

Fuzlul Sarkar, Ph.D.
Director
Molecular Biology Laboratory
Department of Pathology
Harper Hospital
Detroit, Michigan

John D. Taylor, Ph.D.
Professor
Department of Radiation Oncology and Biological Sciences
Wayne State University
Gershenson Radiation Oncology Center
Harper Hospital
Detroit, Michigan

Victor P. Terranova, D.M.D., Ph.D.
Director
Laboratory of Tumor Biology and Connective Tissue Research
Columbia University
New York, New York

Jozef Timar, Ph.D.
Visiting Scientist
Department of Radiation Oncology and Chemistry
Wayne State University
Gershenson Radiation Oncology Center
Harper Hospital
Detroit, Michigan

James Varani, Ph.D.
Professor
Department of Pathology
University of Michigan
Ann Arbor, Michigan

Fernando Vidal-Vanaclocha, Ph.D.
Professor
Department of Cell Biology and Morphological Sciences
School of Medicine and Dentistry
University of the Basque Country
Leioa, Vizcaya
Spain

Mai P. Vu, B.Sc.
Senior Research Assistant I
Department of Anatomy and Stomatology
University of California
San Francisco, California

ACKNOWLEDGMENT

The Editors wish to thank Laura Gamble for her secretarial help in editing and compiling this volume.

TABLE OF CONTENTS

Chapter 1

CHANGES IN THE EXTRACELLULAR MATRIX DURING TRANSFORMATION AND DIFFERENTIATION

James Varani and Subhas Chakrabarty

TABLE OF CONTENTS

I. INTRODUCTION

The events that constitute the metastatic cascade are influenced by properties of both the tumor and the host. For the past several years, investigators have separated the overall process of metastasis into individual steps and have attempted to delineate the specific tumor cell and host properties that influence each individual step. What tumor cell and host properties, for example, are responsible for the initial separation of tumor cells from the primary tumor mass? What underlies the ability of tumor cells to actively invade the surrounding normal tissue and to invade into the vasculature? Is invasion of circulating tumor cells through the vascular wall at secondary sites mediated by the same processes that are involved in invasion at the primary tumor site? By addressing the problem of metastasis in a reductionist manner, it has been possible to elucidate the mechanisms by which many of the individual steps occur. It hardly needs to be stated that multiple mechanisms are available and that different types of tumors as well as different tumors of a single (histological) type may utilize entirely different mechanisms to carry out the same basic processes.

The overall focus of this volume is on the interaction of malignant tumor cells with host elements in the microcirculation. It is generally accepted that once malignant tumor cells enter the circulation, their ability to survive passage through the vasculature and to localize at secondary "fertile" sites requires them to adhere to and interact with host elements in the microvasculature. Endothelial cells of the capillary beds, areas of exposed subendothelial basement membrane, and circulating elements such as platelets, lymphocytes, monocytes, and polymorphonuclear leukocytes are all potential targets. If we are to accept the hypothesis that successful metastatic tumor cells have a unique capacity for adhesion to appropriate host structures, we must rationalize this view with the other well-established observation that malignant cells are much less adhesive than their normal counterpart cells and that it is this loss of adhesiveness that contributes to their capacity for metastasis. In the past few years, there has been an explosion of information on cellular adhesion mechanisms at the cellular, biochemical, and molecular levels. We now understand the biochemical basis for a variety of cell-cell and cell-substrate adhesion reactions. Malignant cells show defects in some but not in all of the molecules that mediate adhesion responses. Thus, it is possible, we believe, for malignant cells to show decreased adhesion under some conditions while at the same time expressing normal or even increased adhesion under other conditions. The focus of this chapter will be on adhesion mechanisms of malignant cells, the differences between malignant cells and their nonmalignant counterparts in regard to these mechanisms, and how alterations in the mechanisms by which malignant tumor cells interact with their substratum and with other cells may contribute to their capacity for metastasis.

II. ALTERATIONS IN CELL-CELL AND CELL-SUBSTRATE ADHESION ACCOMPANYING MALIGNANT TRANSFORMATION

Studies carried out by Coman[1,2] and others[3] in the 1940s and 1950s showed that tumor tissues were often less cohesive than their corresponding normal tissues. It was observed that surgical specimens as well as experimental tumors could be dispersed into single cells by enzymatic or mechanical means much more readily than normal tissues. Low cohesiveness was postulated (quite reasonably) to facilitate separation of tumor cells from the main body of the tumor and to contribute in this way to the formation of distant metastasis. The biochemical and molecular basis for cell-cell and cell-substrate adhesion were unknown at the time. However, a role for divalent cations in adhesive processes was already known, and defects in response to Ca^{2+} were found to be characteristic of malignant cells.[4,5] Not surprisingly, abnormal Ca^{2+} metabolism was postulated to contribute to the adhesive defects in malignant cells.

Although the early studies on whole tumor tissues were crude and open to several interpretations, cell culture studies conducted during the same period provided precise, reliable, and incontrovertable evidence that malignant tumor cells from various sources were often less adherent to glass culture dishes and to assorted other substrata than nonmalignant cells of similar origin.[6-8] Altered adhesion could be detected as either reduced rates of attachment and spreading or as increased sensitivity to release from the substratum by mechanical means, proteolytic enzymes, or in some cases, chelators of divalent cations. How these *in vivo* and *in vitro* observations were related was not fully understood. Abercrombie and his collegues[9] as well as several other investigators[10] tried to relate the phenomena of contact inhibition of growth, contact guidance, and contact inhibition of cell motility to adhesiveness. It was reasoned that alterations in cell-cell and cell-substrate adhesion properties in malignant cells, in addition to facilitating tumor dispersion, also prevented the cells from receiving and properly processing signals that controlled such basic cellular properties as growth, morphology, and motility. While contact inhibition of proliferation and motility were defined on the basis of cell culture observations, loss of growth control and control of motility would have obvious implications for the behavior of cells *in vivo*. While these early studies precisely identified and characterized the biological difference between normal and malignant cells in terms of their adhesive characteristics, the biochemical and molecular basis for these differences remained largely unknown.

III. STRUCTURAL BASIS OF CELL-CELL AND CELL-MATRIX ADHESION

Cell-cell and cell-matrix adhesion properties of cells are critical to virtually every biological process, including fertilization, embryogenesis, parenchymal organ cell morphogenesis, nerve outgrowth, inflammation, and wound healing as well as cancer cell invasion and metastasis. Consequently, cells have evolved a complex series of adhesion receptors and corresponding ligands. Differential regulation of these receptors and ligands provides for a high degree of specificity and sensitivity in the regulations of critical adhesion functions.

A. ADHESION RECEPTORS AND THEIR LIGANDS

Studies from the 1960s and early 1970s showed that many of the major structural components of the extracellular matrix including collagen, fibronectin, fibrinogen/fibrin, and laminin serve as adhesion factors for cells in culture.[11-20] The structure and function of these proteins have been extensively characterized, and good review articles summarizing much of this work are available.[21-32] These large proteins consist of functionally distinct domains that mediate different events. Within domains that are functionally active as mediators of cell-substrate adhesion, there are unique sequences of amino acids that constitute cell-binding domains. The RGD sequence of fibronectin is the best characterized of these sequences.[33-36] The ability of small peptides containing this sequence of amino acids to support directly cell attachment or to inhibit attachment to intact fibronectin shows that binding of the large intact molecule (i.e., fibronectin) depends on the linear sequence of amino acids rather than on secondary or tertiary structure of the molecule and is mediated through a very short segment of amino acids. RGD-containing and non-RGD-containing cell-binding domains from fibronectin and other adhesion proteins also have been elucidated in recent research.[24]

The ability of various extracellular matrix molecules to promote complex biological responses such as cell attachment and spreading suggests the presence of specific cell surface receptors for these moieties. Binding studies with radio-labeled ligands has established that binding of these large adhesion factors occurs in a receptor-like fashion. Binding of matrix components by cells is time- and concentration-dependent, saturable, inhibitable with excess unlabelled ligand, and reversible. Similar kinds of data have been obtained with such diverse molecules as fibronectin, laminin, and thrombospondin.[37-43] In the case of each of these adhesion factors, there is a good relationship between the amount of ligand required to occupy surface receptors and the amount needed to induce adhesion. Antibodies to each ligand interfere with ligand binding and with the adhesion response to a comparable degree without affecting either binding or adhesion mediated by unrelated factors.

Cell surface proteins that constitute receptors for various extracellular matrix molecules have been identified on and isolated from a number of different cells.[44-50] One approach which has been successfully applied involves use of antibodies that interfere with cell-substrate adhesion to isolate cell surface components responsible for antibody binding. Another general approach has been to use the ligand in affinity separation systems. Both approaches have resulted in the isolation of a series of heterodymeric cell surface proteins that function as receptors for adhesion factors. In their native state, the proteins consist of a large (alpha) subunit and a smaller (beta) subunit. A common beta subunit can combine with a number of different alpha subunits. Ligand specificity is determined by the alpha subunit so that a single beta subunit may constitute part of the receptor for a number of different ligands. These heterodymeric receptors for the various extracellular matrix components are members of the integrin supergene family. Leukocyte-endothelial cell adhesion factors constitute another group within this family. It is beyond the scope of this review to discuss the structure of these moieties further, but a number of good recent review articles on the subject are available.[51] It should be pointed out that integrins are not the only moieties capable of binding adhesion factors. Nonintegrin glycoproteins,[38-40,50] proteoglycans,[41,42] and glycolipids[53,54] also serve as biologically important matrix receptors.

B. CONSEQUENCES OF ADHESION RECEPTOR-LIGAND INTERACTIONS

In the simplest systems, an adhesion factor such as fibronectin is adsorbed onto a substratum such as a polystyrene dish. Cells can then be added to the dish, and if they express surface receptors for the fibronectin molecule, they rapidly attach. Normally, in such assays, the polystyrene dishes are coated with a large amount of bovine serum albumin after the adhesion factor has had a chance to bind. This greatly reduces charge-mediated adhesion of cells directly to the polystyrene. Once cells have attached to the adsorbed adhesion factor, the attached cells may flatten out on the substrate. This process of cell spreading occurs because cell surface adhesion receptors are connected via specific proteins such as talin and α-actinin to major cytoskeletal elements.[55,56] Cell-substrate interaction leads to reorganization of the cytoskeleton, which in turn brings about the dramatic changes in cell shape. One of the initial cytoskeletal changes that follow from ligand binding to the cell surface is actin polymerization.[57] In a resting cell, a majority of the actin is monomeric. Polymerization, occurring as a consequence of adhesion factor binding, results in a majority of the cell actin becoming polymerized. It is a critical step in the formation of microfilament bundles. It should be noted that receptors for ligands other than adhesion factors can also lead to actin polymerization. Investigations by Rao and his colleagues[58] have documented actin polymerization as a consequence of the interaction of leukocytic cells with factors that induce activation (i.e., mitogenic lectins, chemotactic factors, phorbol esters, etc.). Not surprisingly, leukocyte activation is almost invariably associated with increased cell-cell and cell-substrate adhesion. Thus, the relationship between alterations in adhesion and cytoskeletal changes are complex and bidirectional. Another consequence of adhesion factor binding to the cell surface is an activation of phospholipid/arachidonic acid metabolism. Studies from our laboratory have shown that murine tumor cells respond to fibronectin or laminin by releasing ^{3}H-arachidonic acid from prelabeled phospholipid pools. Increased arachidonic-acid release is associated with elevated levels of arachidonic acid metabolites in the culture fluids.[59] Further consequences of receptor occupancy with the appropriate adhesion factors are felt in the nucleus. Altered gene transcription occurs, leading to the expression of novel phenotypic characteristics.[60] Thus, the binding of an adhesion factor to its cell surface receptor brings about a cascade of changes in cell behavior rather than simply facilitating cell adhesion to the substratum.

IV. REGULATION OF THE ADHESION RESPONSE IN NORMAL AND MALIGNANT CELLS

Since cell-cell and cell-matrix interactions are critical to virtually every major biological process, they must be closely regulated. This is accomplished through multiple, redundant receptor-ligand combinations that can be functionally inactive or active as the situation warrants. For example, monocytes and polymorphonuclear leukocytes express a repertoire of adhesion receptors which allow them to localize at sites of inflammation. These adhesion receptors are not normally expressed on the surface of resting cells, but are expressed in response to inflammatory stimuli.[61-63] Corresponding ligands on the endothelial cell surface may be simultaneously upregulated under the same conditions.[64-66] Together, this provides a mechanism by which cells that normally circulate in the vasculature can be rapidly mobilized to sites of infection or sites where other inflammatory stimuli are present. Lymphocyte homing to regional lymph nodes is also regulated by controlled expression of a distinct but overlapping repertoire of adhesion receptors.[67]

A. CHANGES IN FIBRONECTIN EXPRESSION DURING TRANSFORMATION AND DIFFERENTIATION

As it relates to the process of malignant transformation, expression of adhesion receptors as well as synthesis of the complementary adhesion ligands may be altered as a result of the malignant transformation process. In particular, it is well-established that the loss of cell-substrate adhesion in rodent mesenchymal cells as a result of transformation by physical, chemical, or viral agents is a direct consequence of decreased fibronectin expression in the matrix.[68-73] In nontransformed cells, immunofluorescence staining with antifibronectin reveals a linear pattern of staining so dense as to often obscure the morphology of the cell layer. Phase-contrast microscopy of the same field reveals a layer of attached and fully spread cells. In contrast, staining of transformed cells in the same manner reveals a complete or almost complete lack of immunoreactive fibronectin. Associated with this is a dramatic change in cell morphology. Instead of the flattened appearance of normal fibroblasts in culture, the transformed cells are round or spindle-shaped. As a result, they project a much more phase-dense image, and techniques such as interference microscopy and electron microscopy confirm the relationship between these features and reduced contact with the substratum. What makes the loss of surface fibronectin so interesting in relation to transformation of mesenchymal cells, particularly those of rodent origin, is its almost universal finding. Further, it is well-established that chemical agents which reverse the transformed phenotype of malignant rodent cells concomitantly restore fibronectin to the surface of treated cells. Agents which do this are referred to as "differentiation agents" and include such diverse chemicals as cAMP, retinoic acid, dexamethazone, sodium dibutyrate, γ-interferon/tumor necrosis factor α, and planar polar compounds such as dimethylsulfoxide and dimethylformamide (DMF).[74-79] Over the past several years, our laboratory has characterized the changes in fibronectin expression by murine AKR fibroblasts under control condition, following transformation with 3-methylcholanthrene and after treatment with DMF to "reverse" the phenotype of the transformed cells.[80-83] Figures 1 and 2 graphically illustrate changes in surface fibronectin that accompany transformation and differentiation in this cell line. Fibronectin can be seen by immunofluorescence in the extracellular matrix of untransformed murine AKR-2B fibroblasts (Figure 1B). In contrast, fibronectin cannot be detected

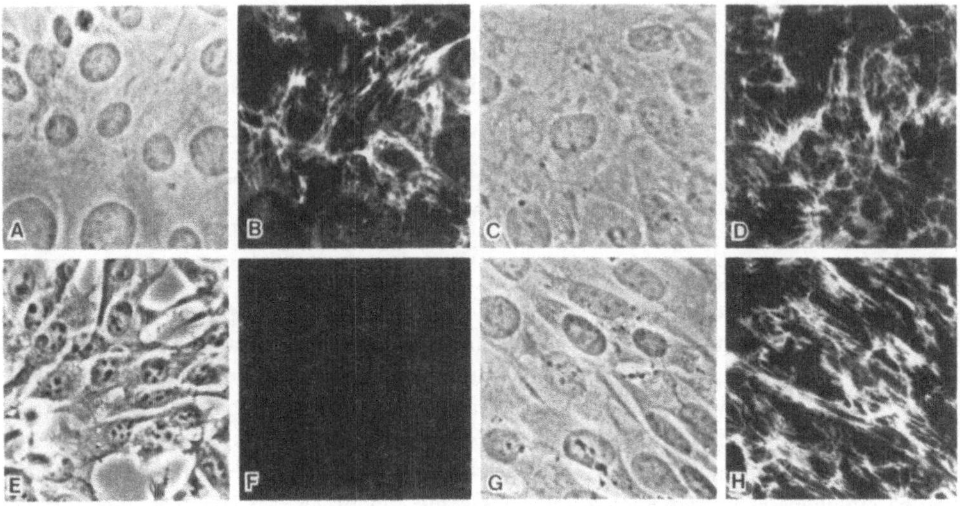

FIGURE 1. Phase contrast images and indirect immunofluorescence staining of AKR-2B and AKR-MCA cells with antifibronectin. (A): Phase-contrast microscopic images of the AKR-2B cells; (C): AKR-2B cells cultured with DMF; (E): AKR-MCA cells; and (G): AKR-MCA cells cultured with DMF. Their corresponding staining patterns with antifibronectin are shown in B, D, F, and H, respectively. (See Reference 77 for details.)

in the same cells after transformation with 3-methylcholanthrene (Figure 1F). While not detectable on the transformed cells under control conditions, treatment of the transformed cells for 4 d with 1% DMF to fully induce differentiation causes a restoration of surface fibronectin (Figure 1H). Treatment of untransformed AKR-2B cells with the same agent has no effect on these cells (Figure 1D). The corresponding morphological changes accompanying transformation and differentiation are shown in the accompanying phase-contrast photomicrographs (Figures 1A,C,E,G).

Another way to visualize the change in surface fibronectin is by Western blotting of purified plasma membrane preparations. Figure 2 shows antifibronectin blotting of purified plasma membranes from control and DMF-treated AKR-2B cells (Lanes 1 and 2) and from control and DMF-treated AKR-MCA cells (Lanes 3 and 4). It is evident that the loss of surface immunofluorescence reflects a loss of plasma membrane-associated fibronectin.

Loss of surface fibronectin following transformation by physical, chemical, and viral agents is well-established.[68-73] Recently, we extended these observations to cells transformed by a single oncogene — Ha-*ras*. Cells transformed with the Ha-*ras* oncogene showed the same loss in surface fibronectin as cells transformed by other means.[84] Interestingly, it was found in the same study that cells transfected with the EGF gene did not show a significant change in surface fibronectin expression. EGF gene-transfected cells showed increased growth potential in soft agar over untransfected control cells and also formed tumors in athymic mice, again in contrast to the untransfected parent cells.[85] However, tumors formed by EGF-transfected cells were well-circumscribed fibromas which did not show evidence of invasion. In contrast, Ha-*ras*-transfected cells were highly invasive and had the capacity to metastasize to distant sites.[85] Thus, the loss of surface fibronectin appears to be associated with acquisition of the fully malignant state rather than with altered growth control, per se.

B. BIOCHEMICAL BASIS FOR ALTERATIONS IN FIBRONECTIN EXPRESSION

Changes in fibronectin expression accompanying transformation and differentiation could result from alterations in endogenous fibronectin synthesis and/or from alterations in fibronectin binding. Altered fibronectin synthesis is at least partially responsible. Decreased

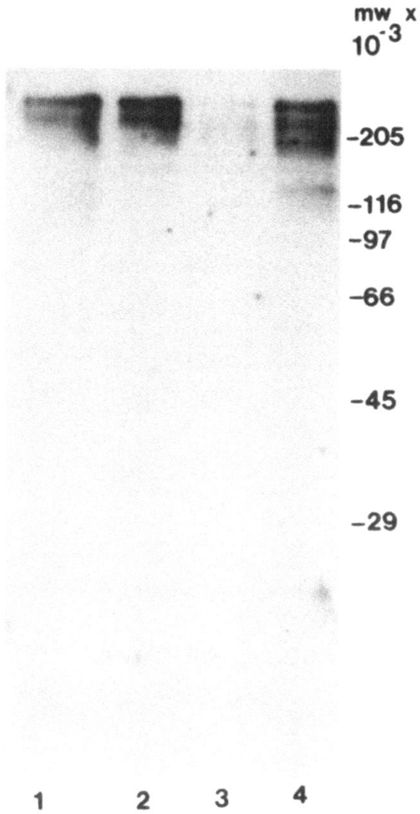

FIGURE 2. Immunoblot of plasma membrane proteins with antifibronectin. Plasma membrane proteins (40 μg) were fractionated by SDS-PAGE and electrophoretically transferred onto nitrocellulose. The antigen-antibody complexes were detected with ^{125}I-protein A. Plasma membranes were prepared from (1) AKR-2B cells, (2) AKR-2B cells cultured with DMF, (3) AKR-MCA cells, and (4) AKR-MCA cells cultured with DMF. (See Reference 77 for details.)

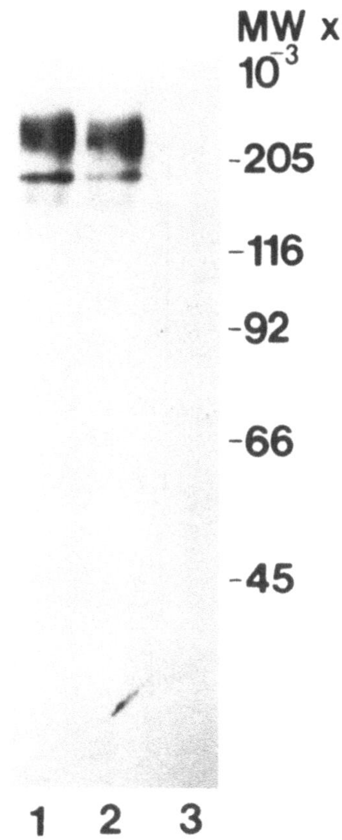

FIGURE 3. Immunoblot of whole cell extracts with antifibronectin. Detergent extracts were prepared from control FR-3T3 fibroblasts (Lane 1) and from FR-3T3 cells transformed with the EGF gene (Lane 2) or with Ha-*ras* (Lane 3), separated by SDS-PAGE, transferred to nitrocellulose, and blotted with antifibronectin and ^{125}I-protein A. (See Reference 84 for details.)

fibronectin biosynthesis by transformed cells has been described in several different cell types.[79,86,87] In the AKR murine fibroblasts, the decrease following transformation with 3-methylcholanthrene may be as great as 90%.[77,88] Likewise, we have found almost complete inhibition of fibronectin synthesis following transformation of FR-3T3 cells with Ha-*ras*.[84] The degree of inhibition observed in FR-3T3 cells following Ha-*ras* transformation, shown in Figure 3, also approaches 90%.

Although reduced fibronectin synthesis following transformation is a common finding, it has not been universal.[68] Additionally, it is difficult to understand how a difference in fibronectin production could, by itself, have such dramatic effects on the behavior of cells grown in the presence of high concentrations of exogenous fibronectin (in the presence of serum). An alternative explanation to account for the loss of surface fibronectin during transformation is failure to bind the ligand. There is, in fact, information to suggest that this is the case. Using antibodies to the α subunit of the fibronectin receptor, Plantefaber and Hynes[89] showed that this moiety was significantly decreased on the surface of several transformed murine cells as compared to their normal counterparts. The loss of the fibronectin receptor appeared to be specific as several other integrins were expressed on the transformed

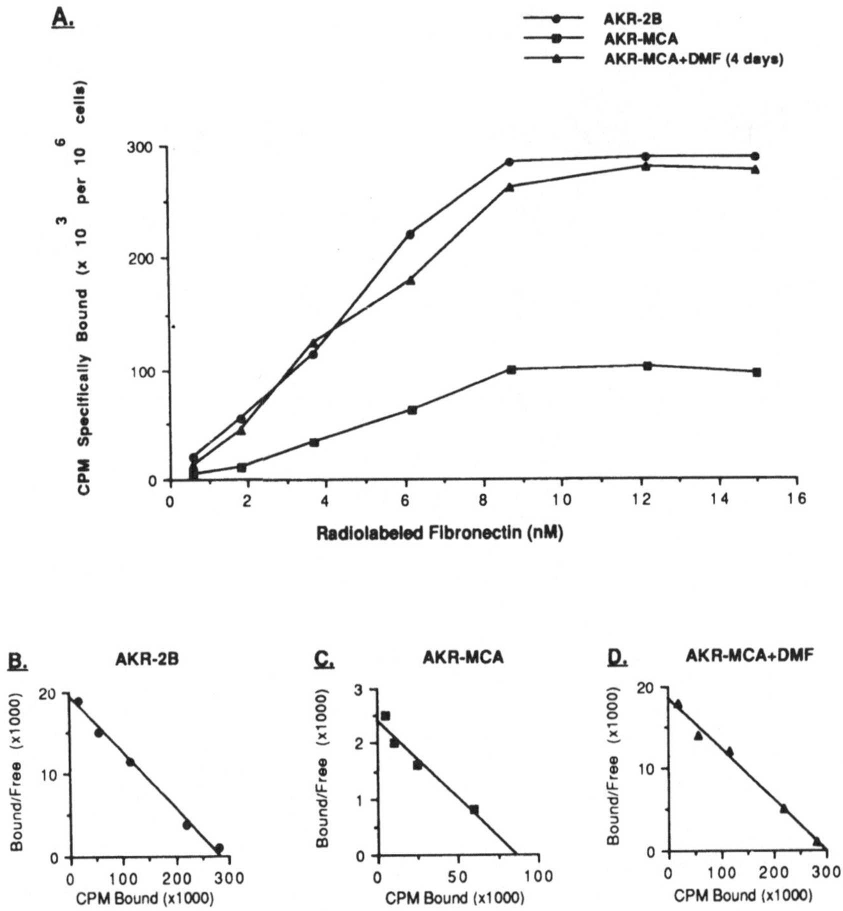

FIGURE 4. Binding studies with ^{125}I-fibronectin. (A): Binding assays were carried out on viable cells in monolayer culture. Nonspecific binding, which routinely accounted for 20 to 25% of the total binding, was determined in the presence of 100-fold excess unlabeled fibronectin and has been subtracted from each data point. (B, C, and D): Scatchard analysis of the binding data. (See Reference 88 for details.)

cells. Since several of the integrins in addition to the fibronectin receptor are capable of binding fibronectin (but with lower affinity), this could explain why fibronectin binding is not completely inhibited following transformation. Under conditions of high exogenous fibronectin, adhesion differences between normal cells and their transformed counterparts tend to be slight. Differences in adhesiveness tend to be much greater at low concentrations of exogeneous fibronectin with the most dramatic difference occurring in the complete absence of exogenous fibronectin. As with other transformed cells, our studies have shown that fibronectin binding is decreased in the AKR fibroblasts following transformation with 3-methylcholanthrene[89] and in the FR-3T3 following Ha-*ras* transfection.[84] Data from whole cell binding studies with the AKR cells is shown in Figure 4.

If loss of fibronectin binding is routinely associated with transformation, then do factors that induce fibronectin re-expression on transformed cells work by inducing receptor expression? We have addressed this question using the AKR fibroblasts. Our studies showed that fibronectin binding activity was expressed on the 3-methylcholanthrene-transformed AKR-fibroblasts within a few hours after exposure to DMF (Figure 4). Our studies also showed that the re-expression of fibronectin binding activity by viable cells was associated with the re-expression of moieties with integrin-like characteristics (Figure 5) and that these moieties

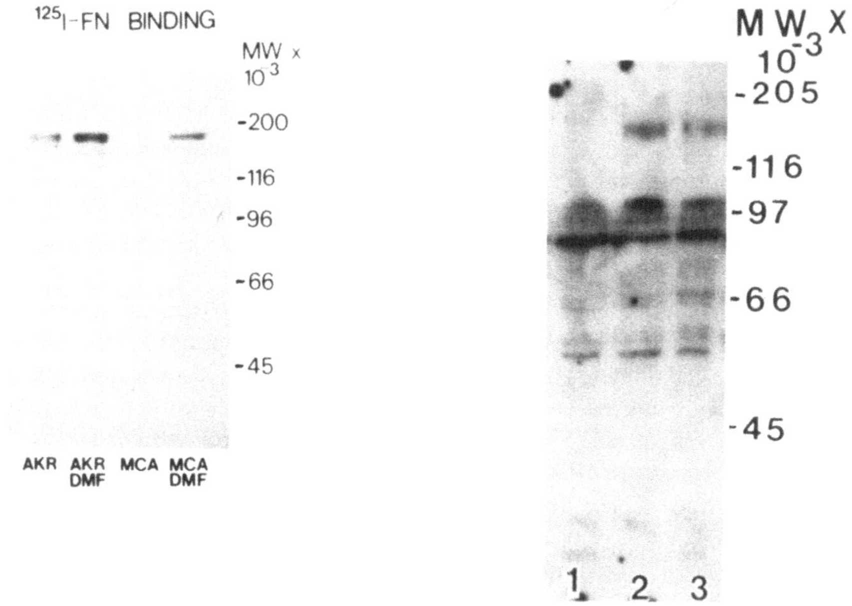

FIGURE 5. ^{125}I-fibronectin binding to cell lysate proteins obtained from AKR-2B and AKR-MCA cells. **Left:** 40 μg of cell lysate protein were used per lane, and each lane was probed with ^{125}I-fibronectin at a concentration of 8 n*M*. Lane 1: AKR-2B; Lane 2: AKR-2B treated with DMF; Lane 3: AKR-MCA; Lane 4: AKR-MCA treated with DMF. **Right:** Immunoblotting of cell lysate proteins obtained from AKR-2B and AKR-MCA cells. Cell lysate proteins were separated by SDS-PAGE, transferred to nitrocellulose, and blotted with antifibronectin receptor and ^{125}I-protein A. Lane 1: AKR-MCA; Lane 2: AKR-MCA treated with DMF; Lane 3: AKR-2B. (See Reference 88 for details.)

were immunologically crossreactive with antibodies to the human fibronectin receptor (Figure 5). The time course for the re-expression of fibronectin receptors paralleled the time course for induction of fibronectin biosynthesis, and both of these were associated closely with the re-acquisition of cell-substrate adhesion capabilities.[77,88] It should be noted that not all cells show decreased expression of fibronectin receptor following transformation. Akiyama, Larjava, Yamada, et al.[91] observed no significant alteration of fibronectin receptor on transformed human fibroblasts; Saga, Chen, and Yamada[90] reported increased fibronectin receptor expression on fibrocytic tumors induced in chickens by Rous sarcoma virus. Not surprisingly, a well-organized fibronectin matrix was associated with these tumors.

These data provide strong support for the idea that fibronectin synthesis and fibronectin receptor expression are co-modulated during transformation and differentiation and that they act together to bring about changes in surface fibronectin. Although not related to transformation per se, Ignotz and Massague[92] and Roberts et al.[93] both observed that transforming growth factor-β (TGFβ) stimulated fibronectin synthesis and fibronectin receptor concomitantly in human fibroblasts. Ryseck et al.[94] observed similar effects in serum-stimulated murine fibroblasts.

C. ALTERATIONS IN LAMININ EXPRESSION DURING TRANSFORMATION AND DIFFERENTIATION

Is the loss of surface fibronectin during transformation a specific consequence of transformation or does it reflect a generalized loss of extracellular matrix components? In some transformed cells, matrix components other than fibronectin are clearly expressed at reduced levels relative to their nontransformed counterparts. For example, Alitalo et al.[73] showed that laminin as well as fibronectin was lost from the pericellular matrix of Rous sarcoma virus-transformed rat kidney cells. Likewise, we observed a low level of laminin expression (in addition to fibronectin) on human colonic carcinoma cells taken from histologically undifferentiated tumors.[95] Further, several histochemical and immunohistochemical studies have demonstrated the lack of intact basement membrane surrounding invasive and metastatic tumor cells *in vivo*.[96-102] These studies have shown that the major components of the basement membrane (e.g., laminin and type IV collagen) are either not present or present but in fragmented basement membrane structures. This last observation has lead to speculation that increased basement membrane degradation rather than reduced synthesis may be the key to understanding basement membrane changes during invasion.

Although these types of studies suggest reduced presence of basement membrane components such as laminin and type IV collagen (as well as fibronectin) in some malignant tumors, the relationship of these changes to the malignant process is not clear. Furthermore, it is evident that *in vitro* at least, laminin expression by malignant cells often is not decreased concomitantly with fibronectin. This has been documented in our own studies as well as in studies by other investigators. Rampoldi et al.[103] used somatic cell hybridization between normal and transformed mouse fibroblasts to demonstrate that tumorigenicity and laminin expression were positively correlated, in contrast to what was observed with fibronectin. Bober, Birk, and Raska[104] used transfection with the adenovirus 12 early region 1 gene to show that sequences which induced transformation (tumorigenicity in athymic mice) caused enhanced expression of surface laminin while nontransforming sequences did not. In addition to these experimental studies in rodents, Brown and Parkinson[105] examined laminin expression by a series of human squamous epithelial cell lines. They reported that laminin expression was positively correlated with a lack of differentiation. Since undifferentiated squamous epithelial tumors tend to be more malignant than their more-differentiated counterparts, this indirectly supports a relationship between laminin expression and malignant capacity.

In our studies, we examined changes in laminin expression along with changes in fibronectin expression during transformation and differentiation. In contrast to the alterations observed with fibronectin, we did not see corresponding changes in laminin. Rather, in rodent cells transformed by a number of different agents, laminin remained visible on the cell surface as indicated by immunofluorescence analysis.[77,84,106] In some cases, an extracellular organization could be seen[77] while in other cases, staining was diffuse.[84] In cells that showed diffuse staining (i.e., after Ha-*ras* transfection), the pattern of fluorescence could indicate changes in either the receptor moieties or in cytoskeletal components. These questions have not been investigated further. Not surprisingly, cells which demonstrated normal levels of surface laminin after transformation were comparable to their nontransformed counterparts in both laminin synthesis and laminin binding.[77,84,106,107]

These data indicate that transformation of rodent cells does not, per se, result in the loss of surface laminin. It is possible, however, to obtain laminin-deficient cells by specifically selecting against cells which have laminin expressed on their surface. This was done by incubating murine fibrosarcoma cells in the presence of complement plus an antibody that recognized laminin.[108-110] In doing this, it was found that virtually 100% of the cells were lysed. The few surviving cells (estimated to be less than 0.01% in the unselected population) were grown to confluency and re-exposed to the antibody plus complement. After four such selection steps, the surviving population of cells was found to be completely resistant to complement-mediated lysis in the presence of antibody to laminin. Immunofluorescence studies revealed that these cells were virtually devoid of surface laminin. Thus, resistance to killing reflected a lack of exposed antigen rather than the development of innate complement resistance. The lack of surface laminin in these cells was associated with decreased laminin production.[106] In contrast, these cells did not show a corresponding reduction in laminin binding. In fact, the laminin-deficient cells bound exogneous laminin as well as or better than their laminin-expressing parental lines.[107] It appears, therefore, in these cells that the loss of surface laminin is related to alterations in biosynthesis/processing rather

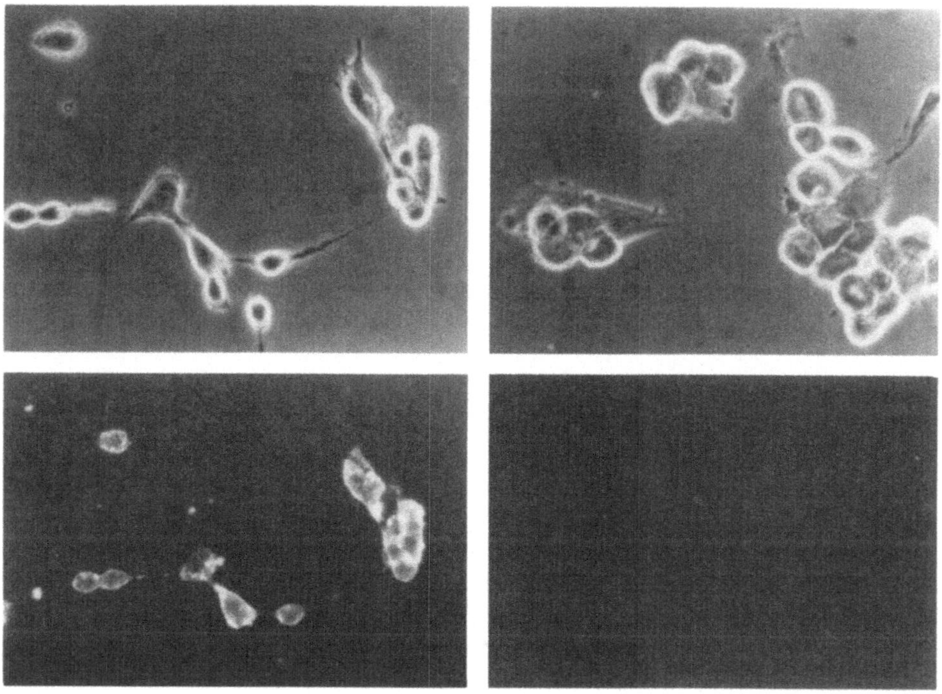

FIGURE 6. Indirect immunofluorescence staining for laminin on the surface of murine fibrosarcoma cells **(left)** and murine fibrosarcoma cells selected for resistance to killing by antilaminin and complement **(right).** (See Reference 106 for details.)

than to a defect in laminin binding. Figure 6 demonstrates the immunofluorescence staining of surface laminin on these transformed murine fibroblasts and the lack of such staining on cells specifically selected for a lack of surface laminin.

V. RELATIONSHIP BETWEEN EXTRACELLULAR MATRIX EXPRESSION AND CELL BEHAVIOR *IN VITRO* AND *IN VIVO*

A. RELATIONSHIP BETWEEN SURFACE FIBRONECTIN/LAMININ AND CELL-SUBSTRATE ADHESION

Are the alterations in surface fibronectin and laminin expression that accompany transformation and differentiation responsible for the alterations in cell-substrate adhesion which also characterize these processes? Although the regulation of adhesion is complex and multifactoral, experimental evidence from several studies suggests that alterations in surface fibronectin and laminin do contribute significantly to the regulation of cell-substrate adhesion. Further, these data suggest that fibronectin and laminin do not participate in adhesion reactions in identical ways, but rather, play complementary roles. The evidence can be summarized as follows:

1. Nontransformed fibroblasts attach and spread more rapidly on fibronectin-coated dishes than their transformed counterparts. Parallel differences are seen in the absence of exogenous fibronectin. Presumably, endogenously-synthesized fibronectin mediates attachment in the absence of exogenous fibronectin since antibodies to fibronectin, antibodies to the fibronectin receptor, and synthetic peptides from the fibronectin cell-binding domain interfere in parallel with attachment to fibronectin-coated dishes and plastic culture dishes.[77,89]

TABLE 1
Relationship Between Fibronectin and Laminin Expression and Adhesion in Murine Mesenchymal Tumor Cells

Group	Surface		Adhesion	
	FN	LN	Early	Late
Normal fibroblast	+ + + +	+ +	Yes	Yes
Transformed fibroblast	—	+ +	No	Yes
Transformed fibroblast (DMF-treated)	+ + + +	+ +	Yes	Yes
Transformed fibroblast (antilaminin resistant)	—	—	No	No

Note: Cells which express surface fibronectin (FN) rapidly attach and spread on plastic culture dishes in the presence of bovine serum albumin while FN-deficient cells do not. FN-deficient cells will attach and spread over a longer time period (4 to 18 h). Cells deficient in laminin (LN) as well as in FN fail to attach and spread even after an extended period. (See References 13 and 77 for details.)

2. Induction of differentiation results in the re-expression of surface fibronectin by transformed cells, and there is a concomitant, parallel re-acquisition of capacity for adhesion to plastic culture dishes and to fibronectin-coated dishes.[77,89] Again, adhesion to the plastic culture dishes as well as to the fibronectin-coated dishes is blocked by antibody to fibronectin or its receptor and by RGDS.
3. Although transformed cells are defective in their initial attachment rates, these cells will often attach and spread on plastic culture dishes over a longer period of time (4 to 18 h). This is due, in part, to the production of laminin by the cells. Evidence for this includes the finding that antibodies to laminin can partially inhibit this process[77] and the finding that cells which are deficient in laminin as well as fibronectin expression do not attach and spread on plastic culture dishes even after longer time periods.[13] These observations are summarized in Table 1.

B. RELATIONSHIP BETWEEN FIBRONECTIN/LAMININ EXPRESSION AND *IN VIVO* BEHAVIOR

Do these alterations in adhesion *in vitro* have *in vivo* counterparts? Does the capacity of the cells to form tumors and to invade and metastasize reflect alterations in adhesion properties identified by these *in vitro* experiments? Data from a large number of studies suggest that the answer to these questions is yes. As already indicated, loss of surface fibronectin is a characteristic feature of rodent cells transformed by a number of agents.[68-73] These tumors are characterized by a high degree of tumorigenicity (tumors can often be induced with as few as 10^2 cells) and a high capacity for invasion and metastasis. However, cells that are lacking both laminin and fibronectin are of low tumorigenicity, and they are much less aggressive in animals.[106-110] Thus, there is a relationship between surface expression of fibronectin and laminin and *in vivo* behavior. Further evidence that a deficiency in surface laminin is related to reduced malignancy comes from the finding that the addition of exogenous laminin to laminin-deficient cells prior to their intravenous injection results in a significantly greater formation of lung colonies.[107,111] These *in vivo* findings are summarized in Table 2.

How can these various data be put together in a meaningful way? We suggest that the loss of surface fibronectin as a consequence of transformation results in an alteration in the way these cells process signals generated by contact with other cells and with the substratum. Because of their abnormal surface architecture, factors that regulate proliferation and motility in normal cells are not properly received and processed. Contact inhibition of growth and contact inhibition of motility are lost. Coupled with these alterations are reduced cell-cell

TABLE 2
Relationship Between Fibronectin and Laminin Expression and *In Vivo* Behavior in Murine Mesenchymal Tumor Cells

Group	Surface FN	Surface LN	Tumorigenicity and metastasis
Normal fibroblast	+ + + +	+ +	No
Transformed fibroblast	—	+ +	High
Transformed fibroblast (anti-LN resistant)	—	—	Reduced
Transformed fibroblast (antilaminin resistant/treated with exogenous laminin)	—	+ +	High

Note: Normal fibroblasts do not form tumors when injected into syngeneic mice. Transformed (3-methylcholanthrene) fibroblasts form tumors at high frequency. The tumors are invasive and highly metastatic. Cells selected for antilaminin (LN) resistance form tumors at a much lower rate and are much less malignant, but become more malignant when exposed to exogenous LN. (See Reference 107 for details.)

and cell-substrate adhesion. Interestingly, it has been shown in several model systems that reduced adhesion to fibronectin is not associated with reduced motility. In fact, a variety of tumor cells are highly responsive to fibronectin in assays that measure chemotaxis and heptotaxis.[112-118] All of these factors together make for a situation in which the forces holding cells localized may be overwhelmed. Although not addressed in this review, additional factors such as enhanced tumor proteolytic enzyme activity and proteolysis mediated by inflammatory cells at the primary tumor site might also contribute to the unstable condition at the primary tumor site.

Simply overcoming the factors that hold cells in place at the primary tumor site is not, obviously, sufficient to produce a fully invasive and metastatic tumor. The released tumor cells must invade the surrounding tissues and eventually gain access to the circulation. Once in the circulation, the cells must be capable of localizing at secondary sites. Adhesion to host endothelial cells or sub-endothelial basement membranes with subsequent local invasion and growth is critical. It might be expected that the reduced adhesiveness of tumor cells would be inhibitory to successful completion of this stage of the metastatic process. As already has been pointed out, however, tumor cells that have the capacity for metastasis formation have not lost all of their adhesion mechanisms. Quite the contrary, adhesion mediated by laminin-laminin receptor interactions are still fully functional in many of these tumor cells. In some cases, they are increased. Thus, adhesive interactions based on laminin-laminin receptors could provide the basis by which cells that have reduced adhesiveness (at the the primary tumor site) interact with endothelial cells or sub-endothelial basement membranes at secondary sites. The large number of studies that have demonstrated a correlation between adhesion to endothelial cells or sub-endothelial matrix and malignant potential among tumor cell variant populations supports such a view.[13,108,119-122]

VI. THE EXTRACELLULAR MATRIX, ADHESION, AND MALIGNANCY IN HUMAN TUMOR CELLS

The matrix changes, alterations in adhesion, and models of metastasis developed above are based largely on findings with murine tumor cells. Are such models valid for tumors from species other than rodent; in particular, for human tumors? The production of various extracellular matrix molecules by human tumor cells has been examined in a number of studies. Reduced fibronectin production has been shown in malignant cells derived from epithelial tumors, tumors of mesenchyme, and tumors of melanocytic origin.[79,86,87] The decreased production relative to the corresponding normal cells has not always been as great, however, as the decrease observed in transformed rodent cells. In contrast to fibronectin, production of other extracellular matrix molecules (i.e., laminin, thrombospondin) does not show a consistent decrease in malignant cells. Rather, production and cell surface expression of extracellular matrix molecules such as laminin and thrombospondin may be either increased or decreased, depending on tumor type and the individual tumor cell line.[20,104,105,123-125]

A. SQUAMOUS EPITHELIAL CELLS

Our laboratory has investigated the role of laminin and thrombospondin in the behavior of human squamous epithelial tumors of the head and neck region. The head and neck squamous epithelial tumors constitute a diverse group of tumors, which may differ considerably in their degree of differentiation and in their degree of malignancy. As a group, these tumors tend to be highly aggressive in terms of local invasion. They expand by direct extension into surrounding normal tissue and in the process create a tremendous amount of tissue damage. Eventually, they gain access to the general circulation (usually the lymphatics) and metastasize widely. Individual tumors vary in their degree of differentiation, and cell lines tend to reflect the degree of differentiation seen in the original tumor.

In a recent study,[123] we examined the production of laminin by a series of squamous epithelial cell lines. Normal epidermal keratinocyte were used for comparison. A number of differences between the normal and malignant cells were seen. First, the molecular forms produced by the normal epithelial cells (as indicated by biosynthetic labeling/immuno precipitation) were identical from patient to patient (Figure 7). This consisted of a chain at approximately 400 kD (equivalent to the A chain of murine laminin) and two chains in the 200 to 240 kD range (consistent with the B_1 and B_2 subunits). In addition, chains at 195, 170, and 160 kD were also consistently observed. The relationship between the three lower molecular weight chains and the standard subunits is not known. They may be unique peptides that associate specifically with squamous epithelial cell laminin. Alternatively, they may be proteolytic fragments of the higher molecular weight laminin forms. These chains do not react with polyclonal antiserum to laminin in Western blot assays. However, the antibodies used in the immunoprecipitation and Western blot studies were prepared against murine laminin and may therefore not contain binding sites reactive with the novel squamous epithelial cell fragments. We have not identified these fragments in tumors derived from teratocarcinomas, melanomas, or colon (adeno) carcinomas.[79,95,123,126] In regards to the possibility that these peptides are proteolytic fragments of laminin, this cannot be ruled out completely. However, it is unlikely that they are produced in the culture fluid because a cocktail of protease inhibitors had no affect on their appearance. Furthermore, culture fluids from these cell lines do not generate similar fragments from purified murine laminin or from laminin obtained from the JAR human choriocarcinoma line. In any event, the molecular forms produced by normal squamous epithelial cells are identical from line to line. In contrast, the molecular forms produced by a series of malignant squamous epithelial cells are unique from line to line (Figure 7). In some lines, one or more of the subunits is absent, and the ratios of the different subunits vary from line to line. Interestingly, we examined cell lines derived from primary and secondary (invasive) tumors from the same patient in four cases. In each case, the patterns in the primary and secondary tumors were identical to each other. This suggests that whatever is responsible for the generation of unique molecular patterns occurs early on, prior to isolation of the first cell line. It is unlikely, therefore, that the unique patterns represent *in vitro* artifacts, generated after the cells have been established in culture.

A second difference between the normal keratinocytes and the malignant squamous epithelial cells is in secretion of laminin. We observed that essentially all of the biosynthesized laminin was incorporated into the cell layer of the normal keratinocytes (a similar finding had been made previously by others.[127]) In contrast, a significant amount of the laminin

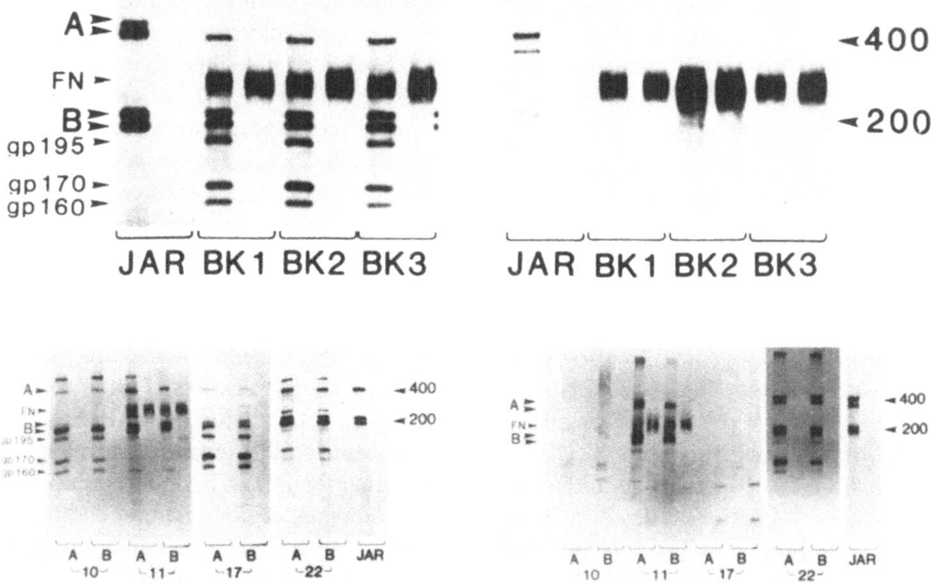

FIGURE 7. Biosynthesis and secretion of immunoreactive laminin forms by human epidermal keratinocytes and human squamous carcinoma cells. **Top left:** Normal keratinocytes (BK1, BK2, and BK3) pulsed for 1 h with ^{35}S-methionine and immunoprecipitated with antilaminin. JAR choriocarcinoma cells are shown for comparison. All three keratinocyte populations show a single A chain, a B doublet, and in addition, chains at 195, 170, and 160 kDa. An intense fibronectin band is also seen, due to direct binding of fibronectin to protein A. **Top right:** Culture fluid from the same cells pulsed for 1 h with ^{35}S-methionine and chased for 4 h with cold methionine. Note the secretion of fibronectin but not of laminin or laminin-associated glycoproteins. **Bottom left:** Squamous carcinoma cells from four different patients pulsed for 1 h with ^{35}S-methionine exactly as above. A and B lines represent cell lines obtained from primary and secondary tumors of the same patient. Note that the laminin chains from each patient are unique and that both cell lines from the same patient are identical. **Bottom right:** Culture fluid from the same cells pulsed for 1 h with ^{35}S-methionine and chased for 4 h with cold methionine. Note the significant amount of secretion with cell lines from two of the tumors. (See Reference 123 for details.)

produced by certain malignant lines was shed into the culture fluid. One possible interpretation for these findings is that the malignant cells are abnormal in their ability to process the biosynthesized molecule and incorporate it into the matrix. Another possibility is that a high level of soluble laminin reflects overproduction by the cells. At present, we cannot fully distinguish between these possibilities. However, it seems unlikely that the presence of soluble laminin in the culture fluid is due simply to improper incorporation into the cell layer. By immunofluorescence, these cells appeared to have as much laminin in the cell layer as the cells that did not shed significant amounts into the culture fluid. Furthermore, when the cells were detergent-lysed and the remaining substrate-bound immunoreactive laminin measured, the cells that had the greatest amount in the culture field also had the most material in the detergent-insoluble layer. Finally, when the cells were examined for attachment and spreading, the cells that released the greatest amount of material into the culture medium were also the ones that attached and spread most rapidly. Our interpretation of these data is that the cells which shed large amounts of laminin do so because they continue to synthesize quantities that are in excess of the amounts that can be incorporated into the matrix rather than because they are incapable of incorporating the material into the matrix.

We have also examined the same squamous carcinoma lines for synthesis of a second extracellular matrix component, thrombospondin. As was seen with laminin, there was a significant degree of variability among the tumor cell lines in the amount of thrombospondin synthesized.[124,125] As was also observed with laminin, normal epidermal keratinocytes synthesized thrombospondin while they were in the undifferentiated state, but ceased production as differentiation occurred.[20] Squamous epithelial cells, both normal and malignant, express surface receptors for thrombospondin, and this molecule serves as an attachment factor for these cells.[41] Among the same squamous carcinoma cells, there appeared to be a direct relationship between thrombospondin synthesis, thrombospondin receptor expression, and thrombospondin-mediated adhesion. Thus, we believe that thrombospondin may serve as an important mediator of squamous epithelial cell adhesion *in vivo,* maintaining cell contact with the basement membrane.

In addition to examining production of these two extracellular matrix components, the same normal and malignant cells also have been examined for fibronectin production. Normal epidermal keratinocytes were found to synthesize and secrete large amounts of fibronectin,[128] as had been previously observed by others.[127] However, among the tumor cell lines, fibronectin synthesis was highly variable. Of interest to note is the fact that several of the malignant lines produced small amounts of fibronectin relative to undifferentiated normal keratinocytes. This includes at least one line which produced large amounts of both laminin and thrombospondin. In contrast, at least one of the cell lines that synthesized large amounts of laminin and thrombospondin also produced a significant amount of fibronectin as well.

These data suggest that extracellular matrix components including laminin and thrombospondin are produced in large amounts by normal, undifferentiated keratinocytes and by a variety of malignant squamous epithelial tumors. In contrast, fibronectin is produced by normal keratinocytes, but may or may not be produced in similar amounts by malignant cells. The production of laminin and thrombospondin is associated with the undifferentiated state in normal keratinocytes. Synthesis of these components is decreased during differentiation, concomitantly with reduced adhesion to the basement membrane. Among malignant cells, the production of these matrix components is also associated with the undifferentiated condition. Since the undifferentiated cells tend to be the most invasive, this may be related to their capacity for interaction with the basement membrane and underlying connective tissue. These changes in extracellular matrix production (i.e., reduced fibronectin production coupled with normal or increased levels of other matrix components) by human squamous epithelial tumor cells are consistent with the changes noted in rodent models. It may be possible to use the rodent models, therefore, to at least partially understand the process of human squamous epithelial cell invasion and metastasis.

B. OTHER HUMAN TUMOR CELLS

While most of our recent work has focused on squamous epithelial tumors of the head and neck, additional studies have been carried out with a series of colon carcinoma cell lines[95,129] and with a series of malignant melanomas.[79] Both of these kinds of tumors behave quite differently from squamous carcinomas. While both are highly metastatic, they tend to show less local tissue invasion/destruction than do the squamous epithelial tumors. Furthermore, these cells behave much differently from squamous carcinomas in culture. Whereas squamous epithelial tumors are highly adherent to the substratum, both colonic carcinomas (which tend to be adenocarcinomas as opposed to squamous carcinomas) and malignant melanomas are much less adhesive than typical squamous epithelial tumors. What accounts for the differences in behavior between these types of tumors and squamous epithelial tumors is not fully understood. However, in cell lines derived from both types of tumors, we have observed changes in the patterns of extracellular matrix expression, which appear to be consistent from line to line and which are different from the patterns observed previously with squamous epithelial tumors. Specifically, the colonic adenocarcinoma lines that we have studied synthesize and express much smaller amounts of laminin and thrombospondin as well as fibronectin than either nonmalignant colon epithelial cells or normal or malignant squamous epithelial cells.[129] Melanoma cells also synthesize lower amounts of fibronectin than their normal counterparts,[79] but produce normal or greater amounts of laminin. Most interestingly, both normal human epidermal melanocytes and several melanoma lines that we examined produced barely detectable amounts of thrombospondin.[79,126] These findings suggest that the patterns of matrix synthesis and expression are dependent to a large extent on the cell type in question as well as on whether the cell is normal or malignant and on the state of differentiation. These findings also suggest that models of metastasis based on changes in the extracellular matrix in murine tumors and human squamous carcinomas may not be directly applicable to other tumors such as adenocarcinomas of the colon or malignant melanomas.

Although these findings attest to the tumor type-specific differences in synthesis/expression of extracellular matrix components, they also attest to the fact that reduced fibronectin production seems to be consistent, at least to some degree, among all of the tumor types examined. Additionally, our studies with colon carcinoma cells and with melanoma cells also have shown a consistent increase in fibronectin expression in these cells following treatment with agents that decrease growth and induce a differentiation-like state. Factors that do this include transforming growth factor-β (TGF-β) in both the colon carcinoma cells and the melanocytic cells[95,126] and combinations of interferon-γ (IFN-γ)/tumor necrosis factor-α (TGF-α) in melanocytic cells.[79] The colon cancer model is particularly interesting in this regard since TGF-β resistant cells were isolated from TGF-β sensitive parental cells.[130] Although these cells did not undergo growth inhibition in response to TGF-β treatment, these cells bound TGF-β with the same characteristics as the parental cells. Furthermore, induction of carcinoembryonic antigen occurred in both the growth-inhibited and growth-not inhibited populations to a similar degree. In contrast, only the growth-inhibited cells demonstrated increased fibronectin expression following treatment. Thus, there appears to be a strong correlation between fibronectin expression and growth inhibition in this model. There is, in fact, no model that we have investigated in which growth inhibition is not accompanied by increased fibronectin expression.

VII. SUMMARY

The process of tumor cell invasion and metastasis is complex, and attempts to focus on one particular aspect may neglect other aspects of the process that are equally important. Certainly, changes in adhesiveness resulting from alterations in the tumor extracellular matrix are not solely responsible for invasion and metastasis. Nonetheless, there is convincing evidence (1) that consistent alterations in the pattern of extracellular matrix expression accompany transformation, (2) that these alterations lead to changes in cell behavior (i.e., adhesiveness), and (3) that changes in adhesion are critical to invasion and metastasis. It is clear, furthermore, that cells have developed multiple overlapping mechanisms of adhesion and that not all of them are defective in malignant cells. This may explain how some adhesive functions, but not all, may be defective in transformed cells and how tumor cells can demonstrate less cohesion than their normal counterpart cells and yet still be capable of adhering to host tissues at critical stages of the invasion and metastatic process.

REFERENCES

1. **Coman, D. R.,** Mechanisms responsible for the origin and distribution of blood-borne tumor cells: a review, *Cancer Res.*, 13, 397, 1953.
2. **McCutcheon, M., Coman, D. R., and Moore, M. B.,** Studies on invasion in cancer: adhesiveness of malignant cells in various human adenocarcinomas, *Cancer,* 1, 460, 1948.
3. **Tjernberg, B. and Zajicek, J.,** Connulation of lymphatics leaving cancerous nodes in studies on tumor spread, *Acta Cytol.*, 9, 197, 1965.
4. **Carruthers, C. and Suntzeff, B.,** Chemical studies on mode of action of methylcholanthrene on mouse epidermis, *Cancer Res.*, 3, 744, 1943.
5. **Carruthers, C. and Suntzeff, B.,** The role of calcium in carcinogenesis, *Science,* 99, 245, 1944.
6. **Sanford, K., Barber, B. E., Woods, M. W., Parshad, R., and Law, L. W.,** Search for indicators of neoplastic conversion *in vitro, J. Natl. Cancer Inst.*, 39, 705, 1967.
7. **Curtis, A. S. G.,** Control of some cell contact reactions in tissue culture, *J. Natl. Cancer Inst.*, 26, 253, 1961.
8. **Pastan, I. and Johnson, G. S.,** Cyclic AMP and the transformation of fibroblasts, *Adv. Cancer Res.*, 19, 303, 1974.
9. **Abercrombie, M. and Heaysman, J. E. M.,** Observations on the social behavior of cells in tissue culture. I. Speed of movement of chick heart fibroblasts in relation to mutual contacts, *Exp. Cell Res.*, 5, 111, 1953.
10. **Projan, A. and Tanneberger, S.,** Some findings on movement and contacts of human normal and tumor cells *in vitro, Eur. J. Cancer,* 9, 703, 1973.
11. **Grinnell, F. and Lamke, C. R.,** Reorganization of hydrated collagen lattices by human skin fibroblasts, *J. Cell Sci.*, 66, 51, 1984.
12. **Murray, J. C., Liotta, L. A., and Terranova, V. P.,** Attachment of metastatic tumor cells to collagen, *Tumor Invasion and Metastasis,* 7, 309, 1982.
13. **Varani, J., Grimstad, I. A., Knibbs, R. N., Hovig, T., and McCoy, J. P.,** Attachment, spreading and growth *in vitro* of highly malignant and low malignant murine fibrosarcoma cells, *Clin. Exp. Metastasis,* 3, 45, 1985.
14. **Vlodavsky, I. and Gospodarowicz, D.,** Respective roles of laminin and fibronectin adhesion of human carcinoma and sarcoma cells, *Nature,* 289, 304, 1981.
15. **Couchman, J. R., Hook, M., Rees, D. A., and Timpl, R.,** Adhesion, growth and matrix production by fibroblasts on laminin substrates, *J. Cell Biol.*, 96, 177, 1983.
16. **Varani, J., Carey, T. E., Fligiel, S. E. G., McKeever, P. E., and Dixit, V.,** Tumor type-specific differences in cell substrate adhesion among human tumor cell lines, *Int. J. Cancer,* 39, 397, 1987.
17. **Roberts, D. D., Sherwood, J. A., and Ginsburg, V.,** Platelet thrombospondin mediates attachment and spreading of human melanoma cells, *J. Cell Biol.*, 104, 131, 1987.
18. **Nozawa, R. T.,** Altered morphology and increased cell adhesiveness of Chinese hamster ovary cells cultured on fibrin, *J. Cell Physiol.*, 90, 351, 1976.
19. **Nozawa, R. T. and Guerrant, R. L.,** Fibrin adherent CHO cell behavior in response to chelators and enterotoxin, *Exp. Cell Res.*, 107, 25, 1977.
20. **Varani, J., Nickoloff, B. J., Riser, B. L., Mitra, R. S., O'Rourke, K., and Dixit, V. M.,** Thrombospondin-induced adhesion of human keratinocytes, *J. Clin. Invest.*, 81, 1537, 1988.
21. **Ruoslahti, E., Engvall, E., and Hayman, E. G.,** Fibronectin: current concepts of its structure and functions, *Coll. Res.*, 1, 95, 1981.
22. **Click, E. M. and Balian, G.,** Domain structure of human plasma and cellular fibronectin; use of a monoclonal antibody and heparin affinity to identify three different subunit chains, *Biochemistry,* 24, 6685, 1985.
23. **Engel, J., Odermatt, E., and Engel, A.,** Shapes, domain organizations and flexibility of laminin and fibronectin, two multifunctional proteins of the extracellular matrix, *J. Mol. Biol.*, 150, 97, 1981.
24. **Yamada, K. M., Akiyama, S. K., Hasegawa, T., Hasegawa, E., Humphries, M. J., Kennedy, D. W., Nagata, K., Urushihara, H., Olden, K., and Chen, W.,** Recent advances in research on fibronectin and other cell attachment proteins, *J. Cell Biochem.*, 28, 79, 1985.
25. **Chung, A. E., Jaffe, R., Freeman, L. L., Vergnes, J. P., Braginski, J. E., and Carlin, B.,** Properties of a basement membrane-related glycoprotein synthesized in culture by a mouse embryonal carcinoma-derived cell line, *Cell,* 16, 277, 1979.
26. **Timpl, R., Rohde, H., Robey, P. G., Rennard, S. I., Foidart, J. M., and Martin, G. R.,** Laminin A glygoprotein from basement membranes, *J. Biol. Chem.*, 254, 9933, 1979.
27. **Baenziger, N., Brodie, G., and Majerus, P.,** A thrombin-sensitive protein of human platelet membranes, *Proc. Natl. Acad. Sci. U.S.A.*, 68, 240, 1971.
28. **Baenziger, N., Brodie, G., and Majerus, P.,** Isolation and properties of a thrombin-sensitive protein of human platelets, *J. Biol. Chem.*, 247, 2723, 1972.

29. **Margossian, S., Lawler, J., and Slayter, H.,** Physical characterization of platelet thrombospondin, *J. Biol. Chem.*, 256, 7495, 1981.
30. **Saglio, S. and Slayter, H.,** Use of radioimmunoassay to quantify thrombospondin, *Blood,* 59, 162, 1982.
31. **Coligan, J. E. and Slayter, H. S.,** Structure of thrombospondin, *J. Biol. Chem.*, 259, 3944, 1984.
32. **Lawler, J., Derick, L. H., Connolly, J. E., Chen, J. H., and Chao, F. C.,** The structure of human platelet thrombospondin, *J. Biol. Chem.*, 260, 3762, 1985.
33. **Pierschbacher, M. D., Hayman, E. G., and Ruoslahti, E.,** Synthetic peptide with cell attachment activity of fibronectin, *Proc. Natl. Acad. Sci. U.S.A.*, 80, 1224, 1983.
34. **Pierschbacher, M. D. and Ruoslahti, E.,** Cell attachment activity of fibronectin can be duplicated by small synthetic fragments of the molecule, *Nature (London),* 309, 30, 1984.
35. **Pierschbacher, M. D. and Ruoslahti, E.,** Variants of the cell recognition site of fibronectin that retain attachment promoting activity, *Proc. Natl. Acad. Sci. U.S.A.*, 81, 5985, 1984.
36. **Ruoslahti, E. and Pierschbacher, M. D.,** Arg-Gly-Asp: a versatile cell recognition signal, *Cell,* 44, 517, 1986.
37. **Akiyama, S. K. and Yamada, K. M.,** The interaction of plasma fibronectin with fibroblastic cells in suspension, *J. Biol. Chem.*, 260, 4492, 1985.
38. **Rao, N. C., Barsky, S. H., Terranova, V. P., and Liotta, L. A.,** Isolation of a tumor cell laminin receptor, *Biochem. Biophys. Res. Comm.*, 111, 804, 1983.
39. **Malinoff, H. L. and Wicha, M. S.,** Isolation of a cell surface receptor protein for laminin from murine fibrosarcoma cells, *J. Cell Biol.*, 96, 1475, 1983.
40. **Silverstein, R. L. and Nachman, R. L.,** Thrombospondin binds to monocytes-macrophages and mediates platelet-monocyte adhesion, *J. Clin. Invest.*, 79, 867, 1987.
41. **Riser, B. L., Varani, J., Carey, T. E., Fligiel, S. E. G., and Dixit, V. M.,** Thrombospondin binding and thrombospondin synthesis by human squamous carcinoma cells: relationship to biological activity, *Exp. Cell Res.*, 174, 319, 1988.
42. **Murphy-Ullrich, J. E., Westrick, L. G., Esko, J. D., and Mosher, D. F.,** Binding of thrombospondin (TSP) to Chinese Hamster Ovary (CHO) cell mutants defective in glycosaminoclycan (GAG) biosynthesis, *J. Cell Biol.*, 104, 93a, 1986.
43. **Murphy-Ullrich, J. E. and Mosher, D. F.,** Interactions of thrombospondin with endothelial cells: receptor-mediated binding and degradation, *J. Cell Biol.*, 105, 1603, 1988.
44. **Giancotti, F. G., Tarone, G., Knudsen, K., Damsky, C., and Comoglio, P. M.,** Cleavage of a 135 Kd cell surface glycoprotein correlates with loss of fibroblast adhesion to fibronectin, *Exp. Cell Res.*, 156, 182, 1985.
45. **Horwitz, A., Duggan, K., Greggs, R., Decker, C., and Buck, C.,** The cell substrate attachment (CSAT) antigen has properties of a receptor for laminin and fibronectin, *J. Cell Biol.*, 101, 2134, 1985.
46. **Pytela, R., Pierschbacher, M. D., and Ruoslahti, E.,** Identification and isolation of a 140 Kd cell surface glycoprotein with properties expected of a fibronectin receptor, *Cell,* 40, 191, 1985.
47. **Knudsen, K., Horwitz, A., and Buck, C. A.,** Monoclonal antibody identifies a glycoprotein complex involved in cell-substratum adhesion, *Exp. Cell Res.*, 157, 218, 1985.
48. **Giancotti, F. G., Comoglio, P. M., and Tarone, G.,** A 135,000 molecular weight plasma membrane glycoprotein involved in fibronectin-mediated cell adhesion, *Exp. Cell Res.*, 163, 47, 1986.
49. **Akiyama, S. K., Yamada, S. S., and Yamada, K. M.,** Characterization of a 140 Kd avian cell surface antigen as a fibronectin-binding molecule, *J. Cell Biol.*, 102, 442, 1986.
50. **Patel, V. P. and Lodish, H. F.,** The fibronectin receptor on mammalian erythroid precursor cells: characterization and developmental regulation, *J. Cell Biol.*, 102, 449, 1986.
51. **Buck, C. A. and Horwitz, A. F.,** Cell surface receptors for extracellular matrix molecules, *Am. Rev. Cell Biol.*, 3, 179, 1987.
52. **Kleinman, H. K., Ogle, R. C., Cannon, F. B., Little, C. D., Sweeney, T. M., and Luckenbill-Edds, L.,** Laminin receptors for neurite outgrowth, *Proc. Natl. Acad. Sci. U.S.A.*, 85, 1282, 1988.
53. **Roberts, D. D., Rao, C. N., Magnani, J. L., Spitalnik, S. L., Liotta, L. A., and Ginsburg, V.,** Laminin binds specifically to sulfated glycolipids, *Proc. Natl. Acad. Sci. U.S.A.*, 82, 1306, 1985.
54. **Roberts, D. D., Haverstick, D. M., Dixit, V. M., Frazier, W. A., Santoro, S. A., and Ginsburg, V.,** The platelet glycoprotein thrombospondin binds specifically to sulfated glycolipids, *J. Biol. Chem.*, 260, 9405, 1985.
55. **Brown, S. S., Malinoff, H. L., and Wicha, M. S.,** Connectin: cell surface protein that binds both laminin and actin, *Proc. Natl. Acad. Sci. U.S.A.*, 80, 5927, 1983.
56. **Cody, R. L. and Wicha, M. S.,** Clustering of cell surface laminin enhances its association with the cytoskeleton, *Exp. Cell Res.*, 165, 107, 1986.
57. **Sugrue, S. P. and Hay, E. D.,** Response of basal epithelial cell surface and cytoskeleton to solubilized extracellular matrix molecules, *J. Cell Biol.*, 91, 45, 1981.
58. **Rao, K. M. K. and Varani, J.,** Actin polymerization induced by chemotactic peptide and concanavalin A in rat neutrophils, *J. Immunol.*, 129, 1605, 1982.

59. **Fligiel, S. E. G., Perone, P., and Varani, J.,** Arachidonic acid metabolism in murine fibrosarcoma cells with differing *in vitro* characteristics, *Int. J. Cancer,* 36, 383, 1985.
60. **Blum, J. L. and Wicha, M. S.,** Role of the cytoskeleton in laminin-induced mammary gene expression, *J. Cell Physiol.,* 135, 13, 1988.
61. **Mentzer, S. J., Herrmann, S. H., Crimmins, M. A. V., Burakoff, S. J., and Faller, D. V.,** The role of CD18 in phorbol ester-induced human monocyte-mediated cytotoxicity, *Cell. Immunol.,* 115, 66, 1988.
62. **Skoglund, G., Patarroyo, M., Forsbeck, K., Nisson, K., and Ingelman-Sundberg, M.,** Evidence for separate control by phorbol esters of CD18-dependent adhesion and translocation of protein kinase C in U-937 cells, *Cancer Res.,* 48, 3168, 1988.
63. **Wencel, M. L., Morganroth, M. L., Schoeneich, S. O., Gannon, D. E., Varani, J., Todd, R. F., Ryan, U. S., and Boxer, L. A.,** Cytoplasts and MO-1 deficient neutrophils pretreated with plasma and LPS induce lung injury, *Am. J. Physiol.,* 256, H751, 1989.
64. **Bevilacque, M. P., Pober, J. S., Wheeler, M. E., Cotran, R. S., and Gimbrone, M. A., Jr.,** Interleukin-1 acts on cultured human vascular endothelium to increase the adhesion of polymorphonuclear leukocytes, monocytes and related leukocyte cell lines, *J. Clin. Invest.,* 76, 2003, 1985.
65. **Pober, J. S., Bevilacqua, M. P., Mendrick, D. L., Lapierre, L. A., Fiers, W., and Gimbrone, M. A.,** Two distinct monokines, interleukin-1 and tumor necrosis factor, each independently induce biosynthesis and transient expression of the same antigen on the surface of cultured human vascular endothelial cells, *J. Immunol.,* 136, 1680, 1986.
66. **Bevilacqua, M. P., Pober, J. S., Majeau, G. R., Fiers, W., Cotran, R. S., and Gimbrone, M. A.,** Recombinant tumor necrosis factor induced procoagulant activity in cultured human vascular endothelial cells: characterization and comparison with the actions of interleukin-1, *Proc. Natl. Acad. Sci. U.S.A.,* 83, 4533, 1986.
67. **Stoolman, L. M.,** Adhesion molecules controlling lymphocyte migration, *Cell,* 56, 907, 1989.
68. **Vaheri, A. and Ruoslahti, E.,** Fibroblast surface antigen produced but not retained by virus-transformed human cells, *J. Exp. Med.,* 142, 530, 1975.
69. **Vaheri, A. and Mosher, D. F.,** High molecular weight cell surface associated glycoprotein (fibronectin) lost in malignant transformation, *Biochem. Biophys. Acta,* 516, 1, 1978.
70. **Hynes, R. O.,** Cell surface proteins and malignant transformation, *Biochem Biophys. Acta,* 458, 73, 1976.
71. **Yamada, K. M., Olden, K., and Pastan, I.,** Transformation sensitive cell surface protein: isolation, characterization and role in cellular morphology and adhesion, *Ann. N.Y. Acad. Sci.,* 312, 256, 1978.
72. **Hayman, E. G., Engvall, E., and Ruoslahti, E.,** Concomitant loss of cell surface laminin and fibronectin from transformed rat kidney celis, *J. Cell Biol.,* 88, 352, 1981.
73. **Alitalo, K., Keski-Oja, J., Hedman, K., and Vaheri, A.,** Loss of different pericellular matrix components of rat cells transformed with a T-class as mutant of Rous sarcoma virus, *Virology,* 119, 347, 1982.
74. **Sporn, M. B. and Roberts, A. B.,** Role of retinoids in differentiation and carcinogenesis, *Cancer Res.,* 43, 3034, 1983.
75. **Hayman, E. G., Engvall, E., and Ruoslahti, E.,** Butyrate restores fibronectin at the cell surface of transformed cells, *Exp. Cell Res.,* 127, 478, 1980.
76. **Milhaud, P., Yamada, K. M., and Gottesman, M. M.,** Sodium butyrate affects expression of fibronectin on CHO cells: specific increase in antibody-mediated cytotoxicity, *J. Cell Physiol.,* 104, 163, 1980.
77. **Chakrabarty, S., Brattain, M. G., Ochs, R. L., and Varani, J.,** Modulation of fibronectin, laminin and cellular adhesion in the transformation and differentiation of murine AKR fibroblasts, *J. Cell. Physiol.,* 133, 415, 1987.
78. **Tanaka, H. and Nishida, T.,** Butyrate stimulates fibronectin synthesis in cultured rabbit cornea, *J. Cell. Physiol.,* 123, 191, 1985.
79. **Varani, J., Mitra, R. S., McClenic, B., Fligiel, S. E. G., Inman, D. R., Dixit, V. M., and Nickoloff, B. J.,** Modulation of fibronectin production in normal human melanocytes and malignant melanoma cells by interferon-γ and tumor necrosis factor-α, *Am. J. Pathol.,* 134, 827, 1989.
80. **Chakrabarty, S., McRae, L. I., Levine, A. E., and Brattain, M. G.,** Restoration of normal growth control and membrane antigen composition in malignant cells by N,N-dimethylformamide, *Cancer Res.,* 44, 2181, 1984.
81. **Chakrabarty, S., Jan, Y., Son, J., Miller, C. A., and Brattain, M. G.,** Selective phosphorylation of cytosol proteins associated with transformation and restoration of normal phenotype in AKR mouse embryo fibroblasts, *Cancer Res.,* 45, 2170, 1985.
82. **Levine, A. E., McRae, L. J., and Brattain, M. G.,** Changes in receptor occupancy and growth factor responsiveness induced by treatment of a transformed mouse embryo cell line with N,N-dimethylformamide, *Cancer Res.,* 45, 6401, 1985.
83. **Marks, M. E., Ziober, B. L., and Brattain, M. G.,** Cell surface features associated with differentiation-induction of methylcholanthrene-transformed AKR-2B fibroblasts by N,N-dimethylformamide, *Cancer Res.,* 45, 1276, 1985.

84. **Chakrabarty, S., Jan, Y., Levine, A. E., McClenic, B., and Varani, J.,** Fibronectin/laminin and their receptors in aberrant growth control in Ha-*ras* oncogene transformed and epidermal growth factor gene transformed FR3T3 cells, *Int. J. Cancer,* 44, 325, 1989.
85. **Stein, D. F., Hare, D. L., Cecchini, M. A., and Weinberg, R. A.,** Construction of a novel oncogene based on synthetic sequence encoding epidermal growth factor, *Science,* 235, 321, 1987.
86. **Taylor-Papadimitriou, J., Burchell, J., and Hurst, J.,** Production of fibronectin by normal and malignant human mammary epithelial cells, *Cancer Res.,* 41, 2491, 1981.
87. **Smith, H. S., Riggs, J. L., and Mosessan, M. W.,** Production of fibronectin by human epithelial cells in culture, *Cancer Res.,* 39, 4138, 1987.
88. **Varani, J. and Chakrabarty, S.,** Modulation of fibronectin synthesis and fibronectin binding during transformation and differentiation of mouse AKR fibroblasts, *J. Cell. Physiol.,* 143, 445, 1990.
89. **Platefaber, L. C. and Hynes, R. O.,** Changes in integrin receptors on oncogenically-transformed cells, *Cell,* 56, 281, 1989.
90. **Saga, S., Chen, W. T., and Yamada, K. M.,** Enhanced fibronectin receptor expression in Rous sarcoma virus-induced tumors, *Cancer Res.,* 48, 5510, 1988.
91. **Akiyama, S. K., Larjava, H., and Yamada, K. M.,** Differences in the biosynthesis and localization of the fibronectin receptor in normal and transformed cultured human cells, *Cancer Res.,* 50, 1601, 1990.
92. **Ignotz, R. A. and Massague, J.,** Cell adhesion protein receptors as targets of transforming growth factor-β action, *Cell,* 51, 189, 1987.
93. **Roberts, C. J., Birkenmeier, T. M., McQuillan, J. J., Akiyama, S. K., Yamada, S. S., Chen, W. T., Yamada, K. M., and McDonald, J. A.,** Transforming growth factor β stimulates the expression of fibronectin and of both subunits of the human fibronectin receptor in cultured human lung fibroblasts, *J. Biol. Chem.,* 263, 4586, 1988.
94. **Ryseck, R. P., McDonald-Bravo, H., Zerial, M., and Bravo, R.,** Coordinate induction of fibronectin, fibronectin receptor, tropomyosin and actin genes in serum-stimulated fibroblasts, *Exp. Cell Res.,* 180, 537, 1989.
95. **Chakrabarty, S., Tobon, A., Varani, J., and Brattain, M. G.,** Induction of carcinoembryonic antigen secretion and modulation of protein secretion/expression and fibronectin/laminin expression in human colon carcinoma cells by transforming growth factor-β, *Cancer Res.,* 48, 4059, 1988.
96. **Babai, F.,** Etude ultrastructurale sur la pathenie de l'invasion du muscle strie' par des tumeurs transplantables, *J. Ultrastruct. Res.,* 56, 287, 1976.
97. **Albrechtsen, R., Nielsen, M., Wewer, U., Engvall, E., and Ruoslahti, E.,** Basement membrane changes in breast cancer detected by immuno-histochemical staining for laminin, *Cancer Res.,* 41, 5076, 1981.
98. **Burtin, P., Chavanel, G., Foidart, J. M., and Martin, E.,** Antigens of the basement membrane and the peritumoral stroma in human colonic adenocarcinomas: an immunofluorescence study, *Int. J. Cancer,* 30, 13, 1982.
99. **Miettinen, M., Foidart, J. M., and Ekblom, P.,** Immunohistochemical demonstration of laminin, the major glycoprotein of basement membranes, as an aid in the diagnosis of soft tissue tumors, *Am. J. Clin. Pathol.,* 79, 306, 1983.
100. **Miettinen, M. and Virtanen, I.,** Expression of laminin in thyroid gland and thyroid tumors: an immunohistologic study, *Int. J. Cancer,* 34, 27, 1984.
101. **Stenback, F., Wasenius, V. M., Risteli, J., and Risteli, L.,** Basement membranes in progressing intraepithelial cervical neoplasia, *Gynecol. Obstet. Invest.,* 20, 158, 1985.
102. **Alon, Y., Horowitz, A. T., Biran, S., Weiss, D. W., and Doljanski, F.,** Immunofluorescent characterization of fibronectin, laminin and keratin in normal and neoplastic human mammary epithelial cells in culture and in breast tissue section, *Int. J. Tissue React.,* 8, 401, 1986.
103. **Rampoldi, E., Larizza, L., Doneda, L., and Barlati, S.,** Fibronectin and laminin in hybrids of rous sarcoma virus transformed and normal mouse fibroblasts, *Tumori,* 71, 419, 1985.
104. **Bober, F. J., Birk, D. E., and Raska, K.,** Expression of varying portions of the adenovirus 12 early region 1 in transformed cells affects tumorigenicity and interaction with extracellular matrix components, *Lab. Invest.,* 56, 37, 1987.
105. **Brown, K. W. and Parkinson, E. K.,** Alteration of the extracellular matrix of cultured human keratinocytes by transformation and during differentiation, *Int. J. Cancer,* 35, 799, 1985.
106. **Varani, J., Lovett, E. J., McCoy, J. P., Shibata, S., Maddox, D. E., Goldstein, I. J., and Wicha, M. S.,** Differential expression of laminin-like substance by high and low metastatic tumor cells, *Am. J. Pathol.,* 111, 27, 1983.
107. **Malinoff, H. L., McCoy, J. P., Varani, J., and Wicha, M. S.,** Metastatic potential of murine fibrosarcoma cells is influenced by cell surface laminin, *Int. J. Cancer,* 33, 651, 1984.
108. **Varani, J., Orr, W., and Ward, P. A.,** Comparison of subpopulations of tumor cells with altered migratory activity, attachment characteristics, enzyme levels and *in vivo* behavior, *Eur. J. Cancer,* 15, 585, 1979.
109. **Varani, J., Orr, W., and Ward, P. A.,** Hydrolytic enzyme activities, migratory activity and *in vivo* growth and metastatic potential of recent tumor isolates, *Cancer Res.,* 39, 2376, 1979.

110. **Varani, J., Lovett, E. J., Wicha, M. S., Malinoff, H., and McCoy, J. P.,** Cell surface α-D-galactopyranosyl end groups: use as a marker in the isolation of murine tumor cell lines with varying cancer-causing potential, *J. Natl. Cancer Inst.*, 71, 1281, 1983.
111. **Barsky, S. H., Rao, C. N., Williams, J. E., and Liotta, L. A.,** Laminin molecular domains which alter metastasis in a murine model, *J. Clin. Invest.*, 74, 843, 1984.
112. **Muller, P. K. and Gauss-Muller, V.,** A study of fibroblast chemotaxis using fibronectin and conditioned medium as chemoattractants, *Eur. J. Cell Biol.*, 29, 268, 1983.
113. **McCarthy, J. B., Palm, S. L., and Furcht, L. T.,** Migration by haptotaxis of a schwann cell tumor line to the basement membrane glycoprotein laminin, *J. Cell Biol.*, 97, 772, 1983.
114. **McCarthy, J. B. and Furcht, L. T.,** Laminin and fibronectin promote the haptotactic migration of B16 mouse melanoma cells *in vitro, J. Cell Biol.*, 98, 1474, 1984.
115. **Situ, R., Lee, E. C., McCoy, J. P., and Varani, J.,** Stimulation of murine tumor cell motility by laminin, *J. Cell Sci.*, 70, 167, 1984.
116. **Varani, J., Fligiel, S. E. G., and Perone, P.,** Directional motility in strongly malignant murine tumor cells, *Int. J. Cancer,* 35, 559, 1985.
117. **Varani, J., Fligiel, S., and Wilson, B.,** Motility of ras^H oncogene transformed NIH-3T3 cells, *Tumor Invasion and Metastasis,* 6, 335, 1986.
118. **Fligiel, S. E. G., Laybourn, K. A., Peters, B. P., Ruddon, R. W., Hiserodt, J. C., and Varani, J.,** Laminin production by murine melanoma cells: possible involvement in cell motility, *Clin. Exp. Metastasis,* 4, 259, 1986.
119. **Nicolson, G. L. and Winkelhake, J. L.,** Organ specificity of blood-borne tumor metastases determined by cell adhesion, *Nature,* 255, 230, 1975.
120. **Briles, E. B. and Kornfeld, S.,** Isolation and metastatic properties of detachment variants of B16 melanoma cells, *J. Natl. Cancer Inst.*, 60, 1217, 1978.
121. **Winkelhake, J. L. and Nicolson, G. L.,** Determination of adhesive properties of variant metastatic melanoma cells to BALB/3T3 cells and their virus-transformed derivatives by a monolayer-attachment assay, *J. Natl. Cancer Inst.*, 56, 285, 1976.
122. **Hart, I. R.,** The selection and characterization of an invasive variant of the B16 melanoma, *Am. J. Pathol.*, 97, 587, 1979.
123. **Frenette, G., Carey, T., Varani, J., Ruddon, R., and Peters, B.,** Comparison of laminin biosynthesis in cultured human basal keratinocytes and malignant keratinocytes derived from primary and metastatic tumors, *Cancer Res.*, 48, 5193, 1988.
124. **Varani, J., Dixit, V. M., Fligiel, S. E. G., McKeever, P. E., and Carey, T. E.,** Thrombospondin-induced attachment and spreading of human squamous carcinoma cells, *Exp. Cell Res.*, 167, 376, 1986.
125. **Varani, J., Riser, B. L., Hughes, L. A., Carey, T. E., Fligiel, S. E. G., and Dixit, V. M.,** Characterization of thrombospondin synthesis, secretion and cell surface expression by human tumor cells, *Clin. Exp. Metastasis,* 7, 265, 1989.
126. **McClenic, B. K., Mitra, R. S., Riser, B. L., Nickoloff, B. J., Dixit, V. M., and Varani, J.,** Production and utilization of extracellular matrix components by human melanocytes, *Exp. Cell Res.*, 180, 314, 1989.
127. **Clark, R. A. F., Nielsen, L. D., Howell, S. E., and Folkvord, J. M.,** Human keratinocytes that have not terminally differentiated synthesize laminin and fibronectin but deposit only fibronectin in the pericellular matrix, *J. Cell Biochem.*, 28, 127, 1985.
128. **Nickoloff, B. J., Mitra, R. S., Riser, B. L., Dixit, V. M., and Varani, J.,** Modulation of keratinocyte motility: correlation with production of extracellular matrix molecules in response to growth promoting and anti-proliferative factors, *Am. J. Pathol.*, 132, 543, 1988.
129. **Varani, J., Schuger, L., and Chakrabarty, S.,** Growth factor induced extracellular matrix production and growth control in human colon carcinoma cells, *J. Cell Biochem.*, (Suppl.) 14A, 183, 1990.
130. **Chakrabarty, S., Jan, Y., Brattain, M. G., Tobon, A., and Varani, J.,** Diverse cellular responses elicited from human colon carcinoma cells by transforming growth factor-β, *Cancer Res.*, 49, 2112, 1989.

Chapter 2

INTERACTIONS OF TUMOR CELLS WITH BASEMENT MEMBRANES

Victor P. Terranova and David E. Maslow

TABLE OF CONTENTS

I. INTRODUCTION

Metastases arise following a complex series of ordered processes, which involve tumor cell attachment to and penetration through the extracellular matrix, motility, and passive transport and invasion and proliferation. The active migration of metastatic cells from the primary bulk tumor is followed by their invasion into the circulatory system. Having entered the circulation, tumor cells arrest in the lumina of small vessels, invade, or rupture the vessel wall, and exit from the circulation. Metastatic lesions result from tumor cell proliferation in the secondary organ. Many of these steps involve the interactions of the tumor cells with basement membrane components that affect and modulate the course of the metastasis.

II. STAGES OF METASTASIS

Tumor cell invasion and metastasis involve specific steps that comprise the metastatic cascade. Understanding the specific steps involved in this process will help to increase our knowledge of the disease process and potential therapies.

A. STAGE I: TUMOR CELL ESCAPE

The first step of the metastatic cascade is tumor cell escape (Figure 1). In order to be successful in forming metastases in distant target organs, tumor cells must possess certain important features that allow them to successfully complete the complex series of events in the metastatic cascade (Table 1). Only a small population of the primary bulk tumor will successfully produce metastases. It is still a matter of some controversy whether the metastases are formed by cells genetically preselected[1-3] to express a metastatic phenotype, or, alternatively, by cells that transiently acquire the properties to survive the many selective pressures that characterize the metastatic cascade.[4-6] These hypotheses are not mutually exclusive as the genetic contribution to cell behavior can never be excluded, and examples of the modulation of expression of genetically determined traits are numerous. Both approaches support the observations that the number of spontaneous metastases formed from a primary tumor is very small despite the large number of cells that enter the vasculature.[7] Although few in number,[8-14] the tumor cells that form metastases must have the capacity to separate from the bulk tumor[15] and attach to, degrade, and invade basement membrane barriers. These cells breach the delineating primary basement membrane of the tumor, migrate toward, and invade vascular basement membrane to enter into the circulation.[1,3,6,8,16,17]

1. Components of Basement Membranes

Basement membranes are composed of a mixture of various components, many of which appear to partially regulate the migration, growth, and differentiation of both normal and tumor cells.[18-38] They are thin sheets of extracellular matrix that separate organ parenchymal cells from interstitial stroma and constitute a major barrier to the spread of metastatic cells.[38-40] Each tissue specific extracellular matrix is composed of characteristic collagens, glycoproteins, and proteoglycans (Table 2). The exact ratio of these components, as well as the presence or absence of fibronectin, is different in basement membranes from various tissues.[26,41-42] Basement membranes are biochemically unique, differing considerably from other types of extracellular matrices such as interstitial stroma or cartilage. In addition, widespread changes have been exhibited during tumorigenesis.[43-45] The specific capacity of invasive tumor cells to metastasize may be related not only to their ability to interact with components of the extracellular matrix, but also to the specific phenotypic response of the cells to extracellular components.

Type IV collagen is a unique collagen specifically associated with basement membranes.[46,47] Comprising 20% of the protein of the basement membrane,[48-49] it serves as a

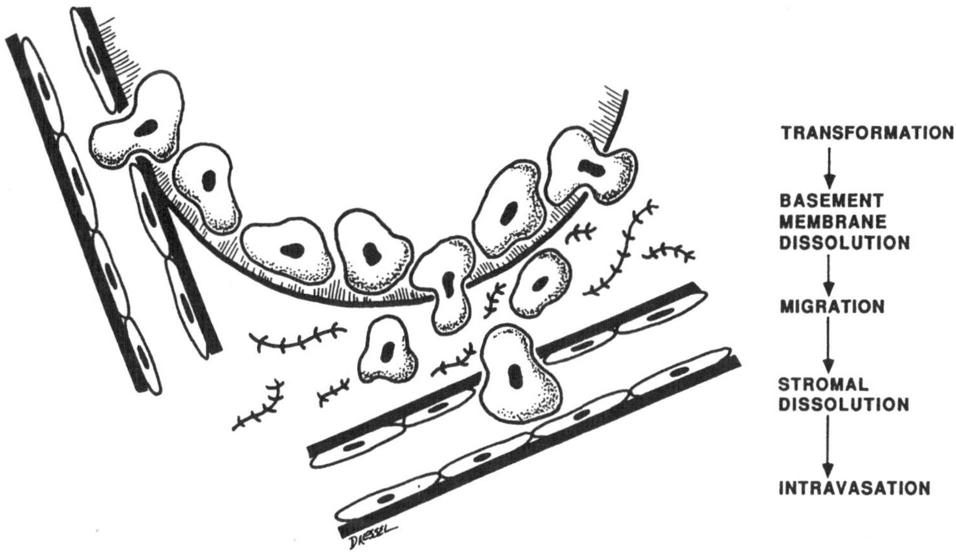

FIGURE 1. Tumor cell escape from the primary tumor. This entails breakdown of an encapsulating basement membrane where both specific and nonspecific enzymes may be employed. Tumor cells not immediately adjacent to a blood vessel migrate through the interstitial stroma while those near a capillary bypass that step. Tumor cell attachment to the stromal matrix is necessary. This process may be mediated by specific attachment factors such as laminin and fibronectin. In addition, proteases are necessary for stromal degradation. Proteolysis may be localized to the tumor cell surface where the concentration of active enzymes is greater than the natural protease inhibitors found in the stroma. Finally, the tumor cells penetrate the capillary basement membrane and enter into the circulation.

TABLE 1
Characteristics of Successfully Metastasizing Cells

Characteristic	Ref.
Transformed	107, 180, 198, 199
Small percentage of total tumor cells	9, 14, 149, 200
Many laminin receptors	6, 37—39, 71, 88, 201—205
High affinity for basement membrane	40, 67, 103
Production and release of type IV and other proteases	120, 155, 174, 206—211
Motile	20, 23, 89, 128—130, 133, 159, 212, 213
Survival and proliferation at target tissue	160, 178, 214

Note: The characteristics listed partially define the metastatic phenotype. Expression of some of these features enables metastatic tumor cells to successfully penetrate basement membrane, affording these cells an advantage in the successful progression along the metastatic cascade. Expression of other features provides advantages at other stages in the process. The end result would be the successful formation and growth of a new lesion.

major structural component.[50-52] The exact size of the collagen molecules in basement membranes is not definitely established. Some studies suggest that the biosynthetic form, type IV procollagen (M_r = 185,000 and 170,000) is converted to a smaller molecule, type IV collagen (M_r = 160,000 and 140,000), which is incorporated into the matrix.[52-53] Other studies suggest that processing of type IV procollagen does not occur and that the biosynthetic form is incorporated into the matrix.[54-59] Type IV differs both chemically and structurally from type I, II, and III, which form fibers in interstitial connective tissues. Unlike the other

TABLE 2
Components of Basement Membrane

Component	Mol. wt.	%	Ref.
Type-IV collagen	185,000—170,000	20	46, 47, 51, 53—59, 68, 215
Laminin	1,000,000	30—50	69—91
Heparan sulfate	110,000—1,000,000	1—2	68, 92—96, 216, 217
Entactin	150,000	<1	97, 98
Nidogen	100,000	<1	68, 218
Fibronectin	220,000	Variable	6, 26, 100—102, 216, 219
Type IV collagen	120,000	Variable	40, 49, 220—224

collagens, type IV collagen contains nonhelical segments[60] and does not form a fibrillar matrix.[61] The nonhelical segments of the molecule confer a greater degree of flexibility and presumably create a more elastic matrix.[62] The arrangement of type IV molecules in basement membrane is unique; the molecules appear to be arrayed in an open network with like ends in opposition and cross-linked.[63-66] This arrangement confers tensile strength on the matrix while also creating an elastic structure. Type IV collagen also contains binding sites for other components of basement membrane, which include heparin sulfate proteoglycan, fibronectin, and laminin, as well as other specific components secreted from the underlying interstitial stroma.[48,49,63,67,68]

Laminin is localized exclusively in basement membranes and is synthesized by cells that normally reside on basement membrane. Laminin is a high molecular weight glycoprotein (M_r = 850,000 to 1,000,000), consisting of two major types of polypeptide chains in a 1:2 ratio. It was first isolated from the Engelbrecht-Holm-Swarm sarcoma, a mouse tumor that produces copious quantities of basement membrane. The A chain, also called GP1 or β-subunit, is represented only once per molecule and has a molecular weight of approximately 440 kilodaltons (kDa). The B chain (GP2 or α-subunit) is present as two or three subunits in close association with the A chain. The B chains have been shown to consist of two polypeptides, termed B_1 and B_2, of closely similar molecular weight (200 kDa and 230 kDa, respectively).[69] A fourth component, derived from placenta and visualized as a 230 to 240 kDa band on sodium dodecylsulfate polyacrylamide gel electrophoresis, has been called the "M" chain.[70] The M chain has not been found in all basement membranes. It has been reported, however, that laminin isolated from some tissues may exhibit distinct antigenic sites not apparent in other basement membranes,[71] the presence of the laminin M chain could account for these findings.

The B_1 chain of mouse laminin has been cloned and shown to consist of 1786 amino acids, comprising seven distinct domains.[72] These include cysteine-rich repeats with homology to epidermal growth factor (EGF), alpha helical and globular domains, and a presumptive signal peptide. The subunits are connected by disulfide bonds to form a cross-shaped structure. The short arms extend approximately 36 nm from the center of the structure, and the long arm is 77 nm in length. A single globular domain caps the long arm of the cross, while the short arms contain two such regions. Alpha-helical segments assembled in coiled-coil structures are located in the rod portion of the long arm of laminin.[73] Despite the proposed model, the precise relationship and interaction of the A, B_1, and B_2 chains await further elucidation.

The native laminin molecule is heavily glycosylated with about 12% of its weight attributed to *N*-linked oligosaccharide chains. Only the AB_1B_2 complex undergoes oligosaccharide side chain processing to produce the mature molecule.[74] Sugar residues that have been identified include fucose, mannose, galactose, glucose, *N*-acetylated hexosamines, sialic acid, and xylose. Biantennary, triantennary, and tetra-antennary high-mannose and complex-type oligosaccharides are present in the molecule, and at least 43 *N*-linkage sites have been described.[75] The globular regions appear enriched in β-D-galactopyranosyl residues while β-D-mannopyranosyl residues may be located in both the globular and rod-like domains.

Exposure of laminin-producing cells to tunicamycin, an inhibitor of *N*-glycosylation, results in decreased laminin secretion. Monensin, a monovalent carboxylic ionophore which disrupts the Golgi complex and reduces intracellular protein transport, inhibits the processing of high-mannose precursors of all three of the major laminin subunits. In the presence of monensin, abnormal laminin molecules sensitive to β-*N*-acetylglucosaminidase H (Endo H) digestion accumulate in the cellular medium, indicating that laminin with incompletely processed oligosaccharide chains is produced by these cells.[76] Such studies suggest that altered laminin may still be secreted by cells, but at an abnormally slow rate. Glycosylation, then, is likely to play some significant role in the normal molecular functions of laminin.

The laminin molecule is known to be synthesized by epithelial and endothelial cells, as well as by muscle cells and some types of fibroblasts, and is perhaps the earliest detectable extracellular matrix protein seen in normal development. The B chain has been identified in the 2-cell mouse embryo,[77] and it appears that only the B_1 and B_2 chains are present from the 4-8 cell stage. From the 16-cell stage onward in development, all three major laminin polypeptides have been identified.[78] Synthesis of the B_2 chain is the rate limiting step for production of native laminin.[74] The molecule has been localized to the lamina densa, lamina rara externa, and lamina rara interna of glomerular basement membrane[79] and has the ability to self-assemble *in vitro*.[80]

Native laminin will bind type IV collagen and protype IV collagen,[81,82] heparan sulfate proteoglycan,[83] heparin,[84] and nidogen.[85] One study[86] has implicated an association of laminin with cytoskeletal components by clustering of connectin, a 70 kDa transmembrane laminin receptor, and "organization" of intracellular actin. Such an interaction could be important in maintenance of epithelial cell polarity.

Partial protease digestion of the native laminin molecule has enabled localization of its binding sites for some basal lamina components (Figure 2). Exposure of laminin to thrombin results in digestion of the laminin long arm to leave a 600,000 kDa fragment, the serine protease resistant α-subunit,[87-88] which will bind tumor cells and type IV collagen. Rotary shadowing of chymotrypsin-treated or pepsin-treated laminin reveals fragments that contain the three short arms without the globular domains; these fragments will bind to cells but not to collagen IV.[88] Trypsin or elastase digestion of the native molecule produces fragments that include the globular domain of the long arm. This region contains a binding site for heparin and possibly also for type IV collagen.[80] The neurite-out-growth promoting activity of murine laminin has been localized to the end of the long arm,[89] while electron microscopy and binding studies reveal that the center of the laminin cross contains a site of attachment for nidogen.[31] A nonapeptide segment of the B_1 chain with homology to epidermal growth factor ("peptide 11") has been shown to be one of the primary sites in laminin mediating cell attachment, migration, and receptor binding.[90-91] Laminin has been shown to regulate several biological functions, including cell (normal and neoplastic) attachment and spreading, tissue remodeling, embryogenesis, cell migration, growth, and differentiation[19,27,31,33,35,82,86,90,103,201,204] (Figure 3).

Heparan sulfate proteoglycans have been isolated from a variety of basement membranes[92-95] These proteoglycans vary in size from M_r = 110,000 to M_r = 10^6. Antibodies prepared against heparan sulfate proteoglycan have revealed a core protein which is glycosylated and sulfated to form a low density form of proteoglycan (M_r = 800,000). This low density proteoglycan is processed proteolytically to form a smaller high density form. The high density proteoglycan is easily extracted from basement membrane producing EHS (Engelbreth-Holm-Swarm) tumors with neutral salt solutions, whereas the larger form (low density) requires urea or guanidine for extraction. This suggests that the low density pro-

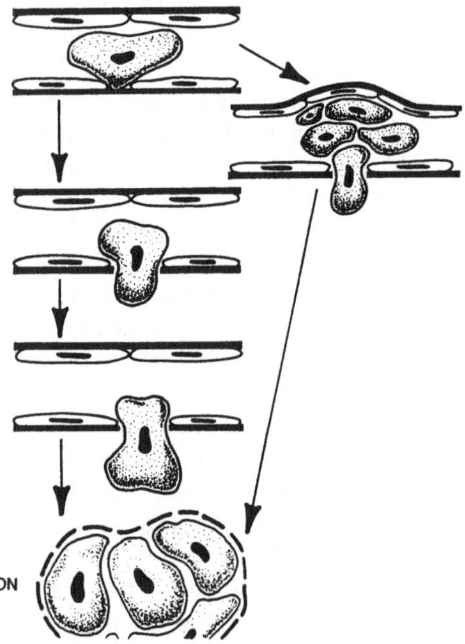

FIGURE 2. Postulated steps in invasion include a sequence of events. Tumor cells lodged in a capillary begin to proliferate or attach to the vascular endothelium and cause retraction of these cells or attach directly to areas of exposed basement membrane. Laminin and the laminin receptor play an important role in this process. After attachment to the subendothelial basement membrane, tumor cell-associated proteases (specifically a type IV collagenase) are released in the microenvironment. This process degrades basement membrane. Migration of the tumor cells through the basement membrane and into the stroma is next hypothesized. Here, target tissue-specific chemoattractants play an important role. Finally, tumor cell proliferation and encapsulation by basement membrane complete the process. The expansive growth of tumor contained within a blood vessel may also rupture it. The new lesion may have cells of increased metastatic propensity due to pressure applied by the host during the entire cascade and the response of the tumor cells to the host environment.

teoglycan is an integral component of the extracellular matrix, whereas the high density form is a degradation product that is loosely associated with the matrix. Type IV collagen, laminin, and fibronectin all bind to heparan sulfate.[52] The role of heparan sulfate in the basement membrane appears to be the formation of an anionically charged barrier to the passage of negatively charged macromolecules.[68,92,93,96]

Entactin is a sulfated glycoprotein (M_r = 150,000) that was first isolated from teratocarcinoma cells and subsequently found to be present in basement membranes of a variety of tissues.[97-98] Its structure and function has not yet been defined, but cell attachment activity has been recorded.[97]

Nidogen is a recently discovered glycoprotein component (M_r = 100,000) of basement membrane.[28] Possessing the capacity to self-aggregate, it is hypothesized that the role of nidogen is to control the initial deposition, as well as the organization, of the basement membrane.[68]

Fibronectin is a large glycoprotein (M_r = 220,000) widely distributed in tissues and blood[25-26] and also comprises a prominent component of basement membranes in developing tissues.[26,99,100] The fibronectin of basement membranes may be produced by adjacent stromal cells or may accumulate there from the circulating fibronectin in the blood.[101] Fibronectin is known to bind type IV collagen,[67,102,103] heparan sulfate,[100] fibrin,[104] and most other glycoproteins of the extracellular matrix.[26]

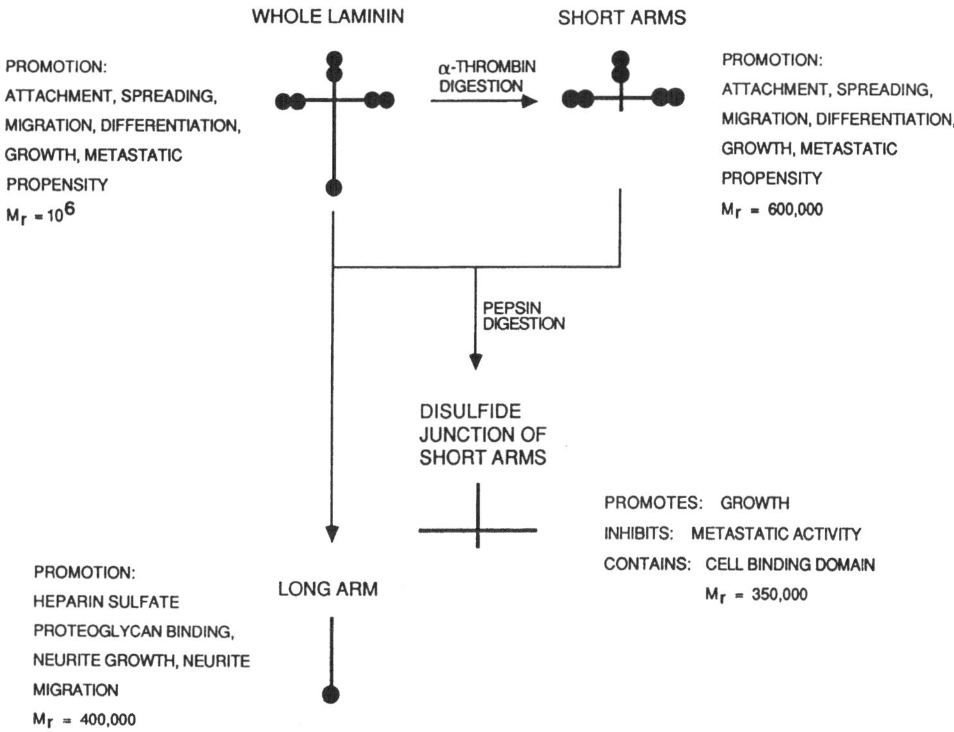

FIGURE 3. The biological function of laminin in relation to metastasis is correlated with the current working hypothesis of the functional domains of the molecule. The whole molecule has a cross-shaped structure with three short arms (35 nm in length) and one long arm (76 nm in length). All of the arms have large globular end-regions that are enriched for carbohydrate. Laminin binding to native type IV collagen is eliminated when the globular end-regions of the short arms are removed by digestion with pepsin. Digestion of the native molecule with alpha-thrombin removes the long arm and the ability of the molecule to bind heparan sulfate proteoglycan. The disulfide junction of the three short arms contains the cell-binding domain. (References are in the text.)

2. Interaction of Tumor Cells with Extracellular Matrix

Local tumor invasion is one of the first steps in the metastatic cascade[3,39,105,106] (Figure 1), following the transformation from *in situ* to invasive carcinoma behavior. The next stage essential in the metastatic cascade involves the entry of tumor cells into the general circulation, a process called intravasation.[107,108] The rate of tumor cell escape into the vasculature is controlled by a number of factors, namely, the tumor vascularity, the number of migrating tumor cells, anatomical factors including the structure of the basement membrane in the tumor capillary bed, and the specific properties of tumor cells[109-112] (Figures 1 and 4). Once in the circulation, tumor cells must successfully evade host defenses, survive the trauma of fluid flow, and arrest in small vessels[2,113-115] (Figures 2 and 4).

The degradation of basement membrane, one mechanism for the intravasation of metastatic tumor cells, most likely occurs in a highly localized region at the point of tumor cell surface-extracellular matrix interface microenvironment. In this region, the concentrations of hydrolytic enzymes expressed by the cell are greater than the concentrations of natural protease inhibitors present in serum or associated with the matrix.[116-118] The ultimate result of this tumor cell-substrate interaction is matrix dissolution (Figures 1, 2, and 4) followed by escape of intravasating cells. A tumor cell may also enter the vasculature through pores in the basement membrane,[119] particularly in blood vessels newly joined in response to angiogenic factors[120] or in areas of change or disorganization of matrix.[121] Additionally, the dissemination of tumor cells can occur through the lymphatic system, a path less complex since, unlike blood capillaries, lymphatic capillaries lack a formed basement membrane.[122]

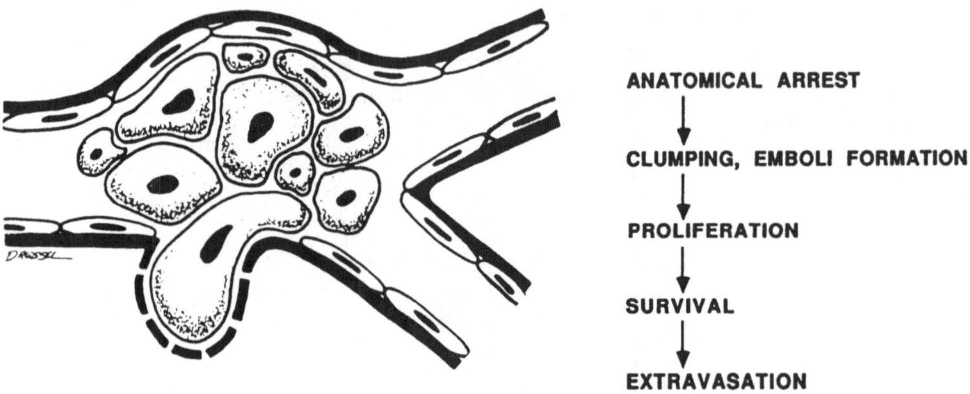

FIGURE 4. Tumor cell arrest may be a function of anatomical entrapment. Other tumor cells or blood cells reach the blocked pathway, and microemboli are formed. The tumor cells then proliferate, giving rise to an ever-increasing bulk of tumor. Extravasation through the vessel wall occurs next.

Highly metastatic cells have a greater capacity to bind to and degrade extracellular matrix *in vitro* (Table 1). However, there is little experimental data on the *in vivo* intravasation of defined tumor cell lines so a definitive correlation between this binding and degrading and *in vivo* cell dissemination cannot be made. The greater capacity to bind to laminin may play an important role in this process, since basement membrane is an initial and ever-present barrier. Also, increased attachment of invasive tumor cells to normal cells and the response of the normal cells may be vital for intravasation. The role of laminin, fibronectin, heparin, and proteases as mediators of intravasation remains to be determined.

There have been a number of techniques described to quantify the motility of tumor cells, including measurements of the invasion of embryonic tissue fragments,[123] the chorioallantoic membrane,[124-126] the human amnion[127] and the vascular endothelium. These natural, heterogeneous materials constitute a less sensitive assay system because of their lack of uniformity and reproducibility. However, experimentation using artificial substrates consisting of unimpregnated cellulose nitrate filters and filters impregnated with matrix constituents has revealed a correlation between spontaneous metastatic behavior of murine malignant cell lines and *in vitro* filter penetration.[128,129] An enhancement of the mobility of some tumor cells following treatment with collagenase (both mammalian and bacterial), independent of matrix degradation, was also reported.[128] The chemotactic effect of these enzymes and their collagen degradation products suggest that the collagenases present in the environment of the invasive cells may be affecting cellular behavior directly in addition to their degradative effects on the matrix[130] (Table 3).

Recently, a method using a biochemically defined barrier to select for highly invasive tumor cells has been developed.[84] The method utilizes a synthetic basement membrane barrier consisting of an overlay of laminin and type IV collagen co-formed and compressed onto a type I collagen matrix. This barrier offers a biochemically defined connective tissue through which tumor cells may penetrate. When the matrix was placed in a modified Boyden Chamber (Figure 5) with tumor cells added to the upper compartment, it was found that the highly metastatic tumor cell lines could penetrate the barrier. When recultured, these tumor cell lines were more invasive and colonizing than those of the parent population. In these experiments, invasiveness was measured by the cells ability to bind to basement membrane, express laminin receptors, degrade basement membrane, and finally, upon intravenous reinjection into animals, produce more lesions. It was found that the addition of specific tissue extracts to the lower compartment of the modified Boyden Chamber stimulated chemotactic migration of tumor cells in a manner corresponding to the distribution of metastases

TABLE 3
Checkerboard Analysis of the Motile Response of Lewis Lung Carcinoma Cells to Type IV Collagenase in the Boyden Chamber Assay

Type IV Collagenase Concentration (μg/ml) Upper Compartment

Type IV Collagenase Concentration (μg/ml) Lower Compartment	0	1	2	3	4	5	10
0	15 ± 4	10 ± 4	11 ± 3	12 ± 3	8 ± 4	12 ± 2	9 ± 1
1	28 ± 5	19 ± 3	16 ± 4	14 ± 4	12 ± 4	10 ± 3	11 ± 2
2	32 ± 4	25 ± 4	21 ± 5	15 ± 4	15 ± 5	16 ± 3	12 ± 2
3	41 ± 5	35 ± 3	24 ± 3	26 ± 5	7 ± 4	10 ± 1	13 ± 2
4	47 ± 6	40 ± 3	31 ± 7	28 ± 6	29 ± 4	17 ± 3	10 ± 2
5	51 ± 6	44 ± 3	41 ± 4	36 ± 4	30 ± 3	33 ± 7	8 ± 1
10	52 ± 6	49 ± 3	51 ± 3	50 ± 5	52 ± 7	50 ± 3	37 ± 5

Mean no. of cells migrated/high power field ± S.D. (3 assays)

Note: The concentration of type IV collagenase was varied systematically over the range 1—10 μg/ml in the upper and lower compartments of a Modified Boyden Chamber (Figure 5). The higher levels of penetration under the conditions of equal collagenase concentration on both sides of the filter (shown along the diagonal of the table) indicates chemokinesis. The increased values generated below the diagonal (positive gradient) represent positive chemotoxis. Thus, type IV collagenase is demonstrated to be a potent chemoattractant with both chemotactic and chemokinetic action.

found *in vivo*.[131,132] It is possible that tissue-specific proteins act as chemoattractants for metastasizing cells. These proteins are thought to exist in sufficient concentrations within tissues to direct target tissue-specific metastasis in the body. Current studies suggest that in different target tissues, the proteins acting as chemoattractants have substantially different molecular weights.[131-132]

B. STAGE II: TUMOR CELL DISSEMINATION AND ARREST

The next stage of the metastatic cascade involves the malignant cells passage from the vicinity of the primary tumor to distant target tissue sites by disseminating throughout the body via blood and, to a lesser extent, the lymphatic circulatory system. This leads to tumor cell interaction with and arrest in the microvasculature.[133]

Factors influencing the ultimate fate and localization of disseminating tumor cells in the body include differences in the exposed cell surface antigens,[134-138] cellular and secreted enzymes, other secreted products,[108] and inflammatory and coagulative responses.[133] Major differences in biological characteristics that also influence dissemination of tumor cells include the capacity of the cells to invade blood vessels and tissues and subsequently to colonize and proliferate within specific target tissues.[1,3,108] Tumor cells also have been shown to affect the adhesive behavior of normal cells.[139]

The host immune system plays an important role in the metastatic process. However, due to the multitude of factors involved, an adequate model system has not been defined. In some tumor systems, suppression of antitumor immune responses results in increased spontaneous or experimental metastasis. In other tumor systems, similar manipulations lead to a decrease or eradication of metastasis. Finally, in still other systems, host immunity appears to have no apparent effect on experimental or spontaneous metastasis.[140-143] It is believed that there may be more than one competing host immune system involved in antitumor responses.[144-147]

The question of variation in the properties of tumor cells derived from primary and secondary lesions is complex and difficult to study. Metastases have been shown to be antigenically and biochemically distinct from their primary tumors,[37,108,148-150] but the relation of these differences to metastasis is unclear. Of course, the differences in tumor age, size, and necrotic component must be considered in any comparisons between a primary tumor and its metastases.

In addition to the possible interaction of tissue basement membrane specific chemoattractants with metastasizing tumor cells, it has been found that tumor cells adhere differentially to capillary endothelial cells *in vitro*.[151] Studies revealed that teratoma tumor cells prelabelled with 3H-thymidine showed preferential adhesion to endothelial capillaries extracted from mouse ovaries, whereas glioma tumor cells showed preferential adhesion to capillary endothelial cells extracted from mouse brain. These experiments suggest that capillary endothelial cells derived from different sources are not alike and that differences expressed at the cell surface of these cells can be distinguished by tumor cells. The endothelial lining of capillaries is the first barrier to penetration of cells that are disseminated through the vascular system.[108,152-157] The capacity of endothelial cells to express different antigens depending on their tissue source is supported by the use of endothelial cells from different tissues to raise specific antisera and monoclonal antibodies.[158] One possible explanation of endothelial cell specificity currently under investigation is that the organ-specific subendothelial basement membrane high affinity chemoattractants modulate the adhesive properties of both capillary endothelial cells and the underlying basement membrane (Figure 6). Perhaps the chemoattractants increase the expression of those endothelial cell surface antigens that are recognized by specific tumor cells. Recently, it has been reported that certain substances functioning as chemoattractants for phagocytes also act as chemoattractants for certain tumor cells. Bombesin, a tetradecapeptide neuronal growth factor, has been found to be a potent chemoattractant for small cell lung carcinoma cells (SCLC) as well as for human monocytes.[159] It is worth noting that leukocytes and spermatozoa are the only cells that utilize chemotactic mechanisms in the course of their normal functions. Metastatic cells may have adopted a chemotactic mechanism similar to that observed in leukocytes.

The preference of many metastasizing tumors for specific secondary sites of proliferation is well documented for tumors of natural[160] and experimental origin.[161-162] The exact mechanism of selective organ tumor growth is not fully understood. Three mechanisms have been proposed, each of which depends on the attachment behavior of disseminating cells within the circulatory system. The first mechanism has been termed the "mechanical" hypothesis.[163] This suggests that tumors will spread locally along the lines of least resistance after dissemination, implying that formation of emboli by tumor cells and other blood components is the important feature in tumor cell arrest (Figure 4). These tumor cell emboli are then trapped. While the trapping of the emboli may be nonspecific, the site of formation of emboli may occur at specific locations. This hypothesis has failed to totally explain several examples of organ-specific metastasis.[164-165] Also a correlation is lacking between the number of emboli formed and the formation of distant metastases.[166,167] The second general mechanism is referred to as the "seed and soil" hypothesis,[168] which suggests that the growth of metastatic lesions appears to be the direct result of the microenvironment provided by the specific organ and the growth preference of the tumor cells. This hypothesis requires the presence of environmental conditions such as released growth factors in target organs that will promote tumor cell survival and proliferation. Growth factors are present throughout

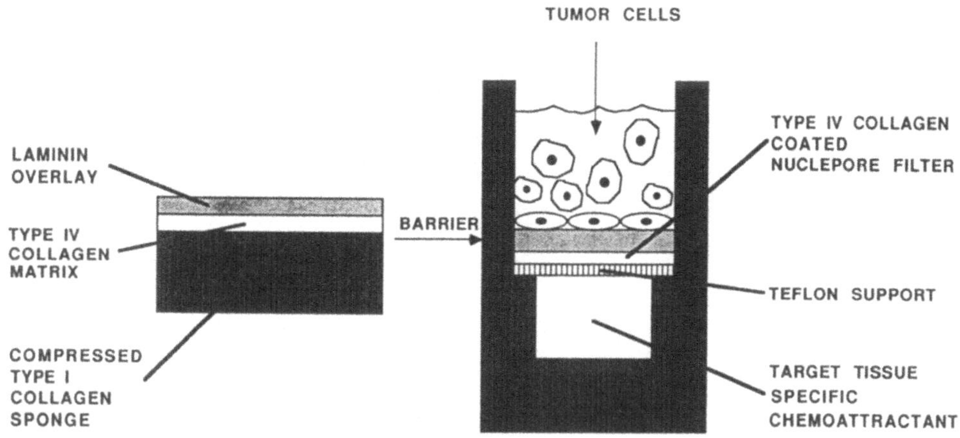

FIGURE 5. Diagram of the chemoinvasion assay using the Modified Boyden Chamber. The synthetic basement membrane-stromal barrier and the assay chamber are depicted.

the body, often specifically localized in specific tissues and organs.[169] The third mechanism suggests the presence of receptors on metastasizing tumor cells that specifically recognize cell surface antigens in cells of the appropriate target organ. This hypothesis does not preclude the existence of recognition molecules in the parenchymal cells.[170] The work of many laboratories indicates that organ-specific metastasis is the result of a combination of these proposed mechanisms.[6,38-40,72,103,110] Currently, small organ-specific polypeptides localized to the subendothelial basement membrane with chemotactive and proliferative capacity are being investigated.

Evidence exists that increased exposure of the subendothelial basement membrane, either by endothelial cell shedding,[108] endothelial cell injury,[171] or active endothelial cell retraction,[16,172,173] plays an important role in the initial adherence and invasion of metastasizing tumor cells. Also of importance are reports that tumor cells, like leukocytes and neutrophils, respond to chemotactic stimuli by showing an increased adhesiveness and subsequent release of hydrolytic enzymes possibly as a result of lysozomal exocytosis. A widening of the vascular endothelial gap could allow the efflux of circulating tumor cells into the interstitium or give tumor cells access to the vascular basement membrane. The microenvironment of the exposed extracellular matrix may contain active levels of potent chemoattractants for tumor cells. Following the attachment of tumor cells to the basement membrane, the tumor cell may respond to the stimuli of organ-derived chemoattractants. These factors may cause the release of hydrolytic enzymes such as type IV collagenase and other neutral proteases to permit extravasation of the tumor cell[174] (Figure 2) or to stimulate growth. These enzymes then may act as a microenvironment-specific chemoattractant. Thus, increased levels of free enzyme in the microenvironment may signal the cell that a specific extracellular matrix has been degraded.

C. STAGE III: TUMOR CELL PROLIFERATION

The final stage in the metastatic process involves target organ colonization by an invading tumor cell, and the survival, proliferation, and formation of secondary tumors at distant locations from that of the primary tumor.

Following tumor cell attachment and migration or invasive growth through the interstitial extracellular matrix, the metastasizing tumor cell eventually lodges in a location with a microenvironment that is optimal for growth (Figure 2). This microenvironment might contain sufficient levels of growth factors to ensure tumor cell proliferation. Matrix lysis occurs in highly localized regions close to the tumor cell surface. Continued invasion within

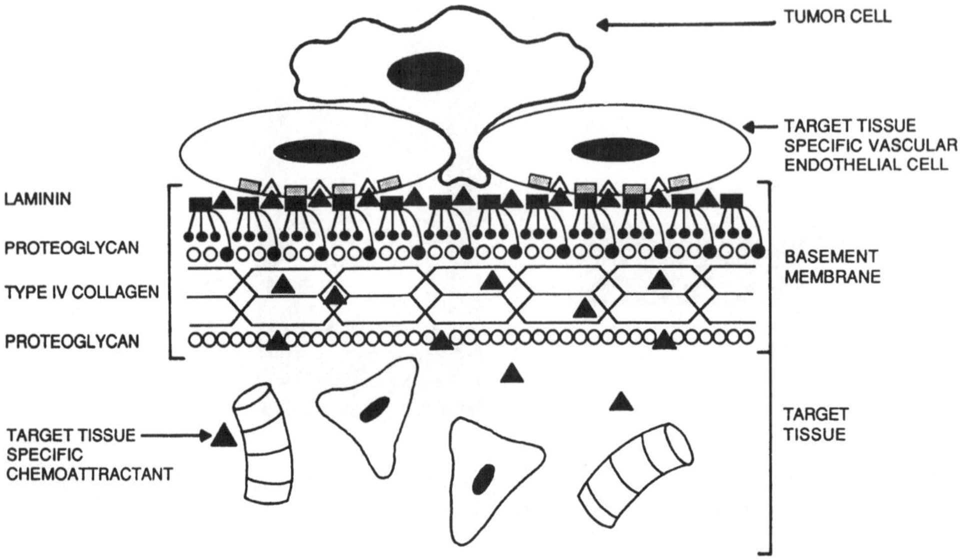

FIGURE 6. Tumor cell-specific attachment to vascular endothelium and basement membrane are shown. Additionally, the target tissue specific factor(s) are shown, and the possible effect on the endothelial and tumor cell is noted. Localization of target tissue-specific chemoattractants to the basement membrane is essential. Tumor cell degradation of the basement membrane and movement into target tissue followed by survival and proliferation could be mediated by these factors.

the secondary site of growth occurs in a process that requires the repetition of attachment, matrix lysis, local cell movement, and cellular proliferation. The proliferation of tumor cells is enhanced by a number of growth factors that are synthesized either exogenously by given tissues, endogenously by the tumor cell, or both. In some situations, there is endogenous and exogenous synthesis, and tumor cell growth is stimulated in both an autocrine and paracrine manner. Autocrine stimulation is a mechanism whereby a cell both produces and utilizes the same hormone.[175-177] It has been proposed that malignant cells may maintain their tumorigenic phenotype by autocrine secretion of transforming growth factors (TGFs).[177-180] TGFs are low-molecular-weight proteins that reversibly induce nonneoplastic cells to lose contact inhibition and undergo anchorage-independent growth.[178] In normal cell lines, such as normal rat kidney (NRK) fibroblasts, TGFs are capable of conferring the transformed phenotype.[187] In tumor cell lines under less stringent growth control, other growth factors along with TGFs can confer anchorage-independent growth. Two types of TGFs have been identified. Type alpha-TGF, originally detected in the conditioned medium of sarcoma-virus transformed cells, is a single chain peptide ($M_r \sim 6{,}000$) that shows sequence homology to epidermal growth factor (EGF).[187] TGF-α competes for the binding of ^{125}I-labelled EGF to the EGF receptor and has mitogenic activity, as does EGF.[178,182] The laminin component of the basement membrane has amino acid sequences which have a large degree of homology with both TGF-α and EGF. Additionally, laminin has been shown to be a mitogen for several tumor cell lines. Type beta-TGF is present in many normal[183] and transformed[184] cells. Platelets act as the major nonneoplastic storage site for the protein.[185] TGF-β has neither a structural nor a functional relationship to EGF or the EGF receptor[183] nor does it induce mitosis.[185-186] Structural studies have shown that this growth factor is composed of two peptide chains, each of 12,500 Da, held together by disulfide bonds.[183,185,197] A synergistic effect of alpha- and beta-TGF is responsible for maximal phenotypic transformation.[185,186] TGF-beta has been shown to increase the number of EGF receptors on the surface of NRK fibroblasts.[188] Platelet derived growth factor (PDGF) has been found to interact in combination with TGF-alpha and TGF-beta to stimulate anchorage-independent growth.[189] Certain melanoma cell lines have been shown to actively secrete TGFs.[189,190] Both EGF and PDGF recently have been demonstrated to enhance cell motility and directed migration,[130] suggesting a role for these factors beyond the control of proliferation.

Recently, it has been shown that the responsiveness of a tumor cell to growth factors correlates with the ability of the cell to express the transformed phenotype.[180,191] The inherent sensitivity of tumor cells to growth factors partially determines whether a particular growth factor can function as a TGF, consequently stimulating the expression of the transformed phenotype. Growth factors that would not otherwise stimulate the transformed phenotype in normal cells may stimulate the proliferation of metastatic tumor cells in secondary lesions.

The contribution of laminin to the formation and proliferation of secondary metastatic lesions has been demonstrated.[6,37,72] The metastatic propensity of a tumor cell has been shown to be related to an increased number of laminin receptors on the cell surface. This relationship may result from the increased ability of metastatic tumor cells both to attach to basement membrane and to respond to laminin as a chemoattractant and growth factor. It is not known whether the levels of expression of any other growth factor receptors on tumor cells correlate with metastatic activity. The promotion of tumor cell growth by laminin[49,67,82,103] may be due to an enhanced deposition of extracellular matrix, which is necessary for the growth of these cells.

Laminin alters the shape and spreading of certain tumor cells, resulting in an alteration of protein and DNA synthesis.[30] It also has a membrane stabilizing effect on epithelial cells.[29,50,192] Laminin has been found in the very early stages of blastula development[59] and shown to promote the growth of fetal hepatocytes.[193] The possibility exists that overexpression of laminin receptors on the cell surface of metastatic tumor cells compares to levels of receptor expression in the embryonic stages of development where laminin may act as both a chemoattractant and growth factor.

Recently, the possibility that the metastatic capacity may be related to expression of distinct oncogenes has been investigated.[175] In experiments using transfected NIH 3T3 cells, Liotta et al.[194] have found that the *ras* oncogene stimulates the expression of the metastatic phenotype. In these transfected cells, the product of the *ras* oncogene (p21 protein) is observed. The increased expression of the metastatic phenotype appears to correlate with increased expression of type IV collagenase.[194] It has been reported that transfection of NIH 3T3 cells with c-Ha-*ras* accelerates the tumorigenicity and enhances the metastatic potential of these cells.[195] Bernstein and Weinberg[196] also reported that metastatic behavior could be induced in *ras*-transformed NIH 3T3 cells by gene transfer of a DNA segment from a human metastatic tumor. However, in all these cases, it was emphasized that the parental or untransfected counterparts of the transfected cells are also tumorigenic and spontaneously metastasize under certain conditions. None of these studies has correlated any specific basement membrane-tumor cell interaction with the increased metastatic potential of the transfected tumor cells. The need for stringent conditions must be adhered to when trying to correlate oncogene activation with the acquisition of specific phenotypic properties.[195] The effect of the *ras* oncogene products on the induction of metastatic phenotype is not thought to be constant in determining the metastatic propensity of cells from different generations. When primary and metastatic human colorectal tumors were examined for p21 *ras* protein expression, highly metastatic tumors appeared to have decreased levels of p21 *ras* protein. The level of p21 *ras* protein in distant metastases was less than in both normal colon tissue and primary tumor tissue.[196] The exact nature of the role of the *ras* oncogene or any defined ''metastatic gene'' in controlling expression of metastatic properties remains to be elucidated. Many interesting questions remain concerning the influence of specific oncogenes on tumor-cell basement membrane interaction.

III. CONCLUSIONS

The ability of metastatic cells to modulate their behavior plays a crucial role in determining the overall success of the potential of a tumor cell to form distant tumors. At each stage in the metastatic cascade, the interaction of tumor cells with matrix components or other environmental factors can potentiate or perturb the ability of the cells to form a metastatic lesion. Tumor cells in the primary tumor interact with basement membrane and extracellular matrix, resulting in matrix degradation. Chemotactic stimulation of motility in response to matrix degradation products, as well as collagenolytic enzymes, affect the intravasation step. The dissemination of the tumor cell is also modulated by plasma fibronectin and prior exposure to laminin. Cellular arrest depends, at least in part, on adhesive interactions with capillary cell walls and may exhibit specificity based on subendothelial basement membrane-specific polypeptides. The specificity of this adhesion is indicated by the observation that many metastatic tumors show a remarkable preference for certain target organs and specific extracellular matrices. Both the adhesive properties of the tumor cells and the matrix constituents at the metastatic sites are of importance. Several components of the basement membrane interact uniquely with tumor cells by glycoprotein receptor molecules exposed on the tumor cell surface. The presence of increased number of laminin receptors correlates with increased metastatic propensity. Fibronectin appears to negatively modulate the expression of laminin receptors in some tumor cells. Thus, the high levels of fibronectin in serum may represent a natural mechanism of defense against the spread and proliferation of certain metastatic tumor cells.

While many aspects of the interactions of tumor cells with basement membrane matrix and other environmental factors have been elucidated, considerably more information from *in vivo* spontaneous metastases must be accumulated to confirm the hypotheses based on the *in vitro* model systems and to take into account the heterogeneity of tumor cells. Further exploitation of molecular, biological, and gene manipulative techniques may permit definitive resolution of some of the issues not yet amenable to analysis *in vivo*. Only then can we hope to transfer this understanding to practical clinical modalities.

ACKNOWLEDGMENT

Work for this project was supported in part by Council For Tobacco Research Grant No. 2093 and Smokeless Tobacco Research Council Grant No. 0164.

REFERENCES

1. **Poste, G.,** Experimental system for analysis of the malignant phenotype, *Cancer Metast. Rev.*, 1, 141, 1982.
2. **Poste, G. and Fidler, I. J.,** The pathogenesis of cancer metastasis, *Nature (London)*, 282, 139, 1980.
3. **Nicolson, G. L. and Poste, G.,** Tumor cell diversity and host responses in cancer metastasis. I. Properties of metastatic cells, *Curr. Probl. Cancer*, 6, 1, 1982.
4. **Weiss, L.,** Random and nonrandom processes in metastasis and metastatic inefficiency, *Invasion Metast.*, 3, 193, 1983.
5. **Harris, J. F., Chambers, A. F., Hill, R. P., and Ling, V.,** Metastatic variants are generated spontaneously at a high rate in mouse KHT tumors, *Proc. Natl. Acad. Sci. U.S.A.*, 79, 5547, 1979.
6. **Terranova, V. P., Williams, J. E., Liotta, L. A., and Martin, G. R.,** Modulation of the metastatic activity of melanoma cells by laminin and fibronectin, *Science*, 226, 982, 1984.
7. **Butler, T. P. and Gullino, P. M.,** Quantitation of cell shedding into efferent blood of mammary adenocarcinoma, *Cancer Res.*, 35, 512, 1975.

8. **Fidler, I. J.**, Selection of successive tumor lines for metastasis, *Nature (London) New Biol.*, 242, 148, 1973.
9. **Fidler, I. J. and Kripke, M. L.**, Metastasis results from pre-existing variant cells within a malignant tumor, *Science*, 197, 893, 1977.
10. **Brattain, M. G., Strobel-Stevens, J., Fine, J., Webb, M., and Sarrif, A. M.**, Establishment of mouse colonic carcinoma cell line with different metastatic properties, *Cancer Res.*, 40, 2142, 1980.
11. **Danielson, K. G., Anderson, H., and Hosick, L.**, Selection and characterization in culture of mammary tumor cells with distinctive growth properties, *in vivo, Cancer Res.*, 40, 1812, 1980.
12. **Miner, K. M., Kawaguchi, T., Uba, G. W., and Nicolson, G. L.**, Clonal drift of cell surface melanogenic and experimental metastatic properties of *in vivo* — selected brain meningescolonizing murine B16 melanoma, *Cancer Res.*, 42, 4631, 1982.
13. **Mayhew, E. and Glaves, D.**, Quantitation of tumorigenic disseminating and arrested cancer cells, *Br. J. Cancer*, 50, 159, 1984.
14. **Weiss, L., Mayhew, E., Rapp, D. G., and Holmes, J. C.**, Metastatic inefficiency in mice bearing B16 melanomas, *Br. J. Cancer*, 45, 44, 1982.
15. **Weiss, L. and Ward, P. M.**, Cell detachment and metastasis, *Cancer Metast. Rev.*, 2, 111, 1987.
16. **Nicolson, G. L. and Poste, G.**, Tumor cell diversity and host response in cancer metastasis. II. Host immune responses and therapy of metastases, *Curr. Probl. Cancer VII*, 7, 3, 1983.
17. **Siegal, G. P., Barsky, S. H., Terranova, V. P., and Liotta, L. A.**, Stages of neoplastic transformation of human breast tissue as monitored by dissolution of the basement, *Invasion Metast.*, 1, 54, 1981.
18. **Kleinman, H. K., Kiebe, R. J., and Martin, G. R.**, Role of collagenous matrices in the adhesion and growth of cells, *J. Cell Biol.*, 88, 473, 1981.
19. **McCarthy, J. B., Palm, S. L., and Furcht, L. T.**, Migration of haptotaxis of a Schwann cell tumor line to the basement membrane glycoprotein laminin, *J. Cell Biol.*, 97, 772, 1983.
20. **Palm, S. L. and Furcht, L. T.**, Production of laminin and fibronectin by Schwannoma cells: cell-protein interactions *in vitro*, *J. Cell Biol.*, 96, 1218, 1982.
21. **Gauss-Muller, V., Kleinman, H. K., Martin, G. R., and Schiffman, E.**, Role of attachment and attractants in fibroblast chemotaxis, *J. Lab. Clin. Med.*, 96, 1071, 1980.
22. **Van-Evercooren, A., Kleinman, H. K., Seppa, H. E. J., Rentier, B., and Dubois-Dalcq, M.**, Fibronectin promotes rat Schwann cell growth and motility, *J. Cell Biol.*, 93, 211, 1982.
23. **Varani, J., Orr, W., and Ward, P. A.**, Comparison of the migration patterns of normal and malignant cells in two assay systems, *Am. J. Pathol.*, 90, 159, 1978.
24. **Mosher, D. F.**, Fibronectin, *Prog. Hemostasis Thromb.*, 6, 111, 1980.
25. **Yamada, K. M.**, Fibronectin and other structure proteins, in Cell Biology of the Extracellular Matrix, E.D., ED., Plenum Press, New York 1985, 95.
26. **Yamada, K. M.**, Cell surface interactions with extracellular matrices, *Ann. Rev. Biochem.*, 52, 761, 1983.
27. **Johannsson, S., Kjellen, J., Hook, M., and Timpl, R.**, Substrate adhesion of rat hepatocytes: a comparison of laminin and fibronectin as attachment proteins, *J. Cell Biol.*, 80, 260, 1981.
28. **Timpl, R., Johansson, S., Van Delden, V., Oberbaumer, I., and Hook, M.**, Characterization of protease-resistant fragments of laminin mediating attachment and spreading of rat hepatocytes, *J. Biol. Chem.*, 258, 8922, 1983.
29. **Sugrue, S. P. and Hay, E. D.**, Response of basal epithelial cell surface and cytoskeleton to solubilized extracellular matrix molecules, *J. Cell Biol.*, 91, 45, 1981.
30. **Gospodarowicz, D., Greenberg, P., and Birdwell, C. R.**, Determination of cellular shape by the extracellular matrix and its correlation with the control of cellular growth, *Cancer Res.*, 38, 4155, 1978.
31. **Gospodarowicz, D., Greenburg, G., Foidart, J. M., and Savion, N.**, The production and localization of laminin in cultured vascular and corneal endothelial cells, *J. Cell Physiol.*, 107, 171, 1981.
32. **Scott, D. M., Murray, J. C., and Barnes, S.** Investigation of the attachment of bovine corneal endothelial cells to collagens and other components of subendothelium role of fibronectin, *Exp. Cell Res.*, 144, 472, 1983.
33. **Carlsson, R., Engvall, E., Freeman, A., and Ruoslahti, E.**, Laminin and fibronectin in cell adhesion: enhanced adhesion of cells from regenerating liver to laminin, *Proc. Natl. Acad. Sci. U.S.A.*, 78, 2403, 1981.
34. **Sell, S. and Ruoslahti, E.**, Expression of fibronectin and laminin in the rat liver after partial hepatectomy, during carcinogenesis and in transplantable hepatocellular carcinomas, *J. Natl. Cancer Inst.*, 69, 1105, 1982.
35. **Macarak, E. J. and Howard, P. S.**, Adhesion of endothelial cells to extracellular matrix proteins, *J. Cell Physiol.*, 116, 76, 1983.
36. **Pearlstein, E. and Gold, L. I.**, High-molecular weight glycoprotein as mediator of cellular adhesion, *Ann. N.Y. Acad. Sci.*, 312, 278, 1978.
37. **Terranova, V. P., Kleinman, H. K., Sultan, L. H., and Martin, G. R.**, Regulation of cell attachment and number by fibronectin and laminin, *J. Cell Physiol.*, 127, 473, 1986.

38. **Terranova, V. P.,** Laminin and fibronectin modulate the metastatic propensity of melanoma cells, in *Cancer Treatment and Research,* Nathanion, L., Ed., Martinus Nihoff, Boston, 1987, 41.
39. **Liotta, L. A., Rao, C. N., and Barsky, S. H.,** Tumor invasion and the extracellular matrix, *Lab. Invest.,* 49, 636, 1983.
40. **Liotta, L. A.,** Tumor invasion and metastases: role of the basement membrane, *Am. J. Pathol.,* 117, 339, 1984.
41. **Roll, R. J., Madri, J. A., Alberta, J., and Furthmayer, H.,** Co-distribution of collagen type IV and AB_2 in basement membranes and mesangium of the kidney: an immunoferritin study of ultra thin frozen sections, *J. Cell Biol.,* 85, 597, 1980.
42. **Yamada, K. M., Hahn, L. H., and Olden, K.,** Structure and function of the fibronectins, *Prog. Clin. Biol. Res.,* 41, 797, 1980.
43. **Liotta, L., Rao, C. N., and Wewer, U. M.,** Biochemical interaction of tumor cells with the basement membrane, *Ann. Rev. Biochem.,* 55, 1037, 1986.
44. **David, G. and Bernfield, M.,** Defective basal lamina formation by transformed mammary epithelial cells: a reduced effect of collagen on basal lamina (heparin-sulfate rich) proteoglycan degradation, *J. Cell Physiol.,* 110, 56, 1985.
45. **Gabbert, H.,** Mechanisms of tumor invasion: evidence from *in vivo* observations, *Metast. Rev.,* 4, 293, 1985.
46. **Kefalides, N. A.,** Isolation of a collagen from basement membrane containing three identical alpha-chains, *Biochem. Biophys. Res. Commun.,* 45, 226, 1971.
47. **Timpl, R., Martin, G. R., Bruckner, P., Wick, G., and Wiedmann, H.,** Nature of the collagenous protein in a tumor basement membrane, *Eur. J. Biochem.,* 84, 43, 1978.
48. **Kleinman, H. K., McGarvey, M. L., Liotta, L. A., Robey, R. G., Tryggason, K., and Martin, G. R.,** Isolation and characterization of type IV procollagen, laminin and heparin sulfate proteoglycan from the EHS sarcoma, *Biochemistry,* 24, 6188, 1982.
49. **Kleinman, H. K., Rohrbach, D. H., Terranova, V. P., Varner, H. H., Hewitt, A. T., Grotendorst, G. R., Wilkes, C. M., Martin, G. R., Seppa, H., and Schiffmann, E.,** Collagenous matrices as determinants of cell function, in *Immunochemistry of the Extracellular Matrix,* Vol. 2, Furthmayer, H., Ed., CRC Press, Boca Raton, FL, 1982, 151.
50. **Hay, E. D.,** *Cell Biology of the Extracellular Matrix,* Plenum Press, New York, 1982.
51. **Hay, E. D.,** Interaction of embryonic surface and cytoskeleton with extracellular matrix, *Am. J. Anat.,* 165, 1, 1982.
52. **Kleinman, H. K., McGarvey, M. L., Hassell, J. R., and Martin, G. R.,** Formation of supramolecular complex is involved in the reconstitution of basement membrane components, *Biochemistry,* 22, 4969, 1983.
53. **Timpl, R., Rohde, H., Robey, P. G., Rennard, S. O., Foidart, J. M., and Martin, G. R.,** Laminin-glycoprotein from basement membranes, *J. Biol. Chem.,* 254, 9933, 1979.
54. **Minor, R., Clark, C. C., Strause, E. L., Koszalka, T. R., Brent, R. L., and Kefalides, N. A.,** Basement membrane procollagen is not converted to collagen in organ cultures of parietal yolk sac endoderm, *J. Biol. Chem.,* 251, 1789, 1976.
55. **Healthcote, J. G., Sear, C. H., and Grant, M. E.,** Studies on the assembly of the rat lens capsule: biosynthesis and partial characterization of collagenous components, *Biochem. J.,* 176, 283, 1978.
56. **Dehm, P. and Kefalides, N. A.,** The collagenous component of lens basement membrane: The isolation and characterization of an alpha chain size collagenous peptide and its relationship to newly synthesized lens components, *J. Biol. Chem.,* 253, 6680, 1978.
57. **Crouch, E. and Bornstein, P.,** Characterization of type IV procollagen synthesized by human amniotic fluid cells in culture, *J. Biol. Chem.,* 254, 4197, 1979.
58. **Karakashian, M. W., Dehm, P., Grambling, T. S., and LeRoy, C.,** Precursor-size components are the basic collagenous subunits of murine tumor basement membrane, *Collagen Relat. Res. Clin. Exp.,* 2, 3, 1982.
59. **Leivo, I. L., Vaheri, A., Timpl, R., and Wartiovaara, J.,** Appearance and distribution of collagens and laminin in the early mouse embryo, *Dev. Biol.,* 76, 100, 1980.
60. **Timpl, R. and Martin, G. R.,** Components of basement membranes, in *Immunochemistry of the Extra-cellular Matrix,* Vol. 2, Furthmayer, H., Ed., CRC Press, Boca Raton, FL, 1985, 125.
61. **Inoue, S., Lebland, C. P., and Laurie, G. W.,** Ultrastructure of Reichert's membrane, a multilayered basement membrane in the parietal wall of the rat yolk sac, *J. Cell Biol.,* 97, 1524, 1983.
62. **Glanville, R. W., Voses, T., and Kuhn, K.,** A comparison of the flexibility of the molecules of basement membrane and interstitial collagens, in *New Trends in Basement Membrane Research,* Kuhn, K., Ed., Raven Press, New York, 1982, 69.
63. **Timpl, R., Weidmann, H., Van Delden, V., Furthmayer, H., and Kuhn, K.,** A network for the organization of type IV collagen molecules in basement membrane, *Eur. J. Biochem.,* 120, 203, 1981.

64. **Timpl, R., Oberbaumer, I., Furthmayer, H., and Kuhn, K.,** Macromolecular organization of type IV collagen, in *New Trends in Basement Membrane Research,* Kuhn, K., Ed., Raven Press, New York, 1982, 57.
65. **Yurchenko, P. D. and Furthmayer, H.,** Self-assembly of basement membrane collagen, *Biochemistry,* 23, 1839, 1984.
66. **Yurchenko, P. D. and Ruben, G. C.,** Basement membrane structure *in situ:* evidence for lateral associations in the type IV collagen network, *J. Cell Biol.,* 105, 2559, 1987.
67. **Terranova, V. P., Rohrbach, D. H., and Martin, G. R.,** The role of laminin in the attachment of PAM_{212} (epithelial) cells to basement membrane collagen, *Cell,* 22, 719, 1980.
68. **Martin, G. R., Kleinman, H. K., Terranova, V. P., Ledbetter, S., and Hassell, J. R.,** The regulation of basement membrane formation and cell matrix interactions by defined supramolecular complexes in *Basement Membranes and Cell Movement,* Ciba Found. Symp., Pitman, London, 1984, 108.
69. **Howe, C. C. and Dietzschold, B.,** Structured analysis of three subunits of laminin from teratocarcinoma-derived parietal endoderm cells, *Dev. Biol.,* 98, 385, 1983.
70. **Dixit, S. N.,** Isolation, purification, and characterization of intact and pepsin-derived fragments of laminin from human placenta, *Connect. Tissue Res.,* 14, 31, 1985.
71. **Wewer, U. M., Liotta, L. A., and Jaye, M.,** Altered levels of laminin receptor mRNA in various human carcinoma cells that have different abilities to bind laminin, *Proc. Natl. Acad. Sci. U.S.A.,* 83, 7137, 1986.
72. **Sasaki, M., Kato, S., Kohno, K., Martin, G. R., and Yamada, Y.,** Sequence of the cDNA encoding the laminin B1 chain reveals a multidomain protein containing cystein rich repeats, *Proc. Natl. Acad. Sci. U.S.A.,* 84, 935, 1987.
73. **Paulsson, M., Deutzmann, R., Timpl, R., Dalzoppo, D., Odermatt, E., and Engel, J.,** Evidence for coiled-coil alpha-helical regions in the long arm of laminin, *EMBO J.,* 4, 309, 1985.
74. **Morita, A., Sugimoto, E., and Kitagawa, Y.,** Post-translational assembly and glycosylation of laminin subunits in parietal endoderm-like F9 cells, *Biochem. J.,* 229, 259, 1985.
75. **Arumugham, R. G., Hsieh, T. C., Tanzer, M. L., and Laine, R. A.,** Structures of the asparagine-linked sugar chains of laminin, *Biochem. Biophys. Acta,* 883, 112, 1986.
76. **Morita, A., Kitagawa, Y., and Sugimoto, E.,** Abnormal laminin secretion from parietal endoderm-like F9 cells in the presence of monensin, *Biochem. J.,* 98, 561, 1985.
77. **Dziadek, M. and Timpl, R.,** Expression of nidogen and laminin in basement membranes during mouse embryogenesis and in teratocarcinoma cells, *Dev. Biol.,* 111, 372, 1985.
78. **Cooper, A. R. and MacQueen, H. A.,** Subunits of laminin are differentially synthesized in mouse eggs and early embryos, *Dev. Biol.,* 96, 467, 1983.
79. **Abrahamson, D. R.,** Post-embedding colloidal gold immunolocalization of laminin to the lamina rara interna, lamina densa, and lamina rara externa of renal glomerular basement membranes, *J. Histochem. Cytochem.,* 34, 847, 1986.
80. **Charonis, A. S., Tsilibary, E. C., Saku, T., and Furthmayr, H.,** Inhibition of laminin self-assembly and interaction with type IV collagen by antibodies to the terminal domain of the long arm, *J. Cell Biol.,* 103, 1689, 1986.
81. **Charonis, A. S., Tsilibary, E. C., Saku, T., and Furthmayr, H.,** Binding of laminin to type IV collagen: a morphological study, *J. Cell Biol.,* 100, 1848, 1985.
82. **Terranova, V. P., Rohrbach, D. H., and Martin, G. R.,** Role of laminin in the attachment of PAM 212 (epithelial) cells to basement membrane collagen, *Cell,* 22, 719, 1980.
83. **Laurie, G. W., Bing, J. T., and Kleinman, H. K.,** Localization of binding sites for laminin, heparan sulfate proteoglycan and fibronectin on basement membrane (type IV) collagen, *J. Mol. Biol.,* 189, 205, 1986.
84. **Ott, U., Odermatt, E., Engel, J., Furthmayr, H., and Timpl, R.,** Protease resistance and conformation of laminin, *Eur. J. Biochem.,* 123, 63, 1982.
85. **Paulsson, M., Aymailley, M., Deutzmann, R., Timpl, R., Beck, K., and Engel, J.,** Laminin-nidogen complex: extraction with chelating agents and structural characterization, *Eur. J. Biochem.,* 166, 11, 1987.
86. **Cody, R. L. and Wicha, M. S.,** Clustering of cell surface laminin enhances its association with the cytoskeleton, *Exp. Cell Res.,* 165, 107, 1986.
87. **Rao, C. N., Margulies, I. M. K., Goldfarb, R. H., Madri, J. A., Woodley, D. T., and Liotta, L. A.,** Differential proteolytic susceptibility of laminin alpha and beta subunits, *Arch. Biochem. Biophys.,* 219, 65, 1982.
88. **Terranova, V. P., Rao, C. N., Kalebic, T., Margulies, I. M., and Liotta, L. A.,** Laminin receptor on human breast carcinoma cells, *Proc. Natl. Acad. Sci. U.S.A.,* 80, 444, 1983.
89. **Engvall, E., Davis, G. E., Dickerson, K., Ruoslahti, E., Varon, S., and Manthorpe, M.,** Mapping of domains in human laminin using monoclonal antibodies: localization of the neurite-promoting site, *J. Cell Biol.,* 103, 2457, 1986.
90. **Graf, J., Iwamoto, Y., Sasaki, M., et al.,** Identification of an amino acid sequence in laminin mediating cell attachment, chemotaxis, and receptor binding, *Cell,* 48, 989, 1987.

91. **Iwamoto, Y., Robey, F. A., Graf, J., et al.,** YIGSR, a synthetic laminin pentapeptide, inhibits experimental metastasis formation, *Science,* 238, 1132, 1987.
92. **Hassell, J. R., Robey, P. G., Barrach, H. J., Wilczek, J., Rennard, S. I., and Martin, G. R.,** Isolation of a heparan sulfate containing proteoglycan from basement membrane, *Proc. Natl. Acad. Sci. U.S.A.,* 77, 4494, 1980.
93. **Kanwar, Y. S., Linker, A., and Farquar, M. G.,** Increased permeability of the glomerular basement membrane to ferritin after removal of glycosaminoglycans (heparin sulfate) by enzyme digestion, *J. Cell Biol.,* 86, 688, 1980.
94. **Kanwar, Y. S., Hacall, V. C., and Farquar, M. G.,** Partial characterization of newly synthesized proteoglycans isolated from glomerular basement membrane, *J. Cell Biol.,* 90, 527, 1981.
95. **Stow, J., Glasgow, E. F., Handley, C. J., and Hascall, V. C.,** Biosynthesis of proteoglycans by isolated rabbit glomeruli, *Arch. Biochem. Biophys.,* 225, 950, 1983.
96. **Hassel, J. R., Leyshon, W. C., Ledbetter, S., Tyree, B., and Kleinman, H. K.,** Isolation of two forms of basement membrane proteoglycan, *J. Biol. Chem.,* 260, 8098, 1985.
97. **Carlin, B., Jaffe, R., Bender, B., and Chung, A. E.,** Entactin: a novel basal lamina-associated sulfated glycoprotein, *J. Biol. Chem.,* 256, 5209, 1981.
98. **Bender, B. L., Jaffe, R., Carlin, B., and Chung, A. E.,** Immunolocalization of entactin, a sulfated basement membrane component, in rodent tissues, and comparison with GP-Z (laminin), *Am. J. Pathol.,* 103, 419, 1981.
99. **Stenman, S. and Vaheri, A.,** Distribution of a major connective tissue protein, fibronectin in normal human tissue, *J. Exp. Med.,* 147, 1054, 1978.
100. **Ruoslahti, E., Engvall, E., and Hayman, E. G.,** Fibronectin: current concepts of its structure and functions, *Collagen Relat. Res.,* 1, 95, 1981.
101. **Oh, E., Pierschbacher, M., and Ruoslahti, R.,** Deposition of plasma fibronectin in tissues, *Proc. Natl. Acad. Sci. U.S.A.,* 78, 3218, 1981.
102. **Dessau, W., Adelmann, B. C., Timpl, R., and Martin, G. R.,** Identification of the sites in collagen and chains that bind serum anti-gelatin factor (cold insoluble globulin), *Biochem. J.,* 169, 55, 1978.
103. **Terranova, V. P., Hujanen, E. S., and Martin, G. R.,** Extracellular matrix influences on tumor cell metastasis, *J. Natl. Cancer Inst.,* 77, 311, 1986.
104. **Sekiguchi, K., Fukuda, M., and Hokomon, Y.,** Domain structure of hamster plasma fibronectin, *J. Biol. Chem.,* 256, 6452, 1981.
105. **Sugarbaker, E. V., Weingrad, D. N., and Roseman, J. M.,** Observations on cancer metastasis in man, in *Tumor Invasion and Metastasis,* Liotta, L. A. and Hart, I. R., Eds., Martinus Nijhoff, Boston, 1982, 427.
106. **Fidler, I. J. and Hart, I. R.,** Biological diversity in metastatic neoplasms: origins and implications, *Science,* 217, 998, 1982.
107. **Hart, I. R.,** Seed and soil revisited: mechanisms of site specific metastasis, *Cancer Metast. Rev.,* 1, 5, 1982.
108. **Nicolson, G. L.,** Cancer metastasis: organ colonization and the cell surface properties of malignant cells, *Biochem. Biophys. Acta,* 695, 113, 1982.
109. **Liotta, L. A., Kleinerman, J., and Saidel, G. M.,** Quantitative relationships of intravascular tumor cells, tumor vessels, and pulmonary metastases following tumor implantation, *Cancer Res.,* 34, 997, 1974.
110. **Glaves, D.,** Correlation between circulating cancer cells and incidence of metastases, *Br. J. Cancer,* 48, 665, 1983.
111. **Tarin, D. and Price, J. E.,** Influence of microenvironment and vascular anatomy on "metastatic" colonization potential of mammary tumors, *Cancer Res.,* 41, 3604, 1981.
112. **Jones, P. A.,** *In vitro* assay of invasion using endothelial and smooth muscle cells, in *Tumor Invasion and Metastasis,* Liotta, L. A. and Hart, I. R., Eds., Martinus Nijhoff, London, 1982, 251.
113. **Frost, P. and Kerbal, R. S.,** Immunology of metastasis: can the immune response cope with dissemination of tumors? *Cancer Metast. Rev.,* 2, 239, 1983.
114. **Weiss, L.,** Metastatic inefficiency, in *Liver Metastasis,* Weiss, L. and Gilbert, P., Eds., G. K. Hall, Boston, 1982, 126.
115. **Weiss, L. and Dimitrov, D. S.,** A fluid mechanical analysis of the velocity, adhesion and destruction of cancer cells in capillaries during metastasis, *Cell Biophys.,* 6, 9, 1984.
116. **Kuettner, K. E., Soble, L., Croxen, R. L., Marczynska, B., Hiti, J., and Harper, E.,** Tumor cell collagenase and its inhibition by a cartilage-derived protease inhibitor, *Science,* 196, 653, 1977.
117. **Reynolds, J. J., Sellers, A., Murphy, G., and Cartwright, E.,** New factor that may control collagen resorption, *Lancet,* 2, 333, 1977.
118. **Wooley, D. E., Tetlow, L. C., Mooney, C. J., and Evanson, J. M.,** Human collagenase and its extracellular inhibitors in relation to tumor invasiveness, in *Proteinases and Tumor Invasion,* Strand, P., Barret, A. H., and Bajei, A., Eds., Raven Press, New York, 1980, 97.

119. **Zweifach, B. W.,** Microvascular aspect of tissue injury in the inflammatory process, Vol. 2, 2nd ed., Zweifach, B. W., Grout, L., McCluskey, R. T., Eds., Academic Press, New York, 1973, 3.
120. **Folkman, J. and Klogsbrun, M.,** Angiogenic factors, *Science,* 235, 442, 1987.
121. **Strauli, P.,** A concept of tumor invasion, in *Proteinases and Tumor Invasion,* Strauli, P., Barret, A. J., and Baici, A., Eds., Raven Press, New York, 1980, 1.
122. **Barsky, S. H., Baker, A., Siegal, G. P., Togo, S., and Liotta, L. A.,** Use of anti-basement membrane antibodies to distinguish blood vessel capillaries from lymphatic capillaries, *Am. J. Surg. Pathol.,* 7, 667, 1983.
123. **Mareel, M. M., Keiler, J. V., Bruyneel, E., Van Cauwenberge, R., and Dragonetti, C.,** Invasiveness of malignant St/A mouse lung cells in vitro, *Virchows Arch. B.,* 38, 101, 1981.
124. **Easty, D. M. and Easty, G. C.,** Measurement of the ability of cells to infiltrate normal tissues *in vitro, Br. J. Cancer,* 29, 36, 1974.
125. **Armstrong, P. B., Quigley, J. P., and Sidebottom, E.,** Transepithelial invasion and intramesenchymal infiltration of check embryo chorioallantois by tumor cell lines, *Cancer Res.,* 42, 1826, 1982.
126. **Poste, G., Doll, J., Hart, I. R., and Fidler, I. J.,** *In Vitro* selection of murine B16 melanoma variants with enhanced tissue invasive properties, *Cancer Res.,* 40, 1636, 1980.
127. **Russo, R. G., Thorgeirsson, U., Liotta, L. A.,** *In vitro* quantitative assay of invasion using human amnion, in *Tumor Invasion and Metastasis,* Liotta, L. A. and Hart, I. R., Eds., Martinus Nijhoff, London, 173, 1982.
128. **Maslow, D. E.,** Collagenase effects on cancer cell invasiveness and motility, *Invasion Metast.,* 7, 297, 1987.
129. **Maslow, D. E. and Goldrosen, M. H.,** Relationship of *in vitro* cell motility and colonization potential in a mouse colon adenocarcinoma (MCA-38) cell line, *Invasion Metast.,* 8, 133, 1988.
130. **Maslow, D. E. and Terranova, V. P.,** Directed migration of cancer cells to collagenase and collagen degradation products, *AACR Proc.,* 28, 76, 1987.
131. **Terranova, V. P., Markus, G., and Maslow, D.,** Directed migration of murine and human tumor cells to collagenases and other proteases, *Cancer Res.,* 49, 4835, 1989.
132. **Hujanen, E. S. and Terranova, V. P.,** Migration of tumor cells to organ-derived chemoattractants, *Cancer Res.,* 45, 3517, 1985.
133. **Weiss, L., Orr, F. W., and Honn, K. V.,** Interactions of cancer cells with the microvasculature during metastasis, *FASEB J.,* 2, 12, 1985.
134. **Dippold, W. G., Lloyd, K. O., Li, L. T. C., Ikeda, H., Oettgen, H. F., and Old, L. J.,** Cell surface antigens of human malignant melanoma: definition of six antigenic systems with monoclonal antibodies, *Proc. Natl. Acad. Sci. U.S.A.,* 77, 6114, 1980.
135. **Johnson, J. P., Demmer-Dieckmann, M., Meo, T., Hadam, M. R., and Reithmuller, G.,** Surface antigens of human melanoma cells defined by monoclonal antibodies. I. Biochemical characterization of two antigens found on cell lines and fresh tumors of diverse tissue origin, *Eur. J. Immunol.,* 11, 825, 1981.
136. **Mitchel, K. F., Fuhrer, J. P., Steplewski, Z., and Koprowski, H.,** Biochemical characterization of human melanoma cell surfaces dissection with monoclonal antibodies, *Proc. Natl. Acad. Sci. U.S.A.,* 77, 7287, 1981.
137. **Natali, P. G., Cavaliere, R., Biogott, A., Nicorta, M. E., Russo, C., Ah Kan, N. G., Giacomini, P., and Ferrone, S.,** Antigenic heterogeneity of surgically removed primary and metastatic human melanoma lesions, *J. Immunol.,* 130, 1462, 1983.
138. **Hollmann, M., Staab, H. J., Spindler, E., Sproll, M., Anderer, F. A., and Furthmayer, H. P.,** Monoclonal antibody defined circulating tumor-associated antigen with epitope shared by normal cells, *Biochem. Biophys. Res. Commun.,* 128, 34, 1985.
139. **Maslow, D. E. and Weiss, L.,** The effects of tumor cells on embryonic cell aggregation, adhesion and detachment, *J. Cell Sci.,* 29, 271, 1978.
140. **Fidler, I. J. and Kripke, M. L.,** Tumor cell antigenicity, host immunity and cancer metastasis, *Cancer Immunol.,* 7, 201, 1980.
141. **Fidler, I. J. and Nicolson, G. L.,** Tumor cell antigenicity, host immunity and cancer metastasis, *Cancer Immunol.,* 7, 201, 1980.
142. **Fidler, I. J. and Nicolson, G. L.,** Immunobiology of experimental metastatic melanoma, *Cancer Biol. Rev.,* 2, 171, 1981.
143. **Stutman, O.,** Immunodepression and malignancy, *Adv. Cancer Res.,* 22, 261, 1975.
144. **Prehn, R. T.,** The immune reaction as a stimulator of tumor growth, *Science,* 176, 170, 1972.
145. **Umiel, T. and Trainin, N.,** Immunological enhancement of tumor growth by syngeneic thymus-derived lymphocytes, *Transplantation,* 18, 244, 1974.
146. **Small, M. and Trainin, N.,** Separation of populations of sensitized lymphoid cells into fractions inhibiting and fractions enhancing syngeneic tumor growth *in vivo, J. Immunol.,* 117, 292, 1976.
147. **Fidler, I. J., Gersten, D. M., and Riggs, C. W.,** Relationship of host immune status to tumor cell arrest, distribution, and survival in experimental metastasis, *Cancer,* 40, 46, 1977.

148. **Sugarbaker, E. V. and Cohen, A. M.,** Altered antigenicity in spontaneous pulmonary metastases from an antigenic murine sarcoma, *Surgery,* 72, 155, 1972.
149. **Hart, I. R. and Fidler, I. J.,** The implications of tumor heterogeneity for studies on the biology and therapy of cancer metastasis, *Biochem. Biophys. Acta,* 37, 651, 1981.
150. **Holzman, B., Johnson, J. P., Kaudewitz, P., and Riethmuller, G.,** *In situ* analysis of antigens on malignant and benign cells of the melanocyte lineage, *J. Exp. Med.,* 161, 366, 1985.
151. **Alby, L. and Auerbach, R.,** Differential adhesion of tumor cells to capillary endothelial cells *in vitro, Proc. Natl. Acad. Sci. U.S.A.,* 81, 5739, 1984.
152. **Kramer, R. M. and Nicolson, G. L.,** Interactions of tumor cells with vascular endothelial cell monolayers: a model for metastatic invasion, *Proc. Natl. Acad. Sci. U.S.A.,* 76, 5704, 1979.
153. **Kramer, R. H. and Nicolson, G. L.,** Invasion of vascular endothelial cell monolayers and underlying matrix by metastatic human cancer cells, in *International Cell Biology,* Schweiger, S., Ed., Springer-Verlag, New York, 794, 1981.
154. **Kefalides, N. A., Alper, R., and Clark, C. C.,** Biochemistry and metabolism of basement membranes, *Int. Rev. Cytol.,* 61, 167, 1979.
155. **Kramer, R. H., Vogel, K. G., and Nicolson, G. L.,** Solubilization and degradation of subendothelial matrix glycoproteins and proteoglycans by metastatic tumor cells, *J. Biol. Chem.,* 257, 2678, 1982.
156. **Nicolson, G. L., Lotan, R., and Rios, A.,** Heterogeneous *in vitro* sensitivities of metastatic B16 melanoma sublines and clones to retinoic acid or BCNU, *Cancer Treat. Rep.,* 65 (Suppl. 2), 71, 1981.
157. **Pearlstein, E. and Hoffstein, S. T.,** Fibronectin-mediated cellular adhesion to vascular subendothelial matrices, *Exp. Cell Res.,* 134, 161, 1981.
158. **Auerbach, R., Alby, L., Morrissey, L. W., Tu, M., and Joseph, J.,** Monoclonal antibodies against tumor specific antigens inhibit metastasis, *Microvasc. Res.,* 17, 311, 1987.
159. **Ruff, M., Schiffmann, E., Terranova, V. P., and Pert, C. B.,** Bonbesin and other neuropeptides are chemoattractants for human monocytes and small cell lung carcinoma cells, *Clin. Immunol. Immunopathol.,* 37, 387, 1985.
160. **Sugarbaker, E. V.,** Patterns of metastasis in human malignancies, in *Cancer Biology Reviews,* Vol. 2, Marchalonis, J. J., Hanna, M. D., and Fidler, I. J., Eds., Marcel-Dekker, New York, 1980.
161. **Fidler, I. J. and Nicolson, G. L.,** Brief communication: organ selectivity for implantation survival and growth of B16 melanoma variant lines, *J. Natl. Cancer Inst.,* 57, 1199, 1976.
162. **Shearman, P. J. and Longenecker, B. M.,** Selection for virulence and organ-specific metastasis of herpes-virus transformed lymphoma cells, *Int. J. Cancer,* 25, 262, 1980.
163. **Ewing, J.,** *Neoplastic Diseases,* 3rd ed., W.B. Saunders, Philadelphia, 1928.
164. **Raz, A. and Hart, I. R.,** Murine melanoma: a model for intracranial metastasis, *Br. J. Cancer,* 42, 331, 1980.
165. **Nicolson, G. L. and Custead, S. E.,** Tumor metastasis is not due to adaption of cells to new organ environment, *Science,* 215, 176, 1982.
166. **Salisbury, A. J.,** The significance of the circulating cancer cell, *Cancer Treat. Rev.,* 2, 55, 1975.
167. **Kieran, M. W. and Longenecker, B. M.,** Organ specific metastasis with special reference to avian systems, *Cancer Metast. Rev.,* 2, 165, 1983.
168. **Paget, S.,** The distribution of secondary growth in cancer of the breast, *Lancet,* 1, 571, 1889.
169. **James, R. and Bradshaw, R. A.,** Polypeptide growth factors, *Annu. Rev. Biochem.,* 53, 259, 1984.
170. **Roos, E., Van De Pavert, I. V., and Middelkoop, D. P.,** Infiltration of tumor into cultures of isolated hepatocytes, *J. Cell Sci.,* 47, 385, 1981.
171. **Fidler, I. J. and Ziedman, I.,** Enhancement of experimental metastasis by x-ray: a possible mechanism, *J. Med.,* 3, 172, 1972.
172. **Warren, B. A., Chauvin, W. J., and Phillips, J.,** Blood-borne tumor emboli and their adherence to vessel walls, in *Cancer Invasion and Metastasis: Biologic Mechanisms and Therapy,* Day, S. D., Laird-Myers, W. P., and Stansly, P., Eds., Raven Press, New York, 1977, 185.
173. **Crissman, J., Slone, B., and Ryan, R.,** Correlation of cathepsin B and metastatic potential in malignant neoplasia, *Lab. Invest.,* Abstr., 50, 13A, 1984.
174. **Liotta, L. A., Tryggvason, K., and Garbisa, S.,** Metastatic potential correlates with the enzymic degradation of basement membrane collagen, *Nature (London),* 284, 67, 1980.
175. **Klein, G. and Klein, E.,** Evolution of tumors and the impact of molecular oncology, *Nature (London),* 315, 190, 1985.
176. **Sporn, M. B. and Todaro, G.,** Autocrine secretion and malignant transformation of cells, *N. Engl. J. Med.,* 303, 878, 1980.
177. **Kaplan, P. L., Anderson, M., and Ozanne, B.,** Transforming growth factor protection enables cells to grow in the absence of serum: an autocrine system, *Proc. Natl. Acad. Sci. U.S.A.,* 71, 485, 1982.
178. **DeLarco, J. E. and Todaro, G. J.,** Growth factors from murine sarcoma virus-transformed cells, *Proc. Natl. Acad. Sci. U.S.A.,* 75, 4001, 1978.

179. **Ozanne, B., Fulton, R. J., and Kaplan, P. L.**, Kirsten murine sarcoma virus transformed cell lines and a spontaneously transformed rat cell line produce transforming factors, *J. Cell Physiol.*, 105, 163, 1980.
180. **Kapan, P. L. and Ozanne, B.**, Cellular responsiveness to growth factors correlates with a cell's ability to express the transformed phenotype, *Cell*, 33, 931, 1983.
181. **Murquardt, H., Hunkapiller, M., Hood, L., Twardzik, K., DeLarco, J. E., Stephenson, J., and Todaro, G. J.**, Transforming growth factors produced by retrovirus-transformed rodent fibroblasts and human melanoma cells: amino acid sequence homology with EGF, *Proc. Natl. Acad. Sci. U.S.A.*, 80, 4684, 1983.
182. **Anzano, M. A., Roberts, A. B., Smith, J. M., Sporn, M. B., and DeLarco, J. E.**, Sarcoma growth factor from conditioned medium of virally transformed cells is composed of both alpha-type and beta-type transforming growth factors, *Proc. Natl. Acad. Sci. U.S.A.*, 80, 6264, 1983.
183. **Roberts, A., Anzano, M., Lamb, L., Smith, J., and Sporn, M.**, New class of transforming growth factors potentiated by epidermal growth factor: isolation from non-neoplastic tissues, *Proc. Natl. Acad. Sci. U.S.A.*, 78, 5339, 1981.
184. **Roberts, A., Anzano, M., Lamb, L., Smith, J., Frolik, C., Murquardt, H., Todaro, G., and Sporn, M.**, Isolation from murine sarcoma cells of novel transforming growth factors potentiated by EGF, *Nature (London)*, 295, 417, 1982.
185. **Assoian, E., Komoriya, A., Meyers, C., and Sporn, M.**, Transforming growth factor-beta in human platelets: identification of a major storage site: purification and characterization, *J. Biol. Chem.*, 258, 715, 1983.
186. **Roberts, A., Anzano, M., Meyers, C., Wideman, J., Blacher, R., Pan, Y.-E., Stein, S., Lehrman, S., Smith, J., Lamb, L., and Sporn, M.**, Purification and properties of type beta transforming growth factor from bovine kidney, *Biochemistry*, 22, 5692, 1983.
187. **Frolik, C., Dart, L., Meyers, C., Smith, D., and Sporn, M.**, Purification and initial characterization of a type beta growth factor from human placenta, *Proc. Natl. Acad. Sci. U.S.A.*, 80, 3676, 1983.
188. **Assoian, R. K., Frolik, C. A., Roberts, A. B., Miller, D. M., and Sporn, M. B.**, Transforming growth factor-beta controls receptor levels for epidermal growth factor in NRK fibroblasts, *Cell*, 36, 35, 1984.
189. **Assoian, R. K., Grotendorst, G. R., Miller, D. M., and Sporn, M. G.**, Cellular transformation by coordinated action of three peptide growth factors from human platelets, *Nature (London)*, 309, 804, 1984.
190. **Kudlow, J. E., Khosravi, M. J., Kobrin, M. S., and Mak, W.**, Inability of anti-epidermal growth factor receptor monoclonal antibody to block "autocrine" growth stimulation in transforming growth factor-secreting melanoma cells, *J. Biol. Chem.*, 259, 11895, 1984.
191. **Lyall, R. M., Huang, J., Gottesman, M. M., and Pastan, I.**, Isolation and genetic characterization of human KB cell lines resistant to epidermal growth factor—pseudomonas exotoxin conjugate, *J. Cell. Physiol.*, 27, 641, 1986.
192. **Sugrue, S. P. and Hay, E. D.**, Interaction of embryonic corneal epithelium with exogenous collagen, laminin and fibronectin: role of endogenous protein synthesis, *Dev. Biol.*, 92, 97, 1982.
193. **Hirta, K., Usul, T., Koshiba, H., Maruyama, Y., Oikawa, I., and Freeman, A. E.**, Effects of basement membrane matrix on the culture of fetal mouse hepatocytes, *Gann*, 74, 687, 1983.
194. **Thorgeirsson, V. P., Turpeenniemi-Hujanen, T., Williams, J. E., Westin, E. H., Heilman, C. A., Talmadge, J. E., and Liotta, L. A.**, NIH/3T3 cells transfected with human tumor DNA containing activated *ras* oncogenes express the metastatic phenotype in nude mice, *Mol. Cell. Biol.*, 5, 259, 1985.
195. **Greig, R. G., Koestler, T. P., Trainer, D. L., Corwin, S. P., Miles, K., Kline, T., Sweet, R., Yokoyama, S., and Poste, G.**, Tumorigenic and metastatic properties of "normal" and *ras*-transfected NIH/3T3 cells, *Proc. Natl. Sci. U.S.A.*, 82, 3698, 1985.
196. **Bernstein, S. C. and Weinberg, R. A.**, Expression of the metastatic phenotype in cells transfected with human metastatic tumor DNA, *Proc. Natl. Acad. Sci. U.S.A.*, 82, 1726, 1985.
197. **Gallick, G. E., Kurzrock, R., Kloetzer, W. S., Arlinghaus, R. B., and Gutterman, J. U.**, Expression of $p21^{ras}$ in fresh primary and metastatic human colorectal tumors, *Proc. Natl. Acad. Sci. U.S.A.*, 82, 1795, 1985.
198. **Vollmers, H. P. and Birchmeier, W.**, Cell adhesion and metastasis: a monoclonal antibody approach, *Trends Biochem. Sci.*, 8, 452, 1983.
199. **Foulds, L.**, The histologic analysis of mammary tumors of mice. II. The histology of responsiveness and progression. The origin of tumors, *J. Natl. Cancer Inst.*, 17, 713, 1976.
200. **Cifone, M. A. and Fidler, I. J.**, Increasing metastatic potential is associated with increasing genetic instability of clones isolated from murine neoplasms, *Proc. Natl. Acad. Sci. U.S.A.*, 78, 6949, 1981.
201. **Varani, J., Lovette, E. J., McCoy, J. P., Shibata, S., Maddox, D., Goldstein, I., and Wicha, M.**, Differential expression of a laminin-like substance by high and low metastatic tumor cells, *Am. J. Pathol.*, 11, 27, 1983.
202. **Malinoff, H. L., McCoy, J. P., Jr., Varani, J., and Wicha, M.**, Metastatic potential of murine fibrosarcoma cells is influenced by cell surface laminin, *Int. J. Cancer*, 33, 651, 1984.
203. **McCoy, J. P., Lloyd, R. V., Wicha, M., and Virani, J.**, Identification of laminin-like substance on the surface of a highly malignant murine fibrosarcoma cell, *J. Cell Sci.*, 65, 139, 1984.

204. **Terranova, V. P., Liotta, L. A., Russo, R. G., and Martin, G. R.,** Role of laminin in the attachment and metastasis of murine tumor cells, *Cancer Res.*, 42, 2265, 1985.
205. **Barsky, S. H., Rao, C. N., Williams, J. E., and Liotta, L. A.,** Domains of laminin which alter metastasis in a murine model, *J. Clin. Invest.*, 74, 843, 1984.
206. **Liotta, L. A., Kleinman, P., Cantanzaro, D., and Rynbrandt, R.,** Degradation of basement membrane by murine tumor cells, *J. Natl. Cancer Inst.*, 58, 1427, 1977.
207. **Nakajima, M., Irimura, T., DiFerrante, N., and Nicolson, G. L.,** Metastatic melanoma cell heparanase: characterization of heparin sulfate degradation fragments produced by B16 melanoma endoglucuronidase, *J. Biol. Chem.*, 259, 2283, 1984.
208. **Strauli, P.,** Proteinase and tumor invasion, in *Proteinases and Tumor Invasion,* Strauli, P., Barrett, A. J., and Baici, A., Eds., Monograph Series of the Europe Organization for Research on Treatment of Cancer, Vol. 6, Raven Press, New York, 1980, 215.
209. **Barsky, S. M., Siegal, G., Jannotta, F., and Liotta, L. A.,** Loss of basement membrane components by invasive but not by their benign counterparts, *Lab. Invest.*, 49, 140, 1983.
210. **Liotta, L. A., Goldfarb, R. H., Brundage, R., Siefal, G. P., Terranova, V. P., and Gargisa, S.,** Effect of plasminogen activator (urokinase) plasmin and thrombin on glycoprotein and collagenous components of basement membranes, *Cancer Res.*, 41, 4629, 1981.
211. **Lam, W. C., Delikatny, E. J., Orr, F. W., Wass, J., Varani, J., and Ward, P. A.,** The chemotactic response of tumor cells: a model for cancer metastasis, *Am. J. Pathol.*, 104, 69, 1981.
212. **Magro, C., Orr, F. W., Manishen, W. J., Sivananthan, K., and Mokashi, S. S.,** Adhesion, chemotaxis and aggregation of Walker carcinosarcoma cells in response to products of resorbing bone, *J. Natl. Cancer Inst.*, 74, 829, 1985.
213. **Holley, R. W.,** Control of animal cell proliferation, *J. Supramol. Struct.*, 13, 191, 1980.
214. **Grant, M. E., Kefalides, N. A., and Prockop, D. J.,** The biosynthesis of basement membrane collagen in embryonic chick lens, *J. Biol. Chem.*, 247, 3539, 1972.
215. **Cohen, M. P. and Sorma, M. L.,** (^{35}S)-Sulfate incorporation into glomerular basement membrane glycosaminoglycans is decreased in experimental diabetes, *J. Lab. Clin. Med.*, 98, 715, 1981.
216. **Ledbetter, S., Hassell, J. R., Horigan, E., Tyree, B., and Martin, G. R.,** Identification of the core protein to a heparin sulfate proteoglycan from basement membrane, in *Proc. 7th Int. Symp. Glycoconjugates,* Chester, M. A. et al., Eds., Lund-Ronneby, Sweden, 1983, 396.
217. **Timpl, R., Dziadek, M., Fujiwara, S., Nowack, H., and Wick, G.,** Nidogen: a new self-aggregating basement membrane protein, *Eur. J. Biochem.*, 137, 455, 1983.
218. **Williams, E. C., Lanmey, P. A., Ferry, J. D., and Mosher, D. F.,** Conformational states of fibronectin, effects of ph, ionic strength and collagen binding, *J. Biol. Chem.*, 257, 14973, 1982.
219. **Bornstein, P. and Sage, H.,** Structurally distinct collagen types, *Ann. Rev. Biochem.*, 49, 957, 1980.
220. **Burgeson, R. E., El Adii, F. A., Kaitila, I. I., and Hollister, D. W.,** Fetal membrane collagens: identification of two new collagen alpha chains, *Proc. Natl. Acad. Sci. U.S.A.*, 73, 2579, 1976.
221. **Fessler, J. H., Bachinger, H., Lunstrum, G., and Fessler, L. I.,** Biosynthesis and processing of some procollagens, in *New Trends in Basement Membrane Research,* Kuhn, K., Schoene, H. M., and Timpl, R., Eds., Raven Press, New York, 1984, 145.
222. **Madri, J. A. and Furthmayer, H.,** Isolation and tissue localization of type AB_2 collagen from lung parenchyma, *Am. J. Pathol.*, 94, 323, 1979.
223. **Rhodes, R. K. and Miller, E. J.,** Physicochemical characterization and molecular organization of collagen A and B chains, *Biochemistry,* 17, 442, 1978.
224. **Sage, H. and Bornstein, P.,** Characterization of a novel collagen chain in human placenta and its relation to AB collagen, *Biochemistry,* 18, 3815, 1979.

Chapter 3

ENDOTHELIAL CELL FUNCTION AND METASTASIS

Michael R. Buchanan and Maria C. Bertomeu

TABLE OF CONTENTS

I. INTRODUCTION

Entry into and subsequent exit out of the vascular bed is a prerequisite for most cancer cells to metastasize from their initial primary tumor. While most of our attention has focused upon the genetic, enzymatic, and biochemical properties unique to cancer cells that facilitate tumor growth and subsequent metastasis, there is an abundance of data which suggest that the endothelial cell lining of blood vessels is also a key player in the metastatic process. Normally, the endothelial cell lining from the large arteries of veins to the minute capillaries plays three major roles in homeostasis. It acts (1) as a selective molecular sieve, regulating the bilateral flow of specific constituents to and from the blood and extracellular tissue, (2) as a specific lining to maintain blood/vessel wall biocompatability, and (3) as a dynamic tissue, producing substances which in turn modulate vessel wall caliber and hemostasis. Not surprisingly, however, many of these functions have significant effects in the development of tumor growth and subsequent metastasis.

In this chapter, we will focus only on those structural/functional properties of the healthy endothelium and its responses to various stimuli, generated during cancer cell/endothelial cell interactions, and examine how these might influence the metastatic process. Subsequent chapters in this book will address specific aspects of these interactions in more detail.

II. THE ENDOTHELIUM AS A TISSUE

The innermost lining of all blood vessels is the endothelium, which is normally biocompatible with the circulating blood, i.e., blood cells and plasma proteins do not adhere to its surface.[1] However, when the endothelium is injured or perturbed, many blood vessel wall interactions occur. In the last 20 years with the development of endothelial cell culture techniques,[2] we have learned that both of these phenomena, namely vessel wall biocompatability and vessel wall responsiveness, are regulated in part by constituents synthesized and/or secreted specifically by endothelial cells.[1,3] The more we learn about the multi-step processes of metastasis, the more we realize that cancer cells are likely to interact at a number of stages during the metastatic process with the vascular endothelium. Consequently, it is possible that any of a number of procoagulant, anticoagulant, fibrinolytic, and enzymatic activities of the endothelium may have a significant effect on the metastatic process.

First, certain physical characteristics of the endothelium should be considered, which emphasize the vast extent of the endothelial cell surface. Endothelial cells are only approximately $20 \times 50\ \mu m^2$ in area and 6 to 8 μm in thickness and cover the entire vascular tree as a single cell layer. Such a thin lining may appear at first to be inconsequential; however, the entire surface area of blood vessels covered by endothelial cells is approximately 1,200 yd^2 or 1,000 m^2. As a mass, the entire endothelium weighs in excess of $^1/_4$ lb or 125 g.[2]

Second, the physical properties of the endothelial cell monolayer differs depending upon the area within the vascular tree. The endothelium is the thickest in the aorta and the thinnest in the capillaries. Most endothelial cell monolayers are continuous such as in the arteries, veins, and capillaries of muscle, but are fenestrated in the capillaries of the viscera.[3] The endothelial cells in arteries and veins align longitudinally according to the direction of blood flow. This pattern is particularly obvious at the orifices and bifurcations of blood vessels where blood flow is turbulent. The endothelial cells in the capillary beds however are more polygonal in shape without any distinct longitudinal orientation.

Most importantly, it should be emphasized that the major proportion of endothelial cells is found in the capillary bed.[3,4] Most cancer cell/endothelial cell interactions take place in the capillaries. This latter point is important to consider, since the surface area to which 1 ml of circulating blood (which may contain cancer cells) is exposed, is more than 1 m^2 in the capillary bed. Thus, at any particular site of blood cell/endothelial cell interaction, the concentration of endothelial cell-secreted constituents, which may be achieved at a local site of interaction, is markedly higher than the concentration measured systemically. These higher concentrations may manifest effects on cancer cells not detected nor thought important from a systemic measurement. In addition, it should be noted that our understanding of endothelial cell function is based predominantly on experimental studies using endothelial cells harvested from large arteries and veins. Therefore, any apparent understanding of the relative importance of various endothelial cell properties or products and/or their regulation must be interpreted with caution, since minimal information has been generated using capillary endothelial cells. The major exception to this is in the area of endothelial cell antigenicity as reviewed by Auerbach in Chapter 11 (which examines the antigenicity of endothelial cells derived from various capillary beds as it relates to tumor cell localization) and in the area of angiogenesis as reviewed by Moses in Chapter 16.

III. ENDOTHELIAL CELL BASEMENT MEMBRANE COMPONENTS

Synthesis of basement membrane components is a prerequisite in the morphogenesis of the endothelial cell monolayer.[5] The basement membrane components provide the foundation upon which the growing monolayer can adhere and maintain its structural integrity. The basement membrane is composed of a variety of components that influence cell adhesion, migration, growth, and differentiation.[5] A number of studies have shown that at least six different types of collagen can be synthesized by endothelial cells: collagen types I, III, IV, V, VI, and VIII.[5-10] *In vitro* studies using cultured endothelial cells indicate that endothelial cells can produce all six collagen types.[8] However, the relative amounts and the type of collagen synthesized appear to depend, in part, upon the source from which the endothelial cells are derived, the passage number, and the culture medium in and the substrate upon which the endothelial cells are grown. Human umbilical vein and vena cava-derived endothelial cells secrete collagen type IV into their ambient surroundings and collagen types IV and V into their underlying basement membrane.[6-9] In contrast, aortic- and pulmonary artery-derived endothelial cells secrete collagen type III into the plasma milieu and collagen types III, IV, and V into their underlying basement membrane.[9] If one assumes that there is a similar *in vivo* difference, one would expect site specificity in regard to the collagen composition of the vessel wall. Whether or not such site specific collagen concentrations are biologically relevant *in vivo,* from the perspective of cancer cell vessel wall interactions, are unclear. However, certain experimental studies suggest that this may have important implications. Cazenave and his colleagues[10] found that when endothelial cells were grown on basement membranes derived from other endothelial cells, the abilities of the newly seeded endothelial cells both to attach to and to grow upon purified collagen type IV were superior to their abilities to attach to it, which in turn was a better substrate than if the cells were plated on collagen type III. In contrast, we found that vascular smooth muscle cells (which synthesize predominantly collagen type III) grew best on collagen type III-rich substrates and did poorly on collagen type IV or authentic endothelial cell basement membrane. Other investigators demonstrated that the ability of smooth muscle cells to migrate and proliferate in a collagen gel was markedly altered when the gel was covered with a monolayer of endothelial cells.[11] These observations provide evidence that the basement membrane collagens synthesized by the different vascular cells facilitate their growth while inhibiting the growth of other cells. Since cancer cells are also required to synthesize basement membrane constituents to facilitate their growth and are required to digest basement membrane components of other cells to metastasize elsewhere in the body, it becomes obvious that the collagenase enzymatic properties of the cancer cells and the collagen make-up of the blood vessels at anatomically different sites may markedly influence the success of cancer cell invasion. Terranova discusses this issue from the perspective of the cancer cells in Chapter 2.

Fibronectin is another major component of the basement membrane underlying endothelial cells.[12] The fibronectin associated with the basement membrane is multimeric in structure, a physical property that enables it to bind both collagen type IV and heparan sulfate, a proteoglycan also produced by endothelial cells and present in the basement membrane.[7,13] Recent histoimmunofluorescent studies indicate that the fibronectin is synthesized and secreted from specific vesicles within the endothelial cells and is only secreted to the underlying basement membrane, since it was not detected on the luminal surface of endothelial cells.[14] A number of other investigators have demonstrated that fibronectin is an important adhesive substrate for cancer cells. Thus, the amount of fibronectin exposed at the site of vessel wall injury influences cancer cell attachment, thereby influencing cancer cell escape into the extravascular tissue.[15-16] Whether endothelial cells synthesize different amounts of fibronectin at different anatomical sites or during different states of vessel wall repair is unclear, but such differences may influence cancer cell attachment.

Laminin is a large glycoprotein (molecular weight 800 to 900 kDa), which is also present in the basement membrane.[7,13,17,18] Cultured endothelial cells secrete large amounts of laminin when they are subconfluent. Therefore, one might expect that endothelial cells, either during division or when spreading over a vessel wall following endothelial injury *in vivo,* deposit greater amounts of laminin in the basement membrane at that site than is normally present in a healthy uninjured vessel wall. Such variation in the basement membrane laminin content may therefore influence cancer cell metastasis since laminin also facilitates cancer cell attachment.

Endothelial cells synthesize and secrete a number of sulfated mucopolysaccharides, as well as their core proteins, into the basement membrane.[19] Recent studies by Alavi et al.[20] demonstrate that the composition of the sulfated polysaccharide in the basement membrane influences subsequent lipid accumulation into the vessel wall. Furthermore, the synthesis of these sulfated polysaccharides change with age.[21]

Thus, a complex basement membrane necessary for normal endothelial growth during angiogenesis or in response to vessel wall injury is formed under the endothelial cell lining. The composition of the basement membrane underlying the endothelium varies significantly, depending upon its location within the vascular tree, the state of vessel wall injury or repair, and the age of the host. It might be expected, therefore, that the relative amounts of the different collagen types, laminin, fibronectin, heparan sulfate, and other proteoglycans will influence significantly the ability of different cancer cells to enter and/or to exit the blood circulation.[22-26] For example, the capacity of different cancer cells to synthesize specific collagenases or chondroitinases, and target organs the cancer cells choose to enter, will depend, in part, upon their ability to transmigrate the endothelial cell basement membrane. This is supported by the observations that the metastatic potential of a variety of cancer cells is dependent, in part, upon their abilities to release heparinases, collagen specific proteases, and cathepsin B to digest the substrates with which they come into contact.[22,24,27,28] When endothelial cells retract, such as in response to certain cytokines or procoagulants, exposing the underlying basement membrane, the composition of the basement membrane exposed will influence which cancer cells can adhere.[26,27] For example, laminin receptors have been found on some cancer cells and are thought to be necessary for their attachment to the basement membrane and for their subsequent migration.[28] Other surface receptors such as the fibronectin receptor, the collagen type I receptor, and the vitronectin receptor may also be involved.[27-29]

In summary, it would appear that, depending upon the anatomical location, the state of endothelial cell integrity, and the specific enzymatic and adhesion receptors of different cancer cells, some cancer cells will be able to locate at specific sites of the vasculature while others will not.

IV. REGULATION OF COAGULATION

The endothelium plays a dual role in coagulation following vessel wall injury and during hypercoagulation.[1,4] Normally, endothelial cells are biocompatible with plasma proteins and only interact with them following stimulation by cytokines released from circulating blood cells, by other procoagulants, or by invasive bacteria and viruses.[32-35] Endothelial cells normally synthesize von Willebrand factor,[2,32-35] which is then released to bind to a smaller component to form factor VIII. von Willebrand factor also binds to specific types of collagens in the de-endothelized vessel wall, both *in vitro* and *in vivo,* which is necessary for platelet adhesion to the injured vessel wall in areas of high shear.[36] When endothelial cells are stimulated, von Willebrand factor is not only secreted into the plasma, but also redistributed within the endothelial cell and secreted into the basement membrane, rendering that surface more adherent.[34] Whether von Willebrand factor also enhances cancer cell attachment is not yet clear, but if so, this could explain the attachment of cancer cells to the vessel wall in areas of high flow. For example, Bastida et al.[15] have demonstrated that fibronectin facilitates tumor cell adhesion to extracellular matrix in an annular flow system. The presence of von Willebrand factor may enhance this process.

The observations that tumor growth is frequently associated with an activation of the coagulation system and that cancer cells rapidly migrate and proliferate into the fibrin mass surrounding cancer cells[39,41] suggest that enhanced coagulation is prometastatic. Thus, any procoagulant activity of endothelial cells in response to cancer cell-released cytokines may enhance metastasis. For example, stimulated endothelial cells express receptors for activated factor V. When activated factor V is bound to the endothelial cell surface, prothrombin activation by factor Xa is accelerated.[38] In addition, when endothelial cells are stimulated by thrombin, endotoxin, or any of a number of cytokines, endothelial cell tissue factor synthesis is increased. Tissue factor is subsequently expressed on the endothelial cell surface[37] and also acts as a receptor for factor VII. The factor VII/tissue factor complex initiates coagulation by activating factor X. These procoagulant reactions are required for optimal thrombin generation.[31,38] Generation of activated factor X on the endothelial cell surface is also associated with the release of endothelial cell mitogenic factors.[39] These latter observations suggest a possible link between the procoagulant activity of endothelial cells (following their activation by cancer cell-derived cytokines) and subsequent metastasis; namely, these mitogenic factors contribute to the metastatic process by stimulating cancer cell proliferation following cancer cell/endothelial cell interactions. In addition, it has also been reported that fibrinogen and fibrin monomers are chemoattractant and chemokinetic for cancer cells.[41]

Clinical evidence showing that enhanced coagulation facilitates metastasis is supported by studies in which cancer patients were treated with warfarin.[42,43] When warfarin was given to patients with small cell carcinoma of the lung, there was prolonged survival and a significant decrease in disease progression. These observations are consistent with earlier animal studies in which warfarin was also effective in preventing tumor growth.[44] It should be noted, however, that warfarin treatment had little or no effect on patients with advanced nonsmall cell lung, head or neck, or prostate cancer. In addition, none of these studies ruled out the possibility that warfarin may affect some but not other tumor cells directly. Nevertheless, these data suggest that enhanced coagulation may be important for the metastasis of some but not other cancer cells. Alternatively, the difference in warfarin effectiveness in the above studies could be simply due to differences in the onset of therapeutic intervention.

When coagulation is enhanced, endothelial cells also express a molecule, thrombomodulin, on their luminal surface.[45] Thrombomodulin binds thrombin and induces a conformational change in the thrombin molecule, which prevents it from activating more thrombin.[46] Instead, thrombomodulin-bound thrombin activates protein C, which downregulates coagulation by forming a complex with a second protein, protein S, to effectively inactivate activated factor V.[46-47]

Thus, the endothelial cell monolayer is an important physiological surface for the up-and-down regulation of coagulation, and in doing so, may also up- or downregulate metastasis. For example, tumor necrosis factor (which is released from cancer cells), downregulates thrombomodulin expression, thereby preventing effective thrombin-mediated-protein C activation. One might expect, therefore, that the normal mechanisms by which endothelial cells downregulate coagulation must be blocked for successful procoagulant-facilitated metastasis, i.e., for cancer cells to escape to fibrin-rich areas at sites of vessel wall injury.

While cancer cells are able to enhance the coagulation at various steps of metastasis, endogenous inhibitors of thrombin such as antithrombin III (a glycoprotein with a molecular weight of 58,000 Da) and heparin cofactor II (a glycoprotein with a molecular weight of 65,000 Da) continuously circulate and inhibit thrombin.[48-52] Specific glycosaminoglycans synthesized by endothelial cells, namely heparan sulfate and dermatan sulfate, catalyse the inhibition of thrombin by antithrombin III and heparin cofactor II, respectively, by at least 1000-fold.[52-57] Recent studies by Okwusidi et al.[58] indicate, however, that when thrombin is bound to a surface e.g., to a thrombus or to the injured vessel wall, the thrombin is resistant to inhibition by the heparin/antithrombin III complexes, whereas thrombin is effectively inhibited by the dermatan sulfate/heparin cofactor II complex. These recent results have rather interesting implications concerning the appropriate anticoagulant strategy to be used as an adjunct therapy in the treatment of cancer. In particular, these observations suggest that a more effective antimetastatic effect with anticoagulant therapy may be better achieved with those agents that effectively inhibit thrombin at specific local surface interfaces rather than by modulating systemic coagulation.

V. ENDOTHELIAL CELL FIBRINOLYSIS AND METASTASIS

While endothelial cells have the ability both to up- and downregulate coagulation effectively in response to the normal wear and tear of the vascular system, this homeostatic balance is frequently offset, resulting in the formation of intravascular thrombi. Not surprisingly, endothelial cells also have the additional capacity to contribute to fibrinolysis or the dissolution of these formed thrombi. When they are stimulated, again by any of a number of procoagulant stimuli, there is a rapid release of tissue plasminogen activator which catalyzes thrombolysis by plasmin.[59] To achieve this effect, tissue plasminogen activator binds to fibrin at the site of the formed thrombus or injured vessel wall, catalyzing the activation of the zymogen plasminogen to plasmin, which in turn, binds to fibrin and digests the thrombus.[59] Interestingly, 4 to 6 h after the onset of tissue plasminogen activator, tissue plasminogen activator levels rapidly decrease. This decrease is paralleled by the *de novo* synthesis and release of a plasminogen activator inhibitor.[59] These observations again emphasize the critical role that the endothelium plays in modulating the pathophysiological responses following blood/vessel wall interactions. From the perspective of fibrinolysis, there appears to be an initial release of fibrinolytic agents that enhance thrombolysis, followed by the release of thrombolytic inhibitors, which turn off the fibrinolytic response, thereby preventing hyperplasminemia. The pro- and antifibrinolytic activities of endothelial cells may also influence metastasis, either by preventing or by assisting cancer cell escape from the circulation. This step also may be influenced by the ability of cancer cells to generate their own tissue plasminogen activators and/or plasminogen activator inhibitors. It is unclear, however, whether or not the plasminogen activator inhibitors released from endothelial cells can downregulate the fibrinolytic constituents secreted by cancer cells, which appear necessary for their escape (see Chapter 3, 4, and 8). Grondahl et al.[61] reported that tissue plasminogen activators were significantly higher in 92 patients with breast cancer as compared to 34 healthy donor controls. Furthermore, there was a positive correlation between the mean tissue plasminogen activator plasma level and the extent of disease and tumor burden in these patients. However, other investigators have reported the opposite, namely that tissue plasminogen activator levels were lower in cancer patients.[62-64] These results may not be contradictory since in neither study, was there any simultaneous measurement of both tissue plasminogen activator and plasminogen activator inhibitor, nor any distinction between vessel wall- and cancer cell-derived fibrinolytic activator. Thus, the apparent increased levels of tissue plasminogen activator in Grondahl's study and the lower levels in Tissot's study may be explained simply on a basis of the time frame when the measurements were made relative to the generation of fibrinolytic activators and/or inhibitors. This notwithstanding, it appears evident that any alteration in the endogenous fibrinolytic system, which is modulated in part by the vessel wall endothelium, plays an important role in subsequent metastasis.

VI. FATTY ACID METABOLISM IN THE ENDOTHELIUM

The influence of fatty acid metabolism by the vessel wall will be discussed in more detail in Chapter 14, however, it is worth mentioning briefly in this chapter the role of certain fatty acid metabolites synthesized by the endothelial cell, which may influence metastasis. Unstimulated endothelial cell rapidly turnover triglycerides, resulting in the synthesis of a monohydroxide, 13-hydroxyoctadecadienoic acid or 13-HODE from the fatty acid, linoleic acid.[65,66] 13-HODE is retained in endothelial cells in specific vesicles that also contain the adhesive molecule, the vitronectin receptor, i.e., at a time when the endothelial cells are nonadhesive.[67] When endothelial cells are stimulated, 13-HODE synthesis ceases,[67] and the vitronectin receptor is expressed on the luminal surface of the endothelial cells, rendering them more adhesive for both platelets and tumor cells.[68-70] Recent studies *in vivo* support the possibility that synthesis of 13-HODE by the vessel wall influences significantly cancer cell adhesion and subsequent metastasis.[71]

The roles of RGD recognizing integrins expressed on the endothelial cell surface are discussed in detail by Kramer in Chapter 10. What has been unclear, however, is, how the expression of these molecules is regulated from the inside of the endothelial cell. This will be addressed in Chapter 14.

It is also well-known that when endothelial cells are stimulated, membrane-associated phospholipases are activated, facilitating the selective liberation of arachidonic acid, which in turn, is metabolized by the cyclooxygenase enzyme into the prostanoid, prostacyclin, or PGI_2.[72] PGI_2 is a potent inhibitor of platelet aggregation and a potent vasodilator. A number of years ago, Honn and colleagues[73] postulated that PGI_2 also may have an important antimetastatic role and may influence cancer cell/platelet interactions. This will be discussed in Chapter 7.

VII. SUMMARY

The biocompatible and permeability properties of the vascular endothelium long have been recognized as essential for normal vascular integrity. However, there are certain functions of the endothelium that may also play an important role in metastasis. Procoagulant and fibrinolytic constituents and their antagonists are also synthesized or regulated by the endothelium. Thus, a battery of pro- and anticoagulant and pro- and antifibrinolytic agents produced by the endothelium play an integral role in actively modulating cellular responses. These properties will be discussed in more detail from the perspective of cancer cells in metastasis in the succeeding chapters. It should also be noted that endothelial cells are capable of an intrinsic modulation of vascular tone by elaborating potent vasoactive substances, including PGI_2 and EDRF and endothelin,[74,75] two potent vasoactive substances that have not been discussed in this chapter, but that are eloquently reviewed by Luscher and Vanhoutte elsewhere.[76]

REFERENCES

1. **Gimbrone, M. A., Jr.,** Vascular endothelium: nature's blood container, in *Vascular Endothelium in Hemostasis and Thrombosis,* Gimbrone, M. A., Jr., Ed., Churchill Livingstone, Edinburg, 1986, 1.
2. **Jaffe, E. A., Nachman, R. L., Becker, C. G., and Minick, C. R.,** Culture of human endothelial cells derived from umbilical cord veins. Identification by morphologic and immunologic criteria, *J. Clin. Invest.,* 52, 2745, 1973.
3. **Thorgeirsson, G. and Robertson, A. L.,** The vascular endothelium-pathobiologic significance, *Am. J. Pathol.,* 93, 803, 1978.
4. **Owen, W. G.,** The control of hemostasis. Role of endothelium in the regulation of inhibitory and catabolic pathways, *Arch. Pathol. Lab. Med.,* 106, 209, 1982.
5. **Leivo, I.,** Structure and composition of early basement membranes: studies with early embryos and teratocarcinoma cells, *Med. Biol.,* 61, 1, 1983.
6. **Mayne, R.,** Collagenous proteins of blood vessels, *Arteriosclerosis,* 6, 585, 1986.
7. **Madri, J. A., Roll, F. J., Furthmayr, H., and Foidart, J. M.,** Ultrastructural localization of fibronectin and laminin in the basement membranes of the murine kidney, *J. Cell. Biol.,* 86, 682, 1980.
8. **Sage, H.,** Collagen synthesis by endothelial cells in culture, in *Biology of Endothelial Cells,* Jaffe, E. A., Ed., Martinus Nijhoff, The Hague, 1984, 161.
9. **Sage, H., Crouch, E. C., and Bornstein, P.,** Collagen synthesis by bovine aortic endothelial cells in culture, *Biochemistry,* 18, 5433, 1979.
10. **Cazenave, J. P.,** personal communication, 1979.
11. **van Buul-Wortelboer, M. F., Brinkman, H. J. M., Dingemans, K. P., de Groot, P. G., van Aken, W. G., and van Mourik, J. A.,** Reconstitution of the vascular wall *in vitro.* A novel model to study interactions between endothelial and smooth muscle cells, *Exp. Cell. Res.,* 162, 151, 1986.
12. **Stenman, S. and Vaheri, A.,** Distribution of a major connective tissue protein, fibronectin, in normal human tissue, *Exp. Med.,* 147, 1054, 1978.
13. **Laurie, G. W., Leblond, C. P., and Martin, G. R.,** Light microscopic immunolocalization of type IV collagen, laminin, heparan sulfate proteoglycan and fibronectin in the basement membranes of a variety of rat organs, *Am. J. Anat.,* 167, 71, 1983.
14. **Aznar-Salatti, J., Bastida, E., Buchanan, M. R., Castillo, R., Ordinas, A., and Escoler, G.,** Differential localization of von Willebrand factor, fibronectin and 13HODE in human endothelial cell cultures, *Histochemistry,* 93, 507, 1990.
15. **Bastida, E., Almirall, L., Bertomeu, M. C., and Ordinas, A.,** Influence of shear stress on tumor cell adhesion to endothelial cell extracellular matrix and its modulation by fibronectin, *Int. J. Cancer,* 43, 1174, 1989.
16. **Terranova, V. P., Hujanen, E. S., Loeb, D. M., Martin, G. R., Thornberg, L., and Glushko, V.,** Use of a reconstituted basement membrane to measure cell invasiveness and select for highly invasive tumor cells, *Proc. Natl. Acad. Sci. U.S.A.,* 83, 465, 1986.
17. **Timpl, R., Rohde, H., Robey, P. G., Rennard, S. I., Foidart, J. M., and Martin, G. R.,** Laminin — a glycoprotein from basement membranes, *J. Biol. Chem.,* 254, 9933, 1979.
18. **Gospodarowicz, D. G., Greenburg, J. M., Foidart, J. M., and Savion, N.,** The production and localization of laminin in culture vascular and corneal endothelial cells, *J. Cell. Physiol.,* 107, 171, 1981.
19. **Oohira, A., Wight, T. N., and Bornstein, P.,** Sulfated proteoglycans synthesized by vascular endothelial cells in culture, *J. Biol. Chem.,* 258, 2014, 1983.
20. **Alavi, Z. M., Richardson, M., and Moore, S.,** The *in vitro* interactions between serum lipoproteins and proteoglycans of the neointima of rabbit aorta after a single balloon catheter injury, *Am. J. Pathol.,* 134, 287, 1989.
21. **Murata, R.,** Distribution of acidic glycosaminoglycans, lipids and water in normal human cerebral arteries at various ages, *Stroke,* 16, 687, 1985.
22. **Liotta, L. A.,** Tumor invasion and membranes. Role of the extracellular matrix, *Cancer Res.,* 46, 1, 1986.
23. **Reich, R., Thompson, E. W., Iwamoto, Y., Martin, G. R., Deason, J. R., Fuller, G. C., and Miskin, R.,** Effects of inhibitors on plasminogen activator, serine proteinases, and collagenase IV on the invasion of basement membranes by metastatic cells, *Cancer Res.,* 48, 3307, 1988.

24. **Liotta, L. A. and Goldfarb, R. H.,** Interactions of tumor cells with the basement membrane of endothelium, in *Hemostatic Mechanisms and Metastasis,* Honn, K. V. and Sloane, B. F., Eds., Martinus Nijhoff, The Hague, 1984, 319.
25. **Albini, A., Iwamoto, Y., Kleinman, H. K., Martin, G. R., Aaronson, S., Kozlowski, J. M., and McEwan, R.,** A rapid *in vitro* assay for quantitating the invasive potential of tumor cells, *Cancer Res.,* 47, 3239, 1987.
26. **Yogeeswaran, G. and Salk, P. L.,** Metastatic potential is positively correlated with cell surface sialylation of cultured murine tumor cell lines, *Science,* 212, 1514, 1981.
27. **Kramer, R. H., Gonzalez, R., and Nicolson, G. L.,** Metastatic tumor cells adhere preferentially to the extracellular matrix underlying vascular endothelial cells, *Int. J. Cancer,* 26, 639, 1980.
28. **Terranova, V. P., Liotta, L. A., Russo, R. G., and Martin, G. R.,** Role of laminin in the attachment and metastasis of murine tumor cells, *Cancer Res.,* 42, 2265, 1982.
29. **Cheresh, D. A., Smith, J. W., Cooper, H. M., and Quaranta, V.,** A novel vitronectin receptor integrin αv βx is responsible for distinct adhesive properties of carcinoma cells, *Cell,* 57, 59, 1989.
30. **Humphries, M. J., Olden, K., and Yamada, K. M.,** Synthetic peptide from fibronectin inhibits experimental metastasis of murine melanoma cells, *Science,* 233, 467, 1986.
31. **Esmon, C. T.,** The regulation of natural anticoagulant pathways, *Science,* 235, 1348, 1986.
32. **Wagner, D. D., Olmsted, J. B., and Marder, V. J.,** Immunolocalization of von Willebrand protein in Weibel Palade bodies of human endothelial cells, *J. Cell. Biol.,* 95, 355, 1982.
33. **Reinders, J. H., de Groot, P. G., Dawes, J., Hunter, W. R., Heugten, H. A. A., van Zandbergen, J., Gonsalves, M. D., and van Mourik, J. A.,** Comparison of secretion and subcellular localization of von Willebrand protein with that of thrombospondin and fibronectin in cultured human vascular endothelial cells, *Biochim. Biophys. Acta,* 84, 306, 1985.
34. **Reinders, J. H., Vervoorn, R. C., Verweij, C. L., van Mourik, J. A., and de Groot, P. E.,** Perturbation of cultured human vascular endothelial cells by phorbol ester or thrombin alters the cellular von Willebrand factor distribution, *J. Cell. Physiol.,* 133, 79, 1987.
35. **Ribes, J. A., Francis, C. W., and Wagner, D. D.,** Fibrin induces release of von Willebrand factor from endothelial cells, *J. Clin. Invest.,* 79, 117, 1987.
36. **Sakariassen, K. S., Bolhuis, P. A., and Sixma, J. J.,** Human blood platelet adhesion to artery subendothelium is mediated by factor VIII-von Willebrand factor bound to the subendothelium, *Nature,* 279, 636, 1979.
37. **Bevilacqua, M. P., Pober, J. S., Majeu, G. R., Fiers, W., Cotran, R. S., and Gimbrone, M. A., Jr.,** Recombinant tumor necrosis factor induces procoagulant activity in culture human vascular endothelium. Characterization and comparison with the actions of Interleukin 1, *Proc. Natl. Acad. Sci. U.S.A.,* 83, 4533, 1986.
38. **Rogers, G. and Shuman, M.,** Prothrombin is activated on vascular endothelial cells by factor Xa and calcium, *Proc. Natl. Acad. Sci. U.S.A.,* 80, 7001, 1983.
39. **Gajdusek, C., Kisiel, W., Nawroth, P., and Stern, D.,** Activation of coagulation released endothelial cell mitogens, *J. Cell Biol.,* 103, 419, 1986.
40. **Dejana, E., Languino, L. R., Polentarutti, N., Balconi, G., Ryckewaert, T. T., Larieu, M. J., Donati, M. B., Mantovani, A., and Marguerie, G.,** Interaction between fibrinogen and cultured endothelial cells. Induction of migration and specific binding, *J. Clin. Invest.,* 75, 11, 1985.
41. **Dvorak, H. F., Dvorak, A. M., Manseau, E. J., Wiberg, L., and Churchill, W. H.,** Fibrin gel investment associated with line 1 and line 10 solid tumor growth, angiogenesis and fibroblasts in guinea pigs. Role of cellular immunity, myofibroblasts, microvascular damage, and infarction in line 1 tumor regression, *J. Natl. Cancer Inst.,* 62, 1459, 1979.
42. **Zacharski, L. R., Henderson, W. G., Rickles, F. R., Forman, W. B., Cornell, C. J., Forcier, R. J., Edwards, R. L., Headley, E., Kim, S., O'Donnell, J. F., O'Dell, R., Tornyos, K., and Kwaan, H. C.,** Effect of sodium warfarin on survival in small cell carcinoma of the lung, VA Cooperative Study #75, *JAMA,* 245, 831, 1981.
43. **Zacharski, L. R., Henderson, W. G., Rickles, F. R., Forman, W. B., Cornell, C. J., Forcier, R. J., Harrower, H. W., and Johnson, R. D.,** Rationale and experimental design for the VA Cooperative Study of anticoagulation (Warfarin) in the treatment of cancer, *Cancer,* 44, 732, 1979.
44. **Hilgard, P., Schulte, H., Wetzig, G., Schmitt, G., and Schmitt, O. G.,** Oral anticoagulation in the treatment of a spontaneously metastatic murine tumor, *Br. J. Cancer,* 35, 78, 1977.
45. **DeBault, L. E., Esmon, N. L., Olson, J. R., and Esmon, C. T.,** Distribution of the thrombomodulin antigen in the rabbit vasculature, *Lab. Invest.,* 54, 172, 1986.
46. **Esmon, C. T., Esmon, N. L., and Harris, K. W.,** Complex formation between thrombin and thrombomodulin inhibits both thrombin-catalyzed fibrin formation and factor V activation, *J. Biol. Chem.,* 257, 7944, 1982.
47. **Esmon, C. T. and Owen, W. G.,** Identification of an endothelial cell cofactor for thrombin-catalyzed activation of protein C, *Proc. Natl. Acad. Sci. U.S.A.,* 78, 2249, 1981.

48. **Downing, M. R., Bloom, J. W., and Mann, K. G.,** Comparison of the inhibition of thrombin by three plasma protease inhibitors, *Biochemistry,* 17, 2649, 1978.
49. **Rosenberg, R. D.,** Chemistry of the hemostatic mechanism and its relationship to the action of heparin, *Fed. Proc.,* 35, 10, 1977.
50. **Hortin, G., Tollefsen, D. M., and Strauss, A. W.,** Identification of two sites of sulfation on human heparin cofactor II, *J. Biol. Chem.,* 261, 15827, 1984.
51. **Rosenberg, R. D. and Damus, P. S.,** The purification and mechanism of action of human antithrombin-heparin cofactor, *J. Biol. Chem.,* 248, 6490, 1973.
52. **Scully, M. F. and Kakkar, V. V.,** Identification of heparin cofactor II as the principal plasma cofactor for the antithrombin activity of pentosan polysulphate (SP54), *Thromb. Res.,* 36, 187, 1984.
53. **Teien, A. N., Abildgaard, U., Hook, M., and Lindahl, U.,** The anticoagulant effect of heparin sulfate and dermatan sulfate, *Thromb. Res.,* 11, 107, 1977.
54. **Wunderwald, P., Schrenk, W. G., and Port, H.,** Antithrombin BM from human plasma: an antithrombin binding moderately to heparin, *Thromb. Res.,* 25, 177, 1982.
55. **Briginshaw, G. F. and Shanberge, J. N.,** Identification of two distinct heparin cofactors in human plasma. II. Inhibition of thrombin and activated factor X, *Thromb. Res.,* 4, 463, 1975.
56. **Ofosu, F. A., Fernandez, F., Gauthier, D., and Buchanan, M. R.,** Heparin cofactor II and other endogenous factors in the mediation of the antithrombotic and anticoagulant effects of heparin and dermatan sulfate, *Semin. Thromb. Hemost.,* 11, 133, 1985.
57. **Ofosu, F. A., Modi, G. J., Smith, L. M., Cerskus, A. L., Hirsh, J., and Blajchman, M. A.,** Heparin sulfate and dermatan sulfate inhibit the generation of thrombin activity in plasmas by complementary pathways, *Blood,* 64, 742, 1984.
58. **Okwusidi, J., Falcone, M., VanRyn-McKenna, J., Hirsh, J., Ofosu, F. A., and Buchanan, M. R.,** *In vivo* catalysis of thrombin inhibition by antithrombin III and heparin cofactor II and antithrombotic effect: differential effects of dermatan sulfate and unfractionated heparin, *Thromb. Hemorrh. Disorders,* vol. 1/2: 77, 1990.
59. **Collen, D.,** On the regulation and control of fibrinolysis, *Thromb. Haemost.,* 43, 77, 1980.
60. **Erickson, L. A., Schleef, R. R., Ny, T., and Loskutoff, D. J.,** The fibrinolytic system of the vascular wall, *Clin. Haematol.,* 14, 513, 1985.
61. **Grondahl, J., Back, F., and Munkholm-Larson, P.,** Tissue type plasminogen activator in plasma from breast cancer patients determined by enzyme-linked immunosorbent assay, *Br. J. Cancer,* 61, 412, 1988.
62. **Duffy, M. J., O'Grady, P., Devaney, D., O'Siorain, L., Fenelly, J. J., and Lijnen, H. R.,** Tissue-type plasminogen activator, a new prognostic marker in breast cancer, *Cancer Res.,* 48, 1348, 1988.
63. **Colombi, M., Barlati, S., Magdelenat, H., and Fiszer-Szafarz, B.,** Relationship between multiple forms of plasminogen activator in human breast tumors and plasma and the presence of metastasis in lymph nodes, *Cancer Res.,* 46, 5743, 1984.
64. **Tissot, J. D., Hauert, J., and Bachmann, F.,** Characterization of plasminogen activator from normal human breast and colon carcinomas, *Int. J. Cancer,* 34, 295, 1984.
65. **Denning, G. M., Figard, P. H., Kaduce, T. L., and Spector, A.,** Role of triglycerides in endothelial cell arachidonic acid metabolism, *J. Lipid Res.,* 24, 1011, 1983.
66. **Buchanan, M. R., Haas, T. A., Lagarde, M., and Guichardant, M.,** 13-Hydroxyoctadecadienoic acid is the vessel wall chemorepellant LOX, *J. Biol. Chem.,* 260, 16056, 1985.
67. **Bertomeu, M. C., Haas, T. A., Eltringham-Smith, L., and Buchanan, M. R.,** Relationship between endothelial cell vitronectin receptor expression and 13-HODE: histoimunofluorescent localization, in *Proc. VIth Int. Symp. Vascular Wall Cells,* Paris, Aug. 27—Sept. 1, 1990, PSIV, 4.
68. **Lauri, D., Bertomeu, M. C., Orr, F. W., Bastida, E., Sauder, D., and Buchanan, M. R.,** Interleukin-1 increases tumor cell adhesion to endothelial cells through an RGD dependent mechanism: *in vitro* and *in vivo* studies, *Clin. Exp. Metast,* 8, 27, 1990.
69. **Buchanan, M. R., Bertomeu, M. C., Brister, S. J., LaFrenie, R. M., Haas, T. H., Orr, F. W., and Bastida, E.,** Vessel wall 13-HODE synthesis, vitronectin expression and metastasis: *in vitro* and *in vivo* studies, in *Proc. 7th Int. Conf. Prostaglandins Related Compounds,* Florence, May 28 to June 1, 1990, 214.
70. **Lafrenie, R. M., Podor, T. J., Buchanan, M. R., and Orr, F. W.,** Interleukin 1α induced vitronectin receptor expression and tumor cell endothelial cell adhesion, *FASEB,* 4, A1134, 1990.
71. **Bertomeu, M. C., Crozier, G. L., and Buchanan, M. R.,** Differential effects of dietary fats on primary tumor growth and secondary metastasis, in *Proc. 7th Int. Conf. Prostaglandins Related Compounds,* Florence, May 28 to June 1, 1990, 277.
72. **Moncada, S., Gryglewski, R. J., Bunting, S., and Vane, J. R.,** An enzyme isolated from arteries transforms prostaglandin endoperoxides to an unstable substance that inhibits platelet aggregation, *Nature,* 263, 663, 1976.
73. **Honn, K. V., Cicone, B., and Skoff, A.,** Prostacyclin a potent antimetastatic agent, *Science,* 212, 1270, 1981.

74. **Brenner, B. M., Troy, J. L., and Ballermann, B. J.,** Endothelium dependent vascular responses. Mediators and mechanism, *J. Clin. Invest.*, 84, 1373, 1989.
75. **Vanhoutte, P. M.,** Endothelium, platelets and vasospasm, in *Blood Cells and Arteries in Hypertension and Atherosclerosis,* Meyer, P. and Marche, P., Eds., Raven Press, New York, 1989, 1.
76. **Luscher, T. F. and Vanhoutte, P. M.,** *The Endothelium: Modulator of Cardiovascular Function,* CRC Press, Boca Raton, FL, 1990.

Chapter 4

PASSAGE ACROSS THE VASCULAR WALL BY MALIGNANT CELLS IN METASTASIS FORMATION

Peter P. H. De Bruyn

The invasive property of malignant growths is manifested in two ways: (1) by their direct penetration into immediately adjacent tissues and organs and (2) by the entry of malignant cells into the vascular system, thus transporting these cells to sites distant from the primary tumor and resulting in secondary growths, i.e., the formation of metastatic tumors. Clinically, the two forms of invasion are of very different importance. It remains, however, uncertain whether the biological mechanisms involved in the cellular invasion of adjacent tissues are the same or different from the movement of malignant cells across the vascular wall. The possibility of such a distinction between these two different manifestations of malignant invasiveness is of interest and has some clinical support: minute malignant tissues may produce widespread metastases, while very large malignant growths do not necessarily result in metastatic dissemination.

The structural events occurring in the cellular interaction during the transmural passage of malignant cells into the circulation have been the object of a number of studies and appear to be structurally well defined. Less is known about the events in the first manifestation of malignancy i.e., in the movement of malignant cells into adjacent anatomical structures. The second manifestation of malignancy, viz, the formation of metastases, consists of two sequential phases: a primary phase which is the entry of malignant cells into the circulation and a secondary phase in which the malignant cells leave the circulation at the site of the future metastasis and then proliferate there extravascularly. The second phase militates against the benefits of surgical removal of the primary tumor and represents, in this respect, the most pernicious aspect of malignancy.

Regarding to the biological mechanisms involved in metastasis formation, the transmural cell movement is of special interest. It is evident that the transmural cell passage into the circulation is a selective event: it is limited to malignant cells; normal stromal or parenchymal cells do not enter the circulation. Clearly, then, there is a specific form of interaction between the malignant cell and the abluminal aspect of the vascular endothelium of the vessel invaded, which allows the malignant cell to enter the vascular lumen. A similar interaction is operating in the transmural movement of the intravascular malignant cell towards the extravascular space in the second phase of metastasis formation. Regarding this specific interaction, knowledge of the pathway of these malignant cells through the vascular wall is of importance. Is the passage of the malignant cell through the vascular wall the result of a localized destructive invasion that occurs in the tumor invasion of neighboring tissues and organs, or does the malignant cell penetrate a functionally and structurally intact wall that takes place in the transmural cell passage generally defined as diapedesis? Furthermore, it is of interest to know whether such transmural passage is through the intercellular clefts of the endothelium which occurs in the diapedesis of blood cells in inflammation[1] or whether the malignant cell penetrates the endothelial cell body in which case the entry of malignant cells into the vascular lumen would be a transcellular process. Each of these two transmural processes can be expected to require a form of cellular interaction different from one another and thus would define differently the nature of cellular malignancy as it relates to metastasis formation.

Light microscopic and fine structural studies on the pathway of malignant cells through the endothelial wall of vessels of malignant tumors have been made on tumors subcutaneously transplanted and known to have at this site metastasis-forming ability. These tumors include

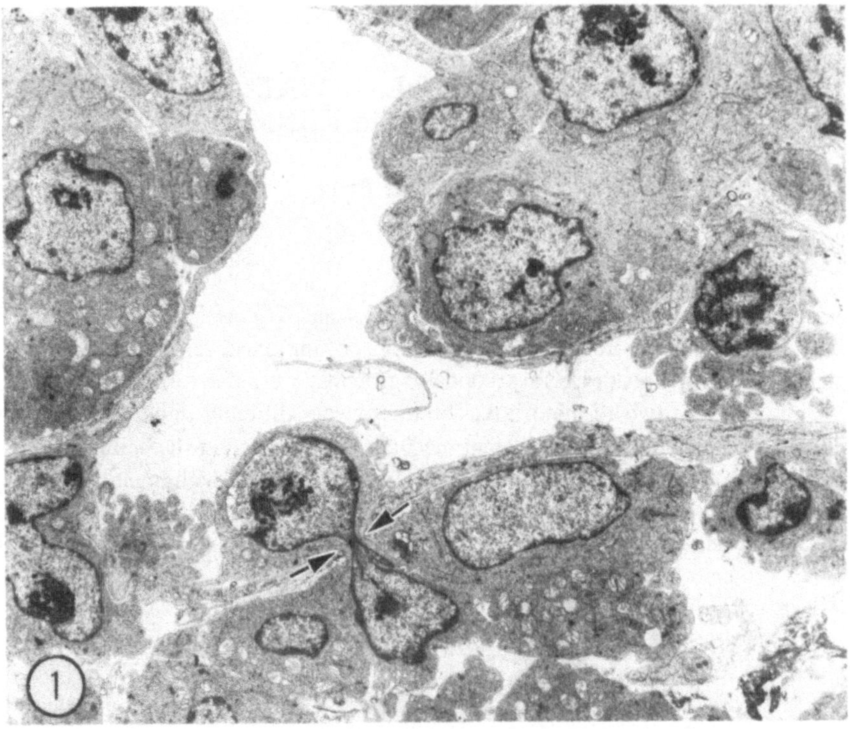

FIGURE 1. Rat tumor cell from a subcutaneously growing myelogenous tumor (Shay) is shown entering a venule (arrows). The venule endothelium is intact. × 4,200.

the allogeneic Shay acute myelogenous leukemia,[2] the syngeneic rat Wistar-Furth acute myelogenous leukemia, and the syngeneic mouse B16 melanoma.[3] They invade the underlying musculature and the subepithelial connective tissue of the skin. They do not, however, enter the surface epithelium. The destructive nature of the transplanted tumors is shown by their penetration into the subcutaneous striated musculature of which there remain at the sites of penetration only dispersed small fragments of degenerated muscle fibers.[3] The transplanted tumors are abundantly supplied with blood vessels induced by the tumor angiogenetic factor of Folkman.[4] Notwithstanding the evident destructive ability of these tumor cells, the continuity of the vasculature remains intact. There are no vacant discontinuities in the endothelial lining of the vessels of the tumor. When the tumor cells are directly deposited on a pre-existing (femoral) vessel, they grew around the arterial and venous vessels and entered the subendothelial venous tissue, but the endothelial lining remained intact and continuous.[3]

The preservation of the endothelial continuity does not, however, prevent the malignant cells from moving across the endothelial barrier and entering the vascular lumen. Light microscopy as well as transmission electron microscopy (Figure 1) and scanning electron microscopy (Figure 2) reveal cells in transmural passage through the vessel endothelium of the tumor. These cells are structurally identical to the tumor cells. The formation of metastasis, the massive presence of malignant cells around the vessels, and the fact that cells in mitosis occur in transmural passage further support the contention that the diapedesing cells are malignant and thus represent the first stage of metastasis formation.

The transmural passage of malignant cells, which correspond structurally to venules, occurs in angiogenically induced vessels, having a relatively wide lumen and being lined solely with a single layer of endothelial cells. Tumor cells, however, may also enter the circulation through the endothelial lining of pre-existing vessels. When tumor cells are

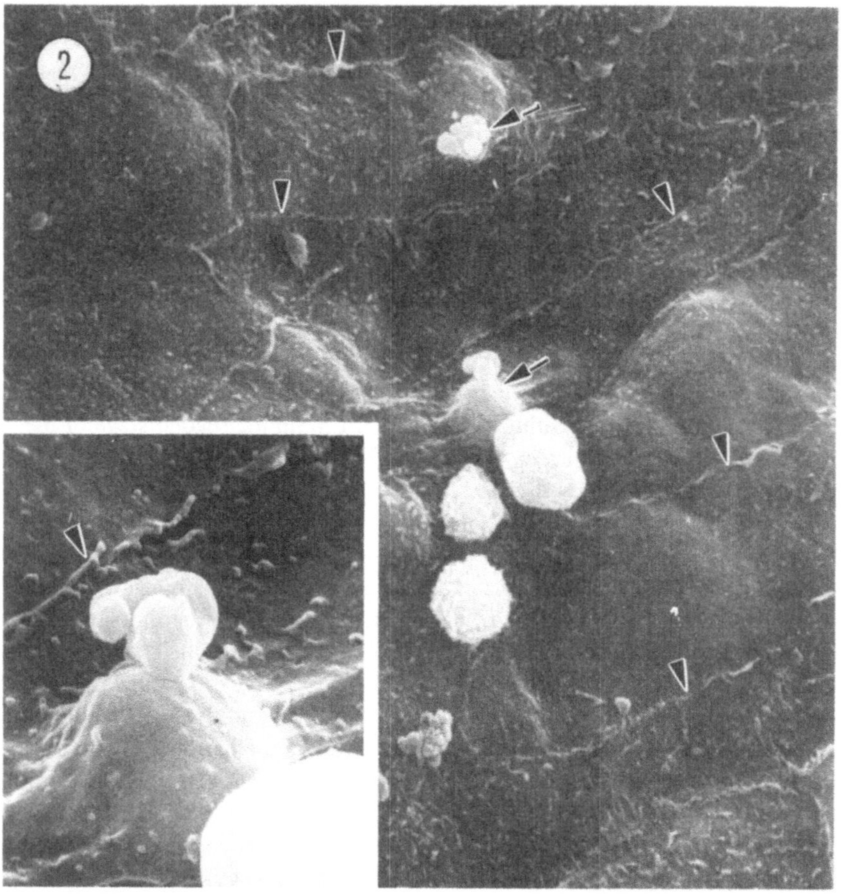

FIGURE 2. Adluminal scanning electron microscopic view of a venule of a subcutaneous Wistar-Furth myelogenous tumor in rat. The endothelium is intact. Two malignant cells (arrows) are entering the vessel lumen independently of the intercellular endothelial junctions (arrowheads). × 1,700. Inset: Enlargement of one of the migrating cells. × 6,000.

directly deposited on the larger branches of inguinal vessels, transmural passage occurs through the penetration by tumor cells of the intact endothelium of the larger veins but not through the arterial vessels.[3]

The pathway of the migrating malignant cell cannot be determined by observations on single sections since they do not reveal the three dimensional relationship between the site of migration and the intercellular endothelial junction. Observations on serial sections have failed to show a relationship between the endothelial migration pore and the intercellular junctions, suggesting that the malignant cells penetrate the endothelial cell body, i.e., through a transcellular pathway in the endothelium.[2,3] Scanning electron microscopy that permits the determination of the position of the migrating cells with regard to the intercellular endothelial junction shows directly that the site of the transmural migration of the malignant cells is independent of the cellular junction, i.e., it is transcellular (Figure 1). Additional structural features of the transcellular malignant cell movement are noted in the figure captions. It is evident that the migration pore made by the malignant cell closes after the passage of the cell since the vascular endothelium remains continuous.

The transmural entry of malignant cells through the temporary migration pore is usually limited to single cells. The simultaneous entry of more than one cell is rare, and multiple entry of malignant cells in the form of sizeable cellular emboli does not seem to occur. The first phase of metastasis formation thus appears to be rather continuous for the transcellular entry of malignant cells into the vascular lumen.

Intravascular infusions of suspensions of malignant cells have been used extensively for studies on metastatic spread.[5] A number of factors involving the properties of tumor cells as well as those of the host tissues and affecting the formation and distribution of metastases have been studied using this experimental model. These aspects of metastasis formation have been reviewed and discussed by Fidler and Nicholson,[6] largely for the B16 melanoma, which has produced the most extensive information on these points. It is to be noted that these are models for the second phase of metastasis formation: the establishment of a secondary malignant locus by circulating malignant cells. Following such procedures, some workers described the transmural passage of malignant cells as occurring through a defect in the vascular wall[7] or as a diapedesis following the intercellular endothelial junction similar to the pathway of migrating leucocytes in inflammation.[8,9] In general such procedures present problems for observations of the cellular events occurring in the second stage of metastasis formation. Such studies, which necessarily must deal with earliest phases of this process, meet with the difficulty of locating the precise site of the future metastatic locus to be formed after the intravascular arrest of the malignant cells.

The intravascular infusion of single cell suspensions of the transplantable Wistar-Furth acute myelogenous leukemia (AML) results in an extravascular malignant myeloid proliferation after the transmural passage. Accepting this as a model for the second stage of metastasis formation, the cellular transmural processes, resulting in the formation of the extravascular tumor, can be studied in their earliest phase.[10] Such experiments have shown that the adhesion of the malignant cells to the adluminal sinus wall and the subsequent penetration of the endothelium occur almost immediately after the presentation of the malignant cells. Intraaortal perfusions of the myeloid tissue, lasting from 2 to 5 min, with tumor cell suspensions derived from ascites tumors showed structural configurations, indicating a specific adhesion of the malignant cells to the adluminal venous sinus wall. Besides images showing a simple random contact, there were configurations that indicated a specific adherence of AML cells to the sinus endothelium. In such instances, the AML cells make contact with the adluminal face of the endothelial sinus surface over a broad base (Figure 3). After longer perfusion times (20 min), the malignant cells penetrated the endothelial cell body (Figure 4) and entered the extravascular parenchyma. Serial sections indicate that the transmural cell passage does not occur through the cell junctions but through the endothelial cell body, i.e., the passage is transcellular. The initial penetration of the endothelial cell body by a malignant cell can occur at multiple points. However, the transcellular passage is through a single pore. Apparently, the supernumerary initial penetrations are aborted, and a single site of entry is selected for the final cell passage.

During this transcellular passage, there are sites of apposition of the two plasmalemmas where the intercellular space is reduced to 2.3 nm, forming a heptalaminar complex similar to intercellular gap junctions (Figures 5 and 6). At these places, the electron lucent intercellular space is interrupted by electron densities with a diameter of 5 nm and 8 nm, from center to center. These densities resemble connexons, which are held to be the functional part of gap junctions and which are sites of intercellular communication, an event requisite for transcellular cell passage. In addition, there are sites of adhesion with an interplasmalemmal spacing of 8 nm (Figure 6). These extend over distances of 800 nm, while the gap junctions cover about 200 nm.

The transcellular movement of malignant cells into the circulation (the first phase of metastasis formation) and from the vascular lumen into the extravascular parenchyma (the second phase of metastasis formation) is selective. The transcellular cell movement into the parenchyma is distinct from the transmural movement of blood cells in inflammation where the exudation of blood cells is intercellular[1] and which does not exhibit cellular selectivity in transmural passage.

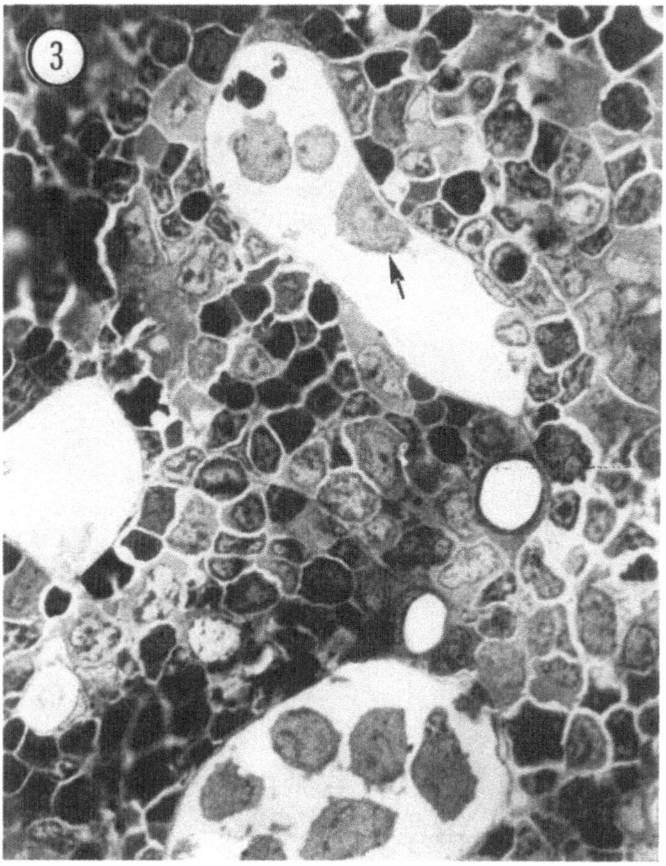

FIGURE 3. Rat bone marrow perfused for 5 min with a suspension of Wistar-Furth tumor cells. The myeloid sinuses contain myeloid tumor cells. One adheres to the sinus wall (arrow). × 1,200.

The above described observations show that a destructive invasion of the vessel wall is not necessary for the entry of malignant cells into the circulation. However, the present observations should not lead to the conclusion that malignant cells cannot, under any circumstances or at any time, destroy walls of blood vessels and release, through such vascular defects, emboli of malignant cells into the vascular lumen. The general conclusion is restricted to the fact that the entry of malignant cells into the circulation, i.e., the first phase of metastasis formation is transcellular, occurs through the penetration of a fully intact endothelial lining. The functional continuity of the endothelial lining is preserved during this process. It is further to be noted that an impairment of the vascular integrity of the tumor circulation might possibly militate against the growth of the tumor.

Selective transcellular cell passage is not limited to metastasis formation, but is of wider occurrence and appears to be essential in the extravascular-intravascular movement of blood cells in normal hematopoiesis. This selective delivery of mature blood cells into the peripheral blood cell pool, while the immature blood cells are retained at the extravascular site, is through a structurally continuous endothelium and through the endothelial cell body, i.e., the delivery is transcellular[11-14] with respect to selectivity and directional movement, a corollary of the first phase of metastasis formation.

In the acute myelogenous leukemia induced by the intravascular administration of Wistar-Furth AML cells, the transformed myeloblasts similarly migrate transcellularly into the myeloid sinus lumen. Apparently, the transformed cells have acquired similar migratory properties as the normal mature blood cells.

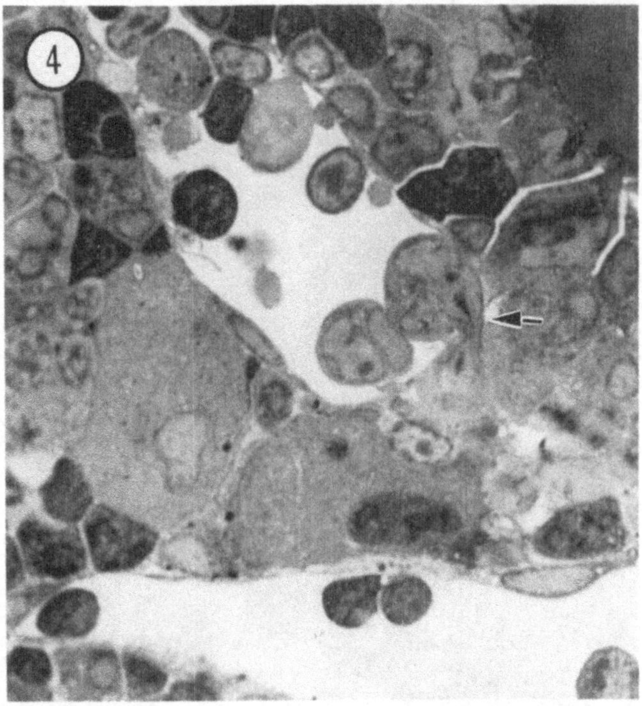

FIGURE 4. Rat bone marrow perfused for 20 min with a suspension of Wistar-Furth tumor cells, one of which is shown in transmural passage entering the parenchyma (arrow). × 1,800.

The presence of cells (lymphocytes) inside other cells has been reported in cell cultures. By means of time cinematography of tissue cultures, living lymphocytes have been seen in malignant cells.[15] This process has been termed *emperipoiesis,* which means "inside round and about wandering." A functional significance for this has not been proposed.

Another instance of selective transcellular cell movement is the passage of intravascular lymphocytes into the lymphatic parenchyma through the high endothelial wall of the postcapillary venules of lymphatic tissues,[16-20] the primary site[16] of the recirculating route of the lymphocytes.[21] This transcellular movement, with respect to its direction of movement and cellular specificity, is a corollary of the second stage of metastasis formation. The interaction between the lymphocytes and the endothelium of the high endothelial postcapillary venules has been extensively investigated largely by means of an *in vitro* model designed by Stampfer and Woodruff.[22] Butcher et al.[23] have shown that the affinity of lymphocytes for the postcapillary venule endothelium as displayed by this *in vitro* model correlates to a high degree with the adherence of lymphocytes to the postcapillary venule endothelium *in vivo.* It was found that the selective affinity involves an interaction between functionally different sets of lymphocytes and the endothelia of the postcapillary venules of different lymphatic organs.[23-25] Specific lymphocyte receptors on the lymphocyte surface are apparently part of the recognition system, directing the lymphocytes to various lymphatic organs.[26,27] This requires the presence of an appropriate specific ligand at the abluminal face of the high endothelial postcapillary venule. Such receptors and ligands have been identified,[28,29] but no such information is yet available for the interaction between malignant cells and the vascular endothelium involved in metastasis formation. It would seem likely that further studies with an *in vitro* model such as the *in vitro* Stamper-Woodruff model might give insight into the malignant cell-endothelium interaction.

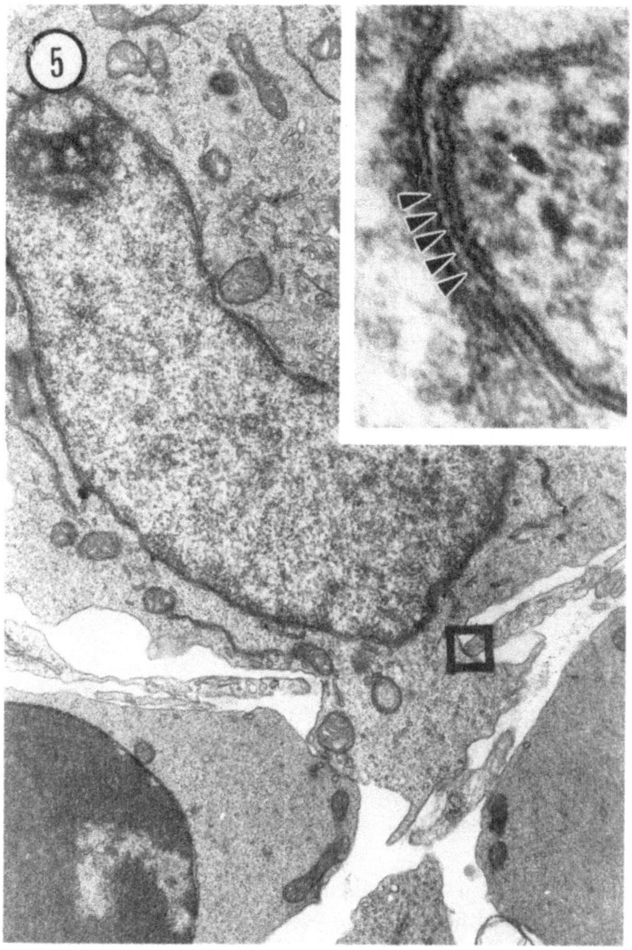

FIGURE 5. Rat bone marrow perfused for 25 min with a suspension of Wistar-Furth tumor cells. A tumor cell penetrates the endothelial cell body and enters the extravascular parenchyma. Inset: The interplasmalemmal space is reduced at one side of the migration pore to 2.4 nm, and a heptalaminar complex similar to gap junctions is formed. The interplasmalemmal space is interrupted by localized areas of increased electron density (arrowheads), which are similar to the connexons of gap junctions. × 15,000. Inset: × 320,000.

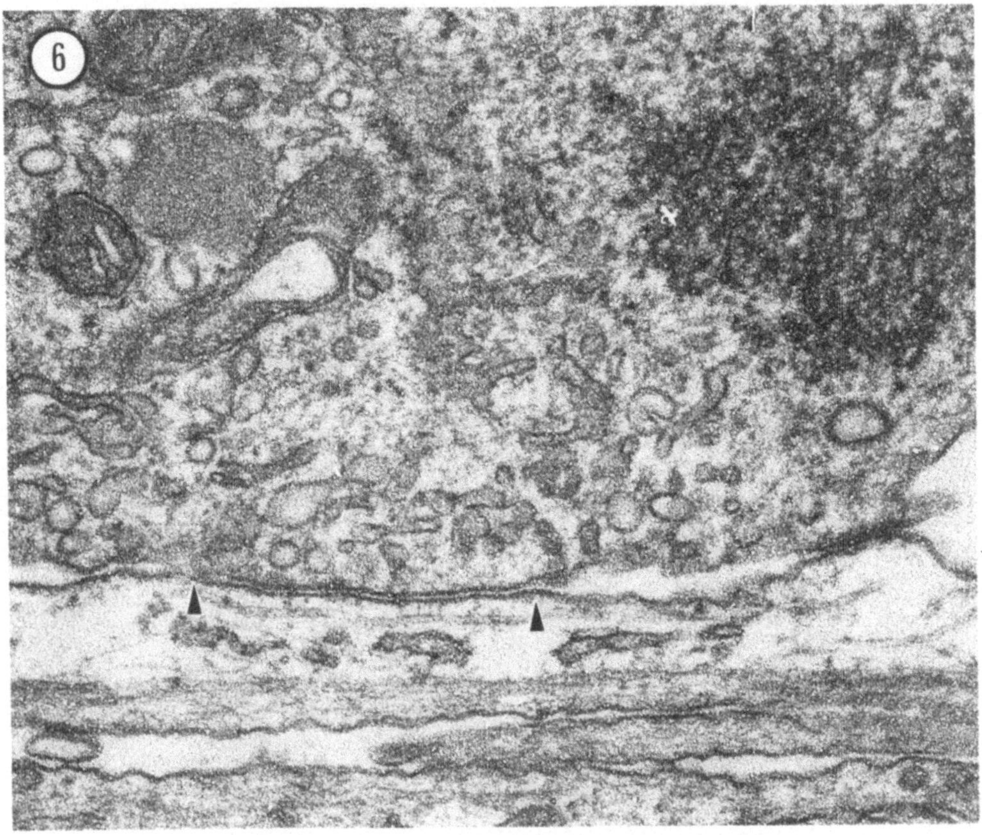

FIGURE 6. Rat bone marrow perfused with AML cells for 20 min. An AML cell makes two contacts with the sinus endothelial cell surface. One (delineated by arrowheads) extends over a distance of 800 nm and has an interplasmalemmal space of 8 nm. The other extends over 190 nm and has an interplasmalemmal space of 2.5 nm. × 63,000.

ACKNOWLEDGMENT

Research by the author and co-workers reported here has been supported by PHS Grant CA 05493.

REFERENCES

1. **Marchesi, V. T.,** The site of leucocyte emigration during inflammation, *Q. J. Exp. Physiol.*, 46, 115, 1961.
2. **De Bruyn, P. P. H. and Cho, Y.,** Entry of metastatic malignant cells into the circulation from a subcutaneously growing myelogenous tumor, *J. Natl. Cancer Inst.*, 62, 1221, 1979.
3. **De Bruyn, P. P. H. and Cho, Y.,** Vascular endothelial invasion via transcellular passage by malignant cells in the primary stage of metastases formation, *J. Ultrastruct. Res.*, 81, 189, 1982.
4. **Folkman, J.,** Tumor angiogenesis, *Adv. Cancer Res.*, 19, 331, 1974.
5. **Fidler, I. J.,** Mechanism of cancer invasion and metastasis. Cancer: a comprehensive treatise, in *Biology of Tumors: Surfaces, Immunology, and Comparative Pathology*, Vol. 4, Becker, F. Y., Ed., Plenum, New York, 1975, 101.

6. **Fidler, I. J. and Nicholson, G. L.,** Immunobiology of experimental metastatic melanoma, in *Cancer Biology Reviews,* Vol. 2, Marchalonis, J. J., Hanna, M. G., Jr., and Fidler, I. J., Eds., Marcel Dekker, New York, 1981, 171.
7. **Chew, E. C., Josephson, R. L., and Wallace, A. C.,** Morphologic aspects of the arrest of circulating cancer cells, in *Fundamental Aspects of Metastasis,* Weiss, L., Ed., Elsevier, New York, 1976, 121.
8. **Warren, B. A.,** Origin and fate of blood borne tumor emboli, in *Cancer Biology Reviews,* Vol. 2, Marchalonis, J. J., Hanna, J. G., Jr., and Fidler, I. J., Eds., Marcel Dekker, New York, 1981, 95.
9. **Sindelar, W. F., Tralka, T. S., and Ketcham, A. S.,** Electron microscopic observations on formation of pulmonary metastases, *J. Surg. Res.,* 18, 137, 1975.
10. **De Bruyn, P. P. H., Cho, Y., and Michelson, S.,** Endothelial attachment and plasmalemmal apposition in the transcellular movement of intravascular leukemic cells entering the myeloid parenchyma, *Am. J. Anat.,* 186, 115, 1989.
11. **De Bruyn, P. P. H., Michelson, S., and Thomas, T. B.,** The migration of blood cells in the bone marrow through the sinusoidal wall, *J. Morphol.,* 133, 417, 1971.
12. **Campbell, F.,** Ultrastructural studies of transmural migration of blood cells in the bone marrow of rats, mice, and guinea pigs, *Am. J. Anat.,* 135, 521, 1972.
13. **Becker, R. P. and De Bruyn, P. P. H.,** The transmural passage of blood cells into myeloid sinusoids and the entry of platelets into the sinusoidal circulation, *Am. J. Anat.,* 145, 183, 1976.
14. **Muto, M. A.,** Scanning and transmission electron microscopic study on rat bone marrow sinuses and transmural migration of blood cells, *Arch. Histol. Jpn.,* 39, 51, 1976.
15. **Humble, J. G., Jayne, W. H., and Pulvertaft, R. J.,** Biological interaction between lymphocytes and other cells, *Int. Rev. Cytol.,* 7, 288, 1958.
16. **Marchesi, V. T. and Gowans, J. L.,** The migration of lymphocytes through the endothelium of venules in lymph nodes: an electron microscope study, *Proc. R. Soc. B,* 159, 283, 1964.
17. **Farr, A. G. and De Bruyn, P. P. H.,** The mode of lymphocyte migration through the postcapillary endothelium in lymph node, *Am. J. Anat.,* 143, 49, 1975.
18. **Cho, Y. and De Bruyn, P. P. H.,** Internal structure of the postcapillary high-endothelial venules of rodent lymph nodes and Peyer's patches and the transendothelial lymphocyte passage, *Am. J. Anat.,* 177, 481, 1986.
19. **Cho, Y. and De Bruyn, P. P. H.,** The endothelial structure of the postcapillary venules of lymph node and the passage of lymphocytes across the venule wall, *J. Ultrastruct. Res.,* 69, 13, 1979.
20. **De Bruyn, P. P. H. and Cho, Y.,** Structure and function of high endothelial postcapillary venules in lymphocyte circulation, in *Current Topics in Pathology: Reaction Patterns of the Lymph Node,* Vol. 84, Grundmann, E. and Vollner, E., Eds., Springer-Verlag, Berlin, 1990.
21. **Gowans, J. L. and Knight, E. J.,** The route of re-circulation of lymphocytes in the rat, *Proc. R. Soc.,* 159, 257, 1964.
22. **Stamper, H. B. and Woodruff, J. J.,** Lymphocyte homing into lymph nodes: *in vitro* demonstration of the selective affinity of recirculating lymphocytes for high endothelial venules, *J. Exp. Med.,* 144, 828, 1976.
23. **Butcher, E. D., Scolley, R. G., and Weissman, I. L.,** Lymphocyte adherence to high endothelial venules: characterization of a modified *in vitro* assay and examination of the binding of syngeneic and allogeneic lymphocyte populations, *J. Immunol.,* 123, 1996, 1979.
24. **Stevens, S. K., Weissman, I. L., and Butcher, E. C.,** Differences in the migration of B and T lymphocytes, organ selectivity and the role of lymphocyte — endothelial cell recognition, *J. Immunol.,* 128, 844, 1982.
25. **Kraal, G., Weissman, I. L., and Butcher, E. C.,** Differences *in vivo* distribution and homing of T cell subsets of mucosal vs. non-mucosal lymphoid organs, *J. Immunol.,* 1330, 1097, 1983.
26. **Gallatin, W. M., Weissman, I. L., and Butcher, E. D.,** A cell surface molecule involved in organ-specific homing of lymphocytes, *Nature,* 304, 30, 1983.
27. **Jalkanen, S. T. and Butcher, E. C.,** *In vitro* analysis of the homing properties of human lymphocytes, developmental regulation of functional receptors for high endothelial venules, *Blood,* 66, 577, 1985.
28. **Streeter, P. R., Berg, E. L., Rouse, B. T. N., Bargatze, R. F., and Butcher, E. C.,** A tissue specific endothelial cell molecule involved in lymphocyte homing, *Nature,* 331, 41, 1988a.
29. **Streeter, P. R., Rouse, B. T. N., and Butcher, E. C.,** Immunohistologic and functional characterization of a vascular addressin, involved in lymphocyte homing into peripheral lymph nodes, *J. Cell Biol.,* 107, 1853, 1988b.

Chapter 5

ENTRY OF CANCER CELLS INTO THE VASCULATURE

Kurt Hellmann

TABLE OF CONTENTS

I. INTRODUCTION

Access by tumor cells to the circulation, whether through lymphatics and blood vessels or by invasion of adjacent tissues, has critical consequences for the patient — the most important being tumor dissemination and the possibility of metastasis formation. Prevention of access, therefore, is an important therapeutic goal. Entry of tumor cells into the circulation can be achieved in two fundamentally different ways. The most common is the active invasion by tumor cells of small veins, venules, or the tumor microvasculature. Less common is the detachment of tumor cells or tumor emboli from the walls of clefts within tumors through which blood flows to join the venous return. In this latter case, access of tumor cells depends on the strength of the adhesion between the tumor cells lining the clefts and the force of the bloodstream through the blood channels formed by the clefts. No invasive activity on the part of the tumor cells is required. Although this method is common for sarcomas, it is not so common for carcinomas.

There is a widespread belief that the entry of tumor cells into the circulation is governed, in the first place, by the development of a tumor neovasculature, which is thought to be formed if tumor growth is to continue beyond an early stage.[1-4]

II. THE DEVELOPMENT OF A NEOVASCULATURE

Several features characterize the tumor neovasculature. The vessels are generally poorly endothelialized and dilated sinusoidal channels.[5] The incomplete endothelial lining of these channels leads to frequent areas of hemorrhage that can be seen by the naked eye and more readily on histology. The vessels, when viewed by contrast angiography, have a characteristic corkscrew appearance, and they are expected to be much more permeable than intact normal vessels.[6] The recognition of these characteristics is important so that the results obtained on what are claimed to be models for tumor angiogenesis can be seen in perspective. Despite the controls that most experiments using such models employ, it is difficult to avoid the conclusion, on seeing the sharp, straight, intact, and well-endothelialized vessels which tumors or tumor cells in such models of tumor angiogenesis induce, that the new vessels in these systems are anything more than inflammatory reactive vessels. A large variety of angiogenic stimulators has been discovered, therefore, it has become difficult to believe that all of them are involved normally in tumor angiogenesis. It is also doubtful whether any of them are specific *tumor* angiogenesis factors.[7-9a]

The questions that have to be answered in defining tumor angiogenesis are not only what (preferably in chemical terms) is the specific stimulus to the development of this process, but also what determines its time course, direction, and sensitivity, and what, if anything, diminishes or stops it.

Antiangiogenesis as a means of inhibiting tumor growth and preventing tumor dissemination is an attractive idea. But since it has become clear that angiogenesis, induced in many highly artifactual experiments, is probably little more than a generalized response to foreign body implantation, this avenue to tumor and especially metastasis inhibition has become much less attractive. This topic will be discussed later at greater length.

It is difficult to know why invoking tumor angiogenesis factors or autocrine growth factors is necessary when rapidly growing tumors are surrounded by one of the most potent stimulators to angiogenesis: hypoxia — known to be a powerful stimulant in the development of a collateral circulation in any hypoxic ischemic area, for example, following myocardial infarction or diabetic retinopathy.[10]

The faster a tumor grows, the more likely it is to develop a rapid angiogenic response. The more rapid this response is, the more imperfect the vasculature that has been induced will be. This conclusion is also reached by the astute and meticulous observer, R. A. Willis, during the course of some 500 cancer postmortems.[11]

III. TUMOR SIZE AND THE NEOVASCULATURE

It has been frequently asserted that the development of a neovasculature is an absolute requirement if tumors are to grow beyond 2 mm. If they fail to develop a blood supply, it has been claimed that growth will stop, and no tumor dissemination can take place.[12]

A. PRIMARY OF UNKNOWN ORIGIN

Such generalizations take no account of the realities of tumor pathology, particularly of the well known, but rarely found primary of unknown origin (PUO), which is generally less than 2 mm and can still rapidly disseminate cells throughout the body. Metastases arising from such PUOs show that this is not the pecularity of one type of tumor, but that the primary can be in any of a number of organs such as the breast, lung, colon, or stomach, whose characteristic secondaries may be found without tracing the primary tumor even after the most diligent searches and investigations both ante- and postmortem. Because the primary cannot be found, nothing can be stated about the way in which the cells from such a tumor enter the circulation except that it is unlikely that they required a tumor neovasculature.[13]

A related problem with PUOs is the question of age of the tumor. It is a widely held belief that the longer a tumor has been growing, the greater its size and the more likely it is to have disseminated. While this may be true, sometimes it is not an absolute rule since a PUO may give rise to metastasis with long intervals between the appearance of the secondaries. Unfortunately, the characteristics of this particular type of tumor seems not to have attracted greater attention or been studied in greater detail, particularly for its experimental, invasive, and disseminating ability. One might predict that a PUO would overcome the difficulty of demonstrating consistent ability to metastasize in human tumors transplanted to nude mice. However, no report of such an experiment seems to have appeared. Furthermore, the invasive properties of this tumor can be confidently predicted to be extremely high, and this, too, would make it a useful experimental model for testing invasive capacity.

The limitation of using secondaries from a PUO is that the age of the primary tumor cannot be determined, and the natural history of the tumor is unknown. It could be that the tumor cells from such a PUO have an inherently high invasive potential *ab initio* and establish themselves effectively and quickly when they are trapped in the distant organs where they form metastases. On the other hand, it could be that they are selected from a large population that grows and dies rapidly. Access to the circulation, therefore, is not necessarily dependent on the size or age of the tumor.

B. KRUKENBERG TUMORS

Another important example which clearly demonstrates that neither size nor the neovasculature of a primary tumor has predictive value for judging the invasive or disseminating character of a tumor is the Krukenberg tumor.[14] This well-known tumor usually has its primary in the wall of the stomach, but may make its first clinical appearance as a tumor of the ovary. The tumors are often bilateral with hemorrhages and small cysts. The primary growth is responsible for these Krukenberg metastases, although frequently a gastric carcinoma of a particularly diffusely infiltrating type may also be from other sites. The primary is so small and inconspicuous that patients have no symptoms or signs referable to the stomach. Even a barium meal may not show any gastric abnormality, and it is, of course, beyond the resolution of computed tomography. Indeed, the primary tumor may be so small as to escape detection altogether. Presumably, if it escapes detection at microscopic level, then it is certainly less than 2 mm, and no special vasculature seems to be required for this tumor to enter the bloodstream and disseminate. Clearly, this is an extreme example of an unusual behavior, but it demonstrates again that no absolutes are possible with malignant tumors.

In this connection, it is also noteworthy that although most gastric neoplasms disseminate to the liver in the case of the Krukenberg metastases, the liver appears to be free of any involvement. It should be emphasized, moreover, that similar Krukenberg tumors can arise from intestinal, biliary, or quite frequently, mammary carcinomas, demonstrating again that neither size of primary tumor nor a tumor neovasculature is a bar to tumor entry into the circulation.

IV. DIRECT VISUALIZATION OF THE TUMOR NEOVASCULATURE

There are major problems when attempting to demonstrate the tumor neovasculature by direct means. Elegant attempts have been made by making casts[15] and examining the casts by electron scanning micrography. The difficulty with this technique is that artifactual impressions can be produced as a result of applying pressures to the permeating fluid used for developing the casts, which are in excess of those that the tumor vasculature would normally experience. This pressure, under *in vivo* conditions, also would be expected to change as the tumor develops, as clearly can be seen from the fact that the central part of most tumors becomes necrotic as a result of their growth and consequent narrowing of the lumen of the vessels, supplying it to the point of total occlusion. This inevitably leads to concomitant opening of collateral channels either through the substance of the tumor or through the opening or growth of the smaller vessels on the periphery of the tumor. This, in turn, has the effect of producing neovascular pathways, forming ultimately peripheral arterio-venous shunts. These changes in the morphology of the neovascular architecture are a dynamic process with constant remodelling that have important consequences for the entry of tumor cells into the vascular system. Casts, on the other hand, are made at one time point in the life of the tumor. It ought to be pointed out at this juncture that no lymph channels with their extremely delicate walls can survive these changes, and none can be demonstrated. Access from tumors into the circulatory system is, therefore, via the bloodstream and may only reach the lymphatics at a later stage.

It is also appropriate to point out at this juncture that new vessel formation by tumors in response to the demands of an increasing cell mass is more likely to come from the arterial system than from the venous. If it comes from the arterioles, direct connections with the venous side through the arterio-venous shunts could develop from the vascular system on the tumor periphery. The existence of the shunts are frequently overlooked by clinicians, but have important therapeutic implications not only for the access of tumor cells into the circulation but also for the access of drugs into the tumor. Labelled anticancer drugs injected into arteries-supplying tumors frequently circulate on the periphery of the tumors, but do not penetrate into their necrotic central areas. However, these necrotic central areas are made up not only of dead, dying, and doomed cancer cells but also of dormant cells, which when transplanted to fresh sites, can grow with great vigor. Thus, once lytic enzymes have reduced the pressure on the central necrotic areas and permit the collapsed blood vessels in these areas to partially re-open, dormant cells can enter the circulation.

V. ADHESION AND THE ACCESS OF TUMOR CELLS INTO THE CIRCULATION

An important factor that influences the access of tumor cells into the neovasculature is the degree of difficulty with which tumor cells detach themselves from the main body of the developing tumor.[16] Much depends on the adhesive forces between the cells of the tumor, and these have been studied in great detail.[17] Most recently, these studies have concerned themselves with the adhesion of tumor cells to preparations of cells from a number of organs and to endothelial cells. Earlier, Coman[18] measured the adhesion between the cells of a tumor mass and the forces required to separate individual cells or clumps of cells from the main body of the tumor. However, the nature of the condition makes it extremely difficult to devise adequate experimental designs to study factors that may influence the weakening or strengthening of the adhesive bonds between the cells in a solid tumor. Biochemical analyses of adhesion has identified a number of substances such as fibronectin, vibronectin, and others to be responsible for the adhesive properties between tumor cells. The leakiness of tumor blood vessels permits fibrinogen and clotting factors to escape and to embed the tumor cells in fibrin.[19] This makes it more difficult for mechanical forces or trauma to dislodge them.

Tumors implanted in a muscle are subjected to constantly changing forces. Under these conditions, although the growth rate of the tumor may not be very different from when it is implanted subcutaneously, the development of lung metastases occurs much more quickly. This observation has been made repeatedly while comparing the times required for lung metastases to appear after implantation of the Lewis lung carcinoma either in the leg muscle or subcutaneously. Although metastases will appear approximately 23 d after subcutaneous implantation, none can be observed if the tumor is excised less than 5 to 6 d after implantation.[20] On the other hand, when tumors are implanted in a leg muscle, excision of the primary implant has to occur within 3 d to avoid lung metastases, indicating the more rapid dissemination from a site of tumor growth where continuing intermittent massage of the tumor is experienced. Similar observations were made many years ago by Tyzzer.[21] Most surgeons believe that undue handling and rough surgical technique of tumors also can be responsible for tumor dissemination; thus, trauma seems to be a factor in assisting the entry of tumor cells into the circulation.

Adhesiveness can be altered by many substances, and among these, EDTA and other chelating agents that remove essential ions required for adhesion can be very effective. It also has been shown that the cyclic AMP inhibitors such as the pyrimido pyrimidines can affect both adhesiveness and invasiveness, thus, preventing cells from gaining access into the circulation. One example of this is the analogue of dipyridamole known as RA233, which has been shown to be an effective inhibitor of invasiveness of a highly metastatic cell line, yet to have no effect in the nonmetastatic variant of the same cell line.[22]

VI. TUMOR EMBOLI AND SINGLE CELL DETACHMENT

It is usually thought that an invasion into the microcirculation appears to be confined to single cancer cells and that the disparity between cancer cell and capillary diameters requires that either the cells and/or the capillaries be deformable.[23] From direct observations, however, it is apparent that although single cells may enter the microcirculation and can be traced in the circulation, few of them survive. A study of circulating Lewis lung tumor cells by Salsbury[24] has shown that clumps consisting of as many as 50 tumor cells may be circulating at any one time and that this is more likely as the tumor grows progressively. The fate of these clumps is not certain. Neither is it certain whether they broke off from the tumor as a clump or whether they aggregated in the bloodstream. However, it would seem possible that in view of the gross appearance of the tumor sinusoids where tumor cells line clefts in the primary tumor, clumps of several tumor cells could have escaped into the circulation without hindrance. If this clump of cells entered the circulation on the postcapillary venous side, then it would be quite easily possible for such a tumor embolus to circulate and reach the lungs, which would be the organ of first encounter.

It is known that the metastatic efficiency for most tumors is extremely low and that most tumor cells injected intravenously will die. What is not clear is why they die in such very large numbers and whether it requires an aggregate or clump of them to survive. It may be that emboli, which go on to form metastases, are aggregates of tumor cells with circulating white blood cells and/or platelets that have special characteristics to allow them to survive. There is, of course, a trapping advantage with cell aggregates as compared with single cells, but this alone cannot account for the greater degree of viability of tumor emboli.

Possibly, one of the reasons why the Lewis lung tumor, in all animals inoculated with a primary implant, regularly and consistently produces lung metastases at the same time and in the same organ is that its growth patterns in the primary implant permit cell clumps to be detached from the primary to reach the lungs intact.

VII. ANTIANGIOGENESIS

If one accepts the claims of Folkman[25] and his collaborators that tumor growth is not possible beyond 2 mm without the development of a neovasculature, then theoretically, prevention or destruction of the angiogenesis process should result in inhibition of tumor growth. Since there would be no channels for dissemination, there would be no tumor metastases. However, the neovasculature, which they have induced and on which the claims are based, seems to have neither morphological nor biochemical similarity with characteristic tumor vessels. They have neither the poorly endothelialized tortuous sinusoidal appearance nor the leaky properties of tumor blood vessels. It also does not resemble in any shape or form the tumor clefts lined by tumor cells. No endothelium, through which blood can flow, carries detached tumor cells or emboli with it. Nevertheless, in view of the problems experienced by most chemotherapeutic agents with hormones and biological response modifers, the idea of influencing tumor growth, invasion, and dissemination with tumor angiogenesis is certainly worthy of serious examination.

The first approach to control of tumor angiogenesis seemed to be very clear. It was the isolation of what was hoped to be a tumor angiogenesis factor (TAF). Although from what has been said above, perhaps it would have been wiser to restrict the concept to the isolation of an angiogenesis factor. The main problem since then, however, has been that too many substances[26] have been found with very effective angiogenesis activity to allow one to believe that they are all specifically involved in tumor angiogenesis. Following the original concept, it would have been more attractive to have isolated a tumor angiogenesis factor than to use it to produce a specific antibody to control tumor angiogenesis. None of this has materialized, and if TAF had been discovered, then it seems doubtful whether an antibody to it would have been effective in controlling the entry of tumor cells into the circulation. As was pointed out earlier, in tumors such as the Krukenberg, massive and destructive dissemination can take place apparently without the necessity of organizing themselves around a tumor neovasculature.

A. HEPARIN AND CORTISONE

More recently Folkman and his group have claimed that tumor proliferation and metastases can be completely prevented by a combined treatment of heparin and cortisone.[27] It is very doubtful, however, whether the doses of heparin and cortisone required for treatment of tumor dissemination in humans could possibly have been reached or maintained. Yet, it has not been possible for other groups[28] to repeat these results, and since then, Folkman has stated that only the special type of heparin used at the time of his experiments could obtain those results. Unfortunately, the batch from which his heparin was derived is no longer available, and Folkman and his group, therefore, have examined other steroids with better characteristics than cortisone.[29] At the present time, it seems improbable that such an approach has anything to offer.

Madarnas used cortisone and maltose tetrapalmitate to prevent tumor growth.[30] They believed that their results were due to the lack of tumor vascularization. Unfortunately, it is not clear, from their experiments, which came first: vascularization inhibition or tumor inhibition. If the combination prevented tumor proliferation per se, angiogenesis clearly also would have ceased.

B. FLAVONE ACETIC ACID

A more recent approach derived from experiments with flavone acetic acid (FAA) was shown to be a highly effective tumor inhibitor in a variety of mouse tumors.[31] Phase 2 studies in humans revealed no activity in any of the tumors tested. Subsequent examination of the reasons for the discrepancy uncovered the fact that FAA rapidly and selectively destroyed the tumor vasculature in the implanted tumors, causing necrosis of the whole tumor.[32] Many questions remain to be answered about this unusual situation; particularly, the role of tumor necrosis factor has yet to be clarified. If destruction of the vasculature were the main mode of action, then the drug should be ineffective in the development of ascitic tumors. If it were given after tumors had disseminated into the bloodstream, then no effect should be seen on the metastases. The results are in line with these expectations.[33] FAA seems to be a member of a new class of drugs that specifically destroy the tumor vasculature. Although not completely clear at this time, it seems that the predilection of FAA is for tumor blood vessels and that normal blood vessels and other tissues are unaffected. It is also not clear on which part of the vascular system or on what components in the system FAA acts. Most importantly, whether it is species-specific is still unclear since the drug has been most disappointing in humans, even though it appears to be one of the more active agents against transplanted solid tumor cells in mice. There is no suggestion that FAA modifies the developing neovasculature; all of the indications are that it destroys the existing tumor vasculature. Therefore, there is no possibility of tumor cells entering the circulation.

C. RAZOXANE

In the course of a series of experiments to discover the mechanism by which razoxane inhibited the development of spontaneous pulmonary metastases from a subcutaneous implant of the Lewis lung carcinoma, razoxane treatment was found to have prevented entry of tumor cells into the circulation and apparently normalized the developing tumor neovasculature.[34-36] At the same time, it appeared to have little influence on the growth of the primary implant. Many substances, of course, will prevent secondaries by their cytotoxic action in an undiscriminating inhibition or destruction of dividing cells. However, razoxane showed, for the first time, that it was possible to delete specifically tumor dissemination and metastases formation without interfering with tumor proliferation and even possibly with invasion by preventing tumor cells from escaping into the circulation. Whether normalization of the developing neovasculature is directly responsible for the failure of the Lewis lung tumor cells to escape remains to be established. No other substance yet has been shown to have a similar inhibitory action, though it is difficult to believe that razoxane is unique in this respect. Failure of tumor cells to enter the circulation could clearly account for the subsequent inhibition of lung metastases. It eliminated the need to consider the possibility of some quite complex interactions between razoxane and circulating malignant cells such as inhibition of aggregation with other tumor cells, platelets, or blood-formed elements. It also eliminated the need to consider the possibility razoxane might have influenced the circulating cells in such a way that it prevented their implantation in the lung. Histological examination of the primary tumor demonstrated, however, that razoxane treatment resulted in a normalization of the developing neovasculature in the primary tumor, which was compatible with the results of direct cytological examination of blood from the ipsilateral draining vein of the primary tumor and which had shown that razoxane treatment prevented escape of tumor cells into the circulation.[35]

Salsbury[34] also examined other tumors before and after razoxane treatment and showed that the sarcoma 180, which disseminates widely, but does not form metastases (probably because of immunological destruction of the disseminating S180 cells), could be influenced by razoxane treatment in an identical fashion to that of the Lewis lung. That there appeared to be a "normalization" of the developing neovasculature is a feature already shown for other tumors by LeServe and Hellmann,[6] using angiographic and other techniques. These authors realized that the normalization of blood vessel development in a tumor could have profound consequences not only for the escape of tumor cells into the circulation but also for the oxygenation of the tumor. However, the more immediate and important questions were whether a normalized tumor neovasculature could prevent the escape of malignant cells from primary and, indeed, secondary tumors, and whether it could prevent the recurrences in patients who had tumors that could not be resected or who had been treated without achieving complete regression. At this time, razoxane has been found to be an effective inhibitor of metastases in 8/10 experimental tumors that metastasized spontaneously.[37] Since it also had shown some effect on advanced colorectal cancer,[38] a fully randomized, prospective clinical trial was set up to see if it prevented recurrences when it was given as adjuvant treatment following surgical resection. Throughout the trial, which was terminated after 7 years, the recurrence-free interval was statistically significantly greater in the razoxane-treated Dukes' C group (44 patients) compared to the controls (44 patients). Survival was also increased, although the statistical significance for this was somewhat less than that for recurrence.[39] Two major conclusions were drawn from this trial. The first conclusion was that only Dukes' C patients benefitted. This patient population faced the greatest risk of recurrence because tumor was almost certainly left behind in some of the draining lymph nodes and then could spread to the liver and also because micrometastases might have been already present at the time of the primary resection. Most patients who recurred with metastases developed them in the liver, but only half of the Dukes' C patients treated with razoxane developed liver metastases as compared to the controls. Those who did develop them took twice as long to do so.[40] The second conclusion was that Dukes' B patients did not benefit. This is not altogether surprising since an unknown number of patients in this category was cured by surgery alone on which no adjuvant treatment could improve. These patients, however, diluted the figures and made comparisons difficult.

D. PIPERAZINEDIONE (593A): A MODIFIER OF THE DEVELOPING NEOVASCULATURE

Another drug with some chemical resemblance to razoxane has been shown to modify the developing neovasculature but has had only very limited Phase I and II examination. Although some responses have been seen in Phase II trials, they have not been enough to encourage the National Cancer Institute (NCI) to promote this compound further. Initially, piperazinedione was found to have exerted a profound effect on the development of the neovasculature of the tumors grown on the chorioallantoic membrane of the chick embryo.[41] Doses that normalized the tumor angioarchitecture were also effective in preventing the growth of metastases in this system. Again, the clear implication is that the normalization of the tumor vasculature prevented the ingress of the tumor cells from the tumor into the circulation of the chick embryo. The development of this drug was essentially as a cytotoxic agent and was abandoned when it did not fulfill the criteria used for these agents.

Despite the different characteristics of tumor blood vessels in different tumors, it may well be useful to try to modify tumor growth and dissemination by influencing tumor blood vessel growth and/or behavior. In the past, a number of attempts were made to selectively shut down or open up the tumor blood supply, but no pharmacological intervention showed any preferential characteristics towards the tumor vasculature.

VIII. CONCLUSIONS

Malignant tumor growth, invasion, and dissemination do not seem to be subjected to a universal law with regard to the vascular system that they organize into themselves. Some tumors cannot grow without this neovasculature, but most can and do find ways of doing so, such as invasion of adjacent tissues, lymph, or blood channels. They may never grow beyond a microscopic collection of cells that proliferate at an unknown rate but that have all the power and malignancy to disseminate widely to kill the host. On the other hand, other tumors need a vasculature in order to grow and to survive. For these tumors, there appears to be tumor growth factors that can prevent their development. Initially, it was thought that there might be a single specific tumor angiogenesis factor (TAF), but such a factor has not been isolated. A variety of angiogenic substances have been isolated, and some of them might play a part in the development of tumor angiogenesis. Several disparate substances have been identified that interfere with or destroy tumor blood vessels, and other substances are able to normalize the development of tumor blood vessel growth. Of this latter group, razoxane has been shown to normalize the neovasculature, resulting in the tumor cells being unable to gain entry into the circulation. Thus, it prevents the primary tumor from disseminating, although the tumor continues to grow. Razoxane is the only drug to date that underwent a clinical trial as an antimetastatic drug. In colorectal cancer, it has shown that it can significantly delay recurrence and increase survival in patients who have the greatest risk of recurrence.

A much larger effort should be made to screen for substances that prevent tumor cells from entering the circulation. This could be done without major technical problems; it might lead to a much more rational and less sterile approach than the current method being used to detect new anticancer drugs. The systems employed for the last 40 years have acted on the uniform assumption that the cancer problem could be solved by finding drugs which could prevent cell division. Theoretically, such a program is almost bound to fail, and this has been borne out by the vast number — possibly more than 1 million new and old chemical entities have been examined without finding a single selective agent. With such a lack of subtlety and fundamental grasp of the pathology of cancer, no doubt this program deserved to fail. Perhaps the President's cancer advisors should ponder over this. It is time to adopt new approaches to cancer research and treatment. Additionally, the discovery of substances that prevent tumor cells from disseminating would be of immense assistance in this respect.

REFERENCES

1. **D'Amore, P. A.,** Growth factors, angiogenesis and metastasis, in *Cancer Metastasis: Experimental and Clinical Strategies,* Alan R. Liss, New York, 1986, 269.
2. **Folkman, J., Long, D. M., and Becker, F. F.,** Growth and metastasis of tumor in organ culture, *Cancer (Philadelphia),* 16, 453, 1963.
3. **Gimbrone, M. A., Aster, R. H., Cotran, R. S., Corkery, J., and Folkman, J.,** Preservation of vascular integrity in organs perfused *in vitro* with a platelet-rich medium, *Nature,* 222, 33, 1969.
4. **Folkman, J.,** How is blood vessel growth regulated in normal and neoplastic tissue? *Cancer Res.,* 46, 467, 1986.
5. **Warren, B. A.,** The vascular morphology of tumors, in *Tumor Blood Circulation,* Peterson, H. I., Ed., CRC Press, Boca Raton, FL., 1979, chaps. 1.
6. **LeServe, A. W. and Hellmann, K.,** Metastases and the normalization of tumour blood vessels by ICRF159: a new type of drug action, *Br. Med. J.,* 1, 597, 1972.
7. **Atherton, A.,** Growth stimulation of endothelial cells by simultaneous culture with Sarcoma 180 cells in diffusion chambers, *Cancer Res.,* 37, 3619, 1977.

8. **Rifkin, D. B., Gross, J. L., Moscatelli, D., and Jaffe, E.,** Proteases and angiogenesis: production of plasminogen activator and collagenase by endothelial cells, in *Pathobiology of the Endothelial Cell,* Nossel, H. L. and Vogel, H. J., Eds., Academic Press, New York, 1982, 191.
9. **Weiss, J. B., Brown, R. A., Kumar, S., and Phillips, P.,** An angiogenic factor isolated from tumours. A potent low-molecular weight compound, *Br. J. Cancer,* 40, 493, 1979.
9a. **Folkman, J. and Klagsbrun, M.,** Angiogenic factors, *Science,* 235, 442, 1987.
10. **Garner, A.,** Ocular angiogenesis, *Int. Rev. Exp. Pathol.,* 28, 249, 1986.
11. **Willis, R. A.,** *The Spread of Tumours in the Human Body,* Butterworth, London, 1972, 113.
12. **Gimbrone, M. A., Leapman, S. B., Cotran, R. S., and Folkman, J.,** Tumor dormancy *in vitro* by prevention of neovascularization, *J. Exp. Med.,* 136, 261, 1972.
13. **Willis, R. A.,** *The Spread of Tumours in the Human Body,* Butterworth, London, 1972, 127.
14. **Krukenberg, F.,** Ueber das Fibrosarcoma ovarii mucocellulare (carcinomatodes), *Arch. Gynaekol.,* 50, 287, 1895.
15. **Grunt, T. W., Larnetschwandtner, A., and Karrer, K.,** The characteristic structural features of the blood vessels of the Lewis lung carcinoma, in *Scanning Electron Microscopy,* SEM, Chicago, 1986, 575.
16. **Weiss, L., Orr, F. W., and Honn, K. V.,** Interactions between cancer cells and the microvasculature: a rate regulator for metastasis, *Clin. Exp. Metast.,* 7, 127, 1989.
17. **Weiss, L., Orr, F. W., and Honn, K. V.,** Interactions of cancer cells with the microvasculature during metastasis, *FASEB J.,* 2, 12, 1988.
18. **Coman, D. R.,** Decreased mutual adhesiveness: a property of cells from squamous cell carcinomas, *Cancer Res.,* 4, 625, 1944.
19. **Nagy, J. A., Brown, L. F., Senger, D. R., Lanir, N., van de Water, L., Dvorak, A. M., and Dvorak, H. F.,** Pathogenesis of tumor stroma generation: a critical role for leaky blood vessels and fibrin deposition, *Biochim. Biophys. Acta,* 948, 305, 1988.
20. **James, S. E. and Salsbury, A. J.,** Effect of (±)-1,2-*Bis*(3,5-dioxopiperazin-1-yl) propane on tumor blood vessels and its relationship to the antimetastatic effect in the Lewis lung carcinoma, *Cancer Res.,* 34, 839, 1974.
21. **Tyzzer, E. E.,** Factors in the production and growth of tumor metastases, *J. Med. Res.,* 23, 309, 1913.
22. **Lichtner, R. B., Erkell, L. J., Schirrmacher, V., and Nicolson, G. L.,** Effects of RA 233 treatment on the adhesive, invasive and metastatic properties of 13762NF rat mammary tumor cells, *Clin. Exp. Metast.,* 7, 175, 1989.
23. **Weiss, L. and Clement, D. S.,** Studies on cell deformability: some rheological considerations, *Exp. Cell. Res.,* 58, 379, 1989.
24. **Salsbury, A. J., Burrage, K., and Hellmann, K.,** Histological analysis of the antimetastatic effect of (±)-1,2-*Bis*(3,5-dioxopiperazin-1-yl) propane, *Cancer Res.,* 34, 843, 1974.
25. **Folkman, J. and Cotran, R.,** Regulation of vascular proliferation to tumor growth, in *International Review of Experimental Pathology,* Richter, G. W. and Epstein, N. A., Eds., Academic Press, New York, 1976, 207.
26. **Kull, F. C., Brent, D. A., Parikh, I., and Cautrecasas, P.,** Chemical identification of a tumor-derived angiogenic factor, *Science,* 236, 843, 1987.
27. **Folkman, J., Langer, R., Linhardt, R., Haudenschild, C., and Taylor, S.,** Angiogenesis inhibition and tumor regression caused by heparin or a heparin fragment in the presence of cortisone, *Science,* (Washington, D.C.), 221, 719, 1983.
28. **Penhaligon, M. and Camplejohn, R. S.,** Combination heparin plus cortisone treatment of two transplanted tumors in C3H/He mice, *J. Natl. Cancer Inst.,* 74, 869, 1985.
29. **Crum, R., Szabo, S., and Folkman, J.,** A new clan of steroids inhibits angiogenesis in the presence of a heparin fragment, *Science,* 230, 1375, 1985.
30. **Madarnas, P., Benrezzak, O., and Nigam, V. N.,** Prophylactic antiangiogenic tumor treatment, Anti-cancer Res., 9, 897, 1989.
31. **Corbett, T. H., Bissery, Y. C., and Woziniak, A.,** Activity of flavone acetic acid (NSC 347512) against solid tumours of mice, *Invest. New Drugs,* 4, 207, 1986.
32. **Bibby, M. C., Double, J. A., Loadman, P. M., and Duke, C. V.,** Reduction of tumor blood flow by flavone acetic acid: a possible component of therapy, J. Natl. Cancer Inst., 81, 216, 1989.
33. **Zwir, L. J., Baguley, B. C., Gavin, J. B., and Wilson, W. R.,** Blood flow failure as a major determinant in the antitumor action of flavone acetic acid, J. Natl. Cancer Inst., 81, 216, 1989.
34. **Salsbury, A. J., Burrage, K., and Hellmann, K.,** Inhibition of metastatic spread by ICRF159: selective deletion of a malignant characteristic, Br. Med. J., 4, 344, 1970.
35. **Hellmann, K. and Burrage, K.,** Control of malignant metastases by ICRF159, *Nature,* 224, 273, 1969.
36. **Hellmann, K., Salsbury, A. J., Burrage, K., LeServe, A. W., and James, S. E.,** Drug induced inhibition of haematogenously spread metastases, in *Chemotherapy of Cancer Dissemination and Metastasis,* Garattini, S. and Franchi, E., Eds., Raven Press, New York, 1973, 355.
37. Editorial, Razoxane, metastasis and adjuvant chemotherapy, Clin. Exp. Metast., 5, 1, 1987.

38. **Marciniak, D. A., Moertel, C. G., and Schutt, A. J.,** Phase II study of ICRF159 (NSC 129943) in advanced colorectal carcinoma, *Cancer Chemother. Rep.*, 59, 761, 1975.
39. **Gilbert, J. M., Hellmann, K., Evans, M., and Cassell, P. G.,** Randomised trial of oral adjuvant razoxane (ICRF159) in resectable colorectal cancer: five year follow-up, *Br. J. Surg.*, 73, 446, 1986.
40. **Hellmann, K., Gilbert, J. M., Evans, M., Cassell, P. G., and Taylor, R.,** Effects of razoxane on metastases from colorectal cancer, *Clin. Exp. Metast.*, 5, 3, 1987.
41. **Gitterman, C. O. and Luell, S.,** Chemotherapeutic studies on metastasis of human epidermoid carcinoma (H.Ep.3) in the embryonated chick egg, in *Chemotherapy of Cancer Dissemination and Metastasis*, Garattini, S. and Franchi, G., Eds., Raven Press, New York, 1973, 279.

Chapter 6

INTERACTIONS BETWEEN CIRCULATING CANCER CELLS AND HOST LEUKOCYTES

Dorothy Glaves

TABLE OF CONTENTS

I. INTRODUCTION

Cancer cells in the microvasculature could encounter almost the full complement of host leukocytes, including T- and B-lymphocytes, killer (K) and natural killer (NK) lymphocytes, and granulocytes and monocytes. All of these leukocytes are capable of interacting with cancer cells *in vitro,* and most can kill malignant cells with varying degrees of efficiency. Cancer cells are free in the circulation for only a few seconds before they become arrested in the microvasculature, and fluid dynamics within the major blood vessels tend to make collisions between cancer cells and leukocytes infrequent. After cancer cells have been arrested, access by leukocytes will be directly via the bloodstream or through the blood vessel wall. If they block the blood vessels, as is likely to occur in the microvasculature, access to cancer cells by leukocytes will be limited.

With the exception of morphologic studies, the most commonly used experimental animal model of the arrest and retention of disseminated cancer cells in the microvasculature involves tracing the fate of radiolabelled cancer cells injected directly into the circulation via the tail vein of rodents. Numerous studies using this model have shown that the vast majority (>90%) of cancer cells are arrested in the microvasculature of the first major organ downstream, which is the lung in this model, in order to interpret intravascular events. The arrested cancer cells subsequently die and are removed from the circulation within 24 h of their arrest, and given the tumoricidal potential of leukocytes, investigators have focussed on their role in this massive cell death. Observations are usually restricted to the 24 h period following injection of cells since extravasation of some of the cancer cells may begin as early as 4 to 6 h postinjection, so that radioactivity counts beyond 24 h will not necessarily reflect events taking place in the microvasculature. Moreover, radioactivity levels often fall close to background levels after 24 h. A fraction of the radiolabel temporarily redistributes to the liver, but the significance of this relocalization is uncertain since it may represent uptake of cell debris by Kupffer cells rather than intact cancer cells. Attempts to assess the overall contribution of intravascular events to the final outcome of metastasis usually involve comparing the short-term survival kinetics (retention patterns) of these radiolabelled cancer cells with the incidence and frequency of tumor nodules that develop after injection of unlabelled cells (organ colonization).

The types of experiments implicating specific leukocyte populations in interactions with cancer cells *in vivo* fall into five main categories:

1. Use of animals with a genetic defect/enhancement in the function of specific leukocytes
2. Use of cancer cells with heightened resistance/sensitivity to specific types of leukocytes
3. Use of animals injected with antisera to deplete specific leukocyte populations
4. Use of animals injected with pharmacologic agents to manipulate the numbers and/or function of specific leukocytes
5. Visual identification of leukocytes in association with cancer cells in the microvasculature (see Chapter 13)

These experimental approaches provide the basis for the discussion in this chapter. While examining the evidence that these approaches provide for the participation of individual types of leukocytes in determining the fate of cancer cells in the microvasculature, it is also important to consider the specificity and sensitivity of the approach used to identify/target the particular leukocyte population.

II. IMMUNOLOGIC INTERACTIONS

Specific antitumor defense factors can influence cancer cell survival in the microvasculature. In some rodent tumor systems, immunologic factors have been shown to be protective and accelerate the intravascular death of radiolabelled cancer cells injected into tumor-sensitized or hyperimmunized hosts.[1-4] In other systems, they had no effect or were self-defeating and actually promoted the retention of cancer cells in the pulmonary vasculature.[1,2,4-6] Of course, the magnitude and quality of tumor-immune responses in these animals may not be equivalent to those in tumor-bearers, but in those studies that have compared the behavior of cancer cells in tumor-bearing and tumor-sensitized hosts, the differences in their retention patterns from normal hosts were similar in both groups.[1,3,6] These alterations in retention patterns in tumor-bearers have at least some immunologic basis, rather than tumor-induced physiologic basis since they were not detected following the injection of antigenically unrelated cancer cells.[2-4]

Unfortunately, there has been little attempt to discriminate between the contribution of cellular, T-lymphocyte-mediated immune responses and humoral antibody, produced by B-lymphocytes, in the clearance of arrested cancer cells. However, only a small fraction of peripheral blood T-lymphocytes can be expected to be specifically sensitized to cancer cells, and it seems more likely that antitumor antibody, the product of B-lymphocytes, was responsible for modulating cancer cell clearance in these experiments. Whether or not such antibodies are directly cytotoxic for cancer cells or mediate antibody dependent cellular cytotoxicity (ADCC) by nonsensitized K-lymphocytes or monocytes has not been addressed. In one attempt to define a role for sensitized lymphocytes during hematogenous metastasis, sub-lines of B16 melanomas were selected by repeated exposure to sensitized lymphocytes.[7] However, these lymphocyte-resistant cells were retained to a greater, rather than lesser, extent in the lungs than their unselected counterparts. Since the retention experiments were apparently made in normal, unsensitized mice, the immunologic significance of these results is unclear and are difficult to explain on a nonspecific defense basis because at least B16F10 and its lymphocyte-resistant sub-line were equally susceptible to NK cells,[8] which could also interact with arrested cancer cells (see below).

Attempts to correlate changes in intravascular survival of cancer cells with the ultimate yield of tumor nodules are difficult in the case of immunologic factors. The effects of sensitization to tumor antigens are prolonged and must be expected to influence the postextravasation behavior of cancer cells. It is only when intravascular retention patterns are altered in a different direction from incidence of tumor nodules in sensitized hosts that definitive statements can be made about the relative contribution of intravascular events. For instance, in one study, the retention of radiolabelled fibrosarcoma cells was decreased in tumor-bearing, tumor-excised, and hyperimmunized rats, and the yield of pulmonary tumor nodules was also decreased in tumor-excised and hyperimmunized rats injected with unlabelled cells.[3] These results would suggest an important role for immunologic factors in intravascular events. However, in other studies, immunization had no effect upon retention of EMT6 mouse mammary carcinoma cells, but decreased the numbers of tumor nodules. More B16 melanoma cells were retained in the lung microvasculature, yet fewer nodules developed in immunized mice. First, it would appear that immunologic responses may influence the survival of cancer cells differently in various anatomic compartments. This is possibly a function of the relative efficiency of humoral factors in the circulation vs. the efficiency of cellular effectors within organ parenchyma. Second, immunologic factors affect individual tumor systems differently. Consequently, it is difficult to predict the net effect of immune responses in the microvasculature upon the overall metastatic potential of disseminated cancer cells — they will certainly have no effect in athymic hosts or upon nonimmunogenic cells that also undergo massive death in the microvasculature. Nevertheless, it is important to remember that many studies of retention patterns have not been made in tumor-bearing animals, so that even potential contributions from immunologic factors are excluded.

III. NONIMMUNOLOGIC INTERACTIONS

Stimulation and inhibition of the reticuloendothelial system (RES) alter the rates at which arrested cancer cells are cleared from the microvasculature. In tumor-bearing animals with depressed RES function, retention of cancer cells is increased.[9] Conversely, administration of RES stimulants, including zymosan,[9] endotoxin,[9,10] glucan,[11,12] *Corynebacterium parvum,*[11,12] and BCG,[11,13] decreases the retention of arrested cancer cells in the lungs. RES stimulation also reduced the numbers of KHT sarcoma cells retained in all major organs examined, including the brain, following systemic dissemination of radiolabelled cells injected into the left ventricle.[14] A functional rather than morphologic definition of the RES, would include not only mobile and fixed monocytes at the vascular endothelium but also polymorphonuclear leukocytes and endothelial cells themselves. However, although RES function was measured prior to cancer cell retention experiments in some studies,[9] the specific leukocytes potentially involved in clearance mechanisms were not identified. Any or all of the three cell types could have been responsible, and both glucan and *C. parvum* are also known to stimulate NK cell activity.[15] Regardless of the specific effectors involved in those studies in which RES function as well as cancer cell retention were both measured, correlations were shown between RES inhibition, increased retention of cancer cells, and increased yield of lung tumors and between RES stimulation, decreased retention, and decreased yields of lung tumors.[9] Interestingly, in mice with zymosan-stimulated RES function,[9] radiolabelled B16 melanoma cells arrested in the lungs were initially cleared faster from the microvasculature than in normal mice, as might be expected. However, by 24 h postinjection, clearance rates had slowed to normal levels with the possibility for further delays beyond the observation period. Moreover, the numbers of melanoma nodules developing in zymosan-stimulated mice were greater than in control animals. RES inhibition and stimulation are acute and chronic sequelae of inflammation, respectively. One of the hallmarks of intravascular inflammation is incidental damage to the vascular endothelium, which can promote metastasis (see Chapter 15). Therefore, RES stimulation appears to be a double-edged sword that may lead on the one hand, to accelerated removal of some cancer cells arrested in the microvasculature, but on the other hand, to the facilitated extravasation of those cells which survive clearance processes.[16] Chapter 15 provides a detailed discussion of the effects of inflammation and microvascular injury upon postdissemination phases of metastasis, but these findings highlight the potential importance of the leukocyte components of the RES in determining the fate of arrested cancer cells. These individual components are discussed separately below.

A. MONONUCLEAR PHAGOCYTES

Two populations of mononuclear phagocytes have the opportunity to interact with disseminated cancer cells. First, circulating monocytes could collide with arrested cancer cells. Second, a proportion of mononuclear phagocytes remains within or alongside the vasculature where they normally function as part of the RES to remove senescent erythrocytes, microorganisms or particulate debris. In the present context, they could interact with arrested cancer cells. Classically, these intravascular populations are found in the liver (Kupffer cells), spleen, and bone marrow. There are indications that there is also a resident population of intravascular macrophages in the lungs of at least sheep, cows, and pigs.[17-19] However, they have not been detected in rats[17], and it is presently unknown if they occur in mice, so that their contribution to lung retention patterns of cancer cells in these commonly used experimental animals is uncertain, if not negligible. It is possible that Kupffer cells participate in the clearance of cancer cells from the liver, which is accelerated in RES-stimulated animals,[9] but only a few studies have addressed directly whether or not particular populations of mononuclear phagocytes are involved in cancer cell interactions in any organ.

Experiments with tumor-bearing mice given the macrophage suppressant, trypan blue,[20] showed that, although the numbers of circulating monocytes were reduced and the numbers and antitumor cytotoxic responses of peritoneal exudate macrophages were less than in controls, the clearance of radiolabelled B16 melanoma cells from the lungs was unexpectedly accelerated. Moreover, fewer melanoma nodules developed in the lungs of trypan blue-treated mice injected with nonradiolabelled cells. By the same token, adoptive transfer experiments in which thioglycollate-elicited macrophages were injected shortly before or shortly after radiolabelled tumor cells showed that macrophages enhanced retention of cells in the lung microvasculature; there was a parallel increase in the numbers of B16 melanoma and Lewis lung carcinoma nodules developing in similarly treated mice given unlabelled cells.[21,22] Co-injection of splenocytes or thymocytes with tumor cells did not modulate retention patterns or nodule incidence. Morphologic observations of arrested cancer cells are discussed in depth in Chapter 13. But briefly, there are a few reports of monocytes/macrophages interacting with cancer cells arrested in the lungs[23] and liver,[24] yet many studies have not reported them on a regular basis.[25-32] Regardless of the mechanisms involved, it appears that mononuclear phagocytes may offer little protection to the host during hematogenous phases of metastasis.

B. NK LYMPHOCYTES

NK cells have been identified by some investigators as primary candidates for effectors of cancer cell clearance from the microvasculature. They are a subpopulation of lymphocytes found predominantly in the spleen and peripheral blood that can be detected in nonimmunized hosts, and they are cytotoxic *in vitro* for a variety of malignant and even normal cells.[33-35] The levels of NK cytotoxicity for tumor cells are genetically controlled and are age-dependent, being low from birth to 3 weeks of age, peaking at 6 to 8 weeks, and then declining to low levels after 12 weeks of age. Levels of NK activity remain high even as adults in athymic, nude mice. The NK compartment can also be modulated *in vivo* by selective depletion with immunopharmacologic agents or by enhancement with biologic response modifiers such as interferon inducers. The availability of animals with variable genetic, age-dependent, and exogenously manipulated defense systems has provided opportunities to examine interactions between NK cells and cancer cells arrested in the microvasculature. Early studies[36] showed that radiolabelled YAC-1[37] and RBL-5[38] lymphoma cells were eliminated faster from both the lungs and the livers of mice with genetically- or age-associated high *in vitro* NK reactivity than from the organs of mice with low *in vitro* levels of NK cytotoxicity against lymphoma cells. Also, elimination of radiolabelled YAC-1[37] lymphoma and H-*ras*-transformed fibrosarcoma cells from the lung microvasculature of athymic mice was accelerated compared with their euthymic counterparts with lower *in vitro* NK activity.

Correlations also have been found between immunopharmacologic enhancement of *in vitro* cytotoxicity of NK cells from mice treated with *C. parvum* or poly I:C and enhanced clearance of lymphoma cells from lungs and liver. Subsequent studies[39,40] confirmed the modulatory effects of *C. parvum* and poly I:C upon both *in vitro* NK cytotoxicity and *in vivo* retention patterns of mouse melanoma cells and showed that accelerated removal of radiolabelled cells from the microvasculature was also correlated with reduced lung colonization by nonradiolabelled melanoma cells. Conversely, pharmacologic suppression of *in vitro* NK activity by treatment of mice with silica was associated with increased retention of lymphoma cells.[36] NK reactivity also can be depressed by the *in vivo* administration of antibody to a glycolipid surface marker on NK cells (asialo-GM1). Injection of this antibody resulted in reduced levels of NK activity expressed by spleen or peripheral blood lymphocytes, increased retention of radiolabelled melanoma cells in the liver and lungs of mice,[40] and increased pulmonary retention of lymphoma cells in rats.[41]

The selectivity of silica as an NK cell inhibitor may be in doubt since it is a well-known macrophage poison,[42] and indeed, it probably mediates its effects on NK cells via macrophages. By the same token, the direct/indirect targets for the stimulatory action of poly I:C include both NK cells and macrophages. Similar comments can be made about anti-asialo GM1 antibody since the glycolipid marker has been detected upon other cells, including macrophages, and injection of the antibody can reduce macrophage-mediated tumoricidal activity under the same conditions that reduce NK activity.[43] However, reconstitution of anti-asialo-GM1 antibody-treated rats with suspensions of lymphocytes enriched for NK cells by removal of nylon wool-adherent cells followed by density gradient centrifugation, at least, partially restored their ability to eliminate radiolabelled lymphoma cells from their lungs.[41] These results would argue against major phagocyte participation in clearance processes, as discussed earlier.

The NK activity of lymphocytes is age-dependent, and in one study,[44] pulmonary retention 24 h after intravenous injection of B16F10^{lr} melanoma cells was 5 times greater in 3-week-old euthymic mice than in 8-week-old animals with lower NK reactivity. Moreover, significantly more nodules developed in the lungs of the younger mice after injection of nonradiolabelled melanoma cells. Similar studies[45] with the parent B16F10 melanoma cells showed that pulmonary retention was increased in 3-week-old athymic mice compared with 8-week-old animals with higher NK reactivity. However, other investigators were unable to confirm this increase in retention of radiolabelled B16F10 melanoma cells in 3-week-old athymic mice and also found no differences in retention patterns of YAC-1 or in three human cell lines between young and adult recipients.[46]

The beige mutation in mice is the homolog of the Chediak-Higashi syndrome (CHS) in humans, which is characterized by abnormal leukocyte lysosomal granulation, defective pigmentation, and depressed phagocyte chemotaxis.[47] Several studies[48-50] have claimed that NK cell activity is selectively depressed in both beige mice and CHS patients, while monocyte, polymorph, and T-lymphocyte tumoricidal activities were relatively normal. As would be predicted from these studies, pulmonary retention of YAC-1 lymphoma cells,[37] as well as cells from a series of H-*ras*-transformed fibroblast lines,[38] has been shown to be greater in beige mice than in their normal counterparts. This increased retention was correlated with greater numbers of tumor nodules in beige recipients. In other studies,[51] the pulmonary retention of NK-sensitive and NK-insensitive B16 melanoma cell lines was compared in beige and normal mice. Approximately 2 to 3 times more NK-sensitive B16 cells were retained in the lungs of beige mice vs. controls, which further implicates NK cells in clearance processes. However, approximately twice as many NK-insensitive B16 cells were also retained in the lungs of beige than of heterozygous mice. Since beige mice had negligible *in vitro* NK tumoricidal activity for both NK-sensitive and -insensitive cells, other factors in addition to NK cells probably participate in tumor cell elimination from the microvasculature. Moreover, these factors are defective in beige mice. Indeed, not all investigators have found the NK defect to be absolute or selective in beige mice. Both suppressed T-cell[52] and delayed macrophage[53] tumoricidal activities have been reported for mice from the same commercial source as the studies cited above,[49] although there is little evidence for their participation in clearance processes, as discussed earlier. A third candidate would be polymorphonuclear leukocytes; many polymorph functions are defective in CHS and beige hosts, but so far, their tumoricidal activities have been reported as normal. Nevertheless, there are indications that polymorphs may contribute to elimination of cancer cells from the microvasculature, as will be discussed later.

The mechanisms and regulation of the tumoricidal activity of natural killer cells have been reviewed in depth elsewhere.[35,54] In the present context of intravascular interactions, not all cancer cells succumb to NK cells. Recent studies[55] have linked pulmonary retention of tumor cells to levels of class I major histocompatibility antigen (MHC) expression such that MHC-positive mouse fibrosarcoma cells were less susceptible to NK cytolysis and were cleared from the microvasculature slower than MHC-deficient cells. However, this inverse correlation between NK cell susceptibility and levels of MHC expression is controversial,[56] and its net contribution to metastasis is uncertain since the MHC-positive survivors of NK cell-mediated clearance processes would be more susceptible to T-lymphocyte attack after extravasation into the lung parenchyma. There is also evidence that coagulation factors may protect tumor cells from destruction by NK cells since treatment of mice with warfarin or heparin abrogated the effects of anti-asialo GM1 antibody on cancer cell retention in the lungs and inhibited NK tumoricidal activity *in vitro*.[40,57] However, the *in vivo* activities of such anticoagulants must be interpreted with caution since heparin, for instance, can stimulate the activities of granulocytes,[58] which may also interact with arrested cancer cells (see below). There is also evidence that tumor cells are less susceptible to NK attack *in vitro* if they are adherent to an endothelial monolayer[59] (see Chapter 11) or coated with the basement membrane glycoprotein, laminin[60] (see Chapter 1).

Much of the evidence for *in vivo* functions of NK cells is indirect and mostly based upon correlations between levels of NK activity of leukocytes measured *in vitro* and tumor cell behavior *in vivo,* and the relative susceptibility of different tumor cell types to NK cells does not always correlate with their organ retention patterns. Correlations that have been found between NK activity and organ retention patterns usually relate to *in vivo* experiments in which the same cell type (constant NK susceptibility) is injected into different strains of animals or into the same strain, treated/untreated with immunopharmacologic agents (variable NK effectors). The lack of absolute correlations raises the possibility, recognized by most investigators, that NK cells are not the exclusive effectors of tumor cell clearance processes. Nevertheless, despite the inherent limitations associated with both the artificialities of the *in vitro* environment and the complexities of *in vivo* interactions, there is a case for involvement of NK cells with cancer cells arrested in the microvasculature.

C. POLYMORPHONUCLEAR LEUKOCYTES

Polymorphonuclear leukocytes (granulocytes) are also candidates for intravascular interactions with cancer cells, especially since the growth of some animal and human tumors is associated with pronounced granulocytosis.[61-65] This expansion of circulating granulocytes may be, in part, a response to hemopoietic colony stimulating factors produced by tumor cells themselves.[62,63,66] The extent of tumor-associated granulocytosis has been correlated with the increasing metastatic potential of a series of rat mammary carcinomas[65] and also with the enhanced development of pulmonary nodules following i.v. injection of fibrosarcoma or melanoma cells into tumor-bearing mice.[62,68] Leukocytosis is also associated with poor prognosis in some cancer patients.[65] These findings implicate polymorphs as promoters of hematogenous metastasis, but their role is controversial since other experimental evidence assigns them both metastasis-promoting and protective functions. For instance, the pulmonary retention of B16 melanoma cells was decreased in mice with trypan blue-induced granulocytosis, and this was correlated with both increased tumoricidal granulocyte activity *in vitro* and with decreased numbers of pulmonary melanomas developing after injection of nonradiolabelled cells into trypan blue-treated mice.[20] Conversely, depleting mice of circulating granulocytes with granulocyte antiserum increased both pulmonary retention and lung colonization by melanoma cells. Similar studies[69] showed a dose-dependent increase in pulmonary 3LL carcinoma nodules in mice injected with granulocyte antiserum, although there was no effect upon lung colonization by an amelanotic variant of the B16 melanoma. Ultrastructural examination showed membrane-membrane interactions taking place between granulocytes and 3LL cells arrested in the microvasculature, and these associations were decreased in granulocyte antiserum-treated mice (see Chapter 13). This protective role of granulocytes against some types of intravascular cancer cells may involve toxic oxygen species since pretreatment of mice with superoxide dismutase (SOD) increased both pulmonary retention and yield of 3LL pulmonary tumor nodules.[70] Whether or not superoxide anion is directly involved in killing of tumor cells, as observed *in vitro*,[71] or exerts its effects indirectly via interactions with other mediators is uncertain.

Evidence that granulocytes could interact with intravascular cancer cells to promote, rather than to inhibit, metastasis comes from studies of acute inflammatory responses in rats[72] (see Chapter 15). Thus, the pulmonary retention of radiolabelled Walker 256 carcinosarcoma cells was three times greater in rats given cobra venom factor to induce complement activation and granulocyte sequestration in the lung microvasculature. This effect could be abrogated by treatment of rats with granulocyte antiserum and appeared to be mediated by activated oxygen species since treatment with catalase to dissipate hydrogen peroxide also abrogated the venom-induced increase in the pulmonary retention of tumor cells, although SOD was ineffective. Aggregates of granulocytes and tumor cells were identified in the lung microvasculature of venom-treated rats, and increased numbers of tumor nodules also developed after venom injections. It was concluded that systemic activation of granulocytes facilitated retention of cancer cells in the lung by inflicting damage to the vascular endothelium and exposing the basement membrane for interaction with tumor cells. These experiments provide the cellular basis for the studies discussed earlier on the tumor cell retention- and growth-promoting effects of acute inflammation induced by zymosan and endotoxin,[9] which were also interpreted as reflections of endothelial damage.[16] In this context, *in vitro* studies[73] have shown that twice as many heterotypic aggregates of tumor cells and granulocytes than homotypic tumor cell aggregates attach to endothelial cell monolayers. Parallel *in vivo* experiments were made, and the authors claimed that the pulmonary retention of radiolabelled heterotypic aggregates was greater than that of homotypic tumor cell aggregates and that this was correlated with higher lung colonization potential by heterotypic aggregates. However, a closer inspection of their data indicates that, although 30% more heterotypic aggregates were retained in the lungs 1 to 4 h postinjection, by 5 h this effect had disappeared and by 24 h there were twice as many homotypic than heterotypic aggregates retained. On this basis, these results are reminiscent of the earlier studies in RES-stimulated mice,[9] in which the retention of tumor cells was decreased in the short term, but the numbers of tumor nodules developed were increased, rather than decreased.

Can the apparent conflicts regarding microvascular granulocyte-cancer cell interactions be resolved? Actually, most of the experimental observations can be reconciled within the framework of the classically dual nature of granulocyte-mediated inflammatory responses, which have both beneficial and harmful components. Thus, on the one hand, the defensive actions of granulocytes would contribute to intravascular cancer cell death, which may be mediated by the products of the respiratory burst. Not all cancer cells may stimulate granulocyte activity or be susceptible to their attack, e.g., the amelanotic B16 melanoma variant[69] and Walker 256 cells,[74] since cells are variably equipped with mechanisms for degradation of toxic oxygen reduction products. On the other hand, interactions between granulocytes and endothelial cells should not be overlooked; it is well known that granulocyte products cause damage to endothelial cells and also to the subsequently exposed basement membrane. Intermediates of oxygen reduction are toxic for endothelial cells and cause structural alterations in collagen composition, protein denaturation, and decomposition of proteoglycans.[75,76] Granulocytes also release proteases capable of degrading basement membrane components. These actions will promote tumor cell attachment to basement membranes and facilitate their survival and extravasation. Also, reactive oxygen species are modulatory — they generate and inactivate chemotactic factors, activate or transform prostaglandins, activate platelets, and inactivate leukotrienes and proteases,[75,76] and they may be modified themselves by such agents as fatty acids.[77] Many of these mediators interact with intravascular cancer cells (see Chapters 1, 2, 7, 11, 14, 15). Given the variety of cancer cell types used in experimental studies, whether or not accessory inflammatory agents are used, and the timing of experiments relative to inflammatory events, it is not surprising that a spectrum of results is observed. Whether or not cancer cells survived intravascular interactions or whether their metastasis-related activities were even promoted depend upon the balance struck between beneficial and harmful effects of granulocyte involvement.

IV. GENERAL COMMENTS

Granulocytes, lymphocytes, and monocytes all have been identified in association with cancer cells arrested in the microvasculature, albeit to varying extents,[23-32,78] and some morphologic studies have failed to identify any leukocytes.[79] However, this discussion has focussed on the evidence for leukocyte-cancer cell interactions provided by a particular experimental model, namely, the intravenous injection of radiolabelled cancer cell suspensions. The numbers of cancer cells used in experiments are governed to some extent by detection limits imposed by the necessity for nontoxic doses of nucleic acid precursor for radiolabelling. How do these cell numbers relate to the numbers of cancer cells actually disseminated from primary tumors? Most experiments have involved injections of 2.5×10^4 to 10^6 radiolabelled cells. The data available for naturally disseminated cancer cells is limited but indicates that in mice, for highly metastatic 3LL carcinomas, the peak circulating level reached a median of approximately 5×10^4/ml, with medians of 2×10^3/ml for B16 melanomas, 6×10^3/ml for B16F10 melanomas, and 6 to 7×10^2/ml for two fibrosarcomas.[80-82] On this basis, investigators may use over two more orders of magnitude cells for retention experiments than would naturally be delivered to the lungs over a period of 1 min. Even though cancer cell release into the circulation occurs throughout tumor growth, it could take 24 h of sustained maximal rates of dissemination to deliver the number of B16 melanoma cells to the lungs that is usually given as a single bolus in retention experiments. The net result of leukocyte activity will depend upon effector:target cell ratios, therefore, it is difficult to estimate the contribution of leukocytes to cancer cell survival in the microvasculature on a precisely quantitative basis.

Arrested cancer cells are potential targets for circulating leukocytes, but some cancer cells are disseminated from the primary lesion with leukocytes already attached to them. For instance, T241 fibrosarcoma cells were detected in tumor-draining blood vessels in close contact with granulocytes and macrophages during early stages of tumor growth and with lymphocytes during later stages.[83] Lymphocytes were also detected attached to circulating 3LL carcinoma and B16 melanoma cells disseminated from intramuscular tumors.[80] Whether or not these leukocytes play an active role in determining the fate of cancer cells when they become arrested in the microvasculature is unknown, but they could certainly play a passive, metastasis-enhancing role since multicell emboli generate disproportionately more tumor nodules than equivalent numbers of single tumor cells — even if the emboli are heterogeneous and contain noncancer cells.[84]

Organ retention patterns of radiolabelled cells grossly underestimate the rate at which cancer cells are functionally inactivated. Radioactivity measurements monitor only the fate of the radiolabel, which is associated with the cell until cytolysis. However, parallel bioassays for tumorigenic cells following i.v. injections have shown that over 80% of 3LL carcinoma and B16 melanoma cells were rendered nontumorigenic, although not lysed, within 5 min of their initial arrest in the lungs.[81,85] Such massive and rapid effects are unlikely to be mediated by leukocytes, and mechanical trauma caused by shear forces imposed on cancer cells as they become impacted in the microvasculature is a likely candidate (see Chapter 9). Leukocyte interactions with surviving cancer cells are superimposed on this catastrophic process while leukocytes and cancer cells are also involved in concomitant interactions with the endothelium, basement membranes, and other vascular elements. The outcome of this interactive cascade may or may not benefit the host.

V. CONCLUSIONS

On the basis of the evidence discussed above, T-lymphocytes do not interact with cancer cells in the microvasculature while humoral antibody produced by B-lymphocytes can promote or inhibit cancer cell survival. Interaction between cancer cells and monocytes is negligible. NK cells may contribute to intravascular cancer cell death, but definitive evidence for an exclusive or major role is presently lacking. Granulocytes interact with cancer cells to the benefit and detriment of the host.

REFERENCES

1. **Weiss, L., Glaves, D., and Waite, D. A.,** The influence of host immunity on the arrest of circulating cancer cells in its modification by neuraminidase, *Int. J. Cancer,* 13, 850, 1974.
2. **Weiss, L. and Glaves, D.,** The immunospecificity of altered arrest pattern of circulating cancer cells in tumor-bearing mice, *Int. J. Cancer,* 18, 774, 1976.
3. **Proctor, J. W., Auclair, B. G., and Rudenstam, C. M.,** The distribution and fate of blood-borne IUDR-labelled tumour cells in immune syngeneic rats, *Int. J. Cancer,* 18, 255, 1976.
4. **Proctor, J. W., Mastromatteo, W. P., Antos, M., and Hedderson, E. D.,** Variations in the level of haematogenous antitumour immunity during progressive tumour growth and spontaneous blood-borne metastatic spread, *Oncology,* 36, 49, 1979.
5. **Brown, J. M. and Parker, E. T.,** Host treatments affecting artificial pulmonary metastases: interpretation of loss of radioactively labeled cells from the lungs, *Br. J. Cancer,* 40, 677, 1979.
6. **Fidler, I. J., Gersten, D. M., and Riggs, C. W.,** Relationship of host immune status to tumor cell arrest, distribution and survival in experimental metastasis, *Cancer,* 40, 46, 1977.
7. **Fidler, I. J., Gersten, D. M., and Budmen, M. B.,** Characterization *in vivo* and *in vitro* of tumor cells selected for resistence to syngeneic lymphocyte-mediated cytotoxicity, *Cancer Res.,* 36, 3160, 1976.
8. **Hanna, N. and Fidler, I. J.,** Relationship between metastatic potential and resistance to natural killer cell-mediated cytotoxicity in three murine tumor systems, *J. Natl. Cancer Inst.,* 66, 1183, 1981.
9. **Glaves, D.,** Metastasis: reticuloendothelial system and organ retention of disseminated malignant cells, *Int. J. Cancer,* 26, 115, 1980.
10. **Glaves, D. and Weiss, L.,** Metastasis and the reticuloendothelial system. II. Effects of triamcinolone acetonide on organ retention of malignant cells in endotoxin-treated mice, *Int. J. Cancer,* 27, 475, 1981.
11. **Proctor, J. W., Stiteler, R. D., Yamamura, Y., Mansell, P. W. A., and Winters, R.,** Effect of glucan and other adjuvants on the clearance of radiolabeled tumor cells from mouse lungs, *Cancer Treat. Rep.,* 62, 1873, 1978.
12. **Stiteler, R. D., Proctor, J. W., Yamamura, Y., and Mansell, P. W. A.,** The effect of glucan on the clearance of intravenously injected tumor cells from the lung, *J. Reticuloendothel. Soc.,* 24, 687, 1978.
13. **Proctor, J. W., Yamamura, Y., DiLuzio, N. R., Mansell, P. W. A., and Harnaha, J.,** Development of a bioassay for the antitumor activity of biologic response modifiers of the reticuloendothelial stimulant class, *Cancer Immunol. Immunother.,* 10, 197, 1981.
14. **Conley, F. K.,** Effect of immunomodulation on the fate of tumor cells in the central nervous system and systemic organs of mice. Distribution of [^{125}I]5-iodo-2′-deoxyuridine-labeled KHT tumor cells after left intracardial injection, *J. Natl. Cancer Inst.,* 69, 465, 1982.
15. **Lotzova, E. and Gutterman, J. U.,** Effect of glucan on natural killer (NK) cells: further comparison between NK cell and bone marrow effector cell activities, *J. Immunol.,* 123, 617, 1979.
16. **Weiss, L. and Glaves, D.,** Cancer cell damage at the vascular endothelium, *Ann. N.Y. Acad. Sci.,* 416, 681, 1983.
17. **Wheeldon, E. B. and Hansen-Flaschen, J. H.,** Intravascular macrophages in the sheep lung, *J. Leuk. Biol.,* 40, 657, 1986.
18. **Rybicka, R., Daly, B. D. T., Miglore, J. J., and Norman, J. C.,** Intravascular macrophages in normal calf lung: an electron microscope study, *Am. J. Anat.,* 139, 353, 1974.
19. **Winkler, G. C. and Cheville, N. F.,** Monocytic origin and postnatal mitosis of intravascular macrophages in the porcine lung, *J. Leuk. Biol.,* 38, 471, 1985.
20. **Glaves, D.,** Role of polymorphonuclear leukocytes in the pulmonary clearance of arrested cancer cells, Invest. Metast., 3, 160, 1983.

21. **Gorelik, E., Wiltrout, R. H., Brunda, M. J., Holden, H. T., and Herberman, R. B.,** Augmentation of metastasis formation by thioglycollate-elicited macrophages, *Int. J. Cancer,* 29, 575, 1982.
22. **Miyaska, M., Takiguchi, T., and Konda, S.,** The paradoxical effects of thioglycollate-induced macrophages on the growth of B16 melanoma cells *in vivo* and *in vitro, Gann,* 71, 293, 1980.
23. **Kinjo, M., Naito, S., and Tanaka, K.,** Fate of intravenously injected rat ascites hepatoma cells in the lungs of congenitally athymic mice, *Acta Pathol. Jpn.,* 32, 437, 1982.
24. **Dingemans, K. P. and Roos, E.,** Ultrastructural aspects of the invasion of liver by cancer cells (II), in *Liver Metastasis,* Weiss, L. and Gilbert, H. A., Eds., G. K. Hall, Boston, 1982, 51.
25. **Ludatscher, R. M., Luse, S. A., and Suntzeff, V.,** An electron microscopic study of pulmonary tumor emboli from transplantable Morris hepatomas 5123, *Cancer Res.,* 27, 1939, 1967.
26. **Dingemans, K. P.,** Behavior of intravenously injected malignant lymphoma cells. A morphologic study, *J. Natl. Cancer Inst.,* 51, 1883, 1973.
27. **Chew, E.-C. and Wallace, A. C.,** Demonstration of fibrin in early stages of experimental metastasis, *Cancer Res.,* 36, 1904, 1976.
28. **Kinjo, M.,** Lodgement and extravasation of tumour cells in blood-borne metastasis: an electron microscope study, *Br. J. Cancer,* 38, 293, 1978.
29. **Bishop, C. J. and Donald, K. J.,** Non-immunological cell death of intravenously injected murine tumor cells, *Br. J. Exp. Pathol.,* 60, 29, 1979.
30. **Hirata, H. and Tanaka, K.,** Fate of intravenously injected human tumor cells in the lungs of nude mice following whole-body-irradiation, *Invas. Metast.,* 5, 61, 1985.
31. **Paku, S., Paweletz, N., Spiess, E., Aulenbacher, P., Werling, H.-O., and Knierim, M.,** Ultrastructural analysis of experimentally induced invasion in the rat lung by tumor cells metastasizing lymphatically, *Anticancer Res.,* 6, 957, 1986.
32. **Crissman, J. D., Hatfield, J. S., Menter, D. G., Sloane, B., and Honn, K. V.,** Morphological study of the interaction of intravascular tumor cells with endothelial cells and sub-endothelial matrix, *Cancer Res.,* 48, 4065, 1988.
33. **Goldfarb, R. H. and Herberman, R. B.,** Characteristics of natural killer cells and possible mechanisms for their cytotoxic activity, *Adv. Inflamm. Res.,* 4, 45, 1982.
34. **Pollack, S. B.,** *In vivo* functions of natural killer cells, *Surv. Synth. Pathol. Res.,* 2, 93, 1983.
35. **Kimber, I. and Moore, M.,** Mechanism and regulation of natural cytotoxicity, *Exp. Cell Biol.,* 53, 69, 1985.
36. **Riccardi, C., Puccetti, P., Santoni, A., and Herberman, R. B.,** Rapid *in vivo* assay of mouse natural killer cell activity, *J. Natl. Cancer Inst.,* 63, 1041, 1979.
37. **Gorelik, E., Wiltrout, R. H., Okumura, K., Habu, S., and Herberman, R. B.,** Role of natural killer cells in the control of metastatic spread and growth of tumor cells in mice, *Int. J. Cancer,* 30, 107, 1982.
38. **Greenberg, A. H., Egan, S. E., Jarolim, L., Gingras, M.-C., and Wright, J. A.,** Natural killer cell regulation of implantation and early growth of H-*ras*-transformed 10T1/2 fibroblasts in mice, *Cancer Res.,* 47, 4801, 1987.
39. **Hanna, N.,** Inhibition of experimental tumor metastasis by selective activation of natural killer cells, *Cancer Res.,* 42, 1337, 1982.
40. **Gorelik, E., Bere, W. W., and Herberman, R. B.,** Role of NK cells in the antimetastatic effect of anticoagulants drugs, *Int. J. Cancer,* 33, 87, 1984.
41. **Barlozzari, T., Reynolds, C. W., and Herberman, R. B.,** *In vivo* role of natural killer cells: involvement of large granular lymphocytes in the clearance of tumor cells in anti-asialoGM1-treated rats, *J. Immunol.,* 131, 1024, 1983.
42. **Allison, A. C., Harrington, J. S., and Birbeck, M.,** An examination of the cytotoxic effects of silica on macrophages, *J. Exp. Med.,* 124, 141, 1966.
43. **Schultz, R. M., Tang, J. C., DeLong, D. C., Ades, E. W., and Altom, M. G.,** Inability of anti-asialoGM1 and 2-chloroadenosine to abrogate maleic anhydride-divinyl ether-induced resistance against experimental murine lung carcinoma metastases, *Cancer Res.,* 46, 5624, 1986.
44. **Hanna, N. and Fidler, I. J.,** Role of natural killer cells in destruction of circulating tumor emboli, *J. Natl. Cancer Inst.,* 801, 809, 1980.
45. **Hanna, N.,** Expression of metastatic potential of tumor cells in young nude mice is correlated with low levels of natural killer cell-mediated cytotoxicity, *Int. J. Cancer,* 26, 675, 1980.
46. **Fodtstad, O., Hansen, C. T., Cannon, G. B., Statham, C. N., Lichtenstein, G. G., and Boyd, M. R.,** Lack of correlation between natural killer activity and tumor growth control in nude mice with different immune defects, *Cancer Res.,* 44, 4403, 1984.
47. **Windhorst, D. B. and Padgett, G.,** The Chediak-Higashi syndrome and the homologous trait in animals, *J. Invest. Dermatol.,* 60, 529, 1973.
48. **Roder, J. C., Haliotis, T., Klein, M., Korec, S., Jett, J. R., Ortaldo, J., Herberman, R. B., Katz, P., and Fauci, A. S.,** A new immunodeficiency disorder in humans involving NK cells, *Nature,* 284, 553, 1980.

49. **Roder, J. C., Lohmann-Matthes, M.-L., Domzig, W., and Wigzell, H.,** The beige mutation in the mouse II: selectivity of the natural killer (NK) cell defect, *J. Immunol.*, 123, 2174, 1979.
50. **Orn, A., Hakansson, E. M., Gidlund, M., Ramstedt, U., Axberg, I., Wigzell, H., and Lundin, L.-G.,** Pigment mutations in the mouse which also affect lysosomal functions lead to suppressed natural killer cell activity, *Scand. J. Immunol.*, 15, 305, 1982.
51. **Talmadge, J. E., Meyers, K. M., Prieur, D. J., and Starkey, J. R.,** Role of natural killer cells in tumor growth and metastasis, *J. Natl. Cancer Inst.*, 65, 929, 1980.
52. **Saxena, R. K., Saxena, Q. B., and Adler, W. H.,** Defective T-cell response in beige mutant mice, *Nature,* 295, 240, 1982.
53. **Mahoney, K. H., Morse, S. C., and Morahan, P. S.,** Macrophage functions in beige (Chediak-Higashi syndrome) mice, *Cancer Res.*, 40, 3934, 1980.
54. **Herberman, R. B., Reynolds, C. W., and Ortaldo, J. R.,** Mechanism of cytotoxicity by natural killer (NK) cells, *Ann. Rev. Immunol.*, 4, 651, 1986.
55. **Algarra, I., Ohlen, C., Perez, M., Ljunggren, H.-G., Klein, G., Garrido, F., and Karre, K.,** NK sensitivity and lung clearance of MHC-class-I-deficient cells within a heterogeneous fibrosarcoma, *Int. J. Cancer,* 44, 675, 1989.
56. **Leiden, J. M., Karpinski, B. A., Gottschalk, L., and Kornbluth, J.,** Susceptibility to natural killer cell-mediated cytolysis is independent of the level of target cell class I HLA expression, *J. Immunol.*, 142, 2140, 1989.
57. **Gorelik, E.,** Augmentation of the antimetastatic effect of anticoagulant drugs by immunostimulation in mice, *Cancer Res.*, 47, 809, 1987.
58. **Cairo, M. S., Allen, J., Higgins, C., Baehner, R. L., and Boxer, L. A.,** Synergistic effect of heparin and chemotactic factor on polymorphonuclear leukocyte aggregation and degranulation, *Am. J. Pathol.*, 113, 67, 1983.
59. **Kaminski, M. and Auerbach, R.,** Tumor cells are protected from NK-cell-mediated lysis by adhesion to endothelial cells, *Int. J. Cancer,* 41, 847, 1988.
60. **Laybourn, K. A., Hiserodt, J. C., Abrozzo, L. V., and Varani, J.,** *In vitro* and *in vivo* interaction between murine fibrosarcoma cells and natural killer cells, *Cancer Res.*, 46, 3407, 1986.
61. **Lee, M., Durch, S., Dale, D., and Finch, C.,** Kinetics of tumor-induced murine neutrophilia, *Blood,* 53, 619, 1979.
62. **Milas, L., Faykus, M. H., McBride, W. H., Hunter, N., and Peters, L. J.,** Concomitant development of granulocytosis and enhancement of metastasis formation in tumor-bearing mice, *Clin. Exp. Metast.*, 2, 181, 1984.
63. **Lee, M. Y., Liu, C. C., Lottsfeldt, J. L., Judkins, S. A., and Howard, G. A.,** Production of granulocyte-stimulating and bone-cell-modulating activities from a neutrophilia hypercalcemia-inducing murine mammary cancer cell line, *Cancer Res.*, 47, 4059, 1987.
64. **Hardy, C. and Balducci, L.,** Hemopoietic alterations of cancer, *Am. J. Med. Sci.*, 290, 196, 1985.
65. **Schoenfeld, Y., Tal, A., Berliner, S., and Pinkhas, J.,** Leukocytosis in non-hematological malignancies — a possible tumor-associated marker, *J. Cancer Res. Clin. Oncol.*, 111, 54, 1986.
66. **Fu, Y., Watson, G., Jiminez, J. J., Wang, Y., and Lopez, D.,** Expansion of immunoregulatory macrophages by granulocyte-macrophage colony-stimulating factor derived from a murine mammary tumor, *Cancer Res.*, 50, 227, 1990.
67. **Aeed, P. A., Nakajima, M., and Welch, D. R.,** The role of polymorphonuclear leukocytes (PMN) on the growth and metastatic potential of 13762NF mammary adenocarcinoma cells, *Int. J. Cancer,* 42, 748, 1988.
68. **Ishikawa, M., Koga, Y., Hosokawa, M., and Kobayashi, H.,** Augmentation of B16 melanoma lung colony formation in C57B1/6 mice having marked granulocytosis, *Int. J. Cancer,* 37, 919, 1986.
69. **Weiss, L., Orr, F. W., and Honn, K. V.,** Interactions of cancer cells with the microvasculature during metastasis, *FASEB J.*, 2, 12, 1988.
70. **Glaves, D.,** Intravascular death of disseminated cancer cells mediated by superoxide anion, *Invas. Metast.*, 6, 101, 1986.
71. **Lichtenstein, A. and Kahle, J.,** Anti-tumor effect of inflammatory neutrophils: characteristics of *in vivo* generation and *in vitro* tumor cell lysis, *Int. J. Cancer,* 35, 121, 1985.
72. **Orr, F. W. and Warner, D. J. A.,** Effects of neutrophil-mediated pulmonary endothelial injury on the localization and metastasis of circulating Walker carcinosarcoma cells, *Invas. Metast.*, 7, 183, 1987.
73. **Starkey, J. R., Liggitt, H. D., Jones, W., and Hosick, H. L.,** Influence of migratory blood cells on the attachment of tumor cells to vascular endothelium, *Int. J. Cancer,* 34, 535, 1984.
74. **Orr, F. W. and Mokashi, S.,** Effect of leukocyte activation on the formation of heterotypic tumor cell aggregates *in vitro, Int. J. Cancer,* 35, 101, 1985.
75. **Rossi, F., Bellavite, P., Berton, G., Czeskowiak, M., and Papini, E.,** Mechanisms of production of toxic oxygen radicals by granulocytes and macrophages and their function in the inflammatory process, *Pathol. Res. Pract.*, 180, 136, 1985.

76. **Fantone, J. C. and Ward, P. A.,** Polymorphonuclear leukocyte-mediated cell and tissue injury, *Human Pathol.,* 16, 973, 1985.
77. **Wong, K. and Chew, C.,** The respiratory burst of human neutrophils treated with various stimulators *in vitro* is dampened by exogenous fatty acids, *J. Cell Physiol.,* 119, 89, 1984.
78. **Skolnik, G., Ericson, L. E., and Bagge, U.,** The effect of thrombocytopenia and antiserotonin treatment on the lodgement of circulating tumor cells, *J. Cancer Res. Clin. Oncol.,* 105, 30, 1983.
79. **Bishop, D. J. and Whiting, V. A.,** The role of natural killer cells in the intravascular death of intravenously injected murine tumour cells, *Br. J. Cancer,* 48, 441, 1983.
80. **Glaves, D.,** Correlation between circulating cancer cells and incidence of metastases, *Br. J. Cancer,* 48, 665, 1983.
81. **Mayhew, E. and Glaves, D.,** Quantitation of tumorigenic disseminating and arrested cells, *Br. J. Cancer,* 50, 159, 1984.
82. **Glaves, D. and Mayhew, E.,** Selective therapy of metastasis. I. Quantitation of tumorigenic circulating and covert cancer cells disseminated from metastatic and non-metastatic tumors, *Cancer Drug Deliv.,* 1, 293, 1984.
83. **Liotta, L. A., Kleinerman, J., and Saidel, G. M.,** Quantitative relationships of intravascular tumor cells, tumor vessels and pulmonary metastases following tumor implantation, *Cancer Res.,* 34, 997, 1974.
84. **Fidler, I. J.,** The relationship of embolic homogeneity, number, size and viability to the incidence of metastasis, *Eur. J. Cancer,* 9, 223, 1973.
85. **Glaves, D.,** Detection of circulating metastatic cells, *Prog. Clin. Biol. Res.,* 212, 151, 1986.

Chapter 7

PLATELETS AND CANCER METASTASIS

Kenneth V. Honn, Irma M. Grossi, Jozsef Timar, Hemi Chopra, and John D. Taylor

TABLE OF CONTENTS

I. INTRODUCTION

The ability to metastasize is a characteristic which usually distinguishes benign from malignant neoplasms. Metastasis can be simply defined as the loss of contiguity between a tumor cell, or a group of tumor cells, with the primary tumor and the successful transfer to and growth of these cells at a spatially separate site. The overall process can be regarded as a series of sequential events (see References 1 and 2 for reviews). During the hematogenous phase of metastasis, the cancer cell can undergo a variety of cell-cell interactions, some of which may be deleterious to the formation of an ultimate metastatic lesion. Examples of these deleterious interactions are interactions with macrophages, NK cells, etc. Other cellular interactions may actually facilitate cancer cell metastasis. One type of cell-cell interaction that may facilitate metastasis is the interaction between the circulating cancer cell and the host platelet. Although a considerable amount of evidence has accumulated over the past 25 years concerning the role of platelets in the metastatic process, this area remains a subject of controversy since no clear mechanism for platelet-enhanced metastasis has been forthcoming (a comprehensive review of the earlier literature can be found in References 3 to 7). In 1962 Gasic and co-workers[8] reported that pretreatment of mice with neuraminadase resulted in a decrease in experimental metastasis following the injection of TA3 ascites cancer cells. These results were initially interpreted as due to the action of neuraminadase on endothelial cell membrane sialic acid. However, in a follow-up study, Gasic et al.[9] demonstrated that neuraminadase-induced thrombocytopenia in mice, suggesting the role of platelets in metastasis. In addition, they demonstrated that platelet antisera also reduced lung colony formation that was abrogated by concomitant platelet infusion. This seminal observation initiated interest in the role of platelets in cancer cell metastasis. Also, hemostatic alterations in cancer patients such as thrombocytopenia, reduction in fibrinogen, and an increase in fibrin-fibrinogen degradation products have been linked to cancer cell metastasis.[10-13] The combination of the earlier preclinical studies and observations in clinical studies have prompted interest in the role played by platelets and the coagulation cascade in the metastatic process. Over the years, numerous human and animal cancer cells were found to be capable of inducing platelet activation.[14-28] However, the interpretation of some studies may be compromised because of the use of heterologous systems of cancer cells and platelets,[17,18,20,28] and the use of mechanically dispersed tumors that may contain host factors (i.e., collagen and ADP from broken cells) and may induce platelet aggregation,[14,15] general lack of standardization with respect to agonist strength, method of platelet preparation (heparinized or citrated plasmas), confluence of cancer cells at harvest, etc. Nevertheless, a correlation has been observed between metastatic potential and the ability to induce platelet activation in some systems;[29-32] however, other studies have demonstrated a lack of such correlation.[28,33] Several mechanisms have been proposed to explain platelet-enhanced metastasis: (1) platelet cancer cell emboli facilitate a mechanical lodging of cancer cells in the microvasculature,[7] (2) platelets-enhanced cancer cells attach to endothelial cells[34,35] and subendothelial matrix,[36-39] (3) platelets form a cocoon around arrested cancer cells, protecting them from destruction by effectors of the cellular immune response,[40,41] (4) platelet derived factors enhance endothelial cell retraction,[42] and (5) growth factors (i.e., platelet derived growth factor) stimulate the proliferation of arrested and extravasated cancer cells.[43]

II. *IN VIVO* STUDIES OF CANCER CELL PLATELET ENDOTHELIAL CELL INTERACTION

Wood[44] first studied cancer cell extravasation using the rabbit V2 carcinoma as observed in rabbit ear chambers. He reported that circulating V2 carcinoma cells were observed to arrest and form platelet thrombi. Following the formation of these thrombi, the cancer cells

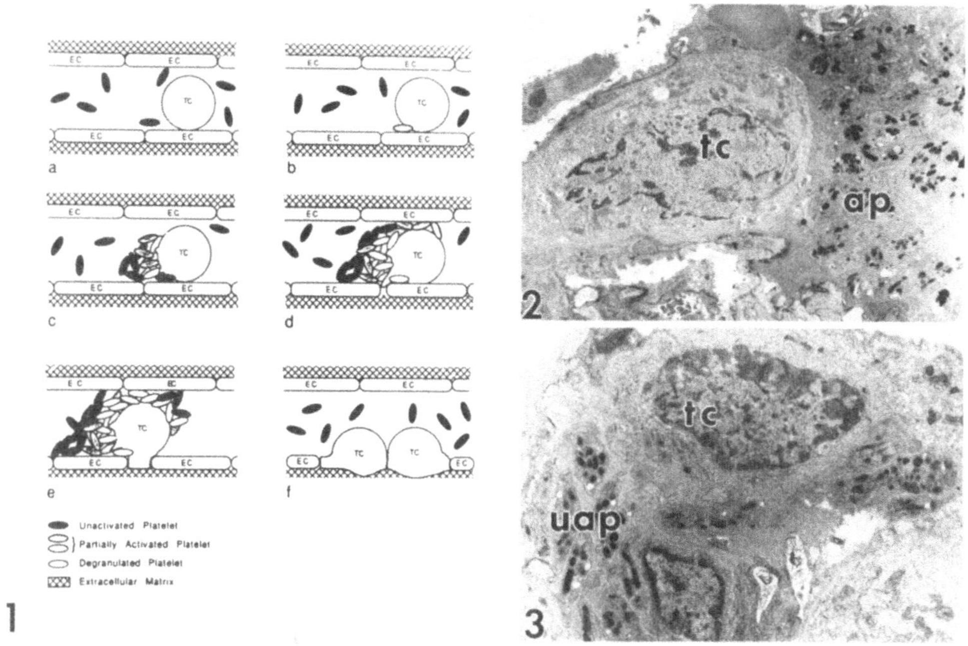

FIGURE 1. (1): Summary of platelet, cancer cell, and endothelial cell interactions during the first 24 hr following arrest; (a) initial arrest, (b) 2 min, (c) 10 min, (d) 1 to 4 hr, (e) 8 hr, (f) 24 hr post arrest. (2): Electron micrograph of a B16a cancer cell (**tc**) arrested in the pulmonary microvasculature 10 min following tail vein injection. Activated platelets (**ap**) formed a focal association with the arrested cancer cell. (3): B16a cancer cell within the pulmonary microvasculature 3 d following arrest. Unactivated platelets (**uap**) are shown in close proximity to the cancer cell plasma membrane.

extravasated from the vascular space in a manner similar to that observed for leukocytes. Other methods of tumor cell extravasation have been reported, such as explosive extravasation of tumor emboli following intravascular proliferation (first reported by Baserga and Safi-Otti[45]), locomotion extravasation in which cancer cells lodged in capillaries migrate into the perivascular space through their own movement, and segregation type extravasation in which cancer cells are segregated from the capillary lumen by endothelial cells that cover the cancer cell emboli.[46] A number of studies conducted in the past 20 years have examined the interaction between the cancer cell and the vessel wall during the arrest and extravasation phase of the metastatic cascade.[47-55] In most of these studies, platelets were reported to be transiently associated with the arrested cancer cell. In a series of *in vivo* studies using three murine cancer cell lines of different histological origin, Crissman and colleagues[51,52,55] examined, at the ultrastructural level, the interactions between cancer cells, platelets, and endothelial cells from 2 min to 192 h following tail vein injection. The results of these studies are summarized in Figure 1.1. In general, these results are in agreement with the morphological studies of other investigators who have reported on platelet interaction with arrested cancer cells. At the earliest time interval examined (i.e., 2 min), cancer cells were found arrested in the vasculature with their plasma membranes juxtaposed to the endothelial cell plasma membrane. Minimal platelet activation was observed at this time interval (Figure 1.1.a). Five to 10 min post arrest-activated platelets were observed generally at the tumor cell-endothelial cell junction (Figure 1.1.b). Platelet activation continued as additional platelets appeared to be recruited to the site of initial platelet activation and degranulation, resulting in a focal aggregate of activated platelets associated with the arrested cancer cell (Figures 1.1.c and 1.1.d). These morphological observations correlate well with *in vitro* observations of a focal platelet interaction with cancer cells.[55-58] Between 2 to 4 h post arrest, endothelial cell retraction was observed, and the capillary lumen was completely occluded by activated and degranulated platelets. Cancer cell pseudopodia were observed in contact with the subendothelial matrix between adjacent endothelial cells (Figure 1.1.d). Eight hours following arrest, the endothelial cells were well retracted, and the cancer cells had firmly established contact with the subendothelial matrix (Figure 1.1.e). In contrast to the observations at the earlier time intervals, 24 h following arrest, there was a complete absence of platelet aggregates associated with the arrested cancer cells, and intravascular cancer cell proliferation was observed (Figure 1.1.f). Figure 1.2 demonstrates an intravascular B16 amelanotic melanoma (B16a) cancer cell with associated activated platelets 10 min following initial arrest. This is compared with an intravascular cancer cell observed 3 d post injection where unactivated platelets are in contact with the cancer cell plasma membrane. Several other investigators have observed both the focal interaction of activated platelets with arrested cancer cells[21,50] and the transient association of activated platelets with the arrested cancer cell.[21,50] In aggregate, these morphological studies suggest that (1) cancer cell arrest in the microvasculature is independent of platelet activation, (2) platelet activation most probably occurs post cancer cell arrest and, in accordance with *in vitro* observations, is localized to specific areas of the cancer cell plasma membrane, (3) endothelial cell retraction occurs concomitant with the presence of activated platelets, (4) platelets are transiently (i.e., 24 to 48 h) associated with intravascular cancer cells, thereby, defining the time interval during which they could potentially enhance cancer cell metastasis, and (5) cancer cells can remain intravascular attached to the subendothelial matrix in the absence of evidence of platelet activation, suggesting that the factors responsible for cancer cell-induced platelet activation are transiently expressed.

III. MECHANISM OF CANCER CELL-INDUCED PLATELET ACTIVATION

Several mechanisms have been proposed to explain cancer cell induced-platelet activation, and a number of factors have been identified or purified to varying extents. In general, aggregation of platelets by cancer cells have been described as being due to the release of ADP,[59,60] to the action of thromboplastic activities present on the cancer cell surface[61-64] or to a sialo-lipoglycoprotein complex.[17,65,66] To date these sialo-lipoprotein complexes and trypsin sensitive surface proteins, which have been reported to be responsible for cancer cell induction of platelet activation, have not been purified to homogeneity or well characterized. Thrombogenic activity by cancer cells has been ascribed to at least four factors. The first is a cancer procoagulant cysteine proteinase first described by Gordon and collaborators.[62] The second is PAA/PCA, which has been purified from murine and rat tumor cells[61] and identified in membrane shed vesicles. The third is tissue factor.[63,67] The fourth is factor Xa bound to the cancer cell surface.[64] A number of investigators have examined co-factors required for platelet activation by cancer cells and, in general, have found requirements for both plasma factors and Ca^{++}.

Despite a number of earlier studies attempting to define the prothrombogenic activities of cancer cells and a detailed morphological study of cancer cell platelet interactions, investigation into specific receptors involved in these cell-cell interactions and the metabolic pathways, activated during cancer cell-platelet interactions, have been only recently investigated. Gasic et al.[68], using the murine 15019A and MCA6 cell lines, demonstrated that trypsin treatment abolished the platelet aggregating ability of these two cancer cell lines. This ability was regained during subsequent incubation by a process that required protein synthesis. Other investigators have reported that platelet aggregating activity is trypsin sensitive.[30] While this trypsin sensitive component may be a prothrombogenic protein or a sialoglycoprotein present on the cancer cell surface, it may equally be a receptor responsible for platelet adhesion to the cancer cell surface. As discussed above, platelet aggregation by cancer cells requires both divalent cations and plasma factors. Honn et al.[56] examined, by transmission and scanning electron microscopy, Walker 256 carcinosarcoma cell interaction with platelets. Their studies demonstrated a focal interaction between platelets and the cancer cell surface. In the absence of plasma factors, no overt platelet aggregation was observed. However, platelets were found to be adherent to the cancer cell plasma membrane with evidence of shape change. In addition, this initial interaction resulted in a rapid disappearance of cancer cell microvilli in areas not involved with platelet contact, suggesting a dynamic interaction between the platelet and the cancer cell. In a series of follow-up studies,[55,57,58] they investigated cancer cell-platelet interactions in samples removed during various phases of the aggregation response. The results demonstrate that cancer cell-platelet interactions involve a series of well defined and sequential events. Initially, one or two platelets adhere to the cancer cell plasma membrane. Additional platelets are then recruited to that initial site as the attached platelets respond to the cancer cell by undergoing shape change, activation, and degranulation.[55,57] This results in the formation of a focal aggregate of activated, degranulated platelets attached to the cancer cell surface.[58] Cancer cells, in turn, respond to activated platelets with a rapid disappearance of microvilli in areas not involved with platelet contact and with the subsequent formation of cellular processes that interdigitate with a focal platelet aggregate.[55,56] These cell surface alterations suggested an involvement of the cancer cell cytoskeleton in mediating their interaction with platelets. Chopra et al.[58] proposed that cancer cell platelet interactions involve at least three distinct events: (1) receptor mediated platelet adhesion to the cancer cell plasma membrane, (2) cancer cell cytoskeletal alterations, and (3) the expression of prothrombogenic activity, resulting in overt platelet aggregation. Chopra et al.[58,69,70] examined the role of the cancer cell cytoskeleton in their interaction with platelets both *in vitro* and *in vivo*. Walker 256 carcinosarcoma (W256) cells were treated with colchicine to disrupt the microtubules, cytochalasin D to disrupt the microfilaments, or cyclohexamide to disrupt the intermediate filaments and were tested for their ability to induce platelet aggregation. Disruption of either the microfilaments or the intermediate filaments inhibited overt platelet aggregation and platelet adhesion to the cancer cell surface as observed by ultrastructural analysis.[58] Colchicine disruption of microtubules also inhibited overt platelet aggregation, however, ultrastructural evidence demonstrated that small focal aggregates of activated platelets were adherent to the cancer cell surface. Colchicine, in some cancer cells[58] and normal cells,[71] has a secondary effect of disrupting intermediate filaments. Therefore, it was not possible to ascribe the colchicine effect to the disruption of microtubules. In a follow-up study[69] using B16a cells in which colchicine does not disrupt intermediate filaments, it was clearly demonstrated that microtubule disruption has no effect on the ability of cancer cells to aggregate platelets, however, intermediate filaments and microfilaments are required.

Several studies have implicated a role for the cancer cell cytoskeleton in metastasis. Hart et al.[72] reported that B16F10 cells pretreated with colchicine and/or cytochalasin B demonstrated decreased lung colonizing ability when compared to solvent treated controls. In addition, cytochalasin B and/or colchicine-treated B16F10 cells demonstrated decreased adhesion to endothelial cell monolayers when compared to untreated controls.[72] Intermediate filaments may also play a role in cancer cell metastasis.[73] Cyclohexamide reduces the synthesis of vimentin, tubulin, and actin by decreasing the concentrations of mRNAs coding for these proteins.[73] However, of these three cytoskeletal elements, only the organization of the intermediate filaments is disrupted by cyclohexamide.[73] B16F10 cells previously treated with cyclohexamide demonstrated a decreased capacity to form lung colonies *in vivo* when compared to untreated cells, and this effect was reversible.[73] These effects of cytoskeletal disruption on lung colonizing ability have been attributed to (1) cancer cell deformability, (2) adhesion, (3) chemotaxis, and (4) invasion. A factor not considered in previous work is the ability of cancer cells to aggregate platelets. Chopra et al.[70] recently investigated the association of B16a cells with platelets *in vivo* following disruption of various cytoskeletal elements. These investigators found that disruption of microfilaments or intermediate filaments, but not microtubules resulted in decreased lung colony formation. Ultrastructural and morphometric analysis revealed no difference in the number of arrested cancer cells in the microvasculature following disruption of microtubules or intermediate filaments when compared to untreated controls. However, while greater than 90% of the control and microtubule disrupted cells were found associated with activated platelets at 10 min following injection, less than 10% of the cells in which the intermediate filaments had been disrupted were found associated with activated platelets. Eight hours following cancer cell injection, there was a significant reduction in the number of intermediate filament disrupted cells remaining in the microvasculature when compared to control or microtubule disrupted cells. However, the cyclohexamide-treated cells observed had regained the ability to activate platelets as evidenced by degranulated platelets in contact with the cancer cell plasma membrane. *In vitro* experiments confirmed a reorganization of intermediate filaments concomitant with the ability to activate platelets 8 h following removal of cyclohexamide. These results suggest that platelets do not play a role in the initial arrest of cancer cells in the microvasculature, but may bc important postarrcst, possibly stimulating cancer cell adhesion to endothelial cells and subendothelial matrix (see below). This conclusion is supported by earlier data in which thrombocytopenia was demonstrated to reduce lung colony formation but not to alter initial cancer cell arrest in the microvasculature.[74] However, the decreased lung colonization by intermediate filament disrupted B16a cells, and the decreased number of these cells in the microvasculature 8 h following injection suggests that the effect of cytoskeletal disruption (i.e., microfilaments and intermediate filaments) on lung colony formation may be related to the decreased ability of cancer cells to interact with platelets *in vivo*.[70]

Recent work has focused on defining both the cancer cell and the platelet receptors responsible for the interaction of these two cell types. The receptors thus far identified are members of a family of adhesive protein receptors termed *integrins*.[75] These receptors play a major role in the cell-cell and cell-matrix interactions.[76] Integrins include the multifunctional platelet receptor $\alpha IIb\beta 3$ and the $\alpha v\beta 3$ receptor on endothelial cells.[77] Normally $\alpha IIb\beta 3$ is found on the surface of platelets and functions as a receptor for fibrinogen, linking platelets during aggregation. In addition, platelets possess another receptor (GpIb), which is demonstrated to bind von Willebrand factor and serve as a receptor for thrombin. Based on these observations, Bastida et al.[78] and Grossi et al.[79] examined the role of GpIb and $\alpha IIb\beta 3$ in the interaction of human cancer cells and human platelets. Using specific antibodies to GpIb, both groups demonstrated partial to full inhibition of cancer cell-induced platelet activation by four distinct human cancer cell lines. These results are consistent with the observation that these cell lines induced platelet aggregation via the generation of thrombin.[78,105] Pretreatment of platelets with monoclonal or polyclonal antibodies against $\alpha IIb\beta 3$ also resulted in an inhibition of platelet aggregation,[78,79] suggesting that the platelet $\alpha IIb\beta 3$ receptor mediates platelet adhesion to the cancer cell surface. Evidence suggests that a related cancer cell receptor may be the counterpart to platelet $\alpha IIb\beta 3$. Grossi et al.[80], using a panel of antibodies specific for human platelet $\alpha IIb\beta 3$, presented the first evidence that cells derived from human solid tumors possess the receptor immunologically related to $\alpha IIb\beta 3$. This protein complex was termed immunologically related (IR) GPIIb/IIIa. Recently, our laboratories expanded these findings, demonstrating that immunoprecipitation of cellular proteins from several murine cancer cell lines yields bands of 125 kDa, 100 kDa, and 24 kDa, all corresponding to similar molecular mass bands from concurrently immunoprecipitated murine and human platelet cell surface proteins.[69] In addition, when mRNA from B16a cells or Lewis lung carcinoma cells were probed with cDNAs for αIIb and $\beta 3$ and analyzed by Northern blot analysis, these probes hybridized to transcripts that corresponded to transcripts found in human erythroleukemia cells,[69,81] which synthesize authentic αIIbβ3.[82] Therefore, we now conclude that the IRGPII/IIIa receptor reported by Grossi et al.[80] is authentic αIIbβ3. This conclusion is supported by other laboratories who reported αIIbβ3-like integrins in cells derived from human tumors.[83-85]

In the studies of Grossi et al.[80], human colon carcinoma cells or cervical carcinoma cells were preincubated with blocking monoclonal or polyclonal antibodies to αIIbβ3. These antibody-pretreated cancer cells were then used to stimulate the aggregation of untreated human platelets. Inhibition of platelet aggregation by antibody-pretreated cancer cells was observed, suggesting that the αIIbβ3-like receptor on cancer cells is the counterpart of platelet αIIbβ3 and mediates the interaction between those two cell types. These results were confirmed by Chopra et al.[69] and Honn et al.[86] who demonstrated that pretreatment of W256, B16a, and Lewis lung carcinoma cells with antibodies to αIIbβ3 inhibited their ability to induce platelet aggregation. Ultrastructural studies confirmed a lack of platelet adhesion to the surface of cancer cells pretreated with antibodies against αIIbβ3, but not with unrelated antibodies or whole serums.[69,86]

Recently, Boukershe et al.[87] also reported that pretreatment of human melanoma cells with an antibody against αIIbβ3 reduced their ability to aggregate human platelets, thereby, lending support to our hypothesis. The identity of the principle linking molecule for platelet adhesion to the tumor cell surface is unknown, although several ligands have been suggested. Karpatkin et al.[83] suggests that von Willebrand factor and fibronectin on the platelet surface may serve as ligands for tumor cell-platelet adhesion. Our laboratories previously suggested that fibrinogen may serve as the linking molecule.[58] The fibrinogen molecule possesses an RGD-dependent and an RGD-independent binding site for platelet αIIbβ3[88] and mediates, in part, platelet-platelet adhesion during aggregation.[89] In addition, αIIbβ3 B16a cancer cell mediates their adhesion to fibrinogen-coated surfaces, which is blocked by monoclonal antibodies against this integrin receptor.[105]

αIIbβ3 is heterogenously distributed on the cancer cell surface. Immunocytochemistry at the ultrastructural level reveals a punctate distribution of reaction product, suggesting clusters of high receptor concentration.[58,80] Recently, we demonstrated that cancer cell αIIbβ3 is sequestered in vesicles located in the Golgi-region of the cell. These vesicles are transported to the cell surface upon stimulation where they fuse with the plasma membrane, resulting in a localized, high concentration of αIIbβ3 in the cancer cell microvilli.[90] These areas of high receptor concentration suggest preferential sites for platelet adhesion to the cancer cell surface. This hypothesis is depicted in Figure 2, which summarizes the ultrastructural results, cytoskeletal results, and integrin receptor results described above.

A. CORRELATION BETWEEN CANCER CELL αIIbβ3 EXPRESSION, PLATELET AGGREGATION, AND METASTASIS

If cancer cell αIIbβ3 is a receptor for platelet adhesion and if this adhesion step is a prerequisite for overt platelet activation, then one may expect a correlation between the surface expression of αIIbβ3 and the ability to induce platelet activation. Onoda et al.[91] reported the separation by centrifugal elutriation of subpopulations of B16a cells that differed in their ability to form lung colonies when injected intravenously. These subpopulations were designated 100, 180, 260, and 340 in increasing order of lung colonizing potential. Cells from each subpopulation did not differ in volume, therefore, the difference in lung colonizing ability could not be attributed to differences in initial arrest.[92] When cells from each of these subpopulations were tested for their ability to aggregate homologous platelets, the lowest lung colonizing subpopulation (i.e., 100) did not demonstrate an ability to aggregate platelets, whereas, the highest lung colonizing subpopulation (i.e., 340) produced the greatest degree of platelet activation[86,93] (Figure 3.1). We compared the ability of aliquots of cells from each of the subpopulations for their ability to (1) form pulmonary tumor

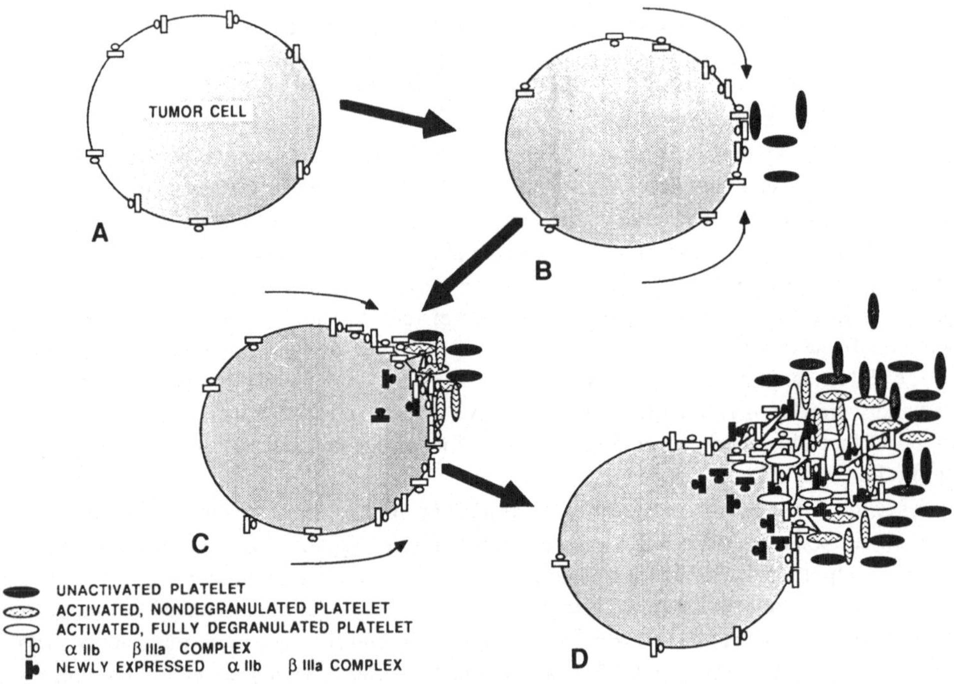

FIGURE 2. Diagramatic representation of events occurring during cancer cell platelet interaction. The $\alpha IIb\beta 3$ integrin is heterogenously expressed on the cancer cell surface (A). Initial contact occurs between the platelets and the cancer cell microvilli,[56] which may contain a high concentration of $\alpha IIb\beta 3$ receptors[90] (B). Following initial contact, additional platelets are recruited to the site of initial contact (C). In addition, there is movement of $\alpha IIb\beta 3$ receptors into the focal area of the cancer cell plasma membrane involved with platelet activation. Cytoplasmic vesicle-derived $\alpha IIb\beta 3$ is newly expressed at the site of platelet activation. Cytoskeletal rearrangement (microfilaments and intermediate filaments) leads to the formation of cellular processes that project into the platelet aggregate (D).

colonies *in vivo,* (2) induce the aggregation of homologous platelets, and (3) express the $\alpha IIb\beta 3$-like integrin. A perfect correlation between the ability of each fraction to induce platelet activation and their ability to form lung colonies *in vivo* was observed (Figure 3.2.a). In addition, a high degree of correlation (R = 0.90) was also observed when the ability to induce platelet activation was compared with the number of cells expressing the $\alpha IIb\beta 3$-like receptor (Figure 3.2.b). Similarly, a high degree of correlation (R = 0.90) was observed between the ability to form pulmonary tumor colonies and the number of cells expressing $\alpha IIb\beta 3$[86,93] (Figure 3.2.c).

IV. PLATELET EICOSANOIDS AND CANCER CELL ADHESION RECEPTORS

Eicosanoids are a group of oxygenated arachidonic acid metabolites that include prostaglandins, thromboxanes, leukotrienes, lipoxins, and various hydroperoxy and hydroxy fatty acids. Two major biosynthetic pathways exist for the formation of eicosanoids. Arachidonic acid is liberated from membrane phospholipids by the action of phospholipase A_2 or from diacylglycerol by diglycerol lipase. Once liberated, arachidonic acid can be converted to a variety of cyclooxygenase (COX) products (i.e., prostaglandins, prostacyclin, and thromboxanes). The first step in this pathway is the conversion of arachidonic acid by the COX component of prostaglandin endoperoxide synthase to the unstable endoperoxide PGG_2. The hydroperoxidase component of PGH synthase then converts this hydroperoxy fatty acid to the corresponding alcohol endoperoxide PGH_2, which is a pivotal intermediate for the

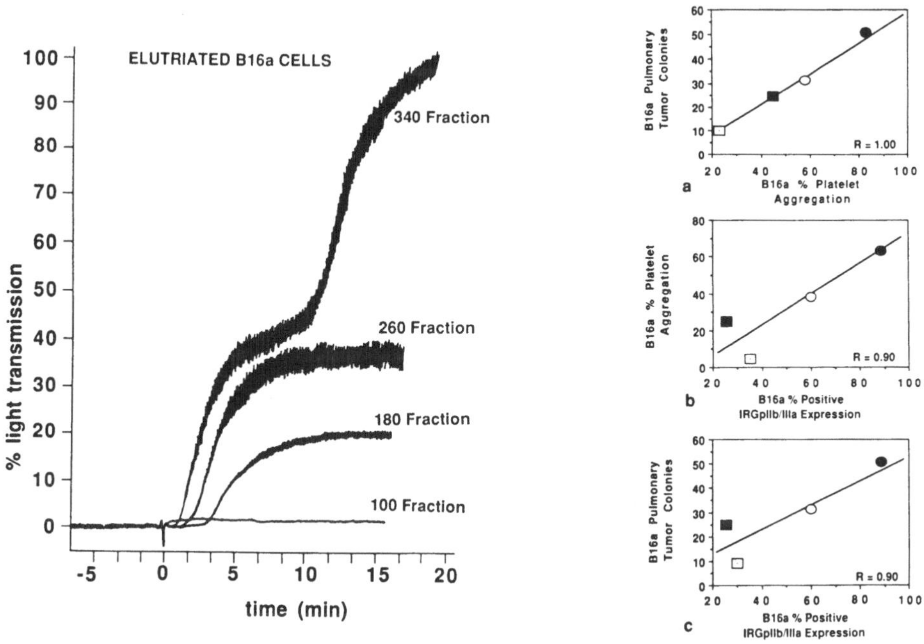

1 2

FIGURE 3. (1): Induction of murine platelet aggregation by elutriated subpopulations of the B16a melanoma (see Reference 93 for experimental details). The 100 fraction exhibits the lowest lung colonizing ability while the 340 fraction represents the highest lung colonizing ability. (2): Elutriated subpopulations (□ = 100; ■ = 180, ○ = 260, ● = 340) were compared for their ability to (a) form pulmonary tumor colonies vs. platelet aggregation, (b) induce platelet aggregation vs. expression of αIIbβ3, and (c) form tumor colonies vs. expression of αIIbβ3.

synthesis of all other COX compounds formed, depending on the enzymatic profile of the given cell type. The second major pathway of arachidonic acid synthesis is lipoxygenation (LOX). Arachidonic acid is metabolized by specific LOX enzymes (i.e., 5-lipoxygenase, 12-lipoxygenase, etc). The highly unstable hydroperoxyeicosatetraenoic acids are converted to the stable monohydroxyeicosatetraenoic acids (mono-HETES). The quantities of mono-HETES varies from cell type to cell type. 5-HPETE, in addition to being a source of 5-HETES, also serves as the intermediate in the generation of the complex HETES termed *leukotrienes* (for review see Reference 94). In addition to the mono-HETEs, a number of dihydroxyacids and trihydroxyacids (lipoxins) are also formed. Products of both the COX and the LOX pathways have been implicated in several aspects of cancer from carcinogenesis to metastasis.

We examined arachidonic acid metabolism by a number of murine tumor cell lines and found evidence for 5-lipoxygenase, 12-lipoxygenase, and 15-lipoxygenase activities.[95,105] However, 12-lipoxygenase appears to be the predominant activity in the cell lines examined thus far. Virtually 100% of the hydroxyeicosatetraenoic acid metabolite formed is the (S) enantiomer.[95] Recent evidence from our laboratories demonstrate that αIIbβ3 expression on the cancer cell surface is enhanced by several stimuli, including 12(S)-HETE, phorbol esters,[96] and platelets interacting with the cancer cell plasma membrane.[106] Similar results have been obtained for B16a cells.[90] This upregulation is dependent upon the intact microfilaments and intermediate filaments that function in the translocation of αIIbβ3-containing vesicles to the plasma membrane.[90] When Lewis lung carcinoma cells were treated with 12(S)-HETE, there was an increased cancer cell adhesion to endothelial cells and subendothelial matrix.[96,97] This enhanced adhesion, not basal cancer cell adhesion, was inhibited with antibodies specific for αIIbβ3 but not with antibodies against unrelated glycoproteins.[96] Since the expression of this receptor on the cancer cell plasma membrane correlates with metastatic potential, the treatment of low metastatic cells with 12(S)-HETE may result in enhanced receptor expression, enhanced ability to aggregate platelets, and enhanced lung colony formation. We previously reported that 12(S)-HETE enhances surface expression of αIIbβ3.[96] Recent data demonstrates that when an elutriated low metastatic subpopulation of B16a cells (i.e., 180) are treated with 12(S)-HETE prior to tail vein injection, an increased number of lung colonies are formed with respect to untreated controls (Figure 4). The biologically inactive enantiomer 12(R)-HETE is ineffective (Figure 4) as are 5, 8, 11, and 15(S)-HETE.[105] In addition, 12(S)-HETE-treated B16a cells (i.e., 180 fraction) have an increased ability to aggregate platelets. This ability is comparable to that observed by 340 fraction cells (Figure 3.2.a). This increased platelet activation is inhibited by pretreatment of the cancer cells with antibodies against αIIbβ3.[105] Similarly, increased lung colony formation by 12(S)-HETE-treated 180 B16a cells is also inhibited, following pretreatment of the cancer cells with antibody to αIIbβ3 prior to tail vein injection.[105] These results suggest that cancer cell metabolism of arachidonic acid to 12(S)-HETE and exogenous 12(S)-HETE both may be important to the ability of cancer cells to aggregate platelets, adhere to endothelium, and form lung colonies *in vivo*. Recently, we reported, using elutriated B16a subpopulations, that the production of 12(S)-HETE in response to arachidonic acid was greater in the 340 fraction than in the 180 fraction,[86] correlating with their differential abilities to form lung colonies and aggregate platelets. In addition to an endogenous metabolism of 12(S)-HETE, exogenously generated 12(S)-HETE may also be important in cancer cell arrest. As discussed above, during cancer cell arrest, there is close apposition of platelets, cancer cells, and endothelial cells. The major lipoxygenase metabolite of platelets is 12(S)-HETE,[98] which is formed during cancer cell-platelet interaction.[99] 12(S)-HETE generated in one cell type may affect adjacent cells by a mechanism known as transcellular metabolism. Marcus and colleagues[100] were the first to demonstrate the transfer of platelet 12-HETE to another cell (i.e., the neutrophil) where it is further metabolized to the novel eicosanoid 12(S)-20-dihydroxy-5, -8, -10, -14-eicosatetraeinoic acid.[101] Transcellular metabolism has been identified in a number of other cell types as well, including a 12(S)-HETE interchange between platelets and endothelial cells.[102] This has lead us to postulate[103] that during cancer cell platelet interaction, platelet 12(S)-HETE may transfer to tumor cells and enhance integrin expression and may also transfer tumor cell adhesiveness to endothelium and subendothelial matrix.

A. PLATELET ENHANCED CANCER CELL INDUCED ENDOTHELIAL CELL RETRACTION

Recently, we reported that 12(S)-HETE induced reversible nondestructive retraction of endothelial cells[42] (Figures 5.A and 5.B). This effect was specific for the (S) enantiomer and was not reproduced by metabolites of either the 5-lipoxygenase or the 15-lipoxygenase pathways. The induction of retraction was both time- and dose-dependent. Scanning electron microscopy confirmed the 12(S)-HETE induced endothelial cell retraction and revealed the collapsed filapodia on the surface of the endothelial cells, the appearance of space between the endothelial cells, and the underlying matrix. Tumor cell adhesion to the endothelial cell monolayers was increased 1 h following the addition of 12(S)-HETE but not 36 h following stimulation with 12(S)-HETE, during which time the monolayers reformed.[42] These results lead us to propose the hypothesis that platelets may be the primary contributors of 12(S)-HETE to cancer cells and endothelial cells during the interaction of these three cell types in the microvasculature. This would lead to (1) retraction and/or detachment of endothelial cells, exposing the subendothelial matrix, and (2) an increase in expression of αIIbβ3 on the cancer cell surface. Recently, we also demonstrated that 12(S)-HETE increases the surface

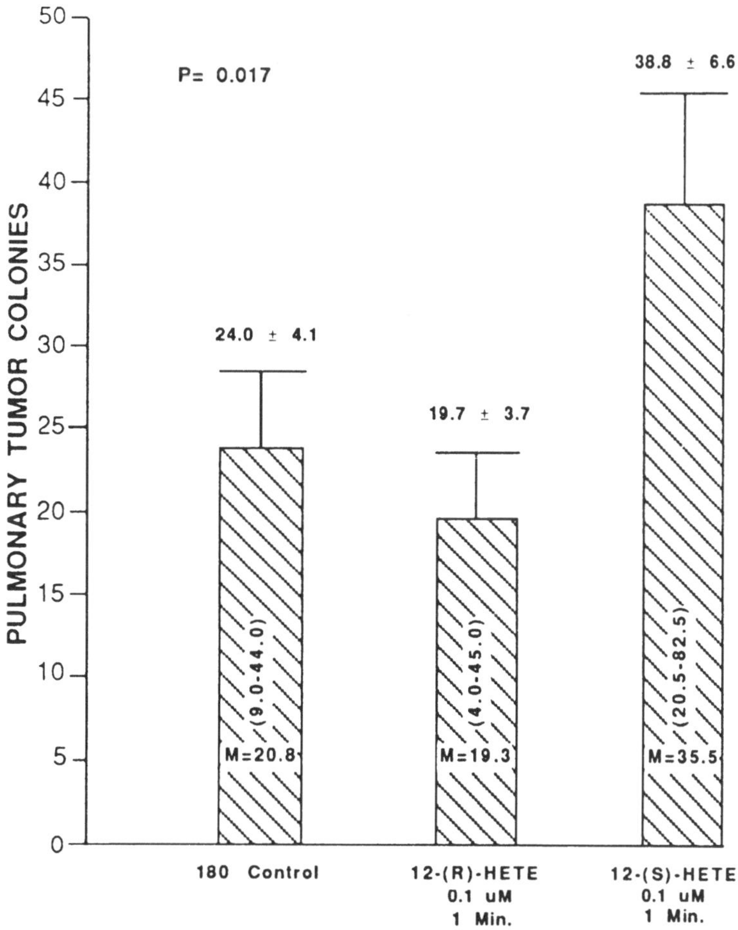

FIGURE 4. Elutriated B16a cells (2.5 × 10^4) from the 180 subpopulation were tail vein injected into C57BL/6J mice and examined for pulmonary tumor colony formation 21 d later. Cells treated (5 min) with 0.1 μM 12(S)-HETE prior to tail vein injection demonstrated increased lung colony formation. 12(R)-HETE was without effect.

expression of the vitronectin receptor on endothelial cells.[103] Since 12(S)-HETE is produced by a number of cancer cells, we initiated studies to determine whether cancer cells use 12(S)-HETE to induce endothelial cell retraction.

Lewis lung carcinoma (3LL) cells produce metabolites of arachidonic acid to 12(S)-HETE as their sole lipoxygenase metabolite.[95] When 3LL cells are added to intact monolayers of murine pulmonary microvessel-derived endothelial cells, they induce endothelial cell retraction evident within 15 min. One hour after plating, 3LL cells on endothelial cell retraction of cell-cell boarders is clearly evident with 3LL cells attached to the subendothelial matrix (Figure 5.C). However, if 3LL cells are previously treated with 1 μM of *n*-benzyl-5-phenylpentanohydroxamic acid (J-KS-122), a newly reported select 12-lipoxygenase inhibitor,[104] then they attach to the endothelial cell surface, but there was no evidence of endothelial cell retraction (Figure 5.D). Honn et al.[42] recently developed an assay to quantitate endothelial cell retraction. This assay is based upon the binding of radiolabeled antibody to type IV collagen to authentic type IV collagen in the subendothelial matrix (for experimental details, see Reference 42). If the 3LL cells were previously treated with 10 μM nordihydroguateric acid (NDGA) prior to plating on endothelial cells, then no retraction was observed (Figure 6.A). Similar results were observed when 3LL cells were preincubated with J-KS-

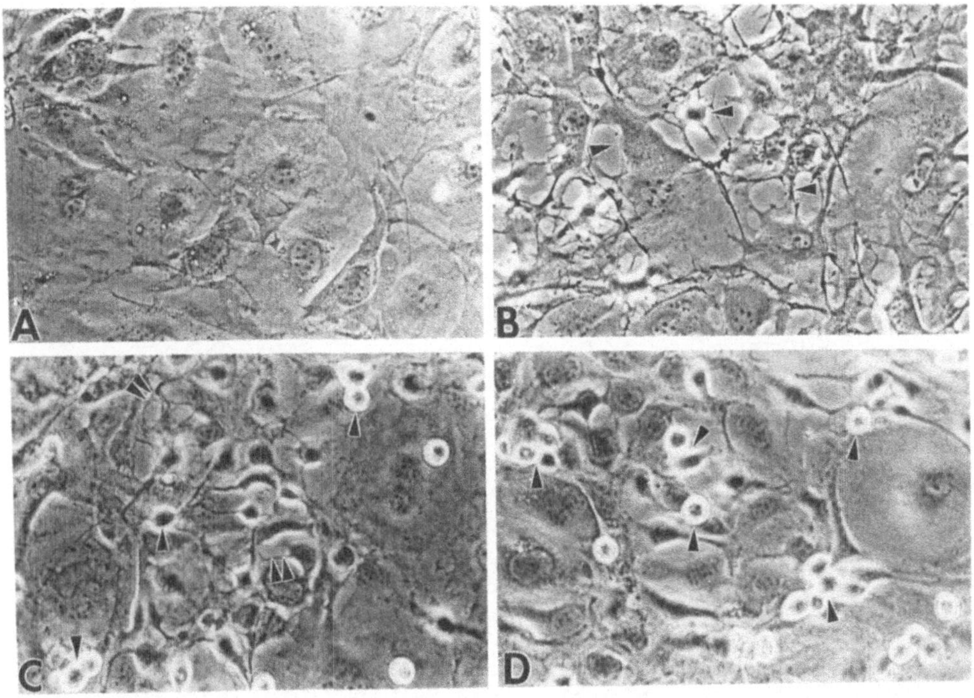

FIGURE 5. (A): Intact monolayer of CD3 murine pulmonary microvessel-derived endothelial cells (see Reference 70 for experimental details) demonstrate normal cobblestoned appearance. (B): Incubation of CD3 cells with 0.1 μ*M* 12(S)-HETE in Dulbecco's minimal essential medium plus 4% bovine serum albumin for 2 h; arrows indicate areas of cell retraction and exposed subendothelial matrix. (C): Incubation of 3LL cells with CD3 monolayers for 60 min in Dulbecco's minimal essential media plus 4% BSA; single arrow = 3LL cells; double arrow = retracted CD3 cell. (D): Incubation of 3LL cells with 1 μ*M* J-KS-122 15 min prior to plating on CD3 monolayer inhibited 3LL induced endothelial cell retraction 60 min postplating.

122, which, alone, had no effect on the retraction of the endothelial cell monolayers (Figure 6.A). In contrast to the results obtained with these two lipoxygenase inhibitors, indomethacin (a cyclooxygenase inhibitor) pretreatment of 3LL cells did not inhibit their ability to induce endothelial cell retraction (Figure 6.A). These results suggest that the induction of endothelial cell retraction by 3LL cells is mediated by a 12-lipoxygenase metabolite. Platelets metabolize arachidonic acid to 12-HETE during activation by cancer cells.[99] When murine platelets[107] are added to murine microvessel endothelial cells, an enhancement of endothelial cell retraction was observed following 1 h of incubation (Figure 6.B). However, when murine platelets and 3LL cells were simulateously added to endothelial cell monolayers, a dose-dependent increase in endothelial cell retraction was observed over that induced by 3LL cells alone or platelets alone (Figure 6.B). Similar to the results described above for pretreatment of 3LL cells with lipoxygenase inhibitors, when platelets are pretreated with a 12-lipoxygenase inhibitor prior to their simultaneous addition with 3LL cells to endothelial monolayers, there was no enhancement of retraction above that observed with 3LL cells alone. Cyclooxygenase inhibitors were without effect.[107]

V. CONCLUSIONS AND HYPOTHESIS

Evidence from our own laboratory as well as an examination of the literature lead us to the conclusion that platelets do not function in the mechanical arrest of cancer cells in the microvasculature. Similarly, the transient association of a platelet thrombi with arrested

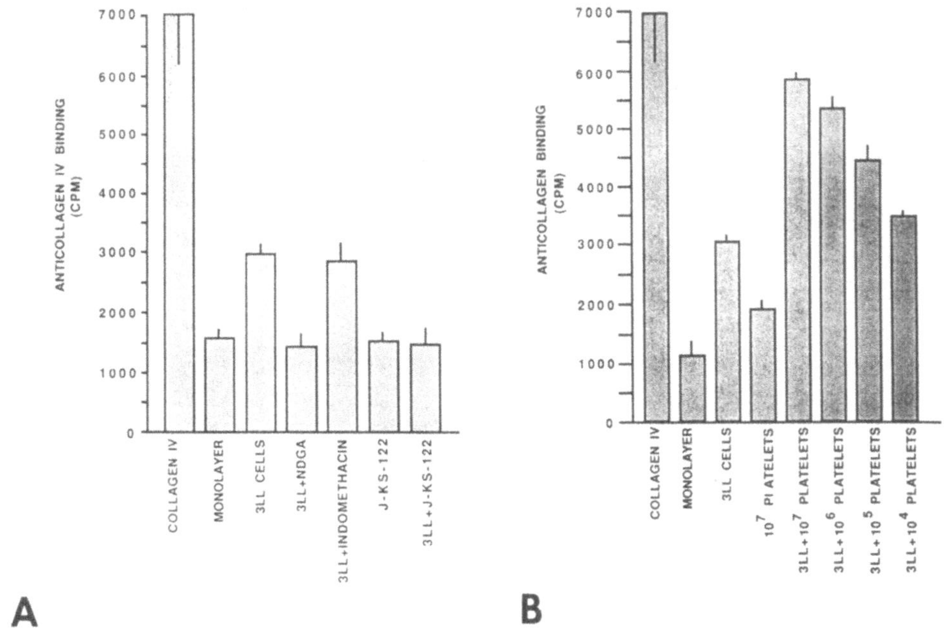

FIGURE 6. (A): Quantitation of endothelial cell retraction using ^{125}I-labelled anticollagen IV antibody (see Reference 42 for experimental details). Pretreatment of 3LL cells with lipoxygenase inhibitors NDGA or J-KS-122 inhibited their ability to induce endothelial cell retraction as evidenced by labelling equal to that observed with intact monolayer alone. Indomethacin pretreatment of 3LL cells was without effect. (B): Dose-dependent increase in endothelial cell retraction obtained, following preincubation of CD3 monolayers with 3LL cells plus increasing doses of washed murine platelets + 0.1% platelet poor plasma.

cancer cells make it unlikely that the protective cocoon mechanism is the principal mechanism of platelet enhanced metastasis. Clearly, platelet derived growth factor is released during the activation of platelets by arrested cancer cells. However, this only may have a transient effect on cancer cell proliferation because of the limited association of activated platelets with arrested cancer cells. The intracellular proliferation of cancer cells and the appearance of mitotic figures following activation of platelets suggest that this may occur.[51,52] The morphological evidence suggests that platelets can form a bridge between the cancer cell and the endothelial cell, stabilizing the bond between these two cell types. But, we believe that platelets function as a rate regulator for metastasis by activating cancer cell adhesion receptor expression, by enhancing the expression of adhesion receptors (i.e., integrins) on cancer cells and endothelial cells immediately following arrest, and by inducing endothelial cell retraction. This hypothesis is depicted in Figure 7. Results from our laboratory suggest that initial cancer cell adhesion to endothelial cells is not mediated by cancer cell integrin receptors as basal adhesion is not blocked by monoclonals specific for $\alpha IIb\beta 3$.[96] However, immediately following cancer cell arrest, there is a focal activation of platelets generally observed at the cancer cell-endothelial cell interface.[51,52] The activation of these platelets by cancer cells results in arachidonic acid metabolism to the cyclooxygenase metabolite thromboxane A2 and the lipoxygenase metabolite 12(S)-HETE. Schafer et al.[102] demonstrated that 12(S)-HETE can transfer from platelets to endothelial cells during their interaction. We postulate that this eicosanoid may also transfer from platelets to cancer cells and to endothelial cells during the interaction of these three cell types (Figure 7). Platelet-derived 12-HETE, in addition to cancer cell 12(S)-HETE, may induce upregulation of $\alpha IIb\beta 3$ (and possibly other integrins) on the cancer cell surface, thereby increasing their binding to endothelial cells. Additionly, 12(S)-HETE increases the expression of at least one receptor (i.e., vitronectin receptor) on endothelial cells,[103] which could serve as receptor counterparts for the

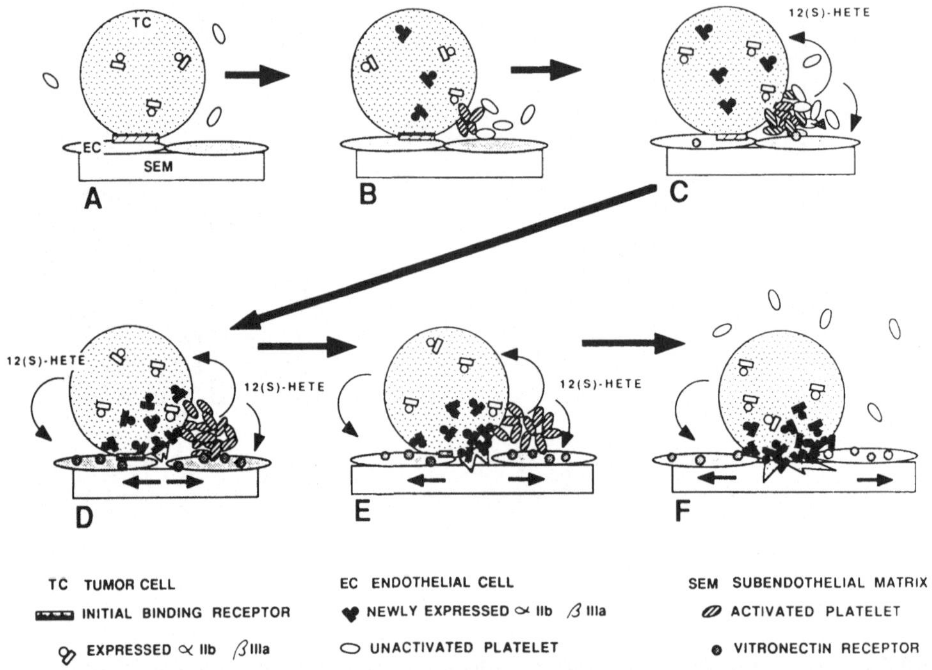

FIGURE 7. Summary of hypothesis suggesting that platelet 12(S)-HETE enhances cancer cell metastasis by (1) increasing integrin receptor expression on cancer cells, (2) increasing integrin receptor expression on endothelial cells, and (3) inducing endothelial cell retraction.

cancer cell integrins. Finally, 12(S)-HETE can induce reversible nondestructive retraction of endothelial cells, allowing the cancer cells to adhere to the subendothelial matrix where the cancer cell can utilize many types of receptors in forming a stable nonreversible bond to the vessel wall.

REFERENCES

1. **Nicolson, G. L.,** Cancer metastasis: tumor cell and host organ properties important in metastasis to specific secondary sites, *Biochim. Biophys. Acta,* 948, 175, 1988.
2. **Weiss, L., Orr, F. W., and Honn, K. V.,** Interactions between cancer cells and the microvasculature: a rate-regulator for metastasis, *Clin. Exp. Metast.,* 7, 127, 1989.
3. **Karpatkin, S. and Pearlstein, E.,** Role of platelets in tumor cell metastases, *Ann. Intern. Med.,* 95, 636, 1981.
4. **Jamieson, G. A., Ed.,** *Interaction of Platelets and Tumor Cells,* Vol. 89, Alan R. Liss, New York, 1982.
5. **Honn, K. V. and Sloane, B. F.,** *Hemostatic Mechanisms and Metastasis,* Martinus Nijhoff, Boston, 1984.
6. **Mehta, P.,** Potential role of platelets in the pathogenesis of tumor metastasis, *Blood,* 63, 55, 1984.
7. **Grignani, G., Pacchiarini, L., and Pagiarino, M.,** The possible role of blood platelets in tumour growth and dissemination, *Haematologica,* 71, 245, 1986.
8. **Gasic, G. J. and Gasic, T. B.,** Removal of sialic acid from the cell coat in tumor cells and vascular endothelium and its effects on metastasis, *Proc. Natl. Acad. Sci. U.S.A.,* 48, 1172, 1962.
9. **Gasic, G. J., Gasic, T. B., and Stewart, C. C.,** Antimetastatic effects associated with platelet reduction, *Proc. Natl. Acad. Sci. U.S.A.,* 61, 46, 1968.
10. **Edwards, R. L. and Rickles, F. R.,** Hemostatic alterations in cancer patients, in *Hemostatic Mechanisms and Metastasis,* Honn, K. V. and Sloane, B. F., Eds., Martinus Nijhoff, Boston, 1984, 342.
11. **Imaoka, S., Sasaki, Y., Iwanaga, T., and Terasawa, T.,** The significance of the fibrin/fibrinogen degradation product in serum of carcinoma patients with hematogenous metastasis, *Cancer,* 58, 1488, 1986.

12. **Blomback, M., Hedlund, P. O., and Sawe, U.**, Changes in blood coagulation and fibrinolysis in patients on different treatment regimens for prostatic cancer — predictors for cardiovascular complications, *Thromb. Res.*, 49, 111, 1988.
13. **Dvorak, H. F.**, Thrombosis and cancer, *Hum. Pathol.*, 18, 275, 1987.
14. **Gasic, G. J., Gasic, T. B., Galanti, N., Johnson, T., Murphy, S.**, Platelet-tumor cell interactions in mice. The role of platelets in the spread of malignant disease, *Int. J. Cancer*, 11, 704, 1973.
15. **Gasic, G. J., Koch, P. A. G., Hsu, B., Gasic, T. B., and Niewiarowski, S.**, Thrombogenic activity of mouse and human tumors: effects on platelets, coagulation, and fibrinolysis, and possible significance for metastases, *Z. Krebsforsch.*, 86, 263, 1976.
16. **Evans, P. M. and Cowie, F. P.**, A species difference in platelet aggregation induced by tumor cells, *Cell Biol. Int. Rep.*, 7, 771, 1983.
17. **Lerner, W. A., Pearlstein, E., Ambrogio, C., and Karpatkin, S.**, A new mechanism for tumor-induced platelet aggregation. Comparison with mechanisms shared by other tumors with possible pharmacologic strategy toward prevention of metastases, *Int. J. Cancer*, 31, 463, 1983.
18. **Karpatkin, S., Smerling, A., and Pearlstein, E.**, Plasma requirement for the aggregation of rabbit platelets by an aggregating material derived from SV40-transformed 3T3 fibroblasts, *J. Lab. Clin. Med.*, 96, 994, 1980.
19. **Bastida, E., Ordinas, A., and Jamieson, G. A.**, Idiosyncratic platelet responses to human tumour cells, *Nature*, 291, 661, 1981.
20. **Grignani, G., Pacchiarini, L., Almasio, P., Pagliarino, M., and Gamba, G.**, Activation of platelet prostaglandin biosynthesis pathway during neoplastic cell-induced platelet aggregation, *Thromb. Res.*, 34, 147, 1984.
21. **Tanaka, N., Ashida, S., Tohgo, A., and Ogawa, H.**, Platelet-aggregating activities of metastasizing tumor cells, *Invasion and Metastasis*, 2, 289, 1982.
22. **Tohgo, A., Tanaka, N., Ashida, S., and Ogawa, H.**, Platelet-aggregating activities of metastasizing tumor cells. II. Variety of the aggregation mechanisms, *Invasion and Metastasis*, 4, 134, 1984.
23. **Eche, N., Sie, P., Jozan, S., Courriere, P., David, J. F.**, Platelet aggregating and procoagulant activities of cultured human breast cancer cells, *Thromb. Res.*, 43, 121, 1986.
24. **Scarlett, J. D., Thurlow, P. J., Connellan, J. M., and Louis, C. J.**, Plasma-dependent and -independent mechanisms of platelet aggregation induced by human tumour cell lines, *Thromb. Res.*, 46, 715, 1987.
25. **Bastida, E., Almirall, L., Jamieson, G. A., and Ordinas, A.**, Cell surface sialylation of two human tumor cell lines and its correlation with their platelet-activating activity, *Cancer Res.*, 47, 1767, 1987.
26. **Panton, R. W., Agarwal, K. C., Robison, B. S., and Parks, R. E.**, Murine tumor-induced platelet aggregation and coagulation: mechanisms, inhibitors, and species difference, *Thromb. Res.*, 46, 65, 1987.
27. **Menter, D. G., Steinert, B. W., Sloane, B. F., Taylor, J. D., and Honn, K. V.**, A new *in vitro* model for investigation of tumor cell-platelet-endothelial cell interactions and concomitant eicosanoid biosynthesis, *Cancer Res.*, 47, 2425, 1987.
28. **Lampugnani, M. G. and Crawford, N.**, Tumour-cell-induced platelet aggregation: studies with cloned metastatic and non-metastatic variants, *Invasion and Metastasis*, 7, 311, 1987.
29. **Pearlstein, E., Salk, P. L., Yogeeswaran, G., and Karpatkin, S.**, Correlation between spontaneous metastatic potential, platelet-aggregating activity of cell surface extracts, and cell surface sialylation in 10 metastatic-variant derivatives of a rat renal sarcoma cell line, *Proc. Natl. Acad. Sci. U.S.A.*, 77, 4336, 1980.
30. **Tohgo, A., Tanaka, N. G., and Ogawa, H.**, Platelet-aggregating activities of metastasizing tumor cells. IV. Effects of cell surface modification on thrombin generation, platelet aggregation and subsequent lung colonization, *Invasion and Metastasis*, 6, 58, 1986.
31. **Sugimoto, Y., Oh-hara, T., Watanabe, M., Saito, H., Yamori, T., and Tsuruo, T.**, Acquisition of metastatic ability in hybridomas between two low metastatic clones of murine colon adenocarcinoma 26 defective in either platelet-aggregating activity or *in vivo* growth potential, *Cancer Res.*, 47, 4396, 1987.
32. **Grignani, G., Pacchiarini, L., Almasio, P., Pagliarino, M., Gamba, G., Rizzo, S. C., and Ascari, E.**, Characterization of the platelet-aggregating activity of cancer cells with different metastatic potential, *Int. J. Cancer*, 38, 237, 1986.
33. **Estrada, J. and Nicolson, G. L.**, Tumor-cell-platelet aggregation does not correlate with metastatic potential of rat 13762NF mammary adenocarcinoma tumor cell clones, *Int. J. Cancer*, 34, 101, 1984.
34. **Honn, K. V., Onoda, J. M., Pampalona, K., Battaglia, M., Neagos, G., Taylor, J. D., Diglio, C. A., and Sloane, B. F.**, Inhibition by dihydropyridine class calcium channel blockers of tumor cell-platelet-endothelial cell interactions *in vitro* and metastasis *in vivo*, *Biochem. Pharm.*, 34, 235, 1985.
35. **Abecassis, J., Millon-Collard, R., Klein-Soyer, C., Nicora, F., Fricker, J.-P., Beretz, A., Eber, M., Muller, D., and Cazenave, J.-P.**, Adhesion of breast cancer cell line MCF-7 to human vascular endothelial cells in culture. Enhancement by activiated platelets, *Int. J. Cancer*, 40, 525, 1987.
36. **Marcum, J. M., McGill, M., Bastida, E., Ordinas, A., and Jamieson, G. A.**, The interaction of platelets, tumor cells, and vascular subendothelium, *J. Lab. Clin. Med.*, 96, 1048, 1980.

37. **Yahalom, J., Eldor, A., Biran, S., Fuks, Z., and Vlodavsky, I.,** Platelet-tumor cell interaction with the subendothelial extracellular matrix: relationship to cancer metastasis, *Radiother. Oncol.*, 3, 211, 1985.
38. **Menter, D. G., Sloane, B. F., Steinert, B. W., Onoda, J., Craig, R., Harkins, C., Taylor, J. D., and Honn, K. V.,** Platelet enhancement of tumor cell adhesion to subendothelial matrix: role of platelet cytoskeleton and platelet membrane, *J. Natl. Cancer Inst.*, 79, 1077, 1987.
39. **Menter, D. G., Steinert, B. W., Sloane, B. F., Gunlach, N., O'Gara, C. Y., Marnett, L. F., Diglio, C., Walz, D., Taylor, J. D., and Honn, K. V.,** Role of platelet membrane in enhancement of tumor cell adhesion to endothelial cell extracellular matrix, *Cancer Res.*, 47, 6751, 1987.
40. **Gorelik, E., Bere, W. W., and Herberman, R. B.,** Role of NK cells in the antimetastatic effect of anticoagulant drugs, *Int. J. Cancer,* 33, 87, 1984.
41. **Gorelik, E.,** Augmentation of the antimetastatic effect of anticoagulant drugs by immunostimulation in mice, *Cancer Res.*, 47, 809, 1987.
42. **Honn, K. V., Grossi, I. M., Diglio, C. A., Wojtukiewicz, M., and Taylor, J. D.,** Enhanced tumor cell adhesion to the subendothelial matrix resulting from 12(S)-HETE-induced endothelial cell retraction, *FASEB,* 3, 2285, 1989.
43. **Hara, Y., Steiner, M., and Baldini, M. G.,** Platelets as a source of growth-promoting factor(s) for tumor cells, *Cancer Res.*, 40, 1212, 1980.
44. **Wood, S., Jr.,** Pathogenesis of metastasis formation observed *in vivo* in the rabbit ear chamber, *Arch. Pathol.*, 667, 550, 1958.
45. **Baserga, R. and Safi-Otti, U.,** Experimental studies on histogenesis of blood-borne metastases, *Arch. Pathol.*, 59, 26, 1955.
46. **Kawaguchi, T. and Nakamura, K.,** Analysis of the lodgement and extravasation of tumor cells in experimental models of hematogenous metastasis, *Cancer Metast. Rev.*, 5, 77, 1986.
47. **Warren, B. A.,** Environment of the blood-borne tumor embolus adherent to vessel wall, *J. Med.*, 4, 150, 1973.
48. **Warren, B. A.,** Some aspects of blood borne tumour emboli associated with thrombosis, *Z. Krebsforsch.*, 87, 1, 1976.
49. **Takanori, K. and Nakamura, K.,** Analysis of the lodgement and extravasation of tumor cells in experimental models of hematogenous metastasis, *Cancer Metast. Rev.*, 5, 77, 1986.
50. **Tanaka, N. G., Tohgo, A., and Ogawa, H.,** Platelet-aggregating activities of metastasizing tumor cells. V. *In situ* roles of platelets in hematogenous metastases, *Invasion and Metastasis,* 6, 209, 1986.
51. **Crissman, J. D., Hatfield, J. S., Menter, D. G., Sloane, B. F., and Honn, K. V.,** Morphological study of the interaction of intravascular tumor cells with endothelial cells and subendothelial matrix, *Cancer Res.*, 48, 4065, 1988.
52. **Crissman, J. D., Hatfield, J. S., Schaldenbrand, M., Sloane, B. F., and Honn, K. V.,** Arrest and extravasation of B16 amelanotic melanoma in murine lungs: a light and electron microscopic study, *Lab. Invest.*, 53, 470, 1985.
53. **Chew, E. C., Josephson, R. I., and Wallace, A. C.,** Morphologic aspects of the arrest of circulating cells, in *Fundamental Aspects of Metastasis,* L. Weiss, Ed., Elsevier, Amsterdam, 1976, 121.
54. **Jones, D. S., Wallace, A. C., and Fraser, E. E.,** Sequence of events in experimental metastases of Walker 256 tumor: light, immunofluorescent, and electron microscopic observations, *J. Natl. Cancer Inst.*, 46, 493, 1971.
55. **Menter, D. G., Hatfield, J. S., Harkins, C., Sloane, B. F., Taylor, J. D., Crissman, J. D., and Honn, K. V.,** Tumor cell-platelet interactions *in vitro* and their relationship to *in vivo* arrest of hematogenously circulating tumor cells, *Clin. Exp. Metast.*, 5, 65, 1987.
56. **Honn, K. V., Menter, D. G., Onoda, J. M., Taylor, J. D., and Sloane, B. F.,** Role of prostacyclin as a natural deterrent to hematogenous tumor metastasis, in *Cancer Invasion and Metastasis: Biologic and Therapeutic Aspects,* G. L. Nicolson and L. Milas, Eds., Raven Press, New York, 1984, 361.
57. **Menter, D. G., Harkins, C., Onoda, J. M., Riorden, W., Sloane, B. F., Taylor, J. D., and Honn, K. V.,** Inhibition of tumor cell induced platelet aggregation by prostacyclin and carbacyclin: an ultrastructural study, *Invasion and Metastasis,* 7, 109, 1987.
58. **Chopra, H., Hatfield, J. S., Chang, Y. S., Grossi, I. M., Taylor, J. D., and Honn, K. V.,** Role of tumor cell cytoskeleton and membrane glycoprotein IRGPIIb/IIIa in platelet adhesion to tumor cell membrane and tumor cell induced platelet aggregation, *Cancer Res.*, 48, 3787, 1989.
59. **Bastida, E., Ordinas, A., and Jamieson, G. A.** Differing platelet aggregating effects by tumor cell lines; absence of role for platelet-derived ADP, *Am. J. Hematol.*, 11, 367, 1981.
60. **Bastida, E., Ordinas, A., Giardina, S. L., and Jamieson, G. A.,** Differentiation of platelet-aggregation effects of human tumor cell lines based on inhibition studies with apyrase, hirudin, and phospholipase, *Cancer Res.*, 42, 4348, 1982.
61. **Cavanaugh, P. G., Sloane, B. F., Bajkowski, A. S., Taylor, J. D., and Honn, K. V.,** Purification and characterization of platelet aggregating activity from tumor cells: copurification with procoagulant activity, *Thromb. Res.*, 37, 309, 1985.

62. **Falanga, A. and Gordon, S. G.,** Isolation and characterization of cancer procoagulant: a cysteine proteinase from malignant tissue, *Biochemistry,* 24, 5558, 1985.
63. **Grignani, G. and Jamieson, G. A.,** Tissue factor-dependent activation of platelets by cells and microvesicles of SK-OS-10 human osteogenic sarcoma cell line, *Invasion and Metastasis,* 7, 172, 1987.
64. **Sakai, T. and Kisiel, W.,** Binding of human factors X and Xa to HepG2 and J82 human tumor cell lines, *J. Biol. Chem.,* 265, 9105, 1990.
65. **Yogeeswaran, E. and Salk, P. L.,** Metastatic potential is positively correlated with cell surface sialylation of cultured murine tumor cell lines, *Science,* 212, 1514, 1981.
66. **Bastida, E., Almirall, L., Jamieson, G. A., and Ordinas, A.,** Cell surface sialylation of two human tumor cell lines and its correlation with their platelet-activating activity, *Cancer Res.,* 47, 1767, 1987.
67. **Bastida, E., Ordinas, A., Escolar, G., and Jamieson, G. A.,** Tissue factor in microvesicles shed from U86MG human glioblastoma cells induces coagulation, platelet aggregation, and thrombogenesis, *Blood,* 64, 177, 1984.
68. **Gasic, G. J., Gasic, T. B., and Jimenez, S. A.,** Platelet aggregating material in mouse tumor cells. Removal and regeneration, *Lab. Invest.,* 36, 413, 1977.
69. **Chopra, H., Hatfield, J. S., Fligiel, S. E. G., Grossi, I. M., Chen, Y. Q., Timar, J., Finch, C. A., Fitzgerald, L. A., Taylor, J. D., and Honn, K. V.,** An *in vitro* study on the role of tumor cell cytoskeleton and integrin ^{a}IIbβ3 in tumor cell platelet interactions, submitted.
70. **Chopra, H., Fligiel, S. E. G., Hatfield, J. S., Nelson, K. K., Diglio, C. A., Taylor, J. D., and Honn, K. V.,** An *in vivo* study of the role of the tumor cell cytoskeleton in tumor cell platelet-endothelial cell interactions, *Cancer Res.,* 50, 7686, 1990.
71. **Henderson, D. and Weber, K.,** Immunoelectron microscopical identification of the two types intermediate filaments in established epithelial cells, *Exp. Cell Res.,* 132, 297, 1981.
72. **Hart, I. R., Raz, A., and Fidler, J. I.,** Effect of cytoskeleton disrupting agents on the metastatic behavior of melanoma cells, *J. Natl. Cancer Inst.,* 64, 891, 1980.
73. **Ben-Ze'ev, A. and Raz, A.,** Relationship between the organization and synthesis of vimentin and the metastatic capability of B16 melanoma cells, *Cancer Res.,* 45, 2632, 1985.
74. **Bagge, U., Skolnik, G., and Ericson, L. E.,** The arrest of circulating tumor cells in the liver microcirculation, *J. Cancer Res. Clin. Oncol.,* 105, 134, 1983.
75. **Hynes, R. O.,** A family of surface receptors, *Cell,* 48, 549, 1987.
76. **Akiyama, S. K., Nagata, K., and Yamada, K. M.,** Cell surface receptors for extracellular matrix components, *Biochem. Biophys. Acta,* 1031, 91, 1990.
77. **Charo, I. F., Fitzgerald, L. A., Steinert, B., Rall, S. C., Bekeart, L. S., Phillips, D. R.,** Platelet glycoproteins IIb and IIIa: evidence for a family of immunologically and structurally related glycoproteins in mammalian cells, *Proc. Natl. Acad. Sci. U.S.A.,* 83, 8351, 1986.
78. **Bastida, E., Almirall, L., and Ordinas, A.,** Tumor-cell-induced platelet aggregation is a glycoprotein-dependent and lipoxygenase-associated process, *Int. J. Cancer,* 39, 760, 1987.
79. **Grossi, I. M., Fitzgerald, L. A., Kendall, A., Taylor, J. D., Sloane, B. F., and Honn, K. V.,** Inhibition of human tumor cell induced platelet aggregation by antibodies to platelet glycoproteins Ib and IIb/IIIa, *Proc. Soc. Exp. Biol. Med.,* 186, 378, 1987.
80. **Grossi, I. M., Hatfield, J. S., Fitzgerald, L. A., Newcombe, M., Taylor, J. D., and Honn, K. V.,** Role of tumor cell glycoproteins immunologically related to glycoproteins Ib and IIb/IIIa in tumor cell-platelet and tumor cell-matrix interactions, *FASEB J.,* 2, 2385, 1988.
81. **Chang, Y. S., Fitzgerald, L. A., Grossi, I. M., Sundram, U., Murray, J. A., Honn, K. V.,** Tumor cell expression of mRNAs coding for integrin receptors, *FASEB J.,* 2, A1406, 1988.
82. **Poncz, M., Eisman, R., Heidenreich, R., Silver, S. M., Vilaire, G., Surrey, S., Schwartz, E., and Bennett, J. S.,** Structure of platelet membrane glycoprotein IIb. Homology to the a subunits of the vitronectin and fibronectin membrane receptors, *J. Biol. Chem.,* 262, 8476, 1987.
83. **Karpatkin, S., Pearlstein, E., Ambrogio, C., and Coller, B. S.,** Role of adhesive proteins in platelet tumor interaction *in vitro* and metastasis formation *in vivo, J. Clin. Invest.,* 81, 1012, 1988.
84. **Knudsen, K. A., Smith, L., Smith, S., Karczews, J., and Tuszynski, G. P.,** Role of IIb-IIIa-like glycoproteins in cell substratum adhesion of human melanoma cells, *J. Cell Phys.,* 136, 471, 1988.
85. **McGregor, B. D., McGregor, J. L., Weiss, L. M., Wood, G. S., Chung-Hong, H., and Warnke, R. A.,** Presence of cytoadhesions (IIb-IIIa-like glycoproteins) on human metastatic melanomas but not on benign melanocytes, *Am. J. Clin. Pathol.,* 92, 495, 1989.
86. **Honn, K. V., Grossi, I. M., Nelson, K. K., Umbarger, L. A., Fitzgerald, L. A., Hatfield, J. S., Fligiel, S. E. G., Steinert, B. W., Diglio, C. A., Taylor, J. D., and Onoda, J. M.,** Correlation among expression of the integrin receptor αIIbβ3, tumor cell induced platelet aggregation, tumor cell adhesion and lung colonization in elutriated subpopulations of the B16 amelanotic melanoma and Lewis lung carcinoma, submitted.
87. **Bourkereche, H., Berthier-Vergnes, O., Tabone, E., Dore, J., Leung, L. L. K., and McGregor, J. L.,** Platelet-melanoma cell interaction is mediated by the glycoprotein IIb-IIIa complex, *Blood,* 74, 658, 1989.

88. **Cheresh, D. A., Berliner, S. A., Vicente, V., and Ruggeri, Z. M.,** Recognition of distinct adhesive sites on fibrinogen by related integrins on platelets and endothelial cells, *Cell,* 58, 945, 1989.
89. **Plow, E. F., Ginsberg, M. H., and Marguerie, G. A.,** Expression and function of adhesive proteins on the platelet surface, in *Biochemistry of Platelets,* Phillips, D. R. and Shuman, A., Eds., Academic Press, Orlando, FL, 1986, 160.
90. **Chopra, H., Timar, J., Rong, X., Grossi, I. M., Fitzgerald, L. A., Taylor, J. D., and Honn, K. V.,** The lipoxygenase metabolite 12(S)-HETE induces an actin- and vimentin-dependent increase in integrin $\alpha IIb\beta 3$ surface expression on melanoma cells, submitted.
91. **Onoda, J. M., Nelson, K. K., Grossi, I. M., Umbarger, L. A., Taylor, J. D., and Honn, K. V.,** Separation of high and low metastatic subpopulations from solid tumors by centrifugal elutriation, *Proc. Soc. Exp. Biol. Med.,* 187, 250, 1988.
92. **Rozhin, J., Gomez, A. P., Ziegler, G. H., Nelson, K. K., Chang, Y. S., Fong, D., Onoda, J. M., Honn, K. V., and Sloane, B. F.,** Correlation of cathepsin B and cysteine proteinase inhibitor activities with metastasis in murine tumor subpopulations, *Cancer Res.,* 50, 6278, 1990.
93. **Honn, K. V., Grossi, I. M., Chopra, H., Steinert, B. W., Onoda, J. M., Nelson, K. K., and Taylor, J. D.,** Role of tumour cell eicosanoids and membrane glycoproteins IRGPIb and IRGPIIb/IIIa in metastasis, in *Eicosanoids, Lipid Peroxidation and Cancer,* Nigam, S. et al., Eds., Springer-Verlag, Berlin, 1988, 29.
94. **Needleman, P., Tork, J., Jackschik, B. A., Morrison, A. R., Lefhonith, J. B.,** Arachidonic acid metabolism, *Ann. Rev. Biochem.,* 55, 69, 1986.
95. **Marnett, L. J., Leithauser, M. T., Richards, K. M., Blair, I., Honn, K. V., Yamamoto, S., Yoshimoto, T.,** Arachidonic acid metabolism of cytosolic fractions of Lewis lung carcinoma cells, in *Advances in Prostacyclin, Thromboxane and Leukotriene Research,* Samuelson, B., Paoletti, R., and Ramwell, P., Eds., Vol. 21, Raven Press, New York, 1991, 895.
96. **Grossi, I. M., Fitzgerald, L. A., Umbarger, L. A., Nelson, K. K., Diglio, C. A., Taylor, J. D., Honn, K V.,** Bidirectional control of membrane expression and/or activation of the tumor cell IRGpIIb/IIIa receptor and tumor cell adhesion by lipoxygenase products of arachidonic acid and linoleic acid, *Cancer Res.,* 49, 1029, 1989.
97. **Honn, K. V., Grossi, I. M., Fitzgerald, L. A., Umbarger, L. A., Diglio, C. A., and Taylor, J. D.,** Lipoxygenase products regulate IRGpIIb/IIIa receptor mediated adhesion of tumor cell to endothelial cells, subendothelial matrix, and fibronectin, *Proc. Soc. Exp. Biol. Med.,* 189, 130, 1988.
98. **Hamberg, M. and Samuelsson, B.,** Prostaglandin endoperoxides: novel transformations of arachidonic acid in human platelets, *Proc. Natl. Acad. Sci. U.S.A.,* 71, 3400, 1974.
99. **Honn, K. V., Steinert, B. W., Moin, K., Onoda, J. M., Taylor, J. D., and Sloane, B. F.,** The role of platelet cyclooxygenase and lipoxygenase pathways in tumor cell induced platelet aggregation, *Biochem. Biophys. Res. Commun.,* 145, 384, 1987.
100. **Marcus, A. J., Safier, L. B., Ullman, H. L., Johan-Broekman, M., Islam, W., Oglesby, T. D., and Goldman, R. R.,** 12(S)-20-Dihydroeicosatetraenoic acid: a new icosanoid synthesized by neutrophils from (12S)-hydroeicosatetraenoic acid produced by thrombin or collagen stimulated platelets, *Proc. Natl. Acad. Sci. U.S.A.,* 81, 903, 1984.
101. **Marcus, A. J., Safier, L. B., Ullman, H. L., Islam, W., Johan-Broekkman, M., Falck, M., Fischer, S., and Vonschacky, C.,** Platelet-neutrophil interaction. 12(S),20-Dihydroeicosatetraen-1, 20-dienoic acid: a new icosanoid synthesized by unstimulated neutrophils from 12(S), 20-Dihydroeicosatetraenoic acid, *J. Biol. Chem.,* 263, 2223, 1988.
102. **Schafer, A. I., Takayama, H., Farrell, S., and Gimborne, M. A., Jr.,** Incorporation of platelet and leukocyte lipoxygenase metabolites by cultured vascular cells, *Blood,* 67, 373, 1986.
103. **Honn, K. V., Grossi, I. M., Diglio, C. A., and Taylor, J. D.,** Role of 12-lipoxygenase metabolites and integrin glycoprotein receptors in metastasis, in *New Concepts in Cancer,* Etievant, C., Cros, J., and Rustum, Y. M., Eds., Vol. 3, Macmillan Press, London, 1990, 42.
104. **Huang, F.-C., Shoupe, T. S., Lin, C. J., Lee, T. D. Y., Chan, W.-K., Tan, J., Schnapper, M., Sun, J. T., Gordon, R. J., Sonnino, P. A., Sutherland, C. A., Van Inwegen, R. G., and Coutts, S. M.,** Differential effects of a series of hydroxamic acid derivatives on 5-lipoxygenase and cyclooxygenase from neutrophils and 12-lipoxygenase from platelets and their *in vivo* effects on inflammation and anaphylaxis, *J. Med. Chem.,* 32, 1836, 1989.
105. **Honn, K. V.,** unpublished observations.
106. **Timar, J. and Honn, K. V.,** unpublished observations.
107. **Grossi, I. M. and Honn, K. V.,** unpublished observations.

Chapter 8

THE THROMBOTIC CONSEQUENCES OF MALIGNANCY

Mohan Chelladurai

TABLE OF CONTENTS

I. INTRODUCTION

An association between coagulation and cancer has been noticed since 1865 and was coined Trousseau's syndrome after its observer who first noted a high incidence of venous thrombosis in a series of patients with gastric carcinoma.[1] There now is documented evidence to support a link between thromboembolic disorders and neoplastic disease. The survival of cancer patients is not only dependent upon the progression of the primary tumor but more so on the successful dissemination of cancer cells via the metastatic cascade. Metastasis is the process whereby a tumor cell growing at a primary site detaches itself, migrates through the body via the vascular or lymphatic system to a secondary site, attaches to the endothelium or subendothelial matrix, and invades the host tissue to start a secondary colony. In order for metastasis to be successful, the tumor cell has to be able to escape from the host's immune system until it can attach to the secondary site. There has been increasing evidence in the past few years that coagulation proteins and platelets can contribute to the protection of the tumor cells from the host immune system and aid in the attachment of tumor cells to damaged endothelial regions to facilitate subsequent intravasation.

In this review, a brief account will be provided of several lines of evidence, suggesting the role of the blood coagulation process in metastasis. A summary is also given of pathways leading to thrombin generation and of some proteins related to the fate of active thrombin. The intimate role of platelets in coagulation and metastasis is also discussed, although superficially, and the reader is referred to Chapter 7 for details. The main focus of this chapter will be placed on tumor-related protein factors that may directly initiate thrombin generation and thus promote the metastatic cascade. Experimental details on a recently detected procoagulant will be presented. Finally, some problems associated with this research area will also be addressed.

II. THE INTERRELATIONSHIP BETWEEN COAGULATION AND CANCER

A. CLINICAL EVIDENCE

Three groups of evidence support an important relationship between blood coagulation and tumor hemostasis: clinical, histologic, and pharmacologic.[2,3] Clinical lines of evidence lie in the observation that there is a high percentage of cancer patients with concurrent thromboembolic disorders. In one study, Ambrus and associates reported that thrombosis and/or bleeding was the second most common cause of death in cancer patients.[4] This increased presence of thromboembolic disorders seen in cancer patients led to the investigation of the possible existence of blood disorders in them. Abnormalities of routine tests of blood coagulation have been reported to occur in as many as 92% of patients with cancer.[5] Elevation of fibrinogen-fibrin degradation products,[5,6] elevation of plasma fibrinogen, Factor V, Factor VIII or other clotting factors,[5,7,8] abnormally rapid fibrinogen turnover, and circulating fibrin monomers are some of the typical characteristics in cancer patients. As a consequence, prolonged prothrombin and thrombin times are observed.[9] This evidence is consistent with the presence in cancer patients of overcompensated intravascular coagulation with fibrinolysis.[10] For example, studies have demonstrated that an upward trend of fibrinopeptide A (FPA) levels appear to parallel progression of clinical disease. A positive correlation has been observed between the elevated levels of FPA and FPB patients with leukemia.[11] FPA is a 16-amino acid peptide cleaved from the a chain of fibrinogen by thrombin. Since the plasma half-disappearance time for FPA is 4 min, plasma levels of the peptide reflect ongoing coagulation.[12] Plasma levels of FPA, therefore, provide a kinetic measure of fibrinogen cleavage. The use of FPA levels, measured by radioimmunoassay, to monitor progress of treatment was contemplated. However, it has become evident that antibodies to the fibrinopeptide crossreacts with fragment of fibrin cleaved by plasmin, hence, raising concern about the specificity of the assay.

Although platelets have yet to be reported in association with extravascular fibrin deposits of solid tumors in animals or humans, there has been a significant amount of evidence to support an important role of platelets in the protection of tumor cells while traversing the circulatory or lymphatic systems as well as in the growth and adhesion of tumor cells to vascular cell matrices.[13-16] Thrombocytopenia, abnormal platelet function, and evidence for *in vivo* activation of platelets all have been reported to occur with increased frequency in cancer patients. Estimates of thrombocytopenia vary from 4% in patients with inoperable lung cancer to 11% in a large series of patients with a variety of tumors.[5,17] In experiments with rabbits, Wood et al. found that tumor cells injected intravenously were trapped in the microvasculature and formed aggregates with platelets and fibrin.[18,19] Several studies have documented either increased platelet destruction or evidence for an *in vivo* platelet activation and release.[20-22] Thrombocytosis that occurs more frequently in untreated patients with cancer may also be explained by the existence of low-grade disseminated intravascular coagulation (DIC), thrombocytolysis, and mechanisms of overcompensation by the host.[23] Thrombopoietic activity has been recovered from serum of patients with cancer and thrombocytosis, suggesting an aberrancy in the usual relationship between platelet count and the production of thrombopoietin in some individuals with cancer.[24]

The mechanisms postulated for the enhancement of metastasis by platelets include promotion of tumor cell clumping with platelets or other blood cells[25,26] and formation of a protective embolus around tumor cells that shields the cells from the host defense system.[27,28] Tumor cells are thought to interact with cytotoxic factors such as macrophages, natural killer cells, or antibody-mediated complement lysis or by shear forces and mechanical trauma and thus are damaged while in passage through the microvasculature. Gorelik et al.[28] have demonstrated that platelets may protect tumor cells from natural killer-cell mediated lysis. Weiss et al.[29] have postulated that friction between the tumor cell periphery and the capillary wall exceeds the critical level for tumor cell rupture. Tumor cells shielded within platelet thrombi may thus be protected from some or all of the above. Finally, platelet mitogenic factors (i.e., platelet derived growth factor) released from activated thrombocytes may enhance tumor cell growth. Platelets also may enhance metastasis by facilitating processes that occur during tumor cell arrest and adhesion;[30,31] whether that includes direct facilitation of adhesion and/or protection of arrested tumor cells from cellular immune destruction[28] is not clear.

In order to form a metastasis, a circulating tumor cell must arrest in the microvasculature, form stable adhesions with attachments to the endothelium or basement membrane, and escape destruction by shear forces or cellular immune mechanisms, all in order to undergo extravasation. Tumor cell adhesion to endothelium and basement membrane are affected by several factors. Irimura and co-workers[32,33] have described a role for surface sialogalactoproteins in tumor cell binding to endothelial cell monolayers, endothelial extracellular matrix, and immobilized fibronectin. Pretreatment of cells with the antibiotic tunicamycin, which inhibits formation of asparagine-linked oligosaccharide chains of glycoproteins,[34,35] results in decreased adhesiveness to the above substrata as well as decreased lung colony formation.[32] Murray and co-workers demonstrated that metastatic tumor cells attach preferentially to type IV collagen.[36] This attachment can be enhanced by laminin and blocked by antilaminin antibody, but cannot be enhanced by fibronectin nor blocked by antifibronectin antibody. In addition, tumor cells that demonstrate laminin-enhanced attachment to type IV collagen produce more pulmonary tumor colonies *in vivo;* this lung colony formation can be decreased by antilaminin antibody.[37] Platelets are now implicated in tumor cell attachment to substrata. Varani and co-workers[38] recently have shown that platelet-released thrombospondin induces attachment and spreading of human carcinomas. Menter et al.[39] and Grossi et al.[40] have suggested that platelets enhance tumor cell adhesion to the endothelial cell matrix probably via glycoproteins Ib and IIb/IIIa. Preferred attachment proteins may vary among tumor types.[41] Schirrmacher et al.[42] have elegantly demonstrated that the metastatic capacity of a range of murine tumor cell lines is regulated by the degree of sialylation of two sugar moieties (*D*-galactose and *N*-acetylgalactosamine) found in animal cell membranes. Clearly, a number of tumor cell surface determinants may be involved in tumor arrest and adhesion to the vessel wall. In addition to these tumor cell surface determinants, the interaction of circulating tumor cells with host platelets and the blood coagulation system is believed to facilitate metastasis. This may be due in part to the ability of platelets to enhance tumor cell adhesion to the vessel wall.[43]

B. HISTOLOGIC EVIDENCE

Secondly, histologic evidence supports a connection between coagulation and cancer. In 1878, Billroth first reported his autopsy observations that human tumor cells were found frequently in association with thrombi.[44] More recent immunochemical and ultrastructural studies have confirmed the presence of fibrin deposition in and around both animal and human tumors.[45] Several observations have been made by examining model systems of tumor cell injections as a function of time. One such example involves the observations made following the implantations of line 1 or the highly malignant line 10 of a bile duct carcinoma in guinea pigs.[46] A gelatinous material rich in fibrin was observed shortly after tumor implantation in the subcutaneous spaces. Initially, the fibrin gel was relatively acellular, but after several days, an infiltrate of neutrophils and monocytes was observed. In the line 1 tumors, an exuberant inflammatory reaction led to the eventual replacement of the fibrin gel by connective tissue and subsequent tumor rejection. In line 10 tumors, the fibrin gel developed to a lesser extent, the inflammatory response was less dramatic, organization did not occur, and the tumor growth was not limited. In experimental situations, similar histologic evidence for the association of platelet thrombi deposited in the vicinity of growing tumor cells supports a possible contributory role for platelets and platelet products in the process of tumor growth.[47-49]

C. PHARMACOLOGIC EVIDENCE

Finally, there is pharmacological evidence that seems to comply with the clinical and histological evidences outlined above. The pharmacologic evidence lies in the effects of anticoagulant and antiplatelet agents on tumor growth and metastasis. Antiplatelet antibodies, capable of inducing thrombocytopenia, can reduce significantly the formation of lung implants following the intravenous infusion of TA3 tumor cells in mice.[50] This protective effect can be reversed with platelet transfusions. Support is also found in studies where thromboxane inhibitors prostacyclin may modulate the growth of B16 amelanotic melanoma cells in syngeneic mice.[51,52] Not all experimental tumors, however, respond to all platelet function inhibitors. For example, negative results have been reported with the use of aspirin for the treatment of VX2 carcinoma in rabbits[53] and with the use of aspirin, RA-223, bencyclan, or cyproheptadine for the treatment of Lewis lung carcinoma in mice.[54] The role of platelets in metastasis therefore needs further resolution before any substantial conclusion can be made.

The inhibitory effects of anticoagulant drugs on various properties of tumor cells have been recognized for at least 30 years since Strauss and Saphir first reported the effects of the vitamin K antagonist dicoumarol on circulating carcinoma cells in rabbits.[55] Coumarin derivatives can inhibit tumor cell locomotion, metabolism, lung colony formation, and the development of spontaneous metastases in various experimental tumor systems.[56-58] Upon recent review, it appears that the effects of coumarin drugs in the treatment of cancer are mediated by their ability to interfere with the utilization of vitamin K[56] since administration of vitamin K promptly reverses the salutary effects. Also experimental vitamin K deficiency provides similar protection from metastasis formation.[57,58] Other inhibitors of blood coagulation have antimetastatic properties in experimental tumor models. For instance, tumor growth suppression has been observed following the use of heparin, which acts presumably by impairing fibrin deposition or accelerating fibrinolysis.[59] The results of one study by the Veterans Administration on the use of warfarin in the treatment of small cell carcinoma of the lung (SCCL) was the first randomized controlled study of this agent as an anticancer drug.[60] The median survival of patients who received warfarin in addition to standard chemotherapy was significantly twofold greater than the median survival of subjects who received chemotherapy alone. Although the data of this study are consistent with the hypothesis that warfarin interferes with local fibrin formation and tumor growth, no consistent relationship was demonstrated between their results and the therapeutic effect. Furthermore, some caution needs to be taken in interpreting the results of this study due to the small sample size and negative results of another randomized study of warfarin treatment of SCCL. While the above pharmacological evidence does not firmly substantiate a connection between the inhibitory effects of antiplatelet and anticoagulant drugs, there is evidence to indicate that such a relationship may exist.

III. THE COAGULATION CASCADE

Before discussing some of the proteins that may contribute to the relationship between coagulation and metastasis, a summary of the coagulant cascade and some regulatory pathways will follow. Details of this pathway have been reviewed elsewhere.[61] The pathway leading to a fibrin clot may be thought of as a zymogen cascade. It contains several proteins that exist in an inactive form until they are proteolytically activated to be capable of carrying out their respective functions. Most of these factors are serine proteases that have serine, aspartate, and histidine associated with their active site pockets. Generally, these enzymes hydrolyze the peptide bond at the carboxy terminal of arginine, thereby, activating their substrate. In most instances, an activation peptide is released. There are at least three protein cofactors that dramatically enhance the rate of coagulation without proteolytic activity. These are FV, FVIII, and tissue factor. A characteristic common to Factors II, V, VII, IX, X, Protein C, and Protein S is their dependence on carboxylation reactions for the formation of an active species. These carboxylation reactions require vitamin K as a cofactor, and the proteins are hence referred to as vitamin K dependent. In the presence of vitamin K, specific glutamic acid residues near the amino terminal end of the proteins are posttranslationally modified to gamma carboxylated residues or "gla" residues. This modification permits the binding of the protein to divalent calcium and aids in bringing into close proximity other coagulant proteins for activation. A surface required for activation is provided either by phospholipids or platelets.

The entire activation sequence is diagramed in Figure 1. There are two major initiating pathways to the entire cascade: the extrinsic and the intrinsic. These two pathways function independently initially but converge at the activation of factors IX and X. The extrinsic involves a combination of tissue factor and FVII involved in the direct activation of FIX or FX. Slight disruption of the cell surface leads to an active expression of tissue factor. The intrinsic pathway can involve either a surface activation (−charge glass, for example) of HMW kininogen, prekallikrein, kallikrein, Factor XIa, or plasmin. The result of this initiation reaction is the production of FXIa. Both pathways result in the activation of FX. Activated FX catalyzes the conversion of prothrombin to thrombin. In the "prothrombinase complex", FXa is accommodated on the platelet surface, presumably on its receptor, the cofactor FVa. Binding is mediated via divalent calcium. This complex then hydrolyzes prothrombin to thrombin. Several coagulation factors, including Factors V and VIII and fibrinogen, are

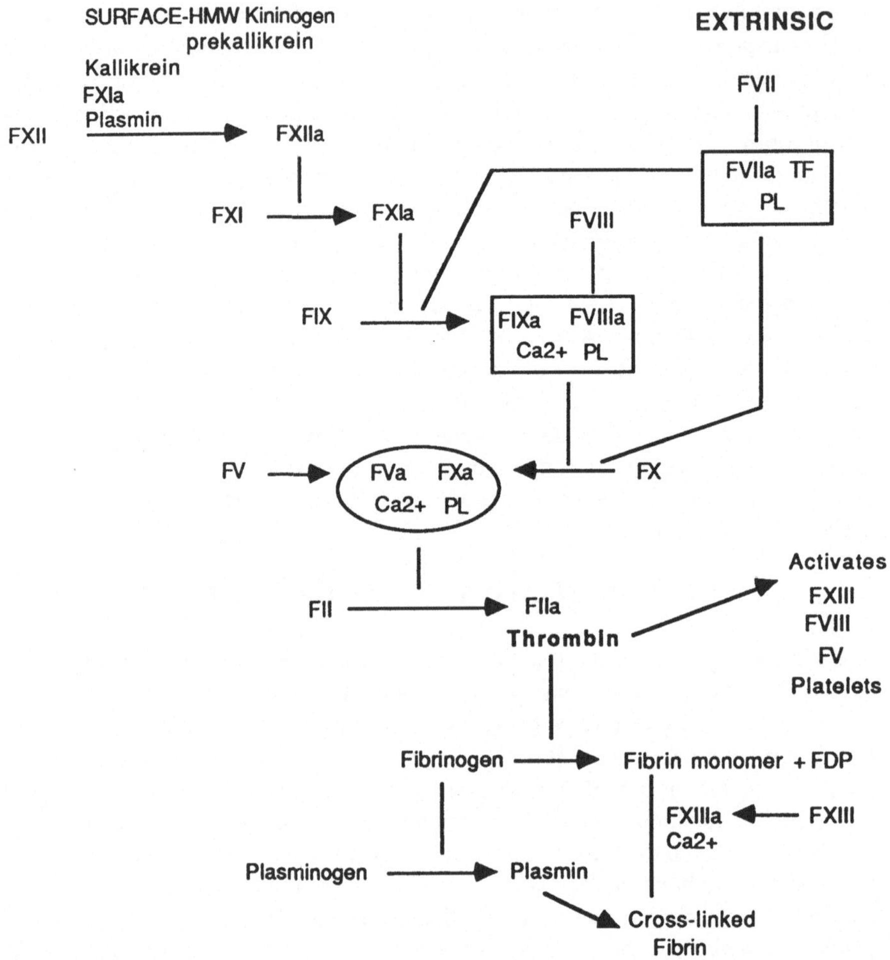

FIGURE 1. The overall scheme of reactions in the coagulation cascade. PL = platelets; a = active form.

secreted from platelet α-granules. Since the platelet arises from megakaryocytes and is unable to synthesize proteins, coagulation proteins may either be synthesized in the liver and taken up into megakaryocytes or synthesized directly in megakaryocytes. Comparisons between the plasma and platelet factors have thus far revealed no differences.

The endothelial cell, on the other hand, has always been thought of as an antithrombogenic agent. The major evidence supporting its anticoagulant properties was the finding of membrane-bound thrombomodulin, a protein that complexes with thrombin to activate protein C.[62] More recently, Stern and co-workers[63] have presented strong support for the idea that the endothelial cell may indeed be thrombogenic. Endotoxin-treated cells[64] have been shown to release tissue factor, and Factor XI may be activated on the endothelial cell surface as easily as on the platelet surface.

The role of tissue factor in coagulation has also been questioned by Zur and co-workers.[65] They have presented convincing evidence that FVII has an inherent capacity to activate FX without tissue factor. FXa would in turn activate more FVII, resulting in a subsequent increased production of FXa.

Thus, once the cascade has been activated, the series of proteolytic reactions that follow lead to the production of the key protein in the entire process: thrombin. Thrombin is the central and multifunctional proteolytic enzyme in the coagulation cascade. There are two major advantages to having several steps in generating thrombin. By virtue of definition, an enzyme, or catalyst, will lower the activation energy in converting a substrate to a product without being immediately used up in the process. Thus, one molecule of Factor XIIa may catalyze the production of, for example, 10 molecules of Factor XIa and so on. This cascade or waterfall hypothesis was first proposed by Davie and Ratnoff[66] and MacFarlane.[67] This amplification will result in the production of a very large amount of thrombin. A second advantage would be an increased opportunity to regulate the generation of thrombin as will become evident later. Thrombin hydrolyzes soluble fibrinogen to insoluble fibrin, which, the end product of the cascade, is then crosslinked by a transglutaminase reaction catalyzed by Factor XIIIa, also activated by thrombin. Monomers of fibrin associate via hydrogen bonding, and these chains of fibrin are readily soluble in 8 *M* urea. Crosslinking by FXIIIa renders the fibrin mesh insoluble to urea. Thrombin may be controlled by one of two ways. Plasma contains several protease inhibitors, including antithrombin and α2-macroglobulin, which may inactivate thrombin. The generation of thrombin in the blood coagulation cascade is controlled by such proteins as FVIII and FV, which are in turn activated by thrombin. Under certain conditions, thrombin will activate anticoagulants that will work to negate its generation. For example, thrombin will bind to thrombomodulin, an endothelial-bound membrane protein. In this form, thrombin will no longer hydrolyze fibrinogen or activate platelets. Instead, the thrombin-thrombomodulin complex will activate protein C in the presence of protein S. Activated protein C will hydrolyze coagulation factors Va[68] and VIIIa,[69] thus inhibiting the production of thrombin. Two proteins also have been isolated from platelets that may regulate thrombin activity.[70,71] These proteins of 74 kDa and 55 kDa individually inhibit thrombin activity, but together, they enhance by twofold the activity of thrombin. Furthermore, these proteins significantly reduce the rate of the inhibition of thrombin by antithrombin.[72] The 74 and 55 kDa proteins also have been detected in plasma and may contribute to the regulation of thrombin in a similar manner. Thus, thrombin's action in blood coagulation may be controlled by autoregulation of its production. (The activities of thrombin are shown in Figure 2.)

IV. TUMOR PROCOAGULANTS

Survival of cancer patients is largely dependent on the events of the metastatic cascade. Metastasis may be described as the sequence of events, whereby a tumor cell growing at a primary site successfully detaches itself, migrates, either singly or in a small group, to a distant part of the body, and sets up a secondary colony. It was initially thought that carcinomas spread via the lymphatic system while tumors of mesenchymal origin metastasized through the vascular system. Hilgard and co-workers[73] showed that tumor cells injected into the lymph eventually reached the bloodstream. It is now generally accepted that tumor cells may move freely between the vascular and lymphatic systems.[74,75] Intravasation and successful transportation through the bloodstream would require some form of protective mechanism since it would be natural for the host cell to recognize the offending tumor cell as nonself. There has been increasing evidence in recent years that platelets and the coagulation cascade contribute to (1) protection of tumor cells from the host immune system and (2) attachment of tumor cells to damaged endothelial regions to facilitate subsequent extravasation. Anticoagulant therapy with warfarin and other coumarins consistently results in a reduction of lung colony formation and spontaneous metastasis, suggesting strongly that components of blood coagulation facilitate metastasis. However, the effect of warfarin on tumor cells, independent of its action as an anticoagulant, should also be considered. O'Meara and his associates were the first to study a tumor-derived procoagulant activity.[76] Four separate factors have since been identified as responsible for the initiation of blood coagulation by tumor cells. The first of these is tissue factor, a lipoprotein also associated with normal tissue.[77,78] The second, cancer procoagulant, is a cysteine proteinase that directly

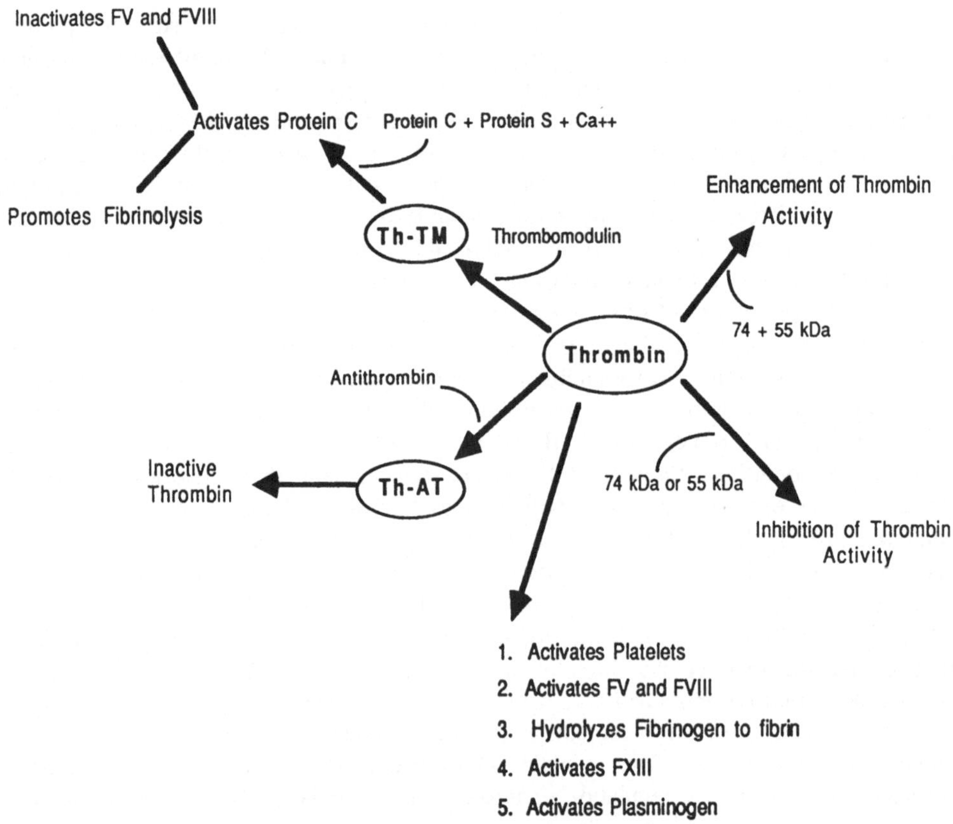

FIGURE 2. The physiologic activities of thrombin.

activates factor X.[79] Fasco and co-workers have described a third Factor X activator activity.[80] The fourth is a platelet aggregating activity/procoagulant activity (PAA/PCA) isolated from solid tumors or from tumor cells grown in culture.[81] Evidence of yet another tumor procoagulant with properties different from those described above will be presented in this paper.

A. TISSUE FACTOR

Several investigators have suggested that the acceleration of coagulation induced by tumor cells may be due to released thromboplastin (tissue factor). The activity of thromboplastin is distinct from other procoagulants in its dependence on coagulation Factor VII for expression of activity.[69] Absence of clotting in Factor VII-deficient plasma has, therefore, been used as the criterion for identifying tumor procoagulant activity as thromboplastin. Based on this criterion, Kinjo et al.,[82] Hudij and Bajaj,[83] Khato et al.,[84] and Dvorak et al.[85] have concluded that tumor cell lines coagulate plasma through a thromboplastin-dependent mechanism. These studies did not take into account the possibility that the cultured tumor cells may themselves have adsorbed Factor VII on their surfaces from the serum used as growth supplement in the tissue culture media. However, Gouault-Heilman et al.[86] have provided substantiative evidence that thromboplastin may indeed be one factor responsible for tumor procoagulant activity by showing that antibodies to human brain thromboplastin neutralize the procoagulant activity of human leukemia promyelocytes. Thromboplastin has not been purified from tumor tissue, making it difficult to compare the various tissue factor-like activities present in normal and tumor tissue. Tissue factor has been purified from normal brain tissue by two groups using Factor VII affinity chromatography.[64,65] It has an apparent molecular weight of 44,000 to 46,000. The protein has an absolute requirement for lipids for activity, operating best at protein:lipids ratios of 1:600. Tissue factor catalyses the hydrolysis of Factor IX and X by Factor VIIa.

B. CANCER PROCOAGULANT

Gordon and co-workers[79,87-91] purified cancer procoagulant (CP) from a soluble extract of rabbit VX2 carcinoma cells, which were extracted at alkaline pH (7.8). The M_r of purified CP is 68,000; the procoagulant activity of CP requires phospholipid. Procoagulant activity of CP is proteolytic as evidenced by the presence of low M_r peptides in SDS-PAGE of incubates of CP with protein substrates. This procoagulant/proteolytic activity can be inhibited with iodoacetamide and mercury and reactivated with potassium cyanide, dithiothreitol, and EDTA, suggesting that CP may be a cysteine proteinase, although no specific cysteine proteinase substrates have been tested. The apparent stability of CP in alkaline pH used during isolation procedures is unusual for lysosomal cysteine proteinases;[92] thus, CP appears to be a nonlysosomal cysteine proteinase. Although tumor-associated cathepsin B has enhanced stability at neutral and alkaline pH,[93] this stability would not be maintained over the extended time required for purification. CP differs in amino acid composition from other known cysteine proteinases.[79] Gordon and co-workers[94] have recently shown that in addition to activation of Factor X, CP will also hydrolytically inactivate Protein S, a cofactor in Protein C activity. Thus, the ability of activated Protein C to inactivate FVa or FVIIIa will be destroyed. The authors suggest that a hypercoagulable state may be present in cancer patients bearing tumors rich in cancer procoagulant activity.

C. FACTOR X ACTIVATOR

Fasco and co-workers[80] have identified a Factor X activator from Lewis lung tumor cells that may play a role in promoting metastasis. Tumor cells grown in normal rodent serum expressed a five- to eightfold higher Factor X activator activity than cells grown in the presence of serum adsorbed with barium sulfate and thus, rendered free of vitamin K-dependent proteins. Injection of Lewis lung tumor cells subcultured in normal serum into recipient C57BL/6J mice gave primary tumors that grew at a linear rate, had good Factor X activator activity, and produced secondary lung foci within 10 d of injection. Lewis lung cells grown in deficient sera did not produce metastatic colonies. Exposure of cells grown in deficient sera to normal mouse serum partially restored both Factor X activator activity as well as metastatic potential. The authors suggest that this Factor X activator may be related to cancer procoagulant. Polyclonal antibodies raised against cancer procoagulant crossreact with a protein from Lewis lung cells as well as from a number of other warfarin-sensitive murine tumors.

D. PLATELET AGGREGATING ACTIVITY/PROCOAGULANT ACTIVITY

Studies by Cavanaugh et al. have shown that yet another procoagulant protein is produced by tumor cells. This protein also expresses platelet aggregatory activity.[81] It appears that the platelet aggregatory activity is induced by thrombin generated by the tumor protein since aggregation of platelets was observed only in the presence of plasma. No aggregation is seen with washed platelets (i.e., in the absence of plasma). Of significance are the observations that the tumor procoagulant (1) does not have any proteolytic activity and (2) induces coagulation in normal plasma and in plasma from patients deficient in any one of the coagulation factors V, VII, VIII, IX, XI and XII. These properties set it apart from cancer procoagulant and from tissue factor.

E. OTHER SOURCES OF TUMOR PROCOAGULANTS

A large number of murine and human tumor cells have been reported to have both procoagulant and platelet aggregatory activity (for example see References 95 to 102). In most instances, intact tumor cells were incubated with either recalcified plasma or with platelets in heparinized plasma. Scarlett and colleagues[95] systematically compared the effect of at least two types of tumor cells with respect to activation of the coagulation process. One set of colon carcinoma cells induced platelet aggregation in heparinized plasma via thrombin generation. This was evidenced by the requirement of Factor VII, suggesting that these cells may produce tissue factor. Another group of cells, however, induced platelet aggregation by a calcium requiring process and was thought to be mediated by ADP since apyrase inhibited the aggregation reaction. At this time, no information is available as to the factor or factors in these tumor cells responsible for activation platelets or the coagulation cascade. Kimura and co-workers[98] found no correlation between experimental metastatic potential and platelet aggregating activity when using melanoma cells in citrated platelet-rich plasma.

As described above, the procoagulant activity associated with tumor cells or attached stromal cells would promote the generation of thrombin, which is a potent and physiologic activator of platelets. It would be intuitive that platelets would be activated in the vicinity of tumor cells. Indeed, intravenously injected tumor cells were observed to induce platelet aggregation.[103] Thrombocytopenia induced by neuraminidase or antiplatelet antiserum results in decreased lung colony formation from tail vein-injected tumor cells,[104-108] and spontaneous metastasis from subcutaneous tumors[106,109] provide additional support for the role of platelets in metastasis.

V. A NOVEL TUMOR PROCOAGULANT AND ITS ROLE IN METASTASIS

Studies carried out by several investigators have shown that platelets and the coagulation cascade probably make a significant contribution towards metastasis. It was the interest of this author to delineate the role of a tumor procoagulant in the overall scheme of metastasis. I have recently identified a procoagulant in murine tumors with properties very different from any of the others described above. Subcellular fractionation of B16 amelanotic melanoma cells has shown that the procoagulant activity of interest resides primarily in the plasma membrane. Since the B16a line is of epithelial origin, fractions from another cell type of the same origin, namely the liver, was also studied. Normal liver tissue also expresses procoagulant activity in the plasma membrane fractions but at much lower specific activities. Furthermore, the malignant counterpart of the liver, the murine hepatoma, has 60,000-fold higher procoagulant activity than normal liver. This suggests that transformation of cells may result in increased expression of the procoagulant protein. The existence of tumor cell heterogeneity combined with one's ability to isolate cells of varying densities by centrifugal elutriation permits the isolation of a number of subpopulations of cells from a single solid tumor. These subpopulations behave differently when tested for their lung colonizing ability. Cells of higher metastatic potential expressed higher specific activities of the tumor procoagulant protein, hence, a positive correlation between metastatic potential and increased expression of tumor procoagulant protein. These studies suggest that a tumor protein with procoagulant activity may promote metastatic events. At this time, it is not clear if the increased activity observed in cells of higher lung colony forming ability is due to increased protein concentration (i.e., antigen concentration) or due to increased surface expression. Increased total procoagulant concentration would mean alteration of transcriptional or translational rates or mechanisms while increased surface expression would suggest an upregulation of the protein. Continued progress in this work lines should enable me to, in the long term, delineate the relationship between the expression of tumor procoagulant protein and tumor cell metastasis. Details of my recent studies are provided below.

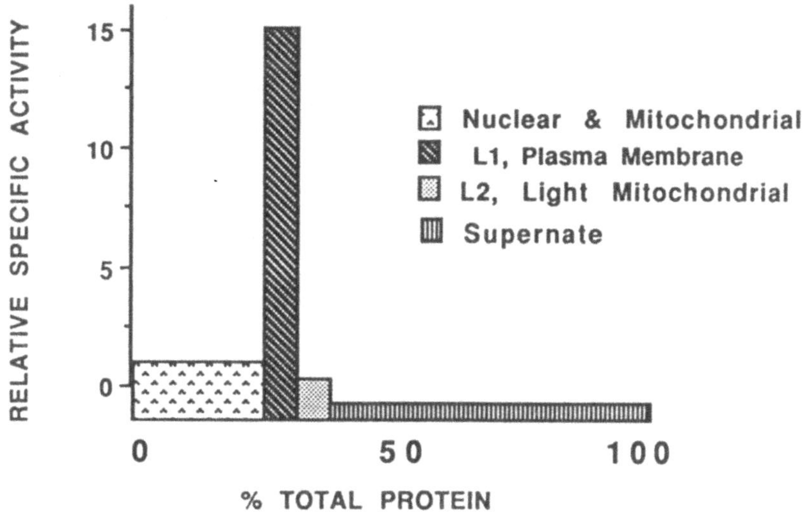

FIGURE 3. Procoagulant activity of B16a tumor cells is localized in the plasma membrane. Results are expressed as relative specific activity with respect to specific activity in tumor homogenates.

A. INTACT TUMOR CELLS WILL INDUCE BLOOD COAGULATION

Intact tumor cells will induce blood coagulation.[81] It has been verified that intact B16a tumor cells either grown in culture or obtained from solid tumors by dispersal and centrifugal elutriation (see below and Reference 110 for isolation of elutriated cells), also enhance coagulation when added to plasma and recalcified. The clotting times are measured in a Sienco sonoclot, which records an increase in the viscosity of the fibrin clot as it forms. In addition, intact cells from two human carcinoma cell lines, the clone A cell line derived from colon tumor and the small cell carcinoma of the lung, also exhibit potent procoagulant activity in this assay. Preliminary assays with normal human melanocytes and a human melanoma (kindly supplied by Dr. Herlyn, Wistar Institute, Philadelphia) show that the activity of procoagulant protein in the melanoma is about 176-fold greater than that in the normal melanocyte. In one experiment, the specific activity of procoagulant protein from normal melanocytes was 12.5 units/10^6 cells while the specific activity from the human melanoma was 2200 units/10^6cells.

B. DISTRIBUTION OF TUMOR PROCOAGULANT IN PLASMA MEMBRANES OF TUMOR CELLS

The observation that intact tumor cells of the B16a cell line are capable of inducing blood coagulation is supported by the finding that the procoagulant activity is localized in the plasma membrane (Figure 3).

Two possible explanations for the observation that intact tumor cells induce coagulation are (1) release of tumor procoagulant from cells and (2) membrane localization of the tumor protein and exposure of the procoagulant to the cell surface exterior. Others[63,111] have reported that tissue factor is released from tumor cells as well as from endothelial cells upon stimulation by endotoxins. In attempts to delineate the distribution of the protein in cells, B16a tumor cells were homogenized, and subcellular fractions were isolated according to the modified[112] method of DeDuve et al.[113] except that the nuclear and mitochondrial fractions were combined. Briefly, the procedure was as follows:

All isolation procedures were carried out at 4°C. Fresh tumors (5 g wet weight) were finely minced with scissors, suspended in 50 ml of 25 m*M* HEPES buffer pH 7.5 containing

TABLE 1
Comparison of Procoagulant Activity in Subcellular Fractions of Various Tissues

Tissue	Homogenate specific activity (units/mg protein)	Subcellular fraction specific activity (units/mg protein)				
		N & M[a]	L[b]	S[c]	L1[d]	L2[e]
B16a melanoma	1,425	649	2,516	276	10,365	824
Mouse liver	0.052	0.036	0.353	0.062	0.539	1.45
Hepatoma	3,173	1,348	98,039	4,760	197,220	204,718

[a] Nuclear and mitochondrial fraction
[b] Light mitochondrial fraction
[c] Supenatant or cytosolic fraction
[d] Plasma membrane fraction
[e] Lysosomal fraction

5% sucrose and 0.9% NaCl (homogenate buffer), and homogenized by ten strokes in a Potter-Elvejheim homogenizer. The cell homogenate was passed through a muslin gauze and an aliquot of filtered homogenate kept for analysis. The filtrate was centrifuged at 6,700 × g for 7 min in a Beckman Ti45 rotor. The pellet that contained the nuclear and mitochondrial fraction was washed once with 20 ml of buffer, and the centrifugation was repeated. The pellet was resuspended and kept aside for analysis. The supernates of these runs were pooled and centrifuged at 15,100 × g for 19 min in the same rotor. The resulting pellet, the light mitochondrial fraction, was resuspended in 9 ml of 30% isotonic percoll and centrifuged at 60,000 × g for 18 min. The light mitochondrial fraction was distributed into two bands; a fluffy band near the top of the centrifuge tube is the plasma membrane or L1 fraction, and the second, close to the bottom of the tube, is the L2 or lysosomal fraction. The bands were separately transferred to Ti 50 tubes, filled with homogenate buffer, and centrifuged at 144,000 × g in a Ti 50 rotor. The L1 and L2 pellets were resuspended in homogenate buffer and kept at 4°C until analysis. As shown in Figure 3, 85% of the specific activity was distributed in the L1 or plasma membrane fraction. Approximately 5.4% of the specific activity was found in the nuclear and mitochondrial fraction, and 6.8% was found in the L2 or lysosomal fraction. For comparison, cells from normal murine liver as well as from murine hepatoma were also fractionated. Specific activities of procoagulant protein in subcellular fractions of all tissues tested are provided in Table 1. While both the B16a and the hepatoma have substantially increased procoagulant activity in the plasma membrane fraction compared to the control, the presence of a large proportion of procoagulant activity in the L2 fraction of the hepatoma is not clear at this time. It is recognized that the subcellular fractions are contaminated with protein from other compartments.[100] Hence, this study was verified with the analyses of several enzymes of known distribution. In addition to measuring the specific activities of tumor procoagulant protein, the specific activities of a variety of enzymes, including β-hexosaminidase, Na+, K+ −ATPase, glucose-6-phosphatase, β-glucuronidase, and galactosyltransferase, were also determined. The results are shown in Table 1. Measurements of all these enzymes confirmed the purity of cellular compartments in this study.

C. PROCOAGULANT ACTIVITY IS PRESENT AT MUCH HIGHER LEVELS IN TUMOR TISSUE COMPARED TO NORMAL CELLS

The melanoma cell originates from the epithelial cell. Therefore, it was appropriate to determine the procoagulant activity in subcellular fractions of normal liver >65% of which are of epithelial origin. The subcellular fractions were prepared as described above. The specific activity of procoagulant activity is about 19,000-fold lower than that found in the

TABLE 2
Specific Activities of Marker Enzymes in Subcellular Fractions of B16 Amelanotic Melanoma

Enzyme	Specific activity[a] (nmol/min/mg protein) Plasma membrane	Lysosomal
Na+/K+ −ATPase	61.2 ± 2.8	13.9 ± 4.9
RSA[b]	3.8	0.7
β-*N*-acetyl-glucosaminidase	8.33 ± 0.1	17.5 ± 1.11
RSA	1.5	3.1
Galactosyltransferase	390 ± 46	2 ± 19
RSA	2.93	0.14
Glucose-6-phosphatase	10.3 ± 0.8	24.5 ± 6.5
RSA	2.3	5.6
β-Glucuronidase	4.46 ± 0.1	11.1 ± 0.52
RSA	1.3	3.4
Tumor procoagulant[c]	639	109
RSA	28	4.8

[a] Specific activity expressed in nmol/min/mg protein; mean ± SE of triplicate.
[b] RSA = Relative Specific Activity; specific activity in fraction/specific activity in total homogenate
[c] Specific activity of tumor procoagulant protein measured as units of activity/mg protein. Activity was measured as described under coagulation assays. Representative data shown, not as mean ± SE.

tumor cells. For example, the specific activity of procoagulant activity in the plasma membrane fraction of tumor cells was 10,365 units/mg protein while in the plasma membrane fraction of normal liver, it was 0.54 units/mg protein. Details of procoagulant activity in subcellular fractions of B16a melanoma cells are compared to fractions from normal liver in Table 2. Since there is no access to normal murine melanocytes, a murine hepatoma line was used for comparison with the normal mouse liver cell. As shown in Table 2, the homogenate of the murine hepatoma contains 61,000 times the activity of the normal liver homogenate.

D. POSITIVE CORRELATION BETWEEN EXPRESSION OF TUMOR PROCOAGULANT ACTIVITY AND LUNG COLONY FORMING ABILITY OF TUMOR CELLS: EVIDENCE FROM CENTRIFUGAL ELUTRIATION STUDIES

The study of isolation of B16a using centrifugal elutriation was carried out in a preliminary form to determine if the tumor procoagulant may, in some manner, be correlated to the metastatic potential of tumor cells. The study utilized monodispersed cells obtained from multiple primary subcutaneous tumors. Cells were obtained by a modification[114] of the procedure previously described by Ryan et al.[110] The subcutaneous tumors used for these isolations were of similar age posttransplantation and of similar weight. Elutriated fractions were homogenized in two volumes of 25 m*M* HEPES buffer pH 7.5 containing 1 m*M* EDTA, 125 m*M* NaCl, and 5% sucrose. Cell suspensions were homogenized at 4°C for 2 min (15 strokes/min) in a Potter Elvehjem vessel. Homogenates were then treated with 0.5%

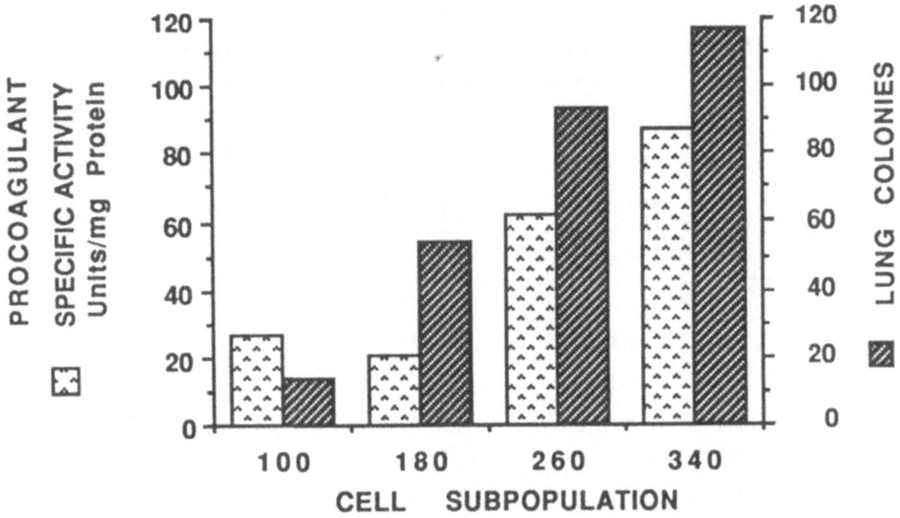

FIGURE 4. Correlation between lung colony formation and expression of tumor procoagulant protein.

CHAPS to solubilize membrane proteins. Protein concentrations were determined according to the Bradford method,[115] and procoagulant activity was determined in coagulation assays as described above.

Studies were carried out to demonstrate a correlation between lung colony forming ability and expression of tumor procoagulant protein in elutriated fractions of B16 amelanotic melanoma. Four fractions were utilized (100, 180, 260, and 340) (Figure 4). An equivalent number (44,500) of cells from each fraction were tail vein injected into C57BL/6J mice and assayed for lung colony forming ability. The 340 fraction produced significantly more lung colonies than the other fractions. It also expressed higher levels of tumor procoagulant protein (Figure 4). These results suggest a positive correlation between lung colony forming ability and metastatic potential. It needs to be emphasized that these studies are very preliminary, and a large number of experiments will have to be carried out to verify the relationship between procoagulant activity and lung colony forming ability.

In summary, a novel procoagulant activity has been identified in tumor cells. The activity is dramatically increased in tumor tissue compared to normal cells. It has no proteolytic activity; in fact, use of protease inhibitors during isolation of membrane fractions has resulted in better recoveries of specific activity. Expression of activity in Factor VII-deficient plasma suggests that the protein is distinct from tissue factor. The finding that the tumor protein is localized almost entirely in the plasma membrane and that a positive correlation exists between the surface expression of the protein and metastatic potential of tumor cells strengthens the hypothesis that the procoagulant activity may contribute to the metastatic cascade. Further studies are underway to delineate the mechanism of action of this procoagulant in generating thrombin and its role in metastasis.

VI. DISCUSSION AND PROBLEM AREAS

There are several areas of difficulties and definitions that need to be addressed, and these are discussed below. Although several investigators are now engaged in this area of coagulation and cancer, the proteins responsible for promoting thrombin generation have yet to be purified from tumor sources in quantities sufficient for sequence analysis. Most of the tumor proteins involved in promoting coagulation are thought to be present on the membrane surfaces of cells or to be released from the cell to carry out a function. Membrane proteins contain large proportions of lipids or carbohydrates. The isolation of proteins from membranes is a new science, and methodologies need to be worked out where lipids and/or carbohydrate moieties have to be removed prior to isolation of the protein of interest. The specific activity of biologic components is extremely high, hence, small amounts of proteins may exert large effects. Thus, contaminants tend to dominate protein preparations. At least three criteria may be used to define a pure protein. These include a single band on gel electrophoresis, a single column chromatography peak, and a single amino-terminal sequence. A single protein band in gel electrophoresis does not necessarily indicate a purified protein with the exception where the band may be extracted from the gel to show a specific bioactivity as high or higher than the starting sample. By far the best definition of a purified protein would be a single amino-terminal sequence. Guha et al.[78] have suggested a combination of limited tryptic digest and gel electrophoresis to demonstrate purity. However, this may give rise to complications where several peptide chains result from hydrolysis as may be true for a large protein.

The activity of tumor procoagulants are accessed either by coagulation assays or in platelet aggregation assays. Coagulation is a process by which thrombin is generated via a cascade of reactions. A major cofactor in these reactions is yet uncharacterized lipids. Cells are a good source of these lipids. A notable example is the positive role platelets play in generating thrombin. Tumor cells possess several proteins and lipids that may also enhance thrombin reaction both *in vivo* and *in vitro*. Lipids, however, are thought to nonspecifically provide a binding surface for the attachment of and to bring into close proximity the enzymes and protein substrates and are, therefore, of little interest. It is essential to differentiate the component under study from lipids when studying tumor procoagulants. Contaminating lipids that contribute to the enhanced activity in assays may be removed either by acetone precipitation or by ethanol or butanol extraction.[96]

Quantitation of activity of procoagulants is also generally lacking. Most of the activity of tumor procoagulants have been carried out using coagulation (one-stage or two-stage) or platelet aggregation assays, which at best are semi-quantitative. Fasco and co-workers[68] have, for example, used an excellent system to quantitate the amount of Factor X activator activity. According to their system, one unit of Factor X activator activity may be described as that amount required to generate sufficient Factor Xa to release 1 μmol of paranitroanilide/g tumor wet weight/min. They have also used a Factor X specific substrate S2222 (*N*-benzoyl-L-isoleucyl-L-glutamylglycyl-L-arginine-*p*-nitroanilide hydrochloride), reducing the possibility of interference from thrombin for which it is a poor substrate.

The question of tumor cell induced platelet aggregation also needs to be addressed. Traditionally, platelet aggregation is carried out using either platelets suspended in citrated plasma, also referred to as platelet-rich plasma, or using gel filtered (or washed) platelets. There is sufficient calcium in the citrated plasma required for platelet aggregation induced by a host of platelet agonists such as thrombin, trypsin, collagen, ADP, wheat germ agglutinin, and ristocetin. Among these, only ADP and ristocetin require plasma for platelet activation. ADP induced platelet aggregation is mediated via fibrinogen, and ristocetin requires von Willebrand factor for activity. Thrombin, collagen, trypsin, and wheat germ agglutinin will all induce platelet aggregation in the presence of low calcium concentrations even when gel filtered platelets are used. One might, therefore, define a platelet agonist as a component that will directly induce platelet aggregation. These agonists would induce platelet aggregation via a platelet receptor — the exception being trypsin, which may induce aggregation by hydrolytic activation of a protein(s) on the platelet surface. Three events occur from the onset of platelet stimulation. Firstly, within the first 10 sec, platelets undergo shape change. Secondly, the contents of the α- and dense granules are secreted, and finally, platelets will aggregate. The secretion products include coagulation factors, fibrinogen, ADP, and serotonin. ADP is thought to contribute to a secondary wave in platelet aggregation, facilitating the completion of aggregation by 2 min. Microscopically, unstimulated platelets are normally discoid in shape and put out long finger-like projections upon stimulation. These projections are thought to be "sticky" and aid the formation of aggregates. When platelet-rich plasma is used, stimulation is also followed by activation of the coagulation cascade with subsequent thrombin generation and hydrolysis of fibrinogen to fibrin. The resulting platelet mesh, therefore, will also contain fibrin.

Tumor cells do not induce platelet aggregation in citrated platelet-rich plasma. In the literature, several papers have shown that tumor cells will induce platelets to aggregate only in heparinized platelet-rich plasma. The question, therefore, may be raised as to the mechanism of action. Another important observation is the need of plasma in these aggregation studies. No aggregation is observed in washed or gel filtered platelets. It also has been shown in some reports that the use of specific thrombin inhibitors such as hirudin,[81] dansyl-arginine *N*-(3-ethyl-1,5-pentanediyl) amide or D-phenylananly-L-propyl-L-arginine chloromethylketone will prevent platelet aggregation as well as inhibit coagulation, which raises the possibility that tumor cells probably induce thrombin generation via their procoagulants and that the generated thrombin causes platelet aggregation. This argument is strengethened by the long lag time, as much as 2 to 5 min for the onset of the aggregation process as opposed to the 30 sec found in traditional aggregation assays. It appears that the thrombin initially generated by tumor cells is consumed by heparin-antithrombin complexes, and only excess thrombin generated may then be available for platelet aggregation.

ACKNOWLEDGMENTS

This work was supported by a grant (CA 49975) from the National Institutes of Health. B16 amelanotic melanoma tumors, hepatomas, and elutriated cells were kindly provided by members of the Cancer Biology Division, Wayne State University. Technical assistance from Elizabeth A. Gordon and Natalie K. Masha is sincerely appreciated.

REFERENCES

1. **Trousseau, A.,** Clinique Medicale de l'Hotel-Dieu de Paris London, New Sydenham Society, 3, 94, 1865.
2. **Rickles, F. R. and Edwards, R. L.,** Activation of blood coagulation in cancer: Trousseau's syndrome revisited, *Blood,* 62, 14, 1983.
3. **Dvorak, H. F.,** Abnormalities of hemostasis in malignancy, in *Thrombosis and Hemostasis,* Colman, R. W., Hirsh, J., Marder, V. J., and Salzman, E. W., Eds., Lippincott, Philadelphis, 1987, 1143.
4. **Ambrus, F. L., Ambrus, C. M., Mink, I. B., and Pickren, J. W.,** Causes of death in cancer patients, *J. Med.,* 6, 6, 1975.
5. **Sun, V. C., McAfee, W. M., Hum, G. J., and Weiner, J. M.,** Hemostatic abnormalities in malignancy, a prospective study in one hundred and eight patients, *Am. J. Clin. Pathol.,* 71, 10, 1979.
6. **Carlsson, S.,** Fibrinogen degradation products in serum from patients with cancer, *Acta Chir. Scand.,* 139, 499, 1973.
7. **Sack, G. H., Jr., Levin, J., and Bell, W. R.,** Trousseau's syndrome and other manifestations of chronic disseminated coagulopathy in patients with neoplasms: clinical, pathologic and therapeutic features, *Medicine,* 56, 1, 1977.
8. **Rasche, H. and Dietrich, M.,** Hemostatic abnormalities associated with malignant disease, *Eur. J. Cancer,* 13, 1053, 1977.
9. **Garrison, S.,** Fibrinogen degradation products in serum from patients with cancer, *Acta Chir. Scand.,* 139, 499, 1973.
10. **Owen, C. A., Jr., and Bowie, E. J. W.,** Chronic intravascular coagulation syndromes, a summary, *Mayo Clin. Proc.,* 49, 673, 1974.
11. **Bauer, K. A. and Rosenberg, R. D.,** Thrombin generation in acute myelocytic leukemia, *Blood,* 64, 791, 1984.

12. **Yoda, Y. and Abe, T.,** Fibrinopeptide A(FPA) level and fibrinogen kinetics in patients with malignant disease, *Thromb. Hemost.*, 1, 1113, 1978.
13. **Weiss, L.,** Overview of the metastatic cascade, in *Hemostatic Mechanisms and Metastasis,* Honn, K. V. and Sloan, B. F., Eds., Martinus Nijhoff, Boston, 1984, 15.
14. **Gasic, G. J., Gasic, T. B., and Stewart, G. J.,** Mechanisms of platelet aggregation by murine tumor cell shedding, in *Hemostatic Mechanisms and Metastasis,* Honn, K. V. and Sloan, B. F., Eds., Martinus Nijhoff, Boston, 1984, 127.
15. **Karpatkin, S., Pearlstein, E.,** Heterogenous mechanisms of tumor cell-induced platelet aggregation with possible pharmacologic strategy toward prevention of metastases, in *Hemostatic Mechanisms and Metastasis,* Honn, K. V. and Sloan, B. F., Eds., Martinus Nijhoff, Boston, 1984, 1.
16. **Sloan, B. F., Cavanaugh, P. G., and Honn, K. V.,** Tumor cysteine proteases, platelet aggregation and metastasis, in *Hemostatic Mechanisms and Metastasis,* Honn, K. V. and Sloan, B. F., Eds., Martinus Nijhoff, Boston, 1984, 170.
17. **Kies, M. S., Posch, J. J., Giolma, J. P., and Rubin, R. N.,** Hemostatic function in cancer patients, *Cancer,* 46, 831, 1980.
18. **Wood, S., Jr.,** Pathogenesis of metastasis formation observed *in vivo* in the rabbit ear chamber, *Arch. Pathol.*, 66, 550, 1950.
19. **Wood, S., Jr., Holyoke, E. D., and Yardley, J. H.,** Mechanisms of metastasis production by blood-borne cancer cells, *Proc. Cancer Res. Conf.*, 4, 167, 1961.
20. **Harker, L. A. and Slichter, S. J.,** Platelet and fibrinogen consumption in man, *N. Engl. J. Med.*, 287, 999, 1972.
21. **Slichter, S. J. and Harker, L. A.,** Hemostasis in malignancy, *Ann. N.Y. Acad. Sci.*, 230, 252, 1974.
22. **Johannson, S., Kutti, J., and Olson, L. B.,** Rapid platelet consumption in a case of metastatic osteogenic sarcoma of the breast, *Acta Pathol. Microbiol. Scand.*, 86, 505, 1978.
23. **Hagedorn, A. B., Bowie, E. J. W., Elveback, L. R., and Owen, C. A.,** Coagulation abnormalities in patients with inoperable lung cancer, *Mayo Clin. Proc.*, 49, 649, 1974.
24. **Saikh, B. S. and Bullard, V.,** Thombopoietic activity in sera of cancer patients, *Blood,* 50, (Suppl. 1), 252, 1977.
25. **Gasic, G. J., Boettiger, D., Catalfamo, J. L., Gasic, T. D., and Stewart, G. J.,** Aggregation of platelets and cell membrane vesiculation by rat cells transformed *in vitro* by Rous sarcoma virus, *Cancer Res.*, 38, 2950, 1978.
26. **Dvorak, H. F., Dvorak, A. M., Manseau, E. J., Wilberg, L., and Churchill, W. H.,** Fibrin-gel investment associated with line 1 and line 10 solid tumor growth, angiogenesis, and fibroplasia in guinea pigs: role of cellular immunity, myofibroblasts, microvascular damage and infarction in line 1 tumor regression, *J. Natl. Cancer Inst.*, 62, 1459, 1979.
27. **Donati, M. B., Poggi, A., and Semeraro, N.,** Coagulation and malignancy, in *Recent Advances in Blood Coagulation,* Poller, L., Ed., Churchill Livingstone, Edinburgh, 1982, 227.
28. **Gorelik, E., Berc, W. W., and Herberman, R. B.,** Role of NK cell in the antimetastatic effect of anticoagulant drugs, *Int. J. Cancer,* 33, 87, 1984.
29. **Weiss, L., Dimitrov, D. S., and Angelova, M.,** The hemodynamic destruction of intravascular cancer cells in relation to myocardial metastasis, *Proc. Natl. Acad. Sci. U.S.A.*, 82, 5737, 1985.
30. **Fidler, I. J.,** The relationship of embolic homogeneity, number, size and viability to the incidence of experimental metastasis, *Eur. J. Cancer,* 9, 223, 1973.
31. **Liotta, L. A., Kleinerman, J., and Saidel, G. M.,** The significance of hematogenous tumor cell clumps in the metastatic process, *Cancer Res.*, 36, 889, 1976.
32. **Irimura, T., Gonzalez, R., and Nicolson, G. L.,** Effects of tunicamycin on B16 metastatic melanoma cell surface glycoproteins and blood-borne arrest and survival properties, *Cancer Res.*, 41, 3411, 1981.
33. **Irimura, T. and Nicolson, G. L.,** The role of glycoconjugates in metastatic melanomna blood-borne arrest and cell surface properties, *J. Supramol. Struct. Cell. Biochem.*, 17, 325, 1981.
34. **Takacz, J. S. and Lampen, J. O.,** Tunicamycin inhibition of polyisoprenyl *N*-acetylglucosaminyl pyrophosphate formation of calf liver microsomes, *Biochem. Biophys. Res. Commun.*, 65, 248, 1975.
35. **Takatsuki, A., Kohno, K., and Tamura, G.,** Inhibition of biosynthesis of polyprenol sugars in chick embryo microsomes by tunicamycin, *Agric. Biol. Chem.*, 39, 2089, 1975.
36. **Murray, J. C., Liotta, L., Rennard, S. I., and Martin, G. R.,** Adhesion characteristics of murine metastatic and nonmetastatic tumor cell lines *in vitro, Cancer Res.*, 40, 347, 1980.
37. **Terranova, V. P., Liotta, L. A., Russo, R. G., and Martin, G. R.,** Role of laminin in the attachment and metastasis of murine tumor cells, *Cancer Res.*, 42, 2265, 1982.
38. **Varani, J., Dixit, V. M., Fligiel, S. E. G., McKeever, P. E., and Carey, T. E.,** Thrombospondin-induced attachment and spreading of human squamous carcinoma cells, *Exp. Cell. Res.*, 167, 376, 1986.
39. **Menter, D. G., Steinert, B. W., Sloane, B. F., Taylor, J. D., and Honn, K. V.,** A new *in vitro* model for investigation of tumor cell-platelet endothelial cell interactions and concomitant eicosanoid biosynthesis, *Cancer Res.*, 47, 2425, 1987.

40. **Grossi, I. M., Menter, D. G., Ohannesian, D., Kendall, A., Onoda, J. M., Sloane, B. F., and Honn, K. V.,** Role of platelet glycoproteins Ib and IIb/IIIa in tumor cell induced platelet aggregation, *Proc. Am. Assoc. Cancer Res.*, 28, 66, 1987.
41. **Vlodavsky, I. and Gospodarowicz, D.,** Respective roles of laminin and fibronectin in adhesion of human carcinoma and sarcoma cells, *Nature (London)*, 289, 304, 1981.
42. **Schirrmacher, V., Altervogt, P., Fogel, M., Dennis, J., Walker, C. A., Barz, D., Schwartz, R., Cheingsong-Popov, R., Springer, G., Robinson, P. J., Nebe, T., Brossmer, W., Vlodavsky, I., Pawelet, N., Zimmermann, H. P., and Uhlenbrach, G.,** Importance of cell surface carbohydrates in cancer cell adhesion, invasion and metastasis: does sialic acid direct metastatic behavior, *Invasion and Metastasis*, 2, 313, 1982.
43. **Menter, D. G., Hatsfield, J. S., Harkins, C., Sloane, B. F., Taylor, J. D., Crissman, J. D., and Honn, K. V.,** Tumor cell-platelet interactions *in vitro* and their relationship to *in vivo* arrest of hematogenously circulating tumor cells, *Clin. Exp. Metastasis*, 5, 65, 1987.
44. **Billroth, T.,** *Lectures on Surgical Pathology and Therapeutics*, 8th ed., (transl.), New Sydenham Society, 1878.
45. **Spar, I. L., Bale, W. F., Marrack, D., Dewey, W. C., McCardle, R. J., and Harper, P. U.,** ^{131}I-labeled antibodies to human fibrinogen. Diagnostic studies and therapeutic trials, *Cancer*, 20, 865, 1967.
46. **Dvorak, H. F., Orenstien, N. S., and Dvorak, A. M.,** Tumor-secreted mediators and the tumor microenvironment: relationship to immunological surveillance, *Lymphokines*, 2, 203, 1981.
47. **Hilgard, P.,** Blood platelets and experimental metastasis, in *Platelets: A Muldisciplinary Approach*, deGaetano, G. and Garattini, S., Eds., Raven Press, New York, 1978, 457.
48. **Marcum, J. M., McGill, M., Bastida, E., Ordinas, A., and Jamieson, G. A.,** The interaction of platelets, tumor cells and vascular subendothelium, *J. Lab. Clin. Med.*, 96, 1046, 1980.
49. **Gasic, G. J., Gasic, T. B., Galanti, N., Johnson, T., and Murphy, S.,** Platelet-tumor cell interactions in mice. The role of platelets in the spread of malignant disease, *Int. J. Cancer*, 11, 704, 1973.
50. **Gasic, G. J., Gasic, T. B., and Stewart, C. C.,** Antimetastatic effects associated with platelet reduction, *Proc. Natl. Acad. Sci. U.S.A.*, 61, 46, 1968.
51. **Honn, K. V., Cicone, B., and Skoff, A.,** Prostacyclin: a potent antimetastatic agent, *Science*, 212, 1270, 1981.
52. **Honn, K. V. and Meter, J.,** Thromboxanes and prostacyclin: positive and negative modulators of tumor growth, *Biochem. Biophys. Res. Commun.*, 102, 1122, 1981.
53. **Wood, S., Hilgard, O.,** Aspirin and tumor metastases, *Lancet*, 2, 1416, 1972.
54. **Hilgard, P., Heller, H., and Schmidt, C. G.,** The influence of platelet aggregation inhibitors on metastasis formation in mice (3LL), *Z. Krebsforsch. Klin. Onkol.*, 86, 243, 1976.
55. **Strauss, J. F. and Saphir, O.,** The possible significance of altered blood coagulability on the spread of carcinoma cells, *Proc. Inst. Med. Chicago*, 17, 263, 1949.
56. **Brown, J. M.,** A study of the mechanism by which anticoagulation with warfarin inhibits blood borne metastases, *Cancer Res.*, 33, 1217, 1973.
57. **Hilgard, P.,** Experimental vitamin K deficiency and spontaneous metastases, *Br. J. Cancer*, 35, 891, 1977.
58. **Hilgard, P. and Maat, B.,** Mechanism of lung tumor colony reduction caused by coumarin anticoagulation, *Eur. J. Cancer*, 15, 183, 1979.
59. **Agostino, D., Grossi, C. E., and Clifton, E. E.,** Effect of heparin on circulating Walker 256 carcinosarcoma cells, *J. Natl. Cancer Inst.*, 27, 17, 1961.
60. **Zacharski, L. R., Henderson, W. G., Rickles, F. R., Forman, W. B., Cornell, C. J., Jr., Forcier, R. J., Edwards, R. L., Headley, E., Kim, S. H., O'Donnell, J. R., O'Dell, R. O., Tornyos, K., and Kwaan, H. C.,** Effect of warfarin on survival in small cell carcinoma of the lung, *JAMA*, 245, 831, 1981.
61. **Mann, K. G., Jenny, R. J., and Krishnaswamy, S.,** Cofactor proteins in the assembly and expression of blood clotting enzyme complexes, *Ann. Rev. Biochem.*, 57, 915, 1988.
62. **Esmon, N. L., Owen, W. G., and Esmon, C. T.,** Isolation of a membrane-bound cofactor from thrombin-catalysed activation of protein C, *J. Biol. Chem.*, 257, 859, 1982.
63. **Stern, D. M., Drillings, M., Kisiel, W., Nawroth, P., Nossel, H. L., and LaGamma, K. S.,** Activation of Factor IX bound to cultured bovine aortic endothelial cells, *Proc. Natl. Acad. Sci. U.S.A.*, 81, 913, 1984.
64. **Stern, D. M., Nawroth, P., Handley, D., and Kisiel, W.,** An endothelial cell-dependent pathway of coagulation, *Proc. Natl. Acad. Sci. U.S.A.*, 82, 2523, 1985.
65. **Zur, M., Radcliff, R. D., Oberdick, J., and Nemerson, Y.,** The dual role of factor VII in blood coagulation: initiation and inhibition of a proteolytic system by a zymogen, *J. Biol. Chem.*, 257, 5623, 1982.
66. **Davie, E. W. and Ratnoff, O. D.,** Waterfall sequence for intrinsic blood clotting, *Science*, 145, 1310, 1964.
67. **MacFarlane, R. G.,** An enzyme cascade in the blood clotting mechanism and its function as a biochemical amplifier, *Nature*, 202, 498, 1964.

68. **Kisiel, W., Canfield, W., Ericsson, L., and Davie, E.,** Anticoagulant properties of bovine plasma protein C following activation by thrombin, *Biochemistry,* 16, 5824, 1977.
69. **Fulcher, C. A., Gardiner, J. E., Griffin, J. H., and Zimmerman, T. S.,** Proteolytic inactivation of human factor VIII procoagulant protein by activated human protein C and its analogy with factor V, *Blood,* 63, 486, 1984.
70. **Chelladurai, M., Fossett, N. G., and Ganguly, P.,** A novel thrombin-reactive protein complex in human platelets, *J. Biol. Chem.,* 258, 1407, 1983.
71. **Chelladurai, M., Fossett, N. G., and Ganguly, P.,** Thrombin-reactive polypeptides of human blood: some biochemical and immunological properties, *Eur. J. Biochem.,* 149, 473, 1985.
72. **Chelladurai, M. and Ganguly, P.,** Thrombin-reactive polypeptides of platelets may regulate inhibition of thrombin by antithrombin, *Biochem. Biophys. Acta,* 870, 204, 1986.
73. **Hilgard, P., Beyerle, L., Hohage, R., Hiemeyer, V., and Kubler, M.,** The effect of heparin on the initial phase of metastasis formation, *Eur. J. Cancer,* 8, 347, 1972.
74. **Fidler, I. J., Gersten, D. M., and Hart, I.,** The biology of cancer invasion and metastasis, *Adv. Cancer Res.,* 28, 149, 1978.
75. **Weiss, L.,** A pathologic overview of metastasis, *Semin. Oncol.,* 4, 5, 1977.
76. **O'Meara, R. A. Q.,** Coagulation properties of cancers, *Irish J. Med. Sci.,* 391, 327, 1958.
77. **Broze, G. J., Leykam, J. E., Schwartz, B. D., and Miletich, J. B.,** Purification of human brain tissue factor, *J. Biol. Chem.,* 260, 10917, 1985.
78. **Guha, A., Bach, R., Konisberg, W., and Nemerson, Y.,** Affinity purification of human tissue factor: interaction of factor VII and tissue factor in detergent micelles, *Proc. Natl. Acad. Sci. U.S.A.,* 83, 299, 1986.
79. **Gordon, S. G. and Lewis, B.,** Comparison of procoagulant activity in tissue culture medium from normal and transformed fibroblast, *Cancer Res.,* 38, 2467, 1978.
80. **Fasco, M. J., Eagan, G. E., Wilson, A. C., Gierthy, J. F., and Lincoln, D. L.,** Loss of metastatic and primary tumor factor X activator capabilities by Lewis lung carcinoma cells cultures in vitamin K-dependent protein deficient serum, *Cancer Res.,* 48, 6504, 1988.
81. **Cavanaugh, P. G., Sloane, B. F., Bajkowski, A. B., Taylor, J. D., and Honn, K. V.,** Purification and characterization of platelet aggregating activity from tumor cells: copurification with procoagulant activity, *Thromb. Res.,* 37, 309, 1985.
82. **Kinjo, M., Oka, K., Naito, S., Kohga, S., Tanaka, K., Oboshi, S., Hayata, Y., and Yasumoto, K.,** Thromboplastic and fibrinolytic activities of cultured human cancer cell lines, *Br. J. Cancer,* 39, 15, 1979.
83. **Hudig, D., Rapaport, S. I., and Bajaj, S. P.,** Tissue factor-like activity of the human monocyte tumor cell line U937, *Thromb. Res.,* 27, 321, 1982.
84. **Khato, J., Suzuki, M., and Sato, H.,** Quantitative study on thromboplastin in various strains of Yoshida ascites hepatoma cells of rat, *GANN,* 65, 284, 1974.
85. **Dvorak, H. F., VanDewater, L., Bitzer, A. M., Dvorak, A., Anderson, D., Harvey, V. S., Bach, R., Davis, G. L., DeWolf, W., and Carvalho, C. A.** Procoagulant activity associated with plasma membrane vesicles shed by cultured tumor cells, *Cancer Res.,* 43, 4334, 1983.
86. **Gouault-Hellmann, M., Chardon, E., Sultan, C., and Josso, F.,** The procoagulant factor of leukemic promyelocytes: demonstration of immunologic cross-reactivity with human brain tissue factor, *Br. J. Haematol.,* 30, 151, 1975.
87. **Gordon, S. G. and Cross, B. A.,** A factor X activating cysteine protease from malignant tissue, *J. Clin. Invest.,* 67, 1665, 1981.
88. **Gordon, S. G., Franks, J. J., and Lewis, B.,** Cancer procoagulant A: a factor X activating procoagulant from malignant tissue, *Thromb. Res.,* 6, 127, 1975.
89. **Gordon, S. G.,** A proteolytic procoagulant associated with malignant transformation, *Histochem. Cytochem.,* 29, 457, 1981.
90. **Gordon, S. G., Franks, J. J., and Lewis, B.,** Comparison of procoagulant activities in extracts of normal and malignant human tissue, *J. Natl. Cancer Inst.,* 62, 773, 1979.
91. **Falanga, A. and Gordon, S. G.,** Isolation and characterization of cancer procoagulant: a cysteine proteinase from malignant tissue, *Biochemistry,* 24, 5558, 1985.
92. **Barrett, A. J., McDonald, J. K., Eds.,** *Mammalian Proteinases — A Glossary and Bibliography Vol. 1: Endopeptidases,* Academic Press, New York, 1980.
93. **Sloane, B. F. and Honn, K. V.,** Cysteine proteinases and metastasis, *Cancer Metast. Rev.,* 3, 249, 1984.
94. **Gordon, S., Marlar, R., Madden, R., and Falanga, A.,** Inactivation of the protein C system by cancer procoagulant, *Thromb. Hemost.,* 62, 40, 1989.
95. **Scarlett, J. D., Thurlow, P. J., Connellan, J. M., and Louis, C. J.,** Plasma-dependent and -independent mechanisms of platelet aggregation induced by human tumour cell lines, *Thromb. Res.,* 46, 715, 1987.
96. **Labateya, N., Thomson, D. M. P., Durko, M., Shenouda, G., Robb, L., and Scanzano, R.,** Extraction of human organ-specific cancer neoantigens from cancer cells and plasma membranes with 1-butanol, *Cancer Res.,* 47, 1058, 1987.

97. **Kitagawa, H., Yamamoto, N., Yamamoto, K., Tanoue, K., Kosaki, G., and Yamazaki, H.,** Involvement of platelet membrane glycoprotein Ib and glycoprotein IIb/IIIa complex in thrombin-dependent and -independent platelet aggregations induced by tumor cells, *Cancer Res.*, 49, 537, 1989.
98. **Kimura, A. K., Metha, P., Xiang, J., Lawson, D., Dugger, D., Kao, K.-J., and Ambrose, L. L.,** The lack of correlation between experimental metastatic potential and platelet aggregating activity of B16 melanoma clones viewed in relation to tumor cell heterogeneity, *Clin. Exp. Metast.*, 5, 125, 1987.
99. **Francis, J. L., El-Baruni, K., Roath, O. S., and Taylor, I.,** Factor X-activating activity in normal and malignant colorectal tissue, *Thromb. Res.*, 52, 207, 1988.
100. **Watanabe, M., Okochi, E., Sugimoto, Y., and Tsuruo, T.,** Identification of a platelet-aggregating factor of murine colon adenocarcinoma 26: M_r 44,000 membrane protein as determined by monoclonal antibodies, *Cancer Res.*, 48, 6411, 1988.
101. **Esumi, N., Todo, S., and Imashuku, S.,** Platelet aggregating activity mediated by thrombin generation in the NCG human neuroblastoma cell line, *Cancer Res.*, 47, 2129, 1987.
102. **Longenecker, G. L., Beyers, B. J., Bowen, R. J., and King, T.,** Human rhabdosarcoma cell-induced aggregation of blood platelets, *Cancer Res.*, 49, 16, 1989.
103. **Gastpar, H.,** Platelet cancer cell interaction in metastasis formation: a possible therapeutic approach to metastasis prophylaxis, *J. Med.*, 8, 103, 1977.
104. **Gasic, G. J., Gasic, T. B., and Stewart, C. C.,** Antimetastatic effects associated with platelet reduction, *Proc. Natl. Acad. Sci. U.S.A.*, 61, 46, 1968.
105. **Gasic, G. J., Gasic, T. B., Galanti, N., Johnson, T., and Murphy, S.,** Platelet-tumor cell interactions in mice. The role of platelets in the spread of malignant disease, *Int. J. Cancer*, 11, 704, 1973.
106. **Pearlstein, E., Ambrogio, C., and Karpatkin, S.,** Effect of anti-platelet antibody on the development of pulmonary metastases following injection of CT26 colon adenocarcinoma, Lewis lung carcinoma and B16 amelanotic melanoma into mice, *Cancer Res.*, 44, 3884, 1984.
107. **Skolnick, G., Ericsson, L. E., and Bagge, U. J.,** The effect of thrombocytopenia and antiserotonin treatment on the lodgement of circulating tumor cells, *Cancer Res. Clin. Oncol.*, 105, 30, 1983.
108. **Ivarrson, L. and Rudenstam, C.-M.,** Trauma, dextran 40 and metastasis formation after intravenous tumor cell injection in rats, *Acta Chir. Scand.*, 142, 226, 1976.
109. **Wood, S., Jr.,** Experimental studies of the intravascular dissemination of ascitic V2 carcinoma cells in the rabbit, with special reference to fibrinogen and fibrinolytic agents, *Bull. Schweiz. Akad. Med. Wiss.*, 20, 92, 1964.
110. **Ryan, R. E., Crissman, J. D., Honn, K. V., and Sloane, B. F.,** Cathepsin B-like activity in viable tumor cells isolated from rodent tumors, *Cancer Res.*, 45, 3636, 1985.
111. **Hara, Y., Steiner, M., and Baldini, M. G.,** Characterization of the platelet aggregating activity of tumor cells, *Cancer Res.*, 40, 1217, 1980.
112. **Rozhin, J., Robinson, D., Stevens, M. A., Lah, T. T., Honn, K. V., Ryan, R. E., and Sloane, B. F.,** Properties of a plasma membrane-associated cathepsin B-like cysteine proteinase in metastatic B16 melanoma variants, *Cancer Res.*, 47, 6620, 1987.
113. **DeDuve, C., Pressman, B. C., Gianetto, R., Wattiaux, R., and Applemans, F.,** Tissue fractionation studies: intracellular distribution patterns of enzymes in rat-liver tissue, *Biochem. J.*, 60, 604, 1955.
114. **Onoda, J. M., Nelson, K. K., Grossi, I. M., Umbarger, L. A., Taylor, J. D., and Honn, K. V.,** Separation of high and low metastatic subpopulations from solid tumors by centrifugal elutriation, *Proc. Soc. Exp. Biol. Med.*, 187, 250, 1988.
115. **Read, S. M. and Northcote, D. H.,** Minimization of variation in the response to different proteins of the coomassie blue G dye-binding assay for proteins, *Anal. Biochem.*, 116, 53, 1981.

Chapter 9

THE BIOMECHANICS OF CANCER CELL TRAFFIC, ARREST, AND INTRAVASCULAR DESTRUCTION

Leonard Weiss

TABLE OF CONTENTS

I. INTRODUCTION

Any phenomenon can be advantageously examined from a multidisciplinary viewpoint. In this chapter, the passage of cancer cells through the microvasculature, their arrest, and the subsequent infliction of lethal trauma on many of them will be described in biomechanical terms.

Because the relevant physical parameters of cancer cells, the microvasculature, the blood, and the surrounding tissues, have not yet been described in sufficient detail, precise analyses are currently impossible. However, in spite of these limitations, some experimentally verifiable general mechanisms can be advanced, which, in addition to revealing hitherto unsuspected processes, complement the morphological and biochemical descriptions of metastasis-related events occurring within the microvasculature.

Although cancer cells are released into the bloodstream both as single cells and as multicellular aggregates, main emphasis will be placed on the interactions between single cells and capillaries.

II. SOME MECHANICAL PROPERTIES OF CANCER CELLS

In common with other animal cells, cancer cells are viscoelastic. Thus, when cells are deformed or recover from deformation, there is a time-dependence due to their viscosity because the dimensions of viscosity are $M.L.^{-1}.T^{-1}$ (M = mass; L = length, and T = time); in isolation, these viscous components are termed Newtonian bodies and are represented in models as fluid-filled dash-pots (Figure 1), in which piston-movement is viscosity-dependent. On account of their elasticity, there is a tendency for deformed cancer cells to recoil into their original shapes when they are no longer subject to deforming forces. Within so-called elastic limits, they behave as Hookean bodies, obeying Hooke's Law (the extent of the deformation is proportional to the forces acting on the body), and are represented in models as springs (Figure 1). The elastic limit, or yield-point, marks the degree of deformation beyond which recovery is not reversible, and elastic deformation is no longer independent of time, but increases slowly under constant force. Bodies exhibiting this yield-point, or plastic deformation, are termed as *St. Venant bodies* and are represented in models as sliding blocks (Figure 1), which on application of force, remain stationary until friction is overcome, and then they move abruptly.

Direct observations on the mesenteric micro-vessels of rodents reveal that cancer cells are deformed into sausage-shapes on entry and passage along them;[1] smaller cells including erythrocytes and leucocytes are deformed less. With certain qualifications, the deformability of cancer cells may be measured by determining the negative pressures required to suck bulges from the cells into micropipettes.[2,3,4] When cancer cells deformed in this manner were expelled from micropipettes by application of positive pressure, the bulges were "resorbed" by the cells within a few seconds; this viscoelastic behavior may be modelled by a combination of Newtonian and Hookean bodies. By application of greater negative pressures, relatively long, sausage-shaped protrusions were sucked from the cancer cells which, after expulsion from the pipettes, were not "resorbed". This represents deformation beyond a yield-point, and rheologic models of these cancer cells must therefore include a St. Venant body.[5] Based on these and other observations, a generalized composite rheologic model for cancer cells was developed,[6] as shown in Figure 1.

None of the current rheologic models based on average, whole cell properties are entirely satisfactory in the context of cancer cell deformation because they do not include details of biologically important hemogeneities generated by the cytoskeleton, organelles, and nucleus. Ultimately, constitutive equations are required for the many different types of cancer cells, which would permit experimentally verifiable, *ab initio* calculations to be made of their

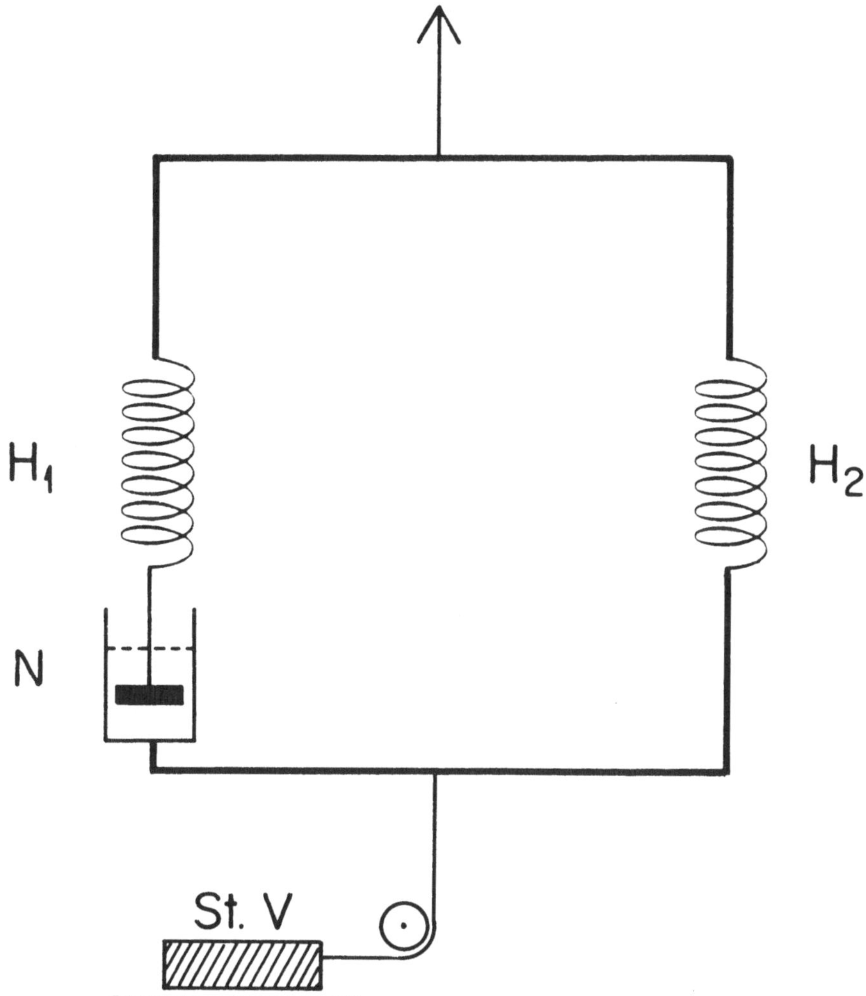

FIGURE 1. Rheologic model of a cancer cell containing two elastic "Hookean" (H) springs, a viscous "Newtonian" (N) dash-pot, and a plastic St. Venant (St. V) sliding block.

interactions with the microvasculature. However, as documented in many of the other chapters, the systems are so complex and dynamic that at present, this is impossible.

It should be noted here that a great deal of work on both theoretical and experimental mechanics has been done on erythrocytes[7,8] and leucocytes;[9,10] some of this work is indubitably relevant to cancer cells.

III. TRANSIT OF CANCER CELLS THROUGH THE CAPILLARIES

Cancer cells entering capillaries are deformed[1] because the capillaries have smaller diameters, which, within limits, are generally, but not invariably less deformable than the cancer cells.[49]

When a cancer cell lies within a tapered vessel of gradually decreasing cross-sectional areas A_1 to A_2 with a taper angle of X°, and the total contact area of the cancer cell with the vessel wall is A_3, then when the blood pressures upstream and downstream of the cell are p_1 and p_2 respectively, the deforming pressure p, acting on the cancer cell, is given by Equation 1, which has been discussed in detail elsewhere:[6]

$$p = (1/\sin x)(1/A_3)(p_1 \cdot A_1 - p_2 \cdot A_2) \tag{1}$$

Thus, the deformation pressure acting on the cancer cell will increase with decreasing taper angle and contact area — increasing pressure gradients between the ends of the cell and increasing disparities between the cross-sectional areas in different parts of the involved vessels. This may account for damage associated with the entry of cancer cells into capillaries from arterioles.

In the case of a single capillary arising from an arteriole, under conditions of unperturbed flow, the density of cancer cells will be lower in the capillary. This is partly due to the geometric entry conditions into the capillary and within an arteriole, partly due to the cell density being near the center of the vessel where blood viscosity is highest and to the cell density being lowest near the wall where the capillary originates.

The passage of cancer cells from arterioles into capillaries may involve their adhesion to the arteriolar wall near the capillary opening, as a preliminary to entry by means of active and/or passive movements. It is known that polymorphs in the bloodstream continuously make collisions with the vessel walls, particularly under conditions of pulsatile flow. The chances that these collisions will result in adhesions depend on the balance between the hemodynamic shear forces, which tend to dislodge the cells, and the strength of the adhesive/cohesive forces at or near the cell/vessel wall interfaces.[11] The effects of velocity gradients within blood flowing through arterioles on erythrocyte movement, deformation, and collisions are discussed in detail by Goldsmith.[12] Shear-induced modifications in erythrocytes affect collisions, and shear-induced and pathologic changes in vessel walls also promote initial contact. Due to streamlining, the more flattened the adherent cells, the less likely they are to be dislodged by flowing blood. It would not be surprising if analogous events occur with circulating cancer cells, bearing in mind their generally larger size and differences in their rheologic properties.

In the context of cancer cell entry, it would be of interest to determine whether there are increased concentrations of adhesive macromolecules and/or receptors at the sites of capillary origin, which could act to trap cancer cells in this location; platelet aggregation occurs preferentially at these sites. Increased entry into capillaries would also be favored by distal, arteriolar obstruction due to the arrest of multicellular emboli.

Only a proportion of single circulating cancer cells within an arteriole are expected to be diverted into any one capillary arising from it, and the capillaries may be bypassed by shunts. However, in situations where arterioles terminate in capillary networks, or where arterioles are blocked, the majority of the cancer cells are expected to enter capillaries.

By analogy with rigorously controlled flow-studies in the field of chemical engineering,[13] it appears probable that having entered a capillary, if other factors remain the same, the transit velocity of a deformed cancer cell will depend on the magnitude of the frictional forces between it and the vessel wall in relation to the blood pressure differentials along the vessel. Friction is reduced by the presence of a "film" of plasma, which is interposed between the cancer cell and the vessel wall and acts as a lubricant. On account of their elastic properties, cancer cells that have been squeezed into the capillaries are now expected to recoil towards the wall, thereby driving out or breaking the lubricating film. One consequence of film loss or thinning is that the distance separating the cancer cell and vessel wall surfaces may decrease to the point at which adhesive bonds may be formed between them, leading to cell arrest. The distances involved in this process are too small to be directly observed in the *in vivo* situation, and reliance is placed on a quasi-theoretical approach.

Formulae permitting the calculation of the rate of approach of the cancer cell surface and the vessel wall (V) (Equation 2) have been derived by Dimitrov[13] and Weiss and Dimitrov[14] and approximate to:

$$V = -dh/dt = Fh^3/2\,\pi\mu R_c L^3 \quad (2)$$

where h is film thickness, t is time, μ is film viscosity, R_c is cell radius, and L is deformed cell length. F is the driving force in the direction of the capillary wall due to the elastic restoring forces, T, in the deformed cancer cell, minus the disjoining pressure, D, of the plasma film (Equation 3):

$$F = 2\,\pi\,TL - 2\,\pi\,R_c LD \quad (3)$$

Estimates of the elastic characteristics of cancer cells are obtained from measurements of the negative pressures required to suck hemispherical bulges from the cancer cells into micropipettes;[2,4] however, these values are certainly over-estimates because they do not take into account surface membrane "excess" (i.e., folding), cytoplasmic elasticity, shear elasticity, and changes in cell diameter during measurements.

Thus, as they are driven along capillaries, cancer cells recoil towards the vessel walls at very approximately calculable rates (V). If the adhesion of the circulating cells to the vessel walls depends on reduction of film thickness to a critical distance h_f, which may be as much as tens of nanometers and which is due to the presence of long-range attractive forces,[15,16] then it is of interest to determine whether or not this film-thinning can occur within the time taken by cells to pass along capillary segments. If it can, then the initial phase of cancer cell arrest/adhesion can be accounted for exclusively in biomechanical terms.

In the *in vitro* system studied by Weiss and Harlos,[17] the rates of adhesion were determined for cancer cells to coverslips when the cells sedimented under the influence of gravity. It was calculated that it took more than 40 min for the cells to descend the final 4 to 8 nm to the coverslips, possibly due to the viscosity of the culture medium lying between them. The driving force *in vivo* within capillaries, as described above, is not gravity, and the time taken to achieve critical film thickness has been computed at several seconds.[18]

At present, no direct measurements of cancer cell transit times through capillaries are available. However, erythrocyte velocities of 0.1 to 0.2 cm/sec have been observed, corresponding to the transit times of 0.5 to 1.0 sec for 0.1 cm capillary length, and leukocytes have lower velocities.[19] On account of their larger size, cancer cells are expected to have lower velocities, and hence longer transit times.

A semiquantitative approach to cancer cell velocity (u) in capillaries has been developed by Weiss et al.[18] (Equation 4):

$$u = phR/2\,\mu L \quad (4)$$

where p is the blood pressure gradient between the ends of a cancer cell of radius R and length L, μ is plasma viscosity, and h is film thickness.

At constant cell volume, L varies inversely with R^2. Therefore, if capillary diameter decreases substantially as in the myocardial capillaries during systole, the corresponding decrease in the radii and increased length of intravascular cancer cells will cause considerable prolongation of transit times. Thus, in diastole, when average myocardial capillary radius is 2.6 μm, cancer cells with an original mean radius of 7.5 μm are calculated to attain velocities of approximately 0.1 cm/sec. During systole, when capillary radius decreases by approximately one third, the transit time is calculated to increase 3 to 4 times. In addition, as the thickness of the lubricating film decreases, cell velocities progressively decrease.[20] The calculated velocities given here are too high even for leukocytes, and are therefore expected to provide gross under-estimates of transit times for cancer cells.

The major problem in interpreting the estimates of rates of elastic recoil of cancer cells towards vessel walls in relation to their transit times lies in estimating the critical distances (h_f) between the cells and vessel walls over which biologically "significant" attractive forces operate. In the present context, "significant" implies that the attractive forces holding the cell to the wall are greater than the distractive shear forces associated with blood flow and tissue movements. If these attractive forces indeed operate "significantly" over tens of nanometers in this situation, then after allowing for the inevitable over-estimates of recoil times and over-estimates of transit times, the initial *arrest* of cancer cells can be explained in biomechanical terms. In addition, *arrest* or *trapping* is expected to be promoted by irregularities in the opposing cancer and endothelial cell surfaces. Thus, according to this approach, subsequent *adhesion* via bridging-molecules (adhesion-molecules) occurs after arrest. This involves the receptors, the integrins, which bind to RGD (arginine-glycine-asparagine)-containing sequences in adhesion proteins (Chapter 10), and serve to stabilize cancer cell/capillary wall encounters, culminating in arrest.

According to the observations and calculations outlined above, arrest of cancer cells is accountable in terms of the rheological properties of cancer cells and plasma and the mechanical properties of the capillaries. This is different from subsequent adhesion *in vivo* and involves different mechanisms from those used in examining cell adhesion to endothelial cell monolayers *in vitro*. At present, there is no experimental evidence correlating differential arrest with different mechanical properties of cancer cells. Therefore, as cancer cell arrest can be described in nonspecific terms of lubrication theory, it appears that the underlying mechanisms for metastatic patterns are to be found in the postarrest phases of metastasis.

In vitro experiments, extensively reviewed by Nicolson,[21] indicate that some types of cancer cells exhibit different adhesive "preferences" for endothelial cell monolayers derived from the microvasculature of different organs. Nicolson considers this to be one basis for organ-specificity in metastasis. Specific adhesion is also explicable in terms of receptor-mediated cell adhesion to surfaces in shear flow, according to a model developed by Hammer and Lauffenburger,[59] (from an earlier model by Bell[60]). In this, initial attachment is considered to occur over a small homogenous region involving receptors in the cancer cell surface and complementary ligands at the endothelial surface. The factors influencing adhesive interactions include bond formation rate, ligand-receptor affinity, receptor mobility, fluid mechanical force, cell deformability, and contact area. The numbers of adhesive bonds formed between the two surfaces during the period of close apposition depend on binding and dissociation rate constants, the rapidity of diffusion of receptors into the contact area, and the size of this area. Cancer cell arrest depends on a positive balance between the numbers of bonds and the distractive forces. Adhesion is controlled by two distinct mechanisms: in the first, the rate of reaction is dominant, and in the second, the ligand receptor affinity is dominant. In this treatment, adhesive molecules are involved in both the arrest and the adhesive processes.

IV. INTRAVASCULAR TRAUMA TO CANCER CELLS

When cancer cells are injected into the lateral tail veins, the portal veins, or the left ventricle of mice, the vast majority (85 to 95%) are lethally traumatized in less than several minutes after arrival in the microvascular beds of the first downstream organ encountered. These and similar observations point to a major component of "metastatic inefficiency" in the intravascular delivery phase of metastasis.[22,23]

A. CANCER CELL PROPERTIES IN RELATION TO MECHANICAL TRAUMA

As discussed earlier, cancer cells are deformed on entering and passing along capillaries. During this period, any deviation from their equilibrium spherical shape mandates increases in their surface areas. For example, at constant cell volume, a cancer cell having an original diameter of 15 μm and being deformed within a 5 μm diameter capillary into a 5 μm diameter cellular cylinder with hemispherical ends, will double its surface area. If the capillary had an internal diameter of less than 1 μm, as in the myocardium during systole, more than a tenfold increase is possible. Calculations of this type assume that the cancer cell is deformed into a regular cylinder. However, if the cancer cell nucleus resists deformation, then the overall demand for increased surface area will be reduced.

Increases in cell surface area may be apparent due to surface membrane unfolding, or the increases may be real due to membrane expansion. The analyses of Evans and Parsegian[24] suggest that in general, the elastic coefficients for surface area expansion are some orders of magnitude greater than those for bending. As a consequence, increase in cell surface area is first expected to be accomplished by unfolding and, if this is insufficient to meet the geometric demands for increase, the next step will involve membrane expansion.

Cancer cell membrane folding and unfolding in itself is expected to be reversible and nonlethal. However, beyond an approximate 5% increase in true surface area, membrane expansion results in rupture, which is irreversible and lethal, as indicated by work on noncancer cell membranes.[25,26,27]

The apparent increases in cell surface area corresponding to the first membrane-unfolding phase of cell shape transition, probably correspond to the low strain deformations, which are expressed as the negative pressures required to suck parts of cells into micropipettes.[2,4,28] The mechanism of increasing apparent cell surface area by membrane unfolding is well-recognized.[29—33]

Experimental data supportive of the two-step, mechanical destruction of cancer cells comes from studies in which analogous changes were produced in membranes by increasing cell volume exposed to hypotonic media. This permitted the effects of shape transitions to be observed in a well-controlled and step-wise manner. In the case of Ehrlich ascites carcinoma (EAT) cells,[34] reversible increases in diameter were recorded over the range of 280 to 70 m*M*/kg with little change in membrane integrity. These reversible increases in volume were accompanied by a smoothing-out of cell surface contours, as assessed by quantitative analysis of electron micrographs. Although the cell swelling itself was virtually nonlethal over this osmolarity-range, under specified conditions, it was associated with a progressive increase in susceptibility to lethal mechanical trauma when cancer cell suspensions were passed through Nuclepore® filters under a positive pressure of 55 cm/H_2O. These data are consistent with the first part of the mechanical trauma hypothesis, demonstrating that reversible shape transitions are associated with surface unfolding, which is not in itself lethal to most cancer cells. The corollary to this is that surface folding provides cells with a buffer against this type of mechanical trauma.[35] Therefore, when surface unfolding determines relative cell deformability, as measured by micropipette experiments, this may well account for the correlation between the ease of deformability and the percentage survival rate of cancer cells passing through the microcirculation.[4]

In contrast to the relatively low degree of trauma inflicted on cancer cells made over the range of 280 to 70 m*M*/kg, abrupt and irreversible trauma occurred over the range of 70 to approximately 40 m*M*/kg due to membrane rupture. Therefore, these results are consistent with the proposed second step in the hypothesis, which indicates that following a reversible unfolding process, irreversible, lethal membrane rupture of surface membranes occurs on their exposure to additional stress.[34]

In vitro studies on the responses of L1210 leukemia cells to hypotonic media revealed significant differences between them and EAT cells.[35] In contrast to the EAT cells, the L1210 cells showed neither a detectable increase in diameter nor evidence of surface unfolding over the osmolarity range of 280 to 70 m*M*/kg. However, electron micrographic evidence was obtained for some sort of nonlethal, ultramicroscopic unfolding/stretching associated with increased susceptibility to mechanical damage on passing through Nuclepore® filters. Thus, of the two cell types examined in detail, both show evidence of susceptibility to mechanical damage in a manner consistent with the two-step hypothesis — one with more evidence of surface unfolding than the other. On the one hand, the survival of L1210 cells within the microcirculation is expected to be greater than EAT cells on account of their smaller diameters (L1210, 10 μm; EAT, 14 μm); on the other hand, their greater potential for surface unfolding is expected to favor the survival of the EAT cells over the L1210.

The differential resistance of cancer cells to mechanical trauma does not depend solely on their diameters and degrees of surface membrane folding, but also on other factors governing their deformability. Thus, in his review of cell mechanics, Elson[36] concludes that cell deformation depends on cytoskeletal mechanics and that measurements of cell deformability yielding well-defined rheologic parameters should provide a useful approach for analysis of this dependence. Experimental evidence for cytoskeletal involvement includes the alignment of microfilaments by tension associated with the relative resistance to distortion by intermediate filaments.[37] Cytoskeletal involvement also is suggested by experiments in which perturbation of microfilaments by cytochalasin B increases fibroblast and B16 melanoma cell deformability.[38] The association of different metastatic potentials with altered cytoskeletal (i.e., actin and vinculin) organization[39] and the alteration of metastatic behavior by cytoskeletal-depolymerizing agents[40] may also be relevant in the present context.

Direct evidence indicating the contributions of the different cytoskeletal components to the resistance of cancer cells to mechanical trauma has been sought in experiments on the effects of cytoskeletal-disrupting agents on the survival of filtered EAT cells. It was first shown by immunocytochemical techniques that cytochalasin D, colchicine, and acrylamide treatment produced disorganization of the microfilaments, microtubules, and the intermediate filaments, respectively. However, on filtration through 8 μm Nuclepore® membranes, only acrylamide-treated cells showed significantly reduced survival; but treatment with this agent alone, in the absence of mechanical trauma, is associated with considerable cell killing. The experiments, therefore, fail to demonstrate a clear cut role for any cytoskeletal elements in EAT cell resistance to mechanical trauma.[41] The roles of the cancer cell surface membrane, cytoskeleton, and nucleus in relation to lethal trauma are currently ill-defined and require further study. It is noteworthy that attempts to identify and isolate subpopulations of L1210 and EAT cancer cells with inherited resistance to mechanical trauma have been unsuccessful.[42]

B. PROPERTIES OF THE MICROVASCULATURE IN RELATION TO MECHANICAL TRAUMA TO CANCER CELLS

In addition to the properties of cancer cells outlined above, any discussion of intravascular trauma must be widened to include the mechanical properties of involved blood vessels and surrounding mechanically-coupled tissues. In order to produce cancer cell deformation, the diameter of a blood vessel must be less than that of the cancer cells, and it must be less deformable. It is reasonably expected that vessels surrounded by thick, dense basement membranes will be less deformable than those with thin or incomplete subendothelial structures. The properties of the tissues surrounding small vessels will also determine their deformability, and in the case of contractile or expansile tissues, contraction or expansion will promote both blood vessel and cancer cell deformation.

1. Cancer Cell Damage in Specific Sites

a. The Myocardium

In the absence of lung metastases, which act as "generalizing" sites for metastasis elsewhere, there is a generally low incidence of myocardial metastasis in humans.[18] Experiments on mice showed that following left ventricular injections (LVI) of cancer cells,

TABLE 1
Intraperitoneal (I.P.) Bioassays on Quadriceps Femoris Muscle[a]

	Muscle Status		
	Flaccid	"Controls"	Contracting
I.P. transplant weights: g ± S.E.(n)	0.633 ± 0.08 (25)	0.028 ± 0.004 (37)	0.001 ± 0.001 (13)
Transplant weight ratios with controls	23:1	1	1:28
Proportion of I.P. "takes"	27/31 (88%)	37/42 (87%)	4/13 (31%)

[a] 65 d after left ventricular injection (L.V.I.) of 5 × 10^5 B16 melanoma cells.[47]

approximately 5% of injected cells were arrested in the myocardial capillaries following delivery via the coronary arteries. In hearts removed 5 min after injection, no intact cancer cells were seen in sections stained by sensitive immunochemical procedures. Three weeks after LVI of melanoma cells, massive deposits of cell-free melanin pigment were found in the myocardium, and since corresponding deposits were not observed in other organs, it was concluded that large numbers of cancer cells were destroyed in the myocardium. In other experiments, hearts, which were coarsely minced and bioassayed in the peritoneal cavities of fresh mice were removed immediately after LVI of cancer cells; bioassay controls consisted of minced hearts, to which known numbers of cancer cells were added just before introduction into the peritoneal cavities. The results showed that 95% of B16 melanoma cells and 80% of EAT cells delivered to the myocardium were killed in less than 5 min and that the killing was associated with delivery to beating hearts. Although estimates of intramyocardial pressures and "hoop" tensions in the myocardium are controversial, even the lowest values are several orders of magnitude higher than those required to rupture unfolded cancer cell membranes.[43] Therefore, the results are consistent with the concept of lethal, intravascular trauma.

b. Skeletal Muscle

In humans, hematogenous metastasis to skeletal muscle is uncommon; collected autopsy data reveals an overall median incidence of approximately 5%.[44] Mice that were given LVI of 10^6 B16 melanoma cells and killed when they became moribund 15 to 16 d later, no tumors were detected in their quadriceps femoris muscles at autopsy, in spite of each muscle receiving 1.5 × 10^3 cancer cells. In other noncontractile organs receiving similar numbers of cancer cells, tumors were detected.[45] In the absence of serial sections of whole muscles, visual inspection only of skeletal muscles may generate false negative reports.[46] Therefore, in additional experiments[47] bioassays were made by introducing into the peritoneal cavities of fresh mice, coarsely minced quadriceps femoris muscles within 5 min after LVI. Cancer cells were delivered via LVI in anesthetized animals with denervated (flaccid) or noncontracting controls, with muscle tone. A third group of mice received cancer cells, and their quadriceps muscles were made to contract by applying an electrical stimulus to the femoral nerve. After 65 d, the end results of the bioassays were expressed in weights of intraperitoneal tumor nodules, corrected for cancer cell content as indicated from planimetry of sections of each nodule. As shown in Table 1, compared with control muscles, significantly more cancer cells survived after delivery to flaccid muscles, and fewer survived when delivery was followed by muscle contraction. The results are consistent with the concept of lethal mechanical trauma.

c. Other Contractile Organs

The intestines, urinary bladder, spleen, and uterus are relatively uncommon sites for hematogenous metastasis. The contributions of mechanical trauma to this situation is currently unknown.

d. The Lungs

The lungs are major sites for both cancer cell delivery and killing during hematogenous metastasis. Many experiments in which known numbers of cancer cells were introduced into the systemic circulation of mice have shown that with few exceptions, more than 95% of cells were arrested in the lungs, and of these, less than 0.1% form tumor colonies.[23] Bioassays indicate that in the lungs, as many as 85% of the trapped cells suffer lethal trauma within 5 min of delivery,[48] and longer term observations indicate that the vast majority of the remainder are killed by slower processes. Considerations of rapid mechanical trauma in the pulmonary capillaries must take into account changes in their tensions during the respiratory cycle. Calculations[49] based on measurements of alveolar wall tensions and elastic moduli for the alveolar wall complex indicate that at the end of expiration, the pulmonary capillaries are much more likely to be deformed by cancer cells than during inspiration when the reverse is the case. These calculations appear reasonable for the alveolar walls, but as described above, the elastic characteristics of the cancer cells are initially over estimates. Thus, at best, calculations of this type indicate the *feasibility* of rapid mechanical trauma to cancer cells in the alveolar capillaries. Indirect evidence for mechanical trauma comes from experiments in which equal numbers of cancer cells were delivered to the lungs of mice via either the bronchial or pulmonary arteries.[50] The resulting tumor burdens were assessed by the numbers of animals with overt pulmonary tumors and by the numbers of tumors per animal. The bronchial arteries have a primarily nutritional function, supplying the bronchi and interlobular alveolar tissue. In contrast, the pulmonary arteries have a primary respiratory function, and they terminate in the capillary networks within the alveolar walls. Therefore, it was expected that cancer cells delivered via the pulmonary arteries would be exposed to more mechanical trauma associated with respiratory movements than cells delivered to less expansile parts of the lungs via the bronchial arteries. The results were in accord with these expectations and showed that greater proportions of B16 and colon-26 cancer cells were killed after tail vein injection and during delivery via the pulmonary arteries than after LVI and during delivery via the bronchial arteries.[50] Although these results are in accord with both the earlier calculations and the concept of mechanical damage to cancer cells, they do not in themselves establish a causal relationship.

e. The Liver

Cancer cell traffic studies in animals reveal that the majority of cancer cells entering the portal circulation are arrested and killed in the liver vasculature and that most of the small minority of cells passing through the liver are lethally damaged and incapable of generating extra-hepatic tumors.[51] Cancer cells entering the portal circulation of mice and rats preferentially survive and grow in the periportal domain of liver acini (acinar zone one), and this is not explicable solely in terms of preferential arrest in this zone.[52] Vital fluorescence microscopy and electron microscopy[20] also have shown the arrest of large numbers of cancer cells in the periportal region of liver sinusoids, where sinusoid diameter is considerably less than cancer cell diameter. As the sinusoids were blocked, but not deformed by arrested cancer cells, it follows that the cancer cells themselves must have been deformed. Scanning electron microscopy of freeze-fractures liver (Figure 2) reveals that 3LL carcinoma cells in transit through sinusoids undergo deformation, resulting in surface unfolding, which *in vitro* studies discussed earlier have associated it with increased susceptibility to mechanical damage.[34] As with other tissues, the key to mechanical intravascular damage in the liver is that

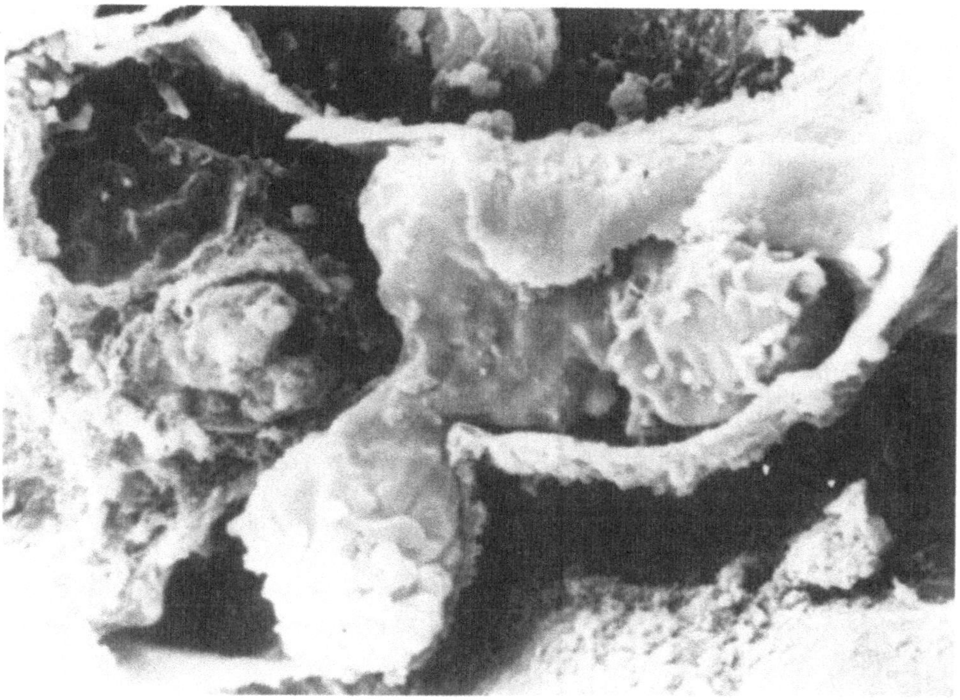

FIGURE 2. A 3LL cell in transit through a liver sinusoid. This scanning electron micrograph shows partial cancer cell surface unfolding. (Courtesy of Dr. F. Vidal-Vanaclocha, University of the Basque Country, Spain.)

the involved blood vessels should be smaller and less deformable than the cancer cells. Therefore, it is of interest that the internal diameter of (rat) liver sinusoids is 6 to 7 μm and that their external surfaces are surrounded by fibroblast-like cells and their products, which include the Space of Disse; the walls and the space constitute the ''blood-hepatocyte barrier''.[53] Unfortunately, no data are currently available on the mechanical properties of these structures. In spite of sparse data, the fact remains that the vast majority of cancer cells arriving in the liver via the portal vein are rapidly destroyed. While the available evidence indicates the feasibility of mechanical trauma playing a role in this destruction, a causal relationship has yet to be determined.

2. ''Hemodynamic'' Trauma

In a single capillary occluded by a cancer cell, the blood pressure gradient originally applied over the entire length of the vessel now will be applied between the ends of the cancer cell. Calculations indicated that under the specific conditions of a single capillary, this blood pressure gradient may increase the tensions to rupture point in the unfolded surface membranes of arrested cancer cells.[14,18,49] However, within a network containing both patent and obstructed capillaries, the pressure between the ends of an arrested cancer cell blocking a vessel would be less than the pressure gradient over the whole network because of the back pressure on the venous side of the cell. Nonetheless, even under these circumstances, a pressure gradient along the cancer cell is expected on account of the viscous pressure drop due to bloodflow in adjacent capillaries.[6] The extent of this ''hemodynamic'' damage is expected to increase with increased proportions of blocked capillaries within networks.

3. Intravascular Mechanical Trauma: Some General Comments

It must be emphasized that rapid mechanical trauma is only one of a number of possible mechanisms for rapid, lethal intravascular trauma to cancer cells. Other nonexclusive mechanisms within this category include injury due to free radicals (see Chapters 6 and 15). In addition, although rapidly inflicted trauma is lethal for the majority of cancer cells delivered to at least some organs and although the majority of the survivors are lethally damaged by slower mechanisms, including the cellular and humoral arms of the inflammatory and immunologic response, in the absence of therapeutic intervention, enough cancer cells survive to kill the patient eventually. Even inefficient processes succeed, if repeated often enough! Therefore, the role of rapid biomechanical trauma is best seen as one of a number of inhibitory rate regulators for hematogenous metastasis, the extent of which varies in different organs. As such, it is a consistently overlooked "soil"-factor underlying the "seed-and-soil" hypothesis for metastatic pattern formation.

C. CANCER CELL CLUMPS

For ease of analysis, discussion so far has been limited to the biomechanical interactions of single cancer cells and capillary walls. It is well-known that in addition to single cells, clumps of cancer cells are also released into the bloodstream from primary lesions. For example, in a study of renal vein blood sampled just prior to nephrectomy in patients with renal cell carcinoma, as many as 20% of the circulating cancer cells were present in multicellular clumps.[54]

The stability of clumps in the larger blood vessels depends on a number of factors, including the dissociative action of blood flow (maximized under conditions of turbulence), the action of collisions with other cells, particularly erythrocytes, and the enzyme activity. Stable clumps will remain confined to the larger vessels and may pass directly through organs.[55] Following the injection of glass spheres into the arterial systems of the spleen, lungs, or portal veins of dogs, cats, or rabbits, spheres having diameters 20 to 40 times that of capillaries were detected in organ venous effluents, indicating their passage through noncapillary arterio-venous shunts (portal-to-hepatic vein in the liver).[56] In isolated human lungs, arterio-venous shunts permitting the passage of 0.5 mm beads were demonstrated.[57]

Emboli consisting of multicellular clumps are ultimately arrested in larger vessels. When they are subjected to the various compressive forces described above, it is expected that pressure relief could be obtained in clusters of cells with heterogenous mechanical properties, by the most susceptible bursting first, thereby, protecting others within the same aggregate from lethal deformation. This expectation is in accord with a number of observations reviewed elsewhere,[58] showing that the metastatic inefficiency of clumps of cancer cells is in fact less than that of corresponding numbers of single cancer cells. It is worthy of comment that in those systems examined, the enhancement of metastatic efficiency by multicellular clumps usually exceeds the enhancement brought about by transfecting cells with genetic material associated with the elusive metastatic phenotype.

V. CONCLUSIONS

Although the biomechanical aspects of cancer cell interactions with the microvasculature will be unfamiliar to most general readers and have received comparatively little attention in the past, they may well serve as major rate regulators of cancer cell arrest and destruction during hematogenous metastasis. Metastatic inefficiency due to biomechanical and other forms of cancer cell trauma may be exploitable by use of regional cancer chemotherapy, as discussed in relation to colorectal carcinoma.[56] While the indirect evidence in favor of the biomechanical hypotheses reviewed here does not provide rigid proof for these hypotheses, this evidence is generally in accord with them and thus supports their *feasibility*. It is hoped that the many deficiencies in identifying and understanding biomechanical interactions presently will be resolved by future iterative experimental and theoretical studies, which are analogous to those that have been successful with erythrocytes and leucocytes.

REFERENCES

1. **Zeidman, I.,** The fate of circulating tumor cells. I. Passage of cells through capillaries, *Cancer Res.*, 21, 38, 1961.
2. **Weiss, L.,** Studies on cell deformability. I. Effect of surface charge, *J. Cell Biol.*, 26, 735, 1965.
3. **Weiss, L.,** Cell deformability: some general considerations, in *Fundamental Aspects of Metastasis,* Weiss, L., Ed., N. Holland, Amsterdam, 1976, 305.
4. **Sato, H. and Suzuki, M.,** Deformability and viability of tumor cells by transcapillary passage with reference to organ affinity in metastasis in cancer, in *Fundamental Aspects of Metastasis,* Weiss, L., Ed., N. Holland, Amsterdam, 1976, 311.
5. **Weiss, L. and Clement, K.,** Studies on cell deformability: some rheological considerations, *Exp. Cell Res.*, 58, 379, 1969.
6. **Weiss, L. and Schmid-Schonbein, G. W.,** Biomechanical interactions of cancer cells with the microvasculature during metastasis, *Cell Biophys.*, 14, 187, 1989.
7. **Fung, Y. C.,** Red blood cells and their deformability, in *Biomechanics,* Springer-Verlag, New York, 1984, 101.
8. **Evans, E. A. and Skalak, R.,** Mechanics and thermodynamics of biomembranes, *CRC Crit. Rev. Bioeng.*, 3, 181, 1979.
9. **Bagge, U., Born, G. V. R., and Gaehtgens, P., Eds.,** *White Blood Cells: Morphology and Rheology as Related to Induction,* Martinus Nijhoff, The Hague, 1983.
10. **Meiselman, H. J., Lichtman, M. A., and LaCelle, P. L., Eds.,** *White Cell Mechanics: Basic Science and Clinical Aspects,* Alan R. Liss, New York, 1984.
11. **McIntire, L. V. and Eskin, S. G.,** Mechanical and biochemical aspects of leukocyte interactions with model vessel walls, in *White Cell Mechanics: Basic Science and Clinical Aspects,* Alan R. Liss, New York, 1984, 209.
12. **Goldsmith, H. L.,** Collisions of circulating cells with the vascular endothelium, in *Fundamental Aspects of Metastasis,* Weiss, L., Ed., N. Holland, Amsterdam, 1976, 99.
13. **Dimitrov, D. S.,** Dynamic interactions between approaching surfaces of biological interest, *Prog. Surface Sci.*, 14, 295, 1983.
14. **Weiss, L. and Dimitrov, D. S.,** A fluid mechanical analysis of the velocity, adhesion, and destruction of cancer cells in capillaries during metastasis, *Cell Biophys.*, 6, 9, 1984.
15. **Israelachvili, J. N. and McGuiggan, P. M.,** Forces between surfaces in liquids, *Science,* 241, 795, 1988.
16. **Helm, C. A., Israelachvili, J. N., and McGuiggan, P. M.,** Molecular mechanisms and forces involved in the adhesion and fusion of amphiliphilic bilayers, *Science,* 246, 919, 1989.
17. **Weiss, L. and Harlos, J. P.,** Some speculations on the rate of adhesion of cells to coverslips, *J. Theor. Biol.*, 37, 169, 1972.
18. **Weiss, L., Dimitrov, D. S., and Angelova, M.,** The hemodynamic destruction of intravascular cancer cells in relation to myocardial metastasis, *Proc. Natl. Acad. Sci. U.S.A.*, 82, 5737, 1985.
19. **Schmid-Schonbein, G. W., Usani, S., Skalak, R., and Chien, S.,** The interaction of leukocytes and erythrocytes in capillary and postcapillary vessels, *Microvasc. Res.*, 19, 45, 1980.
20. **Bagge, U., Skolnik, G., and Ericson, L. E.,** The arrest of circulating tumor cells in the liver microcirculation, *J. Cancer Res. Clin. Oncol.*, 105, 134, 1983.
21. **Nicolson, G. L.,** Organ specificity of tumor metastasis: role of preferential adhesion invasion and growth of malignant cells at specific secondary sites, *Cancer Metast. Rev.*, 7, 143, 1988.
22. **Weiss, L.,** Metastatic inefficiency: causes and consequences, *Cancer Rev.*, 3, 1, 1986.
23. **Weiss, L.,** Metastatic inefficiency, *Adv. Cancer Res.*, 54, 159, 1990.
24. **Evans, E. A. and Parsegian, V. A.,** Energetics of membrane deformation and adhesion in cell and vesicle aggregation, *Ann. N.Y. Acad. Sci.*, 416, 13, 1983.
25. **Kwok, R. and Evans, E.,** Thermoelasticity of large lecithin bilayer vesicles, *Biophys. J.*, 35, 637, 1981.
26. **Wolfe, J., Dowgert, M. F., and Steponkus, P. L.,** Mechanical study of the deformation and rupture of the plasma membranes of protoplasts during osmotic expansions, *J. Membrane Biol.*, 93, 63, 1986.
27. **Evans, E. A., Waugh, R., and Melnik, L.,** Elastic area compressibility modulus of red cell membrane, *Biophys. J.*, 16, 585, 1976.
28. **Mitchison, J. M. and Swann, M. M.,** The mechanical properties of the cell surface: the cell elastimeter, *J. Exp. Biol.*, 31, 443, 1954.
29. **Pulvertaft, R. J. V. and Weiss, L.,** Some effects of microelectrophoresis suspending fluids on tissue cells, *J. Pathol.*, 85, 473, 1963.
30. **Weiss, L.,** Studies on cell deformability. V. Some effects of ribonuclease, *J. Theor. Biol.*, 18, 9, 1968.
31. **Erickson, E. A. and Trinkaus, J. P.,** Microvilli and blebs as sources of reserve membrane during cell spreading, *Exp. Cell Res.*, 99, 375, 1976.
32. **Evans, E. A. and Kukan, B.,** Passive material behaviour of granulocytes based on large deformation and recovery after deformation tests, *Blood,* 64, 1028, 1984.

33. **Mege, J. L., Capo, C., Benoliel, A. M., and Bongrand, P.,** Use of cell contour analysis to evaluate the affinity between macrophages and glutaraldehyde-treated erythrocytes, *Biophys. J.*, 52, 177, 1987.
34. **Weiss, L., Harlos, J. P., and Elkin, G.,** Mechanism of mechanical trauma to Ehrlich ascites tumor cells *in vitro* and its relationship to rapid intravascular death during metastasis, *Int. J. Cancer,* 44, 143, 1989.
35. **Weiss, L., Harlos, J. P., Elkin, G., and Bixler, B.,** Mechanisms for the biomechanical destruction of L1210 leukemia cells: a rate-regulator for metastasis, *Cell Biophys.*, 16, 149, 1990.
36. **Elson, E. L.,** Cellular mechanics as an indicator of cytoskeletal structure and function, *Ann. Rev. Biophys. Chem.*, 17, 397, 1988.
37. **Kolega, J.,** Effects of mechanical tension protrusive activity and microfilament and intermediate filament organization in an epithelium moving in culture, *J. Cell Biol.*, 102, 1400, 1986.
38. **Peterson, N. O., McConnaughey, W. B., and Elson, E. L.,** Dependence of locally measured cellular deformability on position of the cell, temperature and cytochalasin B, *Proc. Natl. Acad. Sci. U.S.A.*, 79, 5327, 1932.
39. **Raz, A. and Geiger, B.,** Altered organization of cell-substrate contacts and membrane-associated cytoskeleton in tumor cell variants exhibiting different metastatic capabilities, *Cancer Res.*, 42, 5183, 1982.
40. **Hart, I. R., Raz, A., and Fidler, I. J.,** Effect of cytoskeletal disrupting agents on the metastatic behaviour of melanoma cells, *J. Natl. Cancer Inst.*, 64, 891, 1980.
41. **Weiss, L., Asch, B., and Elkin, G.,** The contributions of the cytoskeleton of Ehrlich ascites tumor cells to cellular resistance to mechanical trauma, *Invasion and Metastasis,* 1991, in press.
42. **Gabor, H. and Weiss, L.,** Survival of L1210 and Ehrlich ascites cancer cells after mechanical trauma is a random event, *Invasion and Metastasis,* 5, 84, 1985.
43. **Weiss, L.,** Biomechanical destruction of cancer cells in the heart: a rate-regulator for hematogenous metastasis, *Invasion and Metastasis,* 8, 228, 1988.
44. **Weiss, L.,** Biomechanical destruction of cancer cells in skeletal muscle: a rate-regulator for hematogenous metastasis, *Clin. Exp. Metastasis,* 7, 483, 1989.
45. **Weiss, L., Ward, P. M., Harlos, J. P., and Holmes, J. C.,** Target organ patterns of tumors in mice following the arterial dissemination of B16 melanoma cells, *Int. J. Cancer,* 33, 825, 1984.
46. **Weiss, L. and Harlos, J. P.,** The validity of negative necropsy reports for metastases in solid organs, *J. Pathol.*, 148, 203, 1986.
47. **Weiss, L.,** Biomechanical destruction of cancer cells in skeletal muscle: a rate-regulator for hematogenous metastasis, *Clin. Exp. Metastasis,* 7, 483, 1989.
48. **Mayhew, E. and Glaves, D.,** Quantitation of tumorigenic disseminating and arrested cancer cells, *Br. J. Cancer,* 50, 159, 1984.
49. **Weiss, L. and Dimitrov, D. S.,** Mechanical aspects of the lungs as cancer cell-killing organs during hematogenous metastasis, *J. Theor. Biol.*, 121, 307, 1986.
50. **Weiss, L. and Ward, P. M.,** Effects of disseminating route on the liver- and lung-colonizing efficiencies of B16 melanoma and colony-26 carcinoma in mice, *Int. J. Cancer,* 44, 510, 1989.
51. **Weiss, L., Ward, P. M., and Holmes, J. C.,** Liver-to-lung traffic of cancer cells, *Int. J. Cancer,* 32, 79, 1983.
52. **Barbera-Guillem, E., Alonso-Varona, A., and Vidal-Vanaclocha, F.,** Selective implantation and growth in rats and mice of experimental liver metastasis in Acinar Zone One, *Cancer Res.*, 49, 4003, 1989.
53. **Barbera-Guillem, E., Alonso-Varona, A., and Vidal-Vanaclocha, F.,** 5-Inusoidal structure of the liver, *Cell Biol. Rev.*, 16, 1, 1988.
54. **Glaves, D., Huben, R. P., and Weiss, L.,** Haematogenous dissemination of cells from human renal adenocarcinomas, *Br. J. Cancer,* 57, 32, 1988.
55. **Zeidman, I. and Buss, J. M.,** Transpulmonary passage of tumor cell emboli, *Cancer Res.*, 12, 731, 1952.
56. **Prinzmetal, M., Ornitz, E. M., Sinkin, B., and Bergman, H. C.,** Arterio-venous anastomoses in liver, spleen and lungs, *Am. J. Physiol.*, 152, 48, 1948.
57. **Tobin, C. E. and Zariquiez, M. O.,** Arteriovenous shunts in the human lung, *Proc. Soc. Exp. Biol. Med.*, 75, 827, 1950.
58. **Weiss, L.,** Circulating cancer cells, in *Principles of Metastasis,* Academic Press, Orlando, FL, 1985, 139.
59. **Hammer, D. A. and Lauffenburger, D. A.,** A dynamical model for receptor-mediated cell adhesion to surfaces in viscous shear flow, *Cell Biophys.*, 14, 139, 1989.
60. **Bell, G. I.,** Estimate of the sticking probability for cells in uniform shear flow with adhesion caused by specific bonds, *Cell Biophys.*, 3, 289, 1981.

Chapter 10

THE ROLE OF INTEGRIN RECEPTORS IN TUMOR CELL ADHESION TO THE MICROVASCULATURE

Randall H. Kramer, Judy Enenstein, Daniel M. Ramos, Mai P. Vu, and Yao Fen Cheng

TABLE OF CONTENTS

I. INTRODUCTION

Tumor metastasis is a complex and inefficient process that requires a selected population of tumor cells to complete a series of sequential steps.[1] The main events in blood-borne metastasis are intravasation, arrest in the microvasculature, extravasation, and secondary tumor growth. Extravasation is a crucial stage in this cycle; the tumor cells must first arrest in and then penetrate the microvascular wall. This wall is composed of a continuous lining of endothelial cells, joined by tight junctions, and their associated basement membrane, together representing a significant barrier to invasion. Several morphological studies have provided some information about the events of tumor cell arrest and extravasation (see Chapter 13 on the morphology of cancer cell arrest and vascular exit).

Successful implantation and eventual penetration of the vascular wall depend on the tumor cell's forming adhesion contacts with the endothelial cell and/or its basement membrane. The formation of specific adhesion contacts between the arrested tumor cell and the endothelium stabilizes its arrest in the vessel and prevents subsequent detachment. Next, the tumor cell somehow induces the local retraction of neighboring endothelial cells, and thereby penetrates the endothelial cell lining. This exposes the underlying vascular basement membrane, a substrate rich in adhesive extracellular matrix (ECM) molecules. At this point, the tumor cell can establish strong adhesion contacts with the vessel wall that resist detachment. Finally, tumor cell proteases dissolve the basement membrane, and the tumor cell emigrates into the interstitium, where successful growth of a micrometastasis is dependent on neovascularization of the secondary tumor.

The nature of the adhesion receptors on the surfaces of tumor cells that mediate adhesion to the microvasculature awaits characterization, but recent observations indicate that a variety of receptors may be involved.[2] One major class of receptors is the integrin superfamily of heterodimers, which can mediate both cell-cell and cell-matrix adhesion. Other specific receptors, such as the nonintegrin 67 to 72 kDa laminin receptor, also appear to be important.[1,3] Finally, various cell surface adhesion molecules with lectin activities also could be involved.[4]

The integrins are a diverse group of related, noncovalently linked heterodimers that constitute a gene superfamily of receptors (reviewed in References 5 to 9) with a wide phylogenetic distribution. Originally identified in the chick system, the integrins appear to mediate cell adhesion to various ECM proteins, including fibronectin (and other RGD-containing proteins), laminin, and collagen.[10] Integrin complexes have been classified according to the presence of one of six β subunits, which are combined with one of several α subunits (see Table 1). Integrins that interact with the ECM include the β_1 and β_3 complexes (Table 2). Many of the β_1 complexes were first identified as the VLA (very late activation) heterodimers.[11,12] The β_2 subunit associates with a set of unique α chains to form several leukocyte receptors (including LFA-1 [α_l], Mac-1 [α_m], and p150,95 [α_x] that mediate leukocyte cell-cell interactions.[8] The β_3 subunit, which forms complexes that bind ligands such as vitronectin, can combine with one of at least two different α subunits to produce the platelet GP IIb/IIIa and the vitronectin receptor. For all six β subunit families, the ligand specificity appears to be defined by the α chain and the individual β chain to which it is complexed.

From recent evidence, it is clear that cells can express a diverse set of integrin receptors with specificity for particular extracellular matrix components. Certain receptors appear to be widely distributed and are present on a variety of cell types. For example, the fibronectin receptor ($\alpha_5\beta_1$, VLA-5) is present on most cell types (reviewed in Reference 7). Other receptors may have a more restricted expression and may be present only on certain types of differentiated cells or expressed only at specific times. Thus, VLA-1, an integrin-related heterodimer ($\alpha_1\beta_1$) that binds collagen and laminin, is not expressed on quiescent T-lym-

TABLE 1
Integrin Family of Adhesion Receptors

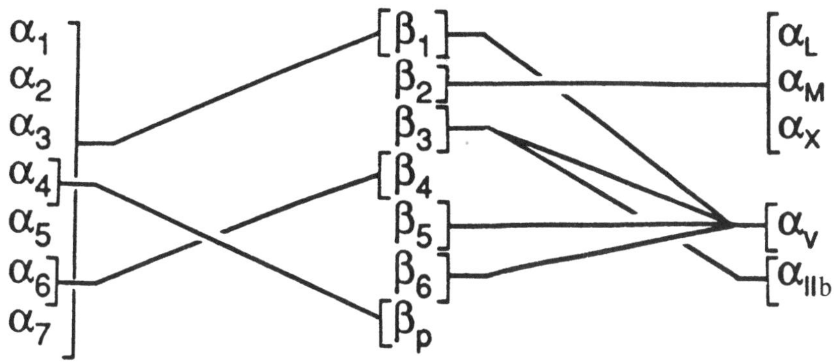

TABLE 2
Ligand Specificity of Integrin Receptors

β Subunit	α Subunit	Ligand
β_1	α_1	Collagen, laminin
	α_2	Collagen, laminin
	α_3	Collagen, laminin, fibronectin
	α_4	Fibronectin
	α_5	Fibronectin
	α_6	Laminin
	α_7	Laminin
β_2	α_L	Leukocyte adhesion
	α_M	Leukocyte adhesion
	α_X	Leukocyte adhesion
β_3	α_V	Vitronectin, von Willebrand factor, fibrinogen, thrombospondin, fibronectin, laminin
	α_{IIb}	Vitronectin, von Willebrand factor, fibrinogen, thrombospondin, fibronectin
β_4	α_6	?
β_5	α_v	Vitronectin, fibronectin
β_p	α_4	High endothelial venules (Peyer's patch)

phocytes, but is induced after activation.[13] In addition, individual integrin receptors may have restricted ligand specificity (e.g., the fibronectin receptor), while others may be promiscuous and have multiple ligand interactions (e.g., $\alpha_1\beta_1$, $\alpha_2\beta_1$, $\alpha_3\beta_1$, $\alpha_{IIb}\beta_3$, $\alpha_v\beta_3$).

In the present survey, we have summarized the nature of the adhesive molecules present in the extracellular matrix of the vessel wall and the corresponding receptors expressed at the tumor cell surface with particular emphasis on the integrin family of receptors. Additional molecules are certain to be identified. It is probable that, like other characteristics of heterogeneous tumor cell populations, the expression of these receptors may vary and could account for differences in the invasive and metastatic potential of individual tumor cells.

II. SURVEY OF ADHESION PROTEINS AND THEIR RECEPTORS

A. TUMOR CELL–ENDOTHELIAL CELL INTERACTIONS

The initial arrest of tumor cells in the microvasculature of the target organ may depend more on simple physical trapping than on specific adhesive interactions because of the rapid passage of cells through the blood vessel.[14] While simple physical trapping of the tumor cells in the small lumen of capillaries is probably sufficient for the initial arrest, secondary mechanisms, such as specific adhesion contacts with the vessel wall and interaction with platelets and fibrin, may also be important.[15] Furthermore, there is evidence to suggest that it is not the initial arrest of the tumor cells that predicts successful metastasis, but rather it is the resistance of tumor cells to detachment from the microvasculature.[1,16] In addition, metastatic patterning, frequently seen for certain tumors, cannot always be explained simply by selective arrest; it probably also reflects successful survival and growth of implanted tumor cells.[17,18] On the other hand, there is evidence that tumor cells can recognize specific determinants expressed on the microvessel endothelium of particular organs. Thus, Auerbach and associates[19] have reported that tumor cells show preferential adhesion to endothelial cells isolated from tissues in which metastases are commonly formed (see Chapter 11).

Tumor cells induce the local displacement of adjacent endothelial cells by mechanisms as yet unknown. While platelet release products may mediate these reactions, other mechanisms must exist, since tumor cells *in vitro* can induce retraction of endothelial cells in the absence of plasma, platelets, or fibrin.[20,21] That endothelial cell retraction occurs at cellular junctions suggests that this process requires active participation of the endothelial cell since retraction requires disruption of both cell-cell adhesions and cell-basement membrane adhesions. The phenomenon of cell-induced contact inhibition of movement[22,23] may play a role in tumor-cell-induced retraction, but as yet we know nothing about the mechanisms responsible. However, the recent identification of "vascular permeability factor"[24] may suggest one mechanism for endothelial cell retraction.

An illustration of cell homing to specific microvasculatures is provided by the binding of lymphoid cells to high endothelial venules of particular organs. The targeting of lymphocyte homing requires the interaction of homing receptors on the lymphocytes with adhesive molecules termed "vascular addressins" on the high endothelial venules.[25-28] A rapidly expanding literature has described homing receptors specific for peripheral lymph nodes, Peyer's patches, and other gut-associated lymphoid tissue as well as less specific receptors. Antibodies to these putative receptors block binding of lymphocytes to high endothelial venules of specific lymphoid tissues *in vivo* and *in vitro*. The peripheral lymph node homing receptor has been shown to bind to the high endothelial venules.

The peripheral lymph node homing receptor, found on mature mouse cortical thymocytes, peripheral blood and lymphoid organ T and B cells, and neutrophils, was first defined by the monoclonal antibody (mAb) MEL-14. The MEL-14 antigen is a single glycoprotein chain of 90 kDa. The sequence of MEL-14 antigen displays a lectin domain, epidermal growth factor domain, and two complement domains.[29] Carbohydrate recognition is dependent on calcium ions.[28] The human equivalent of the mouse homing receptor has been sequenced by several groups.[30-33] This lymphocyte homing receptor shows domain homology to the leukocyte adhesion molecule, ELAM-1, and the granule membrane protein, GMP-140. It exists both as a membrane-bound and a phospholipid-anchored molecule, which may permit it to be rapidly shed, thus facilitating migration. A seemingly unrelated peripheral lymph node homing receptor has been described in the rat.[34]

Murine Peyer's patches homing receptors, isolated by mAb R1-2, are part of the integrin family of adhesion heterodimers.[35] Two homing receptors of normal unstimulated lymphocytes, LPAM-1 and LPAM-2, were isolated and found to have an identical 160 kDa α chain, α_{4m}, and different 130 kDa β chains.[36] LPAM-1 has a unique β chain, β_p, which is unrelated to other integrin β chains, although it maintains the 56 cysteine residues of all integrin β chains. LPAM-2 has a β_1 chain and is homologous to the integrin VLA-4 ($\alpha_4\beta_1$). A mAb that blocked T cell adhesion to fibronectin also immunoprecipitated $\alpha_4\beta_1$.[37] Binding of the α to the β chains is calcium-ion-dependent. Different lymphoma cell lines were shown to express either β_1,β_p, or both β_1 and β_p.[36]

The Hermes-1 antibody defines a nonspecific homing receptor in humans that binds lymphocytes to high endothelial venules of peripheral lymph node, Peyer's patch, mucosa or synovial origin. Hermes antigen is found on lymphocytes, neutrophils, monocytes, and eosinophils. The Hermes-1 antigen, Ip4.2, is 85 to 95 kDa (size varies in different tissues).[38] Although this human homing receptor crossreacts weakly with MEL-14 antibody, the cDNA of the Hermes antigen shows no homology with the MEL-14 antigen.[30,39] Hermes-1 antigen does share homology with cartilage link protein and matrix receptor 3. A related antibody, Hermes-3, defines an antigen of 85 to 95 kDa, which is said to be specific for Peyer's patches and other gut-associated lymphoid tissue.

LFA-1 antigen (CD11a/18), a 180/95 kDa integrin heterodimer, is found on all murine and human leukocytes and on most lymphocytes. Antibodies to LFA-1 partially block lymphocyte adhesion to high endothelial venules.[40] Because the antibodies to LFA-1 were most effective in cell lines that expressed very little MEL-14 antigen, LFA-1 is thought to play an accessory role in lymphocyte homing. LFA-1 recognizes ICAM-1 on endothelial cells, though ICAM-1 may not be the only ligand for LFA-1.

Several vascular addressins have been defined that bind lymphocyte homing receptors. The MECA-79 mouse antigen, 92 kDa in size, is found on the luminal surface of high endothelial venules in peripheral lymph nodes.[27] MECA-79 antibody blocks lymphocyte binding to the peripheral lymph nodes. MECA-367 antigen, a 58 to 67 kDa protein, is found on mucosal lymphoid tissues and high endothelial venules in Peyer's patches.[41] MECA-367 antibody blocks lymphocyte binding to the latter tissue.

Tumor cells may use mechanisms similar to those of lymphocytes to home to specific organs. This would imply that different tissues have different endothelial, basement membrane, or parenchymal antigens, and that the tumor cells themselves bear tissue-specific homing receptors. Microvascular endothelial cells (MEC) of different tissues have been shown to differ in surface antigens[19] and to bind metastatic tumor cells in a site-specific manner (see Chapter 11 on interactions between cancer cells and the endothelium). Both melanoma cells and lymphomas can be selected *in vitro* for enhanced specific homing *in vivo*.[42,43] B16 melanoma cells show enhanced lung metastasis after repeated selection on cryostat lung sections. When lymphoma cells were selected for binding to high endothelial venules, only those lymphoma cells that bound venules *in vitro* spread to all lymph nodes *in vivo* after intramuscular injection. Most lymphoma cells that home to peripheral lymph nodes carry the MEL-14 antigen.[34] It also has been suggested that tumor cell fusion with lymphocytes *in vivo* may produce cells with specific homing capabilities. As mentioned earlier, different lymphomas express β_1 or β_p LPAM integrin. In addition, a cytokine-inducible human endothelial-cell-surface molecule, INCAM-110, appears to support adhesion of melanoma cells.[44] An inducible endothelial cell receptor for neutrophils, ELAM-1, supported colon carcinoma cell adhesion.[44] These last studies give no explanation for directed homing, but do imply that tumor cells might activate receptor expression by endothelium by means of cytokines or that inflamed endothelia would promote tumor adhesion.

Although the apical surface of MEC is a relatively poor substrate for cell adhesion, some attachment does occur. To further define this interaction and to aid in the identification of surface components that are involved in this adhesion, we prepared rabbit antibodies against MEC surface membranes and then evaluated the effect of these antibodies on MeWo cell adhesion to intact MEC monolayers. The antisera were exhaustively absorbed against intact MeWo cells to remove any crossreacting antibodies. When MEC monolayers were preincubated with two different anti-MEC antisera, MeWo cell adhesion was significantly inhibited (Figure 1). This suggests that the antibodies directed against specific MEC surface membrane components can block tumor cell adhesion. We also tested a polyclonal antiserum against the β_1 subunit. This effectively inhibited MeWo cell adhesion to intact MEC monolayers and suggests that tumor cell adhesion to MEC involves this class of integrin receptors.

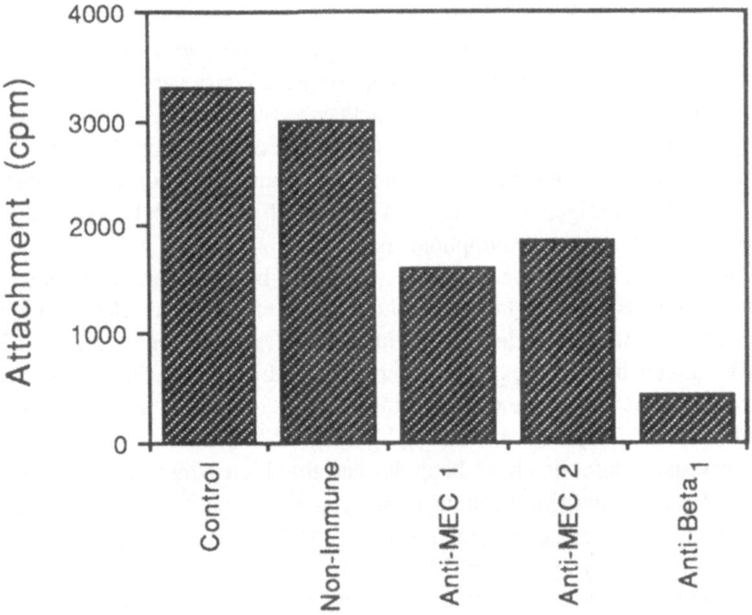

FIGURE 1. The effect of anti-endothelial cell antibodies and anti-β_1 antibodies on the adhesion of melanoma cells to microvascular endothelial cell monolayers. MeWo melanoma cells (radiolabeled with ^{3}H-thymidine) were seeded onto confluent monolayers of microvascular endothelial cells in the presence of polyclonal anti-endothelial cell antibodies (anti-MEC 1 and anti-MEC 2) and anti-β_1 antibodies (all at 1:50 dilution). After 30 min of incubation at 37°C, the number of adherent cells was determined.

B. TUMOR CELL–SUBENDOTHELIAL MATRIX ADHESION

1. Composition of the Vascular Basement Membrane

The vascular basement membrane, once exposed by endothelial cell retraction, is an extremely adhesive substrate (Figure 2). Capillary basement membrane contains type IV collagen, laminin, fibronectin, vitronectin, heparan sulfate proteoglycan, entactin, thrombospondin, and von Willebrand factor.[45,46] Many of these ligands contain a unique binding site, represented by the amino acid sequence Arg-Gly-Asp (RGD), for adhesion receptors. This sequence is present in the cell-binding domain of fibronectin and in other adhesive ligands, including vitronectin, fibrinogen, collagens, entactin, thrombospondin, and laminin. While the RGD site has been shown to be of major importance in cell attachment, many of the protein ligands contain additional domains that could function as adhesion sites for integrin and nonintegrin receptors. Because of the diversity of attachment proteins in this matrix and the multiplicity of surface receptors expressed on the tumor cells, it is likely that the strongest and most durable form of microvessel adhesion occurs between the tumor cell and the subendothelial matrix.

Evidence that metastasis involves interaction with matrix ligand binding is suggested by experiments in which either polypeptide fragments or specific peptides derived from individual ECM proteins were able to block experimental metastasis. Proteolytic fragments of laminin[47] or fibronectin[48,49] have been shown to inhibit metastasis. Specific analogues of RGD peptides were able to inhibit invasion of amnion basement membrane.[50] A sequence

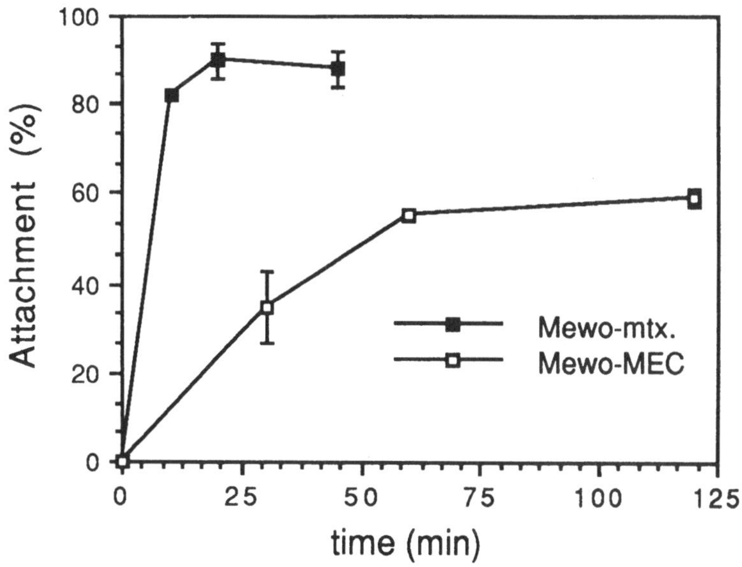

FIGURE 2. Adhesion of MeWo melanoma cells to endothelial cell monolayers and isolated subendothelial extracellular matrix. Confluent MEC monolayers or their matrices (prepared by extraction with hypotonic-NP40 detergent extraction) were seeded with tumor cells. At the indicated times, the number of adherent cells was determined.

derived from the β1 chain of laminin has been shown to inhibit experimental metastasis as well as invasion through the reconstituted basement membrane matrices.[51,52] Recently, synthetic polymers of either RGD or YIGSR (see below) were reported to be much more effective in blocking spontaneous metastasis than the monomer peptides; the polymers also diminished tumor cell arrest and retention in the lungs after i.v. injection.[53] Given the ligand complexities of basement membranes, it is likely that multiple integrin receptors are involved in tumor cell-matrix adhesion. For example, melanoma cells appear to use both the β_1 and β_3 groups of receptors when they adhere to microvascular endothelial cell matrices (Figure 3).

2. Adhesion Proteins and Their Receptors

a. Laminin

Laminin is the major adhesion protein present in basement membranes.[45] As tumor cells adhere to and penetrate basement membranes, it is likely that they will interact with this ligand. Laminin is a large complex glycoprotein (900 kDa) composed of three polypeptide chains (A, B1, and B2) in a cruciform structure. Several unique functional domains in laminin interact with other structural elements of the basement membrane (e.g., type IV collagen, heparan sulfate proteoglycan, and nidogen [explained below]). Laminin has multiple high-affinity cell-binding sites that mediate cell adhesion, but it also contains EGF-like repeats in its short arms that appear to promote cell growth.[54] Different forms of laminin have been identified in the basement membranes of various tissues,[55,56] but the importance or function of these variant forms has not yet been established.

Several radioligand binding studies have shown that laminin fragments 1 and 8 possess cell attachment binding sites[57] with K_Ds of 1 to 10 nM. Since each individual fragment could compete for cell binding, it is likely that the two adhesion sites represent different recognition signals. Fragment 8 contains a high-affinity cell-binding site that promotes neurite outgrowth.[58] Nidogen (entactin) is tightly associated with laminin, and there is evidence that nidogen blocks the expression of a latent cell-binding site on the short arms of laminin.[59,60]

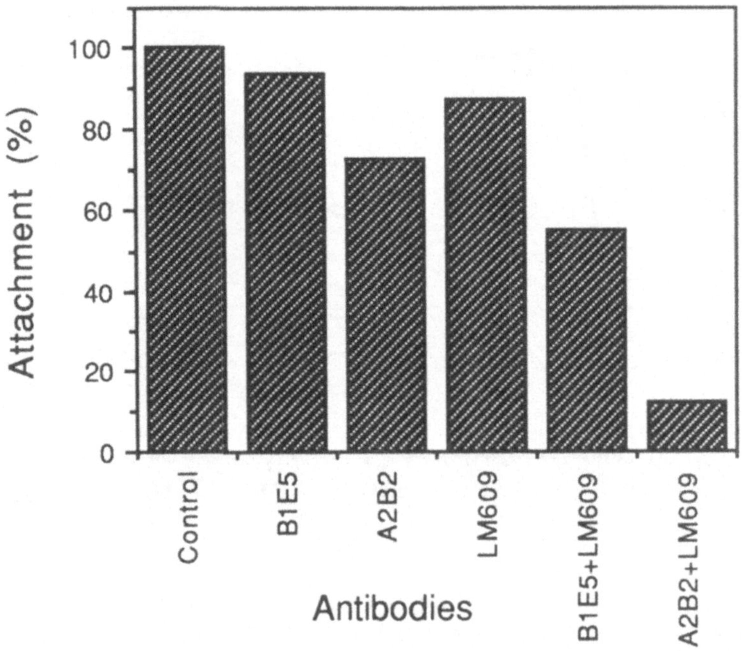

FIGURE 3. Effect of monoclonal antibodies on MeWo melanoma cell adhesion to isolated subendothelial matrix. MeWo cells were allowed to attach to wells containing subendothelial cell matrices in control medium, or in the presence of monoclonal antibodies to the β_1 subunit (A2B2, ascites 1:500), the $\alpha_5\beta_1$ subunit (B1E5, ascites 1:100), or the $\alpha_v\beta_3$ complex (LM609, ascites 1:100) or combinations of these antibodies. The number of adherent cells at the end of the assay (20 min) was then determined.

Receptors for laminin have been implicated in metastasis. Melanoma cells selected for increased attachment to laminin exhibit much higher metastatic potential in lung colonization assays (reviewed in Reference 1). Furthermore, the presence of intact laminin will enhance lung colonization, whereas the C1 proteolytic fragment, which lacks the globular end regions of the short arms of the molecule, inhibits lung arrest.[47] The YIGSR (Tyr-Ile-Gly-Ser-Arg) peptide, a sequence to which the 67 kDa laminin receptor apparently binds, has been shown to inhibit lung colonization by melanoma cells.[52] These and other results strongly suggest that melanoma cells interact with laminin-rich basement membrane and that this interaction facilitates their vascular arrest and colonization of distant sites.

The first laminin-binding protein identified, the 67 to 72 kDa receptor, was extensively studied by several groups (reviewed in References 1 and 61) and has been detected on a variety of cell types. The 67 kDa receptor binds laminin with high affinity and is purported to interact through the specific peptide sequence YIGSR[51] located in the domain III segment of the laminin B1 chain. More recent work by Mecham et al.[3] indicates that hydrophobic peptide sequences in both laminin and elastin are more important for this receptor. Another receptor, a surface galactosyltransferase that binds laminin oligosaccharides, has been identified in B16 melanoma cells.[62] This enzyme appears to be important in cell spreading on laminin, but was not essential during the initial phase of cell attachment.

At least five distinct integrins have laminin-binding activity. Integrin-related complexes that bound to laminin were first identified with the avian-specific monoclonal antibody CSAT (reviewed in Reference 5). Since then, several mammalian laminin-binding integrins ($\alpha_1\beta_1$, $\alpha_2\beta_1$, $\alpha_3\beta_1$, $\alpha_6\beta_1$, $\alpha_7\beta_1$, $\alpha_v\beta_3$) have been identified.[63-67] Wayner and Carter[63] and later, Gehlsen et al.[68] identified a laminin-binding integrin from rat and human cells that corresponds to $\alpha_3\beta_1$. However, recent studies from Carter et al.[69] suggest that $\alpha_3\beta_1$ may be important in the interaction with secreted laminin-containing basement membrane complexes. $\alpha_1\beta_1$ in both rodent and human cells has been shown to be a laminin receptor.[65,70-72] However, $\alpha_1\beta_1$ is also a collagen receptor which preferentially binds to basement membrane type IV collagen rather than to interstitial type I collagen.[70,71,73] Similarly, the integrin receptor $\alpha_2\beta_1$ was initially found to bind to collagen,[63] but has since been shown also to function as a laminin receptor on several cell types, including endothelial cells,[74,75] melanoma cells,[76] and skin keratinocytes.[69]

Originally, $\alpha_6\beta_1$ was defined as the major component of the platelet complex lc/lla.[77] Sonnenberg et al.[78] later showed that the $\alpha_6\beta_1$ complex on platelets and other cell types[79] mediated adhesion to laminin. Ramos et al.[70] identified the $\alpha_6\beta_1$ integrin on murine B16 melanoma cells as the major laminin-binding receptor. Antibodies to $\alpha_6\beta_1$ were able to block melanoma cell attachment to laminin substrates, establishing that this complex is important in mediating the initial adhesion of cells to this substrate. The α_6 subunit can also associate with the β_4 subunit,[80] and this complex has been identified on colon carcinoma cells and other epithelial cells.[81] It has been recently claimed to be a laminin receptor.[82]

Recently, a novel heterodimer complex that contains the β_1 subunit and a unique α subunit was identified on human and mouse melanoma cells;[67,83] this complex binds specifically to laminin-Sepharose columns with moderate affinity, but not to fibronectin- or collagen type I or IV-Sepharose columns. It is electrophoretically and immunochemically distinct from the six currently known β_1 integrins. Following the convention of Hynes,[84] this heterodimer complex has been tentatively designated $\alpha_7\beta_1$. It has restricted tissue distribution and may be specific for melanocyte-derived cells, but has not been detected on cultured primary human melanocytes. Instead, the primary melanocytes appear to use the $\alpha_6\beta_1$ complex to adhere to laminin substrates.[67]

b. Type IV Collagen

Type IV collagen is the major structural component of basement membranes[85,86] and serves as a scaffold for the attachment of epithelial and other cells.[87] By electron microscopy and rotary shadowing, type IV collagen has the appearance of a 390 nm triple-helical rod with a globular carboxyl terminus (NC1 domain) and a disulfide-bond-enriched amino terminus. As a scaffold for attachment, collagen IV possesses binding domains for laminin, fibronectin, proteoglycan, nidogen, and cells.[45] The binding of laminin to collagen IV, mediated by nidogen, is dependent on an intact triple helix in collagen IV. Pepsin digestion studies of collagen IV and rotary shadowing collectively have indicated that laminin binds to type IV collagen at sites 80 nm and 180 nm from the carboxy terminus. Nidogen binds to collagen IV at the same two triple helical sites in collagen IV as does the whole laminin-nidogen complex.[88] The predominant binding sites for heparan sulfate proteoglycan and fibronectin are located within the triple helical regions that are 80 nm and 210 nm away from the NC1 domain.[89] Cell-binding sites are also located in the triple helical region of collagen IV and require an intact triple-helical conformation.[57] Investigations involving fragments have indicated that there are several cell-binding sites in the NC1 and in the triple helical domains.[90-92]

Type IV collagen stimulates the adhesion of a variety of normal and transformed cell types, both by itself and concertedly in the presence of adhesive glycoproteins such as laminin.[87,93-96] Fibrosarcoma cells, such as the HT1080 line, attach specifically to the triple helical domain of type IV collagen.[87] The highly metastatic K1735 M4 melanoma cells have been shown to directly adhere, spread, and migrate in a concentration-dependent manner in response to collagen type IV. The adhesion of these cells to the type IV collagen involves multiple domains of the protein, one of which is RGD-sensitive.[90] Although the triple helix contains many RGD structures,[97] this sequence may not be involved in the adhesion of all cell types.[98] Recently, Chelberg et al.[91] have reported that a specific sequence in the triple-helical domain of type IV collagen that lacks RGD can promote cell attachment. Another cell attachment site has been identified in the α_1 chain of the NC1 domain of type IV collagen.[92] Thus, it is clear that adhesion of cells to type IV collagen, mediated by a multiplicity of potential receptors, occurs in a cell type-specific manner.

Several integrin receptors have been proposed for mediating cell adhesion to type IV collagen. $\alpha_2\beta_1$ was originally shown by Wayner and Carter[63] to bind to interstitial collagens as well as to type IV collagen. $\alpha_1\beta_1$ and $\alpha_2\beta_1$ were shown to bind to type IV collagen by affinity chromatography.[71,73] By affinity chromatography and by anti-integrin antibody experiments, it appears that $\alpha_2\beta_1$ preferentially binds type IV collagen, and $\alpha_1\beta_1$ preferentially binds type I collagen. $\alpha_3\beta_1$ can apparently bind type IV collagen as well as the interstitial collagens.[63,99] In studies with epidermal keratinocytes, Carter et al.[69] have evidence to suggest that this receptor preferentially binds a complex of laminin and type IV collagen.

c. Fibronectin

Discovered in the 1970s, fibronectin was one of the first cell-adhesion proteins to be described and extensively characterized. It is a large, dimeric, multifunctional glycoprotein found both in the extracellular matrix and in plasma (reviewed in Reference 7). It is present in the vascular basement membrane and probably is deposited there by the endothelium and pericytes.[46] Different forms of fibronectin are synthesized by various cell types with regions of alternative splicing of the mRNA constructed from the single fibronectin gene (reviewed in Reference 100). Variations in the sequence of the fibronectin subunit can occur at three sites: extra domains A and B can be included and the IIICS (or variable) region can vary in length.[101] The subendothelial space of blood vessels appears to contain the A form of the molecule.[102,103]

Fibronectin contains a distinct tripeptide sequence, Arg-Gly-Asp (RGD),[7] which is located in the middle of the molecule and appears to mediate many of its adhesive interactions with cells. Many other proteins also contain this or similar sequences that account for various cell-binding activities. The receptor that specifically binds to this site in fibronectin has been identified as an integrin heterodimer composed of the α_5 and β_1 subunits. This complex appears to be highly specific for fibronectin. RGD peptides inhibit cell adhesion to fibronectin substrates, and the same tripeptide also specifically elutes the receptor from fibronectin-Sepharose columns. A monoclonal antibody specific to the receptor will inhibit cell adhesion to immobilized fibronectin. Antireceptor antibodies have localized the receptor in focal adhesion plaques in cells attached to fibronectin substrates.

Melanoma cells and lymphocytes apparently can use two additional adhesion sites produced by alternative splicing within the IIICS (variable region).[48,104,105] The $\alpha_4\beta_1$ complex, which is expressed mainly by lymphoid cells, was found to bind to the CS-1 region of IIICS in fibronectin.[37,106] The β_3-related integrin complexes, including the IIb/IIIa complex ($\alpha_{IIb}\beta_3$) on platelets[107] and the $\alpha_v\beta_5$ complex on epithelial-derived cells,[108,109] also bind fibronectin. In addition, the newly discovered receptor $\alpha_v\beta_1$ also appears to bind fibronectin as well as vitronectin and collagen.[110-112]

d. Vitronectin

Vitronectin is a plasma glycoprotein, consisting of a mixture of a 65 kDa and a 75 kDa polypeptide, that was first identified as a serum spreading factor in cell culture. The 65 kDa protein is derived from the larger precursor. Vitronectin binds to various native collagens, including basement membrane type IV collagen; this binding depends on the collagenous triple helical conformation.[113] Vitronectin also binds strongly to heparan- and chondroitin-sulfated proteoglycans. Based on its affinity for type IV collagen, it would seem likely that vitronectin should associate with the vascular basement membrane. However, immunofluorescence studies indicate that it is concentrated in interstitial structures, particularly elastic fibers and other stromal elements.[114,115] Nevertheless, vitronectin may bind to vascular basement membranes in sufficient amounts to influence tumor cell adhesion to these structures.

Several integrin-related receptors for vitronectin have been identified. Pytela et al.[116] identified an integrin heterodimer on osteosarcoma cells that bound to vitronectin- and RGD-Sepharose columns but not to fibronectin-Sepharose columns. Various other cell types, mostly of mesenchymal origin, were shown to express this vitronectin receptor ($\alpha_v\beta_3$), which is also involved in cell adhesion to fibrinogen and von Willebrand factor. In osteosarcoma cells, the β_3 subunit of the vitronectin receptor is alternatively spliced at its carboxy-terminal end.[117] Platelets express a related receptor, the IIb/IIIa ($\alpha_{IIb}\beta_3$) complex; this receptor is highly promiscuous and binds to various RGD-containing ligands, including vitronectin, fibronectin, fibrinogen, von Willebrand factor, and possibly collagen (reviewed in Reference 118). Whereas fibrinogen binds to the vitronectin receptor only through the RGD site,[108] fibrinogen can bind to platelet IIb/IIIa via the RGD site in the C-terminus of the α-chain or via a site (GGAKQGDV) at the C-terminus of the γ-chain.[108,119]

In contrast to mesenchymal-derived cells, epithelial cells and their malignant counterparts do not express high levels of the $\alpha_v\beta_3$ vitronectin receptor. Instead, epithelial cell types use the α_v subunit complexed to a different subunit, β_5 (β_x).[108] Although it does bind vitronectin, $\alpha_v\beta_5$ differs from the original vitronectin receptor in that it also weakly binds Fn but does not bind fibrinogen or von Willebrand factor. The recently identified $\alpha_v\beta_1$ complex also binds vitronectin.[110-112]

e. von Willebrand Factor

von Willebrand factor (vWF) is responsible for platelet adhesion to components of the subendothelial matrix and may be important in endothelial cell adhesion to the subendothelium. vWF is synthesized by megakaryocytes and endothelial cells as 220,000 MW subunits which form dimers (440 kDa) and large homopolymers (up to 20 mDa).[120] vWF is stored in platelet alpha granules and in the Weibel-Palade bodies of endothelial cells. Endothelial cells secrete variably sized vWF constitutively from secretory granules or secrete high molecular weight vWF from Weibel-Palade bodies upon stimulation. vWF is unusual for its extreme size heterogeneity; endothelial cells produce higher molecular weight forms than do megakaryocytes.[121] A fraction of vWF produced by human umbilical vein endothelial cells is deposited in the extracellular matrix. Matrix contains only the high molecular weight form of vWF. vWF is rich in disulfide bonds (169 half cysteines per subunit), and the loss of even four disulfides per subunit disrupts multimer structure.

Platelets have two receptors for vWF: GP Ib and GP IIb/IIIa. Platelet binding to the subendothelium is extremely rapid (seconds); the initial attachment is via the GP Ib platelet receptor, which binds near the amino terminus of vWF. Spreading of platelets via the GP IIb/IIIa integrin occurs at the RGD site located near the carboxyl terminus of vWF.[120]

Platelets can bind to collagen via vWF. This platelet–collagen binding requires binding of vWF to both GP IIb/IIIa and GP Ib.[122] vWF has two collagen-binding regions: one in the amino terminal region and one in the middle of the vWF molecule. The collagen-binding regions of vWF are structurally similar to the I-domain found in the α_2 subunit of VLA-2, type VI collagen, cartilage matrix protein, complement factors B and C2, and Mac-1.[123-125] Although vWF binds to collagen, it appears to use other molecules to integrate into the matrix, since vWF can bind to subenthothelial matrix even when monoclonal antibodies block the binding of vWF to collagen.[126]

Endothelial cells express the $\alpha_v\beta_3$ vitronectin receptor.[74,127-128] One study showed that antibodies to β_3 did not block initial attachment to the subendothelial matrix, but later induced cell detachment.[129] However, when vWF was used as the substrate, attachment was completely blocked with antibodies to β_3[130] or to the vitronectin receptor.[127] When human umbilical vein endothelial cells were plated on vWF, the β_3 part of the receptor colocalized with the ends of stress fibers and was visible as ovals or "needle eye spots".[130] Tumor cells may also use vWF as an adhesive ligand when expressed on platelets or in the vessel wall.[131]

f. Thrombospondin

Thrombospondin (Tsp) is a 420 kDa, multidomain glycoprotein composed of three disulfide-linked chains. Tsp is synthesized and secreted by a variety of cell types, including endothelial cells, smooth muscle cells, fibroblasts, monocytes, and platelets.[132,133] Its concentration in the circulation is low at 20 ng/ml, but it represents 20 to 30% of protein released from platelets. It is also deposited in extracellular matrix, including the vascular basement membrane.[134] Although its biological function is unknown, there are several important roles it could play in tumor cell arrest and invasion. It has been shown *in vivo* to potentiate experimental tumor metastasis to the lungs.[135]

Thrombospondin is found in alpha granules of platelets and is released along with fibronectin, von Willebrand factor, and platelet factor 4 upon stimulation by thrombin. There are 3100 high-affinity binding sites for Tsp on the surface of inactivated platelets and 35,600 low-affinity sites on the surface of activated platelets. Tsp is thought to act in irreversible platelet aggregation by stabilizing the fibrinogen crossbridges formed during reversible aggregation. Soluble Tsp and antibodies to Tsp each can prevent platelet aggregation. Tsp also has been shown to be the natural lectin of platelets.[136] Tsp binds to platelets via the integrin GP IIb/IIIa; it also binds independently of GP IIb/IIIa. For example, in Glanzmann's thrombasthenia, in which platelets do not express GP IIb/IIIa, they still bind Tsp, but fail to aggregate.[137] Besides GP IIb/IIIa and the $\alpha_v\beta_3$ receptor, an 88 kDa membrane glycoprotein that binds Tsp has been isolated from platelets, endothelial cells, monocytes, and several tumor cells.[138]

Tsp may act indirectly on tumor cell metastasis by altering components of the clotting system. It forms a trimolecular complex with plasminogen and a histidine-rich glycoprotein;[139] this complex can bind heparin and may decrease heparin activity. In addition, Tsp-plasminogen complexes inhibit TPA-induced fibrinolysis. Complexes of Tsp with plasminogen also may provide tumor cells with a source of surface-bound plasminogen.[140]

The direct action of Tsp on endothelium, subendothelial matrix, or the tumor cells themselves may affect the ability of tumor cells to invade. Human endothelial cells attach to (but do not spread on) thrombospondin in a cation-dependent manner that is inhibitable by the peptides RGDSP and GRBDAC.[141] Tsp also promotes the attachment and the spreading of a variety of tumor cell lines, including squamous carcinoma, fibrosarcoma, and melanoma[142-144] and also has been found in the tracks left by migrating cells.[145] It is deposited in the extracellular matrix and can form bonds with other matrix molecules: fibronectin[146] and collagens I, II, III, IV, and V.[147] Tsp colocalizes with cell-surface granules of proteoheparan sulfate. When added to aortic endothelial cells already spread on fibronectin, Tsp reduces the number of focal adhesions present[148] and may thereby modulate all adhesion/migration to extracellular matrices. The amino-terminal domain of Tsp stimulates melanoma cell spreading and chemotaxis while the carboxy-terminal domain of Tsp stimulates haptotaxis.[149] The chemotaxis is inhibitable by heparin, and the spreading is blocked by glucuronosyl-3-sulfate-containing glycolipids.[150,151]

g. Other Ligands

Entactin (nidogen) is a 150 kDa sulfated glycoprotein found ubiquitously in basement membranes (reviewed in Reference 45). Immunostaining has shown entactin to be a component of adult, fetal, and extraembryonic basement membranes. Laminin and nidogen form a highly stable complex that can be extracted from cell culture media and basement membranes.[152] As seen by electron microscopy, the complex is composed of one nidogen molecule bound to one of the short arms of the laminin molecule near the center of the cross.[60] Initial studies suggest that nidogen binds with the highest affinity to the B1 chain of laminin, but also weakly to the B2 and the A chains.[45] In addition, nidogen can directly bind to type IV collagen, thereby increasing the interaction between laminin and type IV collagen.[57]

The function of nidogen is unclear. It is susceptible to proteolysis during extraction, which has complicated its characterization. However, the high sensitivity to proteolysis appears to be essential in the process of remodeling basement membranes.[153] The nidogen molecule has been shown to contain EGF-like cysteine-rich repeats. Both EGF and an EGF-like domain of laminin bind to cell-surface receptors,[154] suggesting a possible role for entactin in either cell adhesion or growth stimulation. A possible role for entactin in cell-ECM interaction is suggested by the presence of the RGD sequence in one of the EGF-type repeats. Durkin et al.[155] demonstrated that a synthetic peptide derived from the RGD site of entactin has cell-binding activity, and that cell attachment to entactin is inhibited by RGD-containing peptides.

Another glycoprotein with widespread distribution in basement membrane and interstitial matrices that may have importance in cell adhesion is SPARC, also called osteonectin or BM-40.[156] It is present in relatively large amounts in basement membranes, but also has been demonstrated in bone and various other ECM in both embryonic and adult tissues. While the functions of this glycoprotein are still a mystery, it is known to specifically bind Ca^{2+}. In addition, it appears that SPARC can modulate adhesion by inhibiting cell spreading and may be important in allowing cells to change their shape when adhering to the ECM.[156]

III. REGULATION OF ADHESION RECEPTOR FUNCTION

A. RECEPTOR FUNCTION IN CELL MOTILITY AND INVASION

Tumor cells must be highly motile in order to detach from the primary tumor and reach neighboring vascular beds for subsequent dissemination. Once the tumor cells have arrested in the microvasculature, they must be able to adhere rapidly to the exposed basement membrane. After penetrating the basement membrane, they must again invade the interstitium to form a new tumor colony. The expression of both high- and low-affinity receptors for the basement membrane substrate may provide malignant cells with a mechanism by which to attach firmly at one time and yet migrate rapidly at another time. The receptors that are involved in cell migration appear to include both integrin and nonintegrin receptors, depending on the cell type and the adhesive ligand. It is now known that stationary cells form stable focal adhesion contacts with the substrate while locomotory cells form weak and transient close contacts.[157] Similarly, integrin adhesion receptors (e.g., the fibronectin receptor) are concentrated in focal contacts when the cells are stationary, but are diffusely distributed in motile cells.[158,159] This capacity of cells to cluster their receptors provides a mechanism to increase the effective avidity of low-affinity receptors by concentrating them into stable focal plaques. In fact, when melanoma cells adhere to the subendothelial matrix produced by microvascular endothelial cells, they form extensive focal adhesion plaques that contain β_1 integrin receptors (Figure 4).

Most of the integrin adhesion complexes bind ECM ligands with only modest affinities. Determinations of binding constants using either intact cells or purified receptors indicate that many of the β_1 class of receptors bind their ligand with K_d in the μM range. This affinity is sufficient for binding, but also provides the cell a mechanism by which it can migrate along tracts of ECM. On the other hand, the nonintegrin 67 kDa receptor, which binds laminin with much higher affinity (K_d in the nM range), may be important for the initial attachment to the vascular basement membrane.

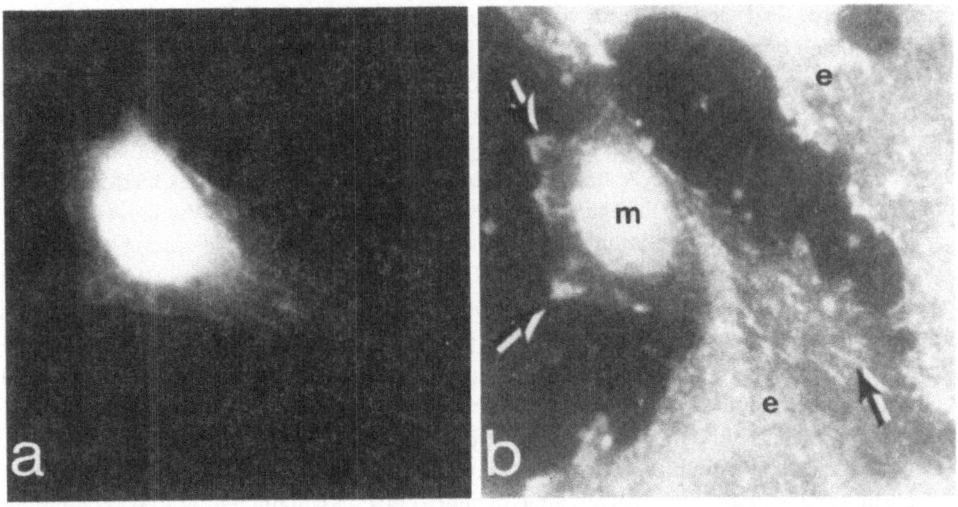

FIGURE 4. Localization of β_1 integrins in focal adhesion plaques of invading melanoma cell. Human MeWo melanoma cells (labeled with fluorescein isothiocyanate) were allowed to attach to confluent cultures of human dermal microvascular endothelial cell monolayers (a). After 3 h of incubation, the cells were fixed and stained with rhodamine-labeled antibody to the β_1 integrin subunit and visualized by immunofluorescence microscopy for fluorescein (a) or rhodamine (b). The melanoma cell (m) has invaded the endothelial cell (e) monolayer and has established focal plaques containing concentrations of β_1 integrin complexes (arrows).

Giancotti and Ruoslahti[160] found that overexpression of the fibronectin receptor ($\alpha_5\beta_1$) induced major changes in cell behavior. The overexpressor cells migrated less than the control cells. Furthermore, the overexpressor cells, in contrast to the control cells, did not grow well in soft agar and failed to form tumors in nude mice. These results suggest that levels of integrin expression can directly modulate not only cell adhesion and migration but also cell growth.

B. MODULATION OF RECEPTOR EXPRESSION AND FUNCTION

The process of malignant transformation results in a profound alteration of the cellular phenotype. Many of these alterations are seen in the behavior of cells toward their adhesive substrates (reviewed in Reference 161). Some of these changes may reflect changes in adhesion receptor function. In particular, the integrin class of receptors have been reported to be modified after transformation. Some of these modifications appear to be a consequence of direct changes in the levels or types of integrin that are expressed. For example, Saga et al.[162] reported that integrins of the β_1 family are increased in Rous sarcoma virus (RSV)-induced tumors. Dedhar and Saulnier[163] recently reported that chemically transformed osteogenic sarcoma cells have increased levels of $\alpha_6\beta_1$, $\alpha_2\beta_1$, and $\alpha_1\beta_1$ whereas $\alpha_5\beta_1$ and $\alpha_3\beta_1$ are unchanged; $\alpha_v\beta_3$ is reduced. Recent work by Hynes and collaborators[164] showed that transformation of rodent cells by RSV results in lower levels of expression of the fibronectin receptor ($\alpha_5\beta_1$) and two other β_1 integrins, while expression of $\alpha_3\beta_1$ remains unchanged. Recently, Peltonen et al.[165] reported that in comparison with normal cells, squamous carcinoma cells appear to have altered expression of β_1 integrins. From these few early studies, it seems that transformation can induce certain changes in integrin expression, but further work is needed to define how universal these alterations are and how they specifically influence the cell phenotype.

Increased phosphorylation of integrins by tyrosine kinases following transformation with oncogenes also has been reported.[166] This increase in phosphotyrosine- and phosphoserine-containing integrins was correlated with decreased condensation of integrin in focal contacts.

Although studies in this area are somewhat contradictory at present, it would appear that increased phosphorylation of integrin results in lowered integrin function. Phosphorylation also resulted in decreased ability to interact with fibronectin and talin.[167]

Certain growth factors have been reported to alter the expression of integrin receptors. In particular, transforming growth factor (TGF-β) has important influences on cell growth, differentiation, and extracellular matrix synthesis and deposition. It has been reported that TGF-β alters expression of $\alpha_1\beta_1$, $\alpha_2\beta_1$, $\alpha_3\beta_1$, $\alpha_5\beta_1$, and $\alpha_v\beta_3$ integrin complexes and that these changes were a result of modified integrin mRNA and protein synthesis.[168-170] Similar upregulation of integrin receptors also was noted with other growth factors, including interleukins. Since cells can receive growth factor stimulation from neighboring host cells or can produce the growth factors directly, this would provide another mechanism by which tumor cells could regulate the amount or type of receptor used for their interaction with the extracellular matrix. The recent observation that certain cytokines induce the expression of an adhesion receptor on endothelial cells that bind tumor cells is an example of how the local environment can influence metastasis in the host.[44]

Whether cells can rapidly modulate the affinity and/or the specificity of adhesion receptors has not yet been determined. However, the function of a specific receptor may vary with cell type. In some cells, $\alpha_2\beta_1$ functions as a laminin receptor, yet in other cells, it acts only as a collagen receptor. For example, $\alpha_2\beta_1$ isolated from endothelial cells, melanoma cells, and platelets bound to collagen I, but only the receptor from endothelial cells and melanoma cells bound to laminin.[76,171] In addition, the $\alpha_2\beta_1$ complex from endothelial cells also bound to the 110 kDa fragment of fibronectin while the platelet receptor did not. These results imply that the activity of individual receptors may be influenced by the cell type on which they are expressed. The mechanism by which this regulation occurs is unknown, but could be alternative splicing, cytoskeletal influences, or glycosylation differences in the lipid environment of the plasma membrane. These modifications of receptor function could occur at the molecular level. Van Kuppevelt et al.[117] reported that the β_3 subunit of the vitronectin receptor can be alternatively spliced at its carboxy-terminal end; this could provide a mechanism by which to regulate the receptor's interaction with the cytoskeleton. Also, alterations in receptor specificity or affinity could be induced by rapid changes in the surface microenvironment. As noted above, the phosphorylation of integrins may provide a means to regulate receptor function from moment to moment.

Another mechanism that may modify receptor expression by tumor cells is mutation or chromosomal loss. It has been established that malignant tumors can be quite heterogenous, particularly in their degree of differentiation, cell morphology, antigenic profiles, and growth rate. Importantly, phenotypic heterogeneity has been demonstrated among primary and metastatic lesions in the same patient and among individual metastases from the same primary tumor. Furthermore, it appears that most malignant tumors evolve in a stepwise pattern. For example, melanomas progress from benign proliferative lesions to invasive melanoma and finally to metastatic melanoma.[172] While it is clear that the phenotypes of tumor cells in different stages of tumor progression exhibit distinct markers, little is known about what changes might occur in the expression of adhesion receptors.

It has been proposed that phenotypic heterogeneity is a consequence of altered gene expression that occurs during normal differentiation. There is evidence that the expression of specific adhesion receptors, such as the 67 kDa high-affinity laminin receptor, is increased on metastatic tumor cells as compared with their normal counterparts (reviewed in Reference 1). Another example of phenotypic heterogeneity is the observation that malignant melanoma cells express high levels of a novel integrin laminin receptor ($\alpha_7\beta_1$) that is not expressed in normal melanocytes.[67,83] That variant tumor cells in a given population may express diverse integrin profiles raises the possibility that a particular set of integrin receptors will enhance the potential of a specific subset of cells for distant metastasis. Thus, a cell that expresses high levels of laminin-binding receptors may be more successful in the initial adherence to the vascular basement membrane.

C. ADHESION RECEPTORS AS SIGNAL TRANSDUCERS

One puzzling question raised from recent work is why there is such a multiplicity of receptors. For example, at least eight different receptors have been reported to bind to laminin. It is important to look beyond the role of a receptor as simply an adhesion molecule. Certainly many of the described receptors perform this function, but it is likely that they have alternative functions in addition to or separate from adhesion. There is some evidence that these receptors act as signaling devices that communicate conditions in the extracellular environment to the cell.[9] This would be particularly important when a cell must respond to the presence of an extracellular matrix by organizing its cytoskeleton and forming actin bundles and focal adhesion contacts. Certain extracellular adhesion proteins have been shown to modulate cell phenotype as well as differentiation. For example, myogenic differentiation is induced by a laminin but not by a fibronectin substrate; anti-integrin antibody blocks this differentiation step.[173]

An example of how surface receptors may act as signal transducers is the observation that laminin can induce tumor cells to upregulate their expression of type IV collagenase through its interaction with the 67 kDa laminin receptor.[174] In contrast, fibronectin failed to produce any inductive effect on proteinase expression. This result suggests that tumor cell adhesion to basement membrane substrates initiates a cellular response that provides for subsequent invasion of this structure. Recent work by Werb et al.[175] provides an interesting example of how integrin adhesion receptors may act as signal transducers. When cells that were adherent to fibronectin substrates were treated with antibodies against the fibronectin receptor complex, metalloproteinase (collagenase and stromelysin) expression was induced; alternatively, fragments of fibronectin containing the RGD sequence also could initiate the induction. These results imply that a specific integrin receptor, when appropriately manipulated, can act as a signal transducer that results in specific gene expression of proteolytic enzymes involved in invasion.

REFERENCES

1. **Liotta, L. A., Rao, C. N., and Wewer, U. M.,** Biochemical interactions of tumor cells with the basement membrane, *Annu. Rev. Biochem.*, 55, 1037, 1986.
2. **Juliano, R. L.,** Membrane receptors for extracellular matrix macromolecules: relationship to cell adhesion and tumor metastasis, *Biochim. Biophys. Acta*, 907, 261, 1987. (Review)
3. **Mecham, R. P., Hinek, A., Griffin, G. L., Senior, R. M., and Liotta, L.,** The elastin receptor shows structural and functional similarities to the 67-kDa tumor cell laminin receptor, *J. Biol. Chem.*, 264, 16652, 1989.
4. **Lotan, R. and Raz, A.,** Lectins in cancer cells, *Ann. N. Y. Acad. Sci.*, 551, 385, 1988.
5. **Buck, C. A. and Horwitz, A. F.,** Cell surface receptors for extracellular matrix molecules, *Ann. Rev. Cell Biol.*, 3, 179, 1987.
6. **Hynes, R. O.,** Integrins: a family of cell surface receptors, *Cell*, 48, 549, 1987.
7. **Ruoslahti, E.,** Fibronectin and its receptors, *Ann. Rev. Biochem.*, 57, 375, 1988.
8. **Springer, T. A.,** Adhesion receptors of the immune system, *Nature*, 346, 425, 1990.
9. **Hemler, M. E.,** VLA proteins in the integrin family: structures, functions, and their role on leukocytes, *Annu. Rev. Immunol.*, 8, 365, 1990.
10. **Horwitz, A., Duggan, K., Greggs, R., Decker, C., and Buck, C.,** The cell substrate attachment (CSAT) antigen has properties of a receptor for laminin and fibronectin, *J. Cell Biol.*, 101, 2134, 1985.
11. **Hemler, M. E., Huang, C., and Schwarz, L.,** The VLA protein family. Characterization of five distinct cell surface heterodimers each with a common 130,000 molecular weight β subunit, *J. Biol. Chem.*, 262, 3300, 1987.

12. **Takada, Y., Strominger, J., and Hemler, M.,** The very late antigen family of heterodimers is part of superfamily of molecules involved in adhesion and embryogenesis, *Proc. Natl. Acad. Sci. U.S.A.*, 84, 3239, 1987.
13. **Hemler, M. E., Jacobson, J. G., and Strominger, J. L.,** Biochemical characterization of VLA-1 and VLA-2. Cell surface heterodimers on activated T cells, *J. Biol. Chem.*, 260, 15246, 1985.
14. **Weiss, L., Orr, F. W., and Honn, K. V.,** Interactions of cancer cells with the microvasculature during metastasis, *Faseb J.*, 2, 12, 1988.
15. **Gasic, J., Tuszynski, G. P., and Gorelik, E.,** Interaction of hemostatic and immune systems in the metastatic spread of tumor cells, *Int. Rev. Exp. Pathol.*, 29, 173, 1986.
16. **Fidler, I. J.,** Origin of cancer metastases and its implications for therapy, *Isr. J. Med. Sci.*, 24, 456, 1988.
17. **Cavanaugh, P. G. and Nicolson, G. L.,** Purification and some properties of a lung-derived growth factor that differentially stimulates the growth of tumor cells metastatic to the lung, *Cancer Res.*, 49, 3928, 1989.
18. **Fornabaio, D. M., Alterman, A. L., and Stackpole, C. W.,** Metastatic dissemination of B16 melanoma: evidence that metastases can result from nonspecific trapping of disseminated tumor cells, *Invas. Met.*, 8, 1, 1988.
19. **Auerbach, R., Alby, L., Morrissey, L. W., Tu, M., and Joseph, J.,** Expression of organ-specific antigens on capillary endothelial cells, *Microvasc. Res.*, 29, 401, 1985.
20. **Kramer, R. H., Gonzalez, R., and Nicolson, G. L.,** Metastatic tumor cells adhere preferentially to the extracellular matrix of vascular endothelial cells, *Int. J. Cancer*, 26, 639, 1980.
21. **Kramer, R. H., Vogel, K. G., and Nicolson, G. L.,** The solubilization and degradation of subendothelial matrix glycoproteins and proteoglycans by metastatic tumor cells, *J. Biol. Chem.*, 257, 2678, 1982.
22. **Abercrombie, M. and Heaysman, J. E.,** Observations on the social behavior of cells in tissue culture. II. Monolayering of fibroblasts, *Exp. Cell Res.*, 6, 293, 1954.
23. **Kramer, R. H. and Nicolson, G. L.,** Interaction of tumor cells with vascular endothelial cell monolayers: a model for metastatic invasion, *Proc. Natl. Acad. Sci. U.S.A.*, 76, 5704, 1979.
24. **Keck, P. J., Hauser, S. D., Krivi, G., Sanzo, K., Warren, T., Feder, J., and Connolly, D. T.,** Vascular permeability factor, an endothelial cell mitogen related to PDGF, *Science*, 246, 1309, 1989.
25. **Duijvestin, A. and Hamann, A.,** Mechanism and regulation of lymphocyte migration, *Immunology Today*, 10, 23, 1989.
26. **Stoolman, L. M.,** Adhesion molecules controlling lymphocyte migration, *Cell*, 56, 907, 1989.
27. **Streeter, P. R., Rouse, B. T. N., and Butcher, E. C.,** Immunohistologic functional characterization of a vascular addressin involved in lymphocyte homing into peripheral lymph nodes, *J. Cell Biol.*, 107, 1853, 1988.
28. **Yednock, T. A. and Rosen, S. D.,** Lymphocyte homing, *Adv. Immunol.*, 44, 313, 1989.
29. **Lasky, L. A., Singer, M. S., Yednock, T. A., Dowbenko, D., Fennie, C., Rodriguez, H., Nguyen, T., Stachel, S., and Rosen, S. D.,** Cloning of a lymphocyte homing receptor reveals a lectin domain, *Cell*, 56, 1045, 1989.
30. **Bowen, B. R., Nguyen, T., and Lasky, L. A.,** Characterization of a human homologue of the murine peripheral lymph node homing receptor, *J. Cell Biol.*, 109, 421, 1989.
31. **Siegelman, M. H. and Weissman, I. L.,** Human homologue of mouse lymph node homing receptor: evolutionary conservation at tandem cell interaction domains, *Proc. Natl. Acad. Sci. U.S.A.*, 86, 5562, 1989.
32. **Tedder, T. F., Isaacs, C. M., Ernst, T. J., Demetri, G. D., Adler, D. A., and Disteche, C. M.,** Isolation and chromosomal localization of cDNA's encoding a novel human lymphocyte cell surface molecule, LAM-1, *J. Exp. Med.*, 170, 123, 1989.
33. **Camerini, D., James, S. P., Stamenkovic, I., and Seed, B.,** Leu-8/TQ1 is the human equivalent of the MEL-14 lymph node homing receptor, *Nature*, 342, 78. 1989.
34. **Sher, B. T., Bargatze, R., Holzmann, B., Gallatin, W. M., Matthews, D., Wu, N., Picker, L., Butcher, E. C., and Weissman, I. L.,** Homing receptors and metastasis, *Adv. Cancer Res.*, 51, 361, 1988.
35. **Holzmann, B. and Weissman, I.,** Integrin molecules involved in lymphocyte homing to Peyer's patches, *Immunol. Rev.*, 108, 45, 1989.
36. **Holzmann, B. and Weissman, I. L.,** Peyer's patch-specific lymphocyte homing receptors consist of a VLA-4-like α chain associated with either of two integrin β chains, one of which is novel, *EMBO J.*, 8, 1735, 1989.
37. **Wayner, E. A., Garcia-Pardo, A., Humphries, M. J., McDonald, J. A., and Carter, W. G.,** Identification and characterization of the T lymphocyte adhesion receptor for an alternative cell attachment domain (CS-1) in plasma fibronectin, *J. Cell Biol.*, 109, 1321, 1989.
38. **Jalkanen, S., Jalkanen, M., Bargatze, R., Tamme, M., and Butcher, E. C.,** Biochemical properties of glycoproteins involved in lymphocyte recognition of high endothelial venules in man, *J. Immunol.*, 141, 1615, 1988.

39. **Goldstein, L. A., Zhou, D. F. H., Picker. L. J., Minty, C. N., Bargatze, R. F., Ding, J. F., and Butcher, E. C.,** A human lymphocyte homing receptor, the Hermes antigen, is related to cartilage proteoglycan core and link proteins, *Cell,* 56, 1063, 1989.
40. **Hamann, A., Jablonski-Westrich, D., Duijvestijn, A., Butcher, E. C., Baisch, H., Harder, R., and Thiele, H.-G.,** Evidence for an accessory role of LFA-1 in lymphocyte-high endothelium interactions during homing, *J. Immunol.,* 140, 693, 1988.
41. **Streeter, P. R., Berg, E. L., Rouse, B. T. N., Bargatze, R. F., and Butcher, E. C.,** A tissue-specific endothelial cell molecule involved in lymphocyte homing, *Nature,* 331, 41, 1988.
42. **Netland, P. A. and Zetter, B. R.,** Organ-specific adhesion of metastatic tumor cells *in vitro, Science,* 224, 1113, 1984.
43. **Bargatze, R. F., Wu, N. W., Weissman, I. L., and Butcher, E. C.,** High endothelial venule binding as a predictor of the dissemination of passaged murine lymphomas, *J. Exp. Med.,* 166, 1125, 1987.
44. **Rice, E. G. and Bevilacqua, M. P.,** An inducible endothelial cell surface glycoprotein mediates melanoma adhesion, *Science,* 246, 1303, 1989.
45. **Timpl, R.,** Structure and biological activity of basement membrane proteins, *Eur. J. Biochem.,* 180, 487, 1989.
46. **Kramer, R. H., Karasek, M. A., and Bensch, K. G.,** Isolation and characterization of human vascular endothelial cells with application to studies of the subendothelial matrix, in *Cell Separation: Methods and Selected Applications,* Vol. 5, Pretlow, T. G. and Pretlow, T. P., Eds, Academic Press, New York, 1987, 1.
47. **Bartsky, S. H., Rao, C. N., Williams, J. E., and Liotta, L. A.,** Laminin molecular domains which alter metastasis in a murine model, *J. Clin. Invest.,* 74, 843, 1984.
48. **McCarthy, J. B., Hagen, S. T., and Furcht, L. T.,** Human fibronectin contains distinct adhesion- and motility-promoting domains for metastatic melanoma cells, *J. Cell Biol.,* 102, 179, 1986.
49. **Terranova, V. P., Williams, J. E., Liotta, L. A., and Martin, G. R.,** Modulation of the metastatic activity of melanoma cells by laminin and fibronectin, *Science,* 226, 982, 1984.
50. **Gehlsen, K. R., Argraves, W. S., Pierschbacher, M. D., and Ruoslahti, E.,** Inhibition of *in vitro* tumor cell invasion by Arg-Gly-Asp-containing synthetic peptides, *J. Cell Biol.,* 106, 925, 1988.
51. **Graf, J., Iwamoto, M., Sasaki, S., Martin, G. R., Kleinman, H., Robey, F. A., and Yamada, Y.,** Identification of an amino acid sequence in laminin mediating cell attachment, chemotaxis, and receptor binding, *Cell,* 48, 989, 1987.
52. **Iwamoto, Y., Robey, F. A., Graf, J., Sasaki, M., Kleinman, H. K., Yamada, Y., and Martin, G. R.,** YIGSR, a synthetic laminin pentapeptide, inhibits experimental metastasis formation, *Science,* 238, 1132, 1987.
53. **Saiki, I., Murata, J., Lida, J., Sakurai, T., Nishi, N., Matsuno, K., and Azuma, I.,** Antimetastatic effects of synthetic polypeptides containing repeated structures of the cell adhesive Arg-Gly-Asp (RGD) and Tyr-Ile-Gly-Ser-Arg (YIGSR) sequences, *Br. J. Cancer,* 60, 722, 1989.
54. **Panayotou, G., End, P., Aumailley, M., Timpl, R., and Engel, J.,** Domains of laminin with growth-factor activity, *Cell,* 56, 93, 1989.
55. **Hunter, D. D., Shah, V., Merlie, J. P., and Sanes, J. R.,** A laminin-like adhesive protein concentrated in the synaptic cleft of the neuromuscular junction, *Nature,* 338, 229, 1989.
56. **Ehrig, K., Leivo, I., Argraves, W. S., Ruoslahti, E., and Engvall, E.,** Merosin, a tissue-specific basement membrane protein is a laminin-like protein, *Proc. N. Y. Acad. Sci.,* 87, 3264, 1990.
57. **Aumailley, M., Nurcombe, V., Edgar, D., Paulsson, M., and Timpl, R.,** The cellular interactions of laminin fragments: cell adhesion correlates with two fragment-specific high affinity binding sites, *J. Biol. Chem.,* 262, 11532, 1987.
58. **Edgar, D., Timpl, R., and Thoenen, H.,** The heparin binding domain of laminin is responsible for its effect on neurite outgrowth and neuronal survival, *EMBO J.,* 3, 1463, 1984.
59. **Nurcombe, V., Aumailley, M., Timpl, R., and Edgar, D.,** The high affinity binding of laminin to cells. Assignation of a major cell-binding site to its short arms, *Eur. J. Biochem.,* 180, 9, 1989.
60. **Paulsson, M., Aumailley, M., Deutzmann, R., Timpl, R., and Beck, K.,** Laminin-nidogen complex. Extraction with chelating agents and structural characterization, *Eur. J. Biochem.,* 166, 11, 1987.
61. **von der Mark, K. and Risse, G.,** Isolation and characterization of laminin receptors, *Methods Enzymol.,* 144, 490, 1987.
62. **Runyan, R. B., Versalovic, J., and Shur, B. D.,** Cell adhesion and spreading: the requirement for surface galactosyltransferase in cell spreading, *J. Cell Biol.,* 107, 1863, 1988.
63. **Wayner, E. A., and Carter, W. G.,** Identification of multiple cell adhesion receptors for collagen and fibronectin in human fibrosarcoma cells possessing unique α and common β subunits, *J. Cell Biol.,* 105, 1873, 1987.
64. **Gehlsen, K. R., Dilner, L., Engvall, E., and Ruoslahti, E.,** The human laminin receptor is a member of the integrin family of cell adhesion receptors, *Science,* 241, 1228, 1988.

65. **Ignatius, M. J. and Reichardt, L. F.,** Identification of a neuronal laminin receptor: an M_r 200 K/120 K integrin heterodimer that binds laminin in a cation divalent dependent manner, *Neuron,* 1, 713, 1988.
66. **Kramer, R. H., McDonald, K. A., Crowley, E., Ramos, D. M., and Damsky, C. H.,** Melanoma cell adhesion to basement membrane mediated by integrin-related complexes, *Cancer Res.,* 49, 393, 1989.
67. **Kramer, R. H., Vu, M. P., Cheng, Y. F., and Ramos, D.,** Novel melanoma laminin-binding integrin is poorly expressed on normal melanocytes, *Proc. Am. Assoc. Cancer Res.,* 31, 67, 1990.
68. **Gehlsen, K. R., Dickerson, K., Argraves, W. S., Engvall, E., and Ruoslahti, E.,** Subunit structure of a laminin-binding integrin and localization of its binding site on laminin, *J. Biol. Chem.,* 264(32), 19034, 1989.
69. **Carter, W. G., Wayner, E. A., Bouchard, T. S., and Kaur, P.,** The role of integrins $\alpha_2\beta_1$ and $\alpha_3\beta_1$ in cell-cell and cell-substrate adhesion of human epidermal cells, *J. Cell Biol.,* 110(4), 1387, 1990.
70. **Ramos, D. M., Berston, E. D., and Kramer, R. H.,** Identification of integrin receptors for laminin and type IV collagen on metastatic B16 melanoma cells, *Cancer Res.,* 50, 728, 1990.
71. **Clyman, R. I., Turner, D. C. and Kramer, R. H.,** An $\alpha_1\beta_1$-like integrin receptor on rat aortic smooth muscle cells mediates adhesion to laminin and collagen types I and IV, *Arteriosclerosis,* 10, 402, 1990.
72. **Hall, D. E., Reichardt, L. F., Crowley, E., Holley, B., Moezzi, H., Sonnenberg, A., and Damsky, C. H.,** The alpha-1 beta-1 and alpha-6 beta-1 integrin heterodimers mediate cell attachment to distinct sites on laminin, *J. Cell Biol.,* 110, 2175, 1990.
73. **Kramer, R. H. and Marks, N.,** Identification of integrin collagen receptors on human melanoma cells, *J. Biol. Chem.,* 264, 4684, 1989.
74. **Kramer, R. H., Cheng, Y.-F., and Clyman, R. I.,** Human microvascular endothelial cells use β_1 and β_3 integrin complexes to attach to laminin, *J. Cell Biol.,* 111, 1233, 1990.
75. **Languino, L. R., Gehlsen, K. R., Wayner, E., Carter, W. G., Engvall, E., and Ruoslahti, E.,** Endothelial cells use $\alpha_2\beta_1$ integrin as a laminin receptor, *J. Cell Biol.,* 109, 2455, 1989.
76. **Elices, M. J. and Hemler, M. E.,** The human integrin VLA-2 is a collagen receptor on some cells and a collagen/laminin receptor on others, *Proc. Natl. Acad. Sci. U.S.A.,* 86, 9906, 1989.
77. **Sonnenberg, A., Janssen, H., Hogervorst, F., Calafat, J., and Hilgers, J.,** A complex of platelet glycoproteins Ic and IIa identified by a rat monoclonal antibody, *J. Biol. Chem.,* 262, 10376, 1987.
78. **Sonnenberg, A. J., Modderman, P. W., and Hogervorst, F.,** Laminin receptor on platelets is the integrin VLA-6, *Nature (London),* 336, 487, 1988.
79. **Sonnenberg, A., Linders, C. J., Moderman, P. W., Damsky, C. H., Aumailley, M., and Timpl, R.,** Integrin recognition of different cell-binding fragments of laminin (P1, E3, E8) and evidence that $\alpha_6\beta_1$ but not $\alpha_6\beta_4$ functions as a major receptor for fragment E8, *J. Cell Biol.,* 110, 2145, 1990.
80. **Kajiji, S., Tamura, R. N., and Quaranta, V.,** A novel integrin ($\alpha_E\beta_4$) from human epithelial cells suggests a fourth family of integrin adhesion receptors, *EMBO J.,* 8, 673, 1989.
81. **Hemler, M., Crouse, C., and Sonnenberg, A.,** Association of the VLA α_6 subunit with a novel protein, *J. Biol. Chem.,* 264, 6529, 1989.
82. **Lotz, M., Korzelius, C., and Mercurio, A. M.,** Human colon carcinoma cells use multiple receptors to adhere to laminin: involvement of $\alpha_6\beta_4$ and $\alpha_2\beta_1$ integrins, *Cell. Regul.,* 1, 249, 1990.
83. **Kramer, R. H., McDonald, K. A., and Vu, M. P.,** Human melanoma cells express a novel integrin receptor for laminin, *J. Biol. Chem.,* 264, 15642, 1989.
84. **Hynes, R. O.,** Integrins: a family of cell surface receptors, *Cell,* 48, 549, 1987.
85. **Timpl, R., Wiedemann, H., van Delden, V., Furthmayr, H., and Kuhn, K.,** A network model for the organization of type IV collagen molecules in basement membrane, *Eur. J. Biochem.,* 139, 401, 1984.
86. **Yurchenco, P. D. and Ruben, G. C.,** Basement membrane structure *in situ:* evidence for lateral associations in the type IV collagen network, *J. Cell Biol.,* 105, 2559, 1987.
87. **Aumailley, M. and Timpl, R.,** Attachment of cells to basement membrane collagen type IV, *J. Cell Biol.,* 103, 1569, 1986.
88. **Aumailley, M., Widemann, H., Mann, K., and Timpl, R.,** Binding of nidogen and the laminin-nidogen complex to basement membrane collagen type IV, *Eur. J. Biochem.,* 184, 241, 1989.
89. **Laurie, G. W., Bing, J. T., Kleinman, H. K., Hassell, J. R., Aumailley, M., Martin, G. R., and Feldmann, R. J.,** Localization of binding sites for laminin, heparan sulfate proteoglycan and fibronectin on basement membrane (type IV) collagen, *J. Mol. Biol.* 189, 205, 1986.
90. **Chelberg, M. K., Tsilibary, E. C., Hauser, A. R., and McCarthy, J. B.,** Type IV collagen-mediated melanoma cell adhesion and migration: involvement of multiple, distinct domains of the collagen molecule, *Cancer Res.,* 19, 1798, 1989.
91. **Chelberg, M. K., McCarthy, J. B., Skubitz, A. P., Furcht, L. T., and Tsilibary, E. C.,** Characterization of a synthetic peptide from type IV collagen that promotes melanoma cell adhesion, spreading, and motility, *J. Cell Biol.,* 111, 261, 1990.
92. **Tsilibary, E. C., Reger, L. A., Vogel, A. M., Koliakos, G. G., Anderson, S. S., Charonis, A. S., Allegre, J. N., and Furcht, L. T.,** Identification of a multi-functional, cell-binding peptide sequence from the al(NC1) of type IV collagen, *J. Cell Biol.,* 111, 1583, 1990.

93. **Terranova, V. P., Rohrbach, D. H., and Martin, G. R.,** Role of laminin in the attachment of PAM 212 (epithelial) cells to basement membrane collagen, *Cell,* 22, 719, 1980.
94. **Sugrue, S. P.,** Isolation of collagen binding proteins from embryonic chicken corneal epithelial cells, *J. Biol. Chem.,* 262, 3338, 1987.
95. **Dedhar, S., Ruoslahti, E., and Pierschbacher, M. D.,** A cell surface receptor complex for collagen type I recognizes the Arg-Gly-Asp sequence, *J. Cell Biol.,* 104, 585, 1987.
96. **Herbst, T. J., McCarthy, J. B., Tsilibary, E. C., and Furcht, L. T.,** Differential effects of laminin, intact type IV collagen, and specific domains of type IV collagen on endothelial cell adhesion and migration, *J. Cell Biol.,* 106, 1365, 1988.
97. **Brazel, O., Oberbäumer, I., Dieringer, H., Babel, W., Gianville, R. W., Deutzmann, R., and Kuhn, K.,** Completion of the amino acid sequence of the α_1 chain of human basement membrane collagen (type IV) reveals 21 non-triplet interruptions located within the collagenous domain, *Eur. J. Biochem.,* 168, 529, 1987.
98. **Tomaselli, K. J., Damsky, C. H., and Reichardt, L. F.,** Interactions of a neuronal cell line (PC 12) with laminin, collagen IV, and fibronection: identification of integrin-related glycoproteins involved in attachment and process outgrowth, *J. Cell Biol.,* 105, 2347, 1987.
99. **Takada, Y., Wayner, E. A., Carter, W. G., and Hemler, M. E.,** Extracellular matrix receptors, ECMRII and ECMRI, for collagen and fibronectin correspond to VLA-2 and VLA-3 in the VLA family of heterodimers, *J. Cell. Biochem.,* 37, 385, 1988.
100. **Hynes, R. O.,** Fibronectins: a family of complex and versatile adhesive glycoproteins derived from a single gene, *Harvey Lect.,* 81, 133, 1985.
101. **Schwarzbauer, J. E., Spencer, C. S., and Wilson, C. L.,** Selective secretion of alternatively spliced fibronectin variants, *J. Cell Biol.,* 109, 3445, 1989.
102. **Glukhova, M. A., Frid, M. G., Shekhonin, B. V., Vasilevskaya, T. D., Grunwald, J., Saginati, M., and Koteliansky, V. E.,** Expression of extra domain A fibronectin sequence in vascular smooth muscle cells is phenotype dependent, *J. Cell Biol.,* 109, 357, 189.
103. **Glukhova, M. A., Frid, M. G., Shekhonin, B. V., Balabanov, Y. V., and Koteliansky, V. E.,** Expression of fibronectin variants in vascular and visceral smooth muscle cells in development, *Dev. Biol.,* 141, 193, 1990.
104. **Humphries, M. J., Akiyama, S. K., Komoriya, A., Olden, K., and Yamada, K. M.,** Identification of an alternatively spliced site in human plasma fibronectin that mediates cell type-specific adhesion, *J. Cell Biol.,* 103, 2637, 1986.
105. **Humphries, M. J., Komoriya, A., Akiyama, S. K., Olden, K., and Yamada, K. M.,** Identification of two distinct regions of the type III connecting segment of human plasma fibronectin that promote cell type-specific adhesion, *J. Biol. Chem.,* 262, 6886, 1987.
106. **Garcia-Pardo, A., Wayner, E. A., Carter, W. G., and Ferreira, O. C.,** Human B lymphocytes define an alternative mechanism of adhesion to fibronectin. The interaction of the $\alpha_4\beta_1$ integrin with the LHGPEILDVPST sequence of the type III connecting segment is sufficient to promote cell attachment, *J. Immunol.,* 144(9), 3361, 1990.
107. **D'Souza, S. E., Ginsberg, M. H., Burke, T. A., Lam, S. C., and Plow, E. F.,** Localization of an Arg-Gly-Asp recognition site within an integrin receptor, *Science,* 242, 91, 1988.
108. **Cheresh, D. A., Smith, J. W., Cooper, H. M., and Quaranta, V.,** A novel vitronectin receptor integrin ($\alpha_v\beta_x$) is responsible for distinct adhesive properties of carcinoma cells, *Cell,* 57, 59, 1989.
109. **Smith, J. W., Vestal, D. J., Irwin, S. V., Burke, T.A., and Cheresh, D. A.,** Purification and functional characterization of integrin $\alpha_v\beta_5$, an adhesion receptor for vitronectin, *J. Biol. Chem.,* 265, 11008, 1990.
110. **Bodary, S. C. and McLean, J. W.,** The integrin β_1 subunit associates with the vitronectin receptor α_v subunit to form a novel vitronectin receptor in a human embryonic kidney cell line, *J. Biol. Chem.,* 265, 5938, 1990.
111. **Vogel, B. E., Tarone, G., Giancotti, F. G., Gailit, J., and Ruoslahti, E.,** A novel fibronectin receptor with an unexpected subunit composition ($\alpha_v\beta_1$), *J. Biol. Chem.,* 265, 5934, 1990.
112. **Dedhar, S. and Gray, V.,** Isolation of a novel integrin receptor mediating Arg-Gly-Asp-directed cell adhesion to fibronectin and type I collagen from human neuroblastoma cells. Association of a novel beta-1-related subunit with αv, *J. Cell Biol.,* 110, 2185, 1990.
113. **Gebb, C., Hayman, E. G., Engvall, E., and Ruoslahti, E.,** Interaction of vitronectin with collagen, *J. Biol. Chem.,* 261, 16698, 1986.
114. **Reilly, J. T. and Nash, J. R.,** Vitronectin (serum spreading factor): its localisation in normal and fibrotic tissue, *J. Clin. Pathol.,* 41, 1269, 1988.
115. **Loridon-Rosa, B., Vielh, P., Cuadrado, C., and Burtin, P.,** Comparative distribution of fibronectin and vitronectin in human breast and colon carcinomas. An immunofluorescence study, *Am. J. Clin. Pathol.,* 90, 7, 1988.
116. **Pytela, R., Pierschbacher, M. D., and Ruoslahti, E.,** Identification and isolation of a 140 kD cell surface glycoprotein with properties expected of a fibronectin receptor, *Cell,* 40, 191, 1985.

117. **van Kuppevelt, T. H. M. S. M., Languino, L. R., Gailit, J. O., Suzuki, S., and Ruoslahti, E.,** An alternative cytoplasmic domain of the integrin β_3 subunit, *Proc. Natl. Acad. Sci, U.S.A.*, 86, 5415, 1989.
118. **Ginsberg, M. H., Loftus, J. C., and Plow, E. F.,** Cytoadherens, integrins, and platelets, *Thromb. Haemos.* 159, 1, 1988.
119. **Tranqui, L., Andrieux, A., Hudry Glergeon, G., Ryckewaert, J. J., Soyez, S., Chapel, A., Ginsberg, M. H., Plow, E. F., and Marguerie, G.,** Differential structural requirements for fibrinogen binding to platelets and to endothelial cells, *J. Cell Biol.*, 108, 2519, 1989.
120. **Handin, R. I. and Wagner, D. D.,** Molecular and cellular biology of von Willebrand factor, *Prog. Hemost. Thromb.*, 9, 233, 1989.
121. **Tannenbaum, S. H., Rick, M. E., Shafer, B., and Granick, H. R.,** Subendothelial matrix of cultured endothelial cells contains fully processed high molecular weight von Willebrand factor, *J. Lab. Clin. Med.*, 113, 372, 1989.
122. **Fressinaud, E., Baruch, D., Girma, J. P., Sakariassen, K., Baumgartner, H., and Meyer, D.,** von Willebrand factor-mediated platelet adhesion to collagen involves platelet membrane glycoprotein IIb-IIIa as well as glycoprotein Ib, *J. Lab. Clin. Med.*, 112, 58, 1988.
123. **Takada, Y. and Hemler, M. E.,** The primary structure of the VLA-2/collagen receptor $\alpha 2$ subunit (platelet GP1a): homology to other integrins and the presence of a possible collagen-binding domain, *J. Cell Biol.*, 109, 397, 1989.
124. **Pytela, R.,** Amino acid sequence of the murine Mac-1 α chain reveals homology with the integrin family and an additional domain related to von Willebrand factor, *EMBO J.*, 7, 1371, 1988.
125. **Bonaldo, P., Russo, V., Bucciotti, F., Bressan, G. M., and Colombatti, A.,** α_1 chain of chick type VI collagen, *J. Biol. Chem.*, 264, 5575, 1989.
126. **de Groot, P. G., Ottenhof-Rovers, M., van Mourik, J. A., and Sixma, J. J.,** Evidence that the primary binding site of von Willebrand factor that mediates platelet adhesion on subendothelium is not collagen, *J. Clin. Invest.*, 82, 65, 1988.
127. **Cheresh, D. A.,** Human endothelial cells synthesize and express an Arg-Gly-Asp-directed adhesion receptor involved in attachment to fibrinogen and von Willebrand factor, *Proc. Natl. Acad. Sci, U.S.A.*, 84, 6471, 1987.
128. **Plow, E. F., Pierschbacher, M. D., Ruoslahti, E., Marguerie, G. A., and Ginsberg, M. H.,** The effect of Arg-Gly-Asp-containing peptides on fibrinogen and von Willebrand factor binding to platelets, *Proc. Natl. Acad. Sci. U.S.A.*, 82, 8057, 1985.
129. **Chen, C. S., Thiagarajan, P., Schwartz, S. M., Harlan, J. M., and Heimark, R. L.,** The platelet glycoprotein IIb/IIIa-like protein in human endothelial cells promotes adhesion but not initial attachment to extracellular matrix, *J. Cell Biol.*, 105, 1885, 1987.
130. **Dejana, E., Lampugnani, M. G., Giorgio, M., Gaboli, M., Federici, A. B., Ruggeri, Z. M., and Marchisio, P. C.,** von Willebrand factor promotes endothelial cell adhesion via an Arg-Gly-Asp-dependent mechanism, *J. Cell Biol.*, 109, 367, 1989.
131. **Karpatkin, S., Pearlstein, E., Ambrogio, C., and Coller, B. S.,** Role of adhesive proteins in platelet tumor interaction *in vitro* and metastasis formation *in vivo*, *J. Clin. Invest.*, 81, 1012, 1988.
132. **Mosher, D. F., Doyle, M. J., and Jaffe, E. A.,** Synthesis and secretion of thrombospondin by cultured human endothelial cells, *J. Cell Biol.*, 93, 343, 1982.
133. **Silverstein, R. L., Leung, L. L. K., and Nachman, R. L.,** Thrombospondin: a versatile multifunctional glycoprotein, *Arteriosclerosis*, 6, 245, 1986.
134. **Wight, T. N., Raugi, G. J., Mumby, S. M., and Bornstein, P.,** Light microscopic immunolocation of thrombospondin in human tissues, *J. Histochem. Cytochem.*, 33, 291, 1985.
135. **Tuszynski, G., Gasic, T., Rothman, V. L., Knudsen, K., and Gasic, G. J.,** Thrombospondin: a potentiator of tumor cell metastasis, *Cancer Res.*, 47, 4130, 1987.
136. **Jaffe, E. A., Leung, L. L. K., Nachman, R. L., Levin, R., and Mosher, D. F.,** Thrombospondin is the endogenous lectin of human platelets, *Nature*, 195, 246, 1982.
137. **Hourdille, P., Hasitz, M., Belloc, F., and Nurden, A. T.,** Immunocytochemical study of the binding of fibrinogen: thrombospondin to ADP, and thrombin-stimulated human platelets, *Blood*, 65, 912, 1985.
138. **Asch, A. S., Barnwell, J., Silverstein, R. L., and Nachman, R. L.,** Isolation of the thrombospondin membrane receptor, *J. Clin. Invest.*, 79, 1054, 1987.
139. **Silverstein, R. L., Leung, L. L. K., Harpel, P. C., and Nachman, R. L.,** Platelet thrombospondin forms a trimolecular complex with plasminogen and histidine-rich glycoprotein, *J. Clin. Invest.*, 75, 2065, 1985.
140. **Asch, A. S. and Nachman, R. L.,** Thrombospondin: phenomenology to function, *Prog. Hemost. Thromb.*, 9, 157, 1989.
141. **Lawler, J., Weinstein, R., and Hynes, R. O.,** Cell attachment to thrombospondin: the role of Arg-Gly-Asp, calcium and integrin receptors, *J. Cell Biol.*, 107, 2351, 1988.
142. **Varani, J., Dixit, V., Fligiel, S., McKeever, P., and Carey, T. E.,** Thrombospondin-induced attachment and spreading of human squamous carcinoma cells, *Exp. Cell Res.*, 167, 376, 1986.

143. **Varani, J., Riser, B. L., Hughes, L. A., Carey, T. E., Fliegel, S. E. G., and Dixit, V. M.,** Characterization of thrombospondin synthesis, secretion and cell surface expression by human tumor cells, *Clin. Exp. Metastasis,* 7, 265, 1989.
144. **Roberts, D. D., Sherwood, J. A., and Ginsberg, V.,** Platelet thrombospondin mediates attachment and spreading of human melanoma cells, *J. Cell Biol.,* 104, 131, 1987.
145. **Vischer, P., Völker, W., Schmidt, A., and Sinclair, N.,** Association of thrombospondin of endothelial cells with other matrix proteins and cell attachment sites and migration tracks, *Eur. J. Cell Biol.,* 47, 36, 1988.
146. **Lahav, J., Lawler, J., and Gimbrone, M. A.,** Thrombospondin interactions with fibronectin and fibrinogen, *Eur. J. Biochem.,* 145, 151, 1984.
147. **Galvin, N. J., Vance, P. M., Dixit, V. M., Fink, B., and Frazier, W. A.,** Interaction of human thrombospondin with types I-V collagen: direct binding and electron microscopy, *J. Cell Biol.,* 104, 1413, 1987.
148. **Murphy-Ullrich, J. E. and Höök, M.,** Thrombospondin modulates focal adhesions in endothelial cells, *J. Cell Biol.,* 109, 1309, 1989.
149. **Taraboletti, G., Roberts, D. D., and Liotta, L.,** Thrombospondin-induced tumor cell migration: haptotaxis and chemotaxis are mediated by different molecular domains, *J. Cell Biol.,* 105, 2409, 1987.
150. **Roberts, D. D.,** Interactions of thrombospondin with sulfated glycolipids and proteoglycans of human melanoma cells, *Cancer Res.,* 48, 6785, 1988.
151. **Roberts, C. J., Birkenmeier, T. M., McQuillan, J. J., Aliyama, S. K., Yamada, S. S., Chen, W. T., Yamada, K. M., and McDonald, J. A.,** Transforming growth factor beta stimulates the expression of fibronectin and of both subunits of the human fibronectin receptor by cultured human lung fibroblasts, *J. Biol. Chem.,* 263, 4586, 1988.
152. **Carlin, B., Durkin, M., Bender, B., Jaffe, R., and Chung, A.,** Synthesis of laminin and entactin by F9 cells induced with retinoic acid and dibutryrl cyclic AMP, *J. Biol. Chem.,* 258, 7729, 1983.
153. **Dziadek, M., Paulsson, M., and Timpl, R.,** Identification and interaction repertoire of the large forms of the basement membrane protein nidogen, *EMBO J.,* 4, 2513, 1985.
154. **Apella, E., Weber, I., and Blasi, F.,** Structure and function of epidermal growth factor-like regions in proteins, *FEBS Lett.,* 231, 1, 1988.
155. **Durkin, M., Chakravarti, S., Bartos, B., Liu, S. H., Friedman, R., and Chung, A.,** Amino acid sequence and domain structure of entactin. Homology with epidermal growth factor precursor and low density lipoprotein receptor, *J. Cell Biol.,* 107, 2749, 1988.
156. **Sage, H., Vernon, R. B., Funk, S. E., Ever, H. E. A., and Angello, J.,** SPARC, a secreted protein associated with cellular proliferation, inhibits cell spreading *in vitro* and exhibits Ca^{+2}-dependent binding to the extracellular matrix, *J. Cell Biol.,* 109, 341, 1989.
157. **Burridge, K. and Fath, K.,** Focal contacts: transmembrane links between the extracellular matrix and the cytoskeleton, *Bioessays,* 10, 104, 1989.
158. **Duband, J. L., Nuckolls, G. H., Ishibara, A., Hasegawa, T., Yamada, K. M., Thiery, J. P., and Jacobson, K.,** Fibronectin receptor exhibits high lateral mobility in embryonic locomoting cells but is immobile in focal contacts and fibrillar streaks in stationary cells, *J. Cell Biol.,* 107, 1385, 1988.
159. **Akiyama, S. K., Yamada, S. S., Chen, W. T., and Yamada, K. M.,** Analysis of fibronectin receptor function with monoclonal antibodies: roles in cell adhesion, migration, matrix assembly, and cytoskeletal organization, *J. Cell Biol.,* 109, 863, 1989.
160. **Giancotti, F. G. and Ruoslahti, E.,** Elevated levels of the $\alpha_5\beta_1$ fibronectin receptor suppress the transformed phenotype of Chinese hamster ovary cells, *Cell,* 60, 849, 1990.
161. **Nicolson, G. L.,** Cancer metastasis: organ colonization and the cell-surface properties of malignant cells, *Biochim. Biophys. Acta,* 695, 113, 1982.
162. **Saga, S., Chen, W., and Yamada, K. M.,** Enhanced fibronectin receptor expression in Rous sarcoma virus-induced tumors, *Cancer Res.,* 48, 5510, 1988.
163. **Dedhar, S. and Saulnier, R.,** Alternations in integrin receptor expression on chemically transformed human cells: specific enhancement of laminin and collagen receptor complexes, *J. Cell Biol.,* 110, 481, 1990.
164. **Plantefaber, L. C. and Hynes, R. O.,** Changes in integrin receptors on oncogenically transformed cells, *Cell,* 56, 281, 1989.
165. **Peltonen, J., Larjava, H., Jaakkola, S., Gralnick, H., Akiyama, S. K., Yamada, S. S., Yamada, K. M., and Uitto, J.,** Localization of integrin receptors for fibronectin, collagen, and laminin in human skin, *J. Clin. Invest.* 84, 1916, 1989.
166. **Hirst, R., Horwitz, A., Buck, C., and Rohrschneider, L.,** Phosphorylation of the fibronectin receptor complex in cells transformed by oncogenes that encode tyrosine kinases, *Proc. Natl. Acad. Sci. U.S.A.,* 83, 6470, 1986.
167. **Tapley, P., Horwitz, A., Buck, C., Duggan, K., and Rohrschneider, L.,** Integrins isolated from Rous sarcoma virus-transformed chicken embryo fibroblasts, *Oncogene,* 4, 325, 1989.

168. **Heino, J., Ignotz, R. A., Hemler, M. E., Crouse, C., and Massagué, J.,** Regulation of cell adhesion receptors by TGF-β concomitant regulation of integrins that share a common β_1 subunit, *J. Biol. Chem.*, 264, 380, 1989.
169. **Ignotz, R. A. and Massagué, J.,** Cell adhesion protein receptors as targets for transforming growth factor-β action, *Cell,* 51, 189, 1987.
170. **Ignotz, R. A., Heino, J., and Massagué, J.,** Regulation of cell adhesion receptors by transforming growth factor-β, *J. Biol. Chem.,* 264, 389, 1989.
171. **Kirchhofer, D., Languino, L. R., Ruoslahti, E., and Pierschbacher, M. D.,** $\alpha_2\beta_1$ integrins from different cell types show different binding specificities, *J. Biol. Chem.,* 265, 615, 1990.
172. **Herlyn, M., Clark, W. H., Rodeck, U., Mancianti, M. L., Jambrosic, J., and Koprowski, H.,** Biology of tumor progression in human melanocytes, *Lab. Invest.,* 56, 461, 1987.
173. **Menko, A. S. and Boettiger, D.,** Occupation of the extracellular matrix receptor, integrin, is a control point for myogenic differentiation, *Cell,* 51, 51, 1987.
174. **Turpeenniemi-Hujanen, T., Thorgeirsson, U. P., Rao, C. N., and Liotta, L. A.,** Laminin increases the release of type IV collagenase from malignant cells, *J. Biol. Chem.,* 261, 1883, 1986.
175. **Werb, Z., Tremble, P. M., Behrendtsen, O., Crowley, E., and Damsky, C.,** Signal transduction through the fibronectin receptor inducers, collagenase and stromelysin gene expression, *J. Cell Biol.,* 109, 877, 1989.

Chapter 11

INTERACTIONS BETWEEN CANCER CELLS AND THE ENDOTHELIUM

Robert Auerbach

TABLE OF CONTENTS

I. INTRODUCTION

For many years experienced clinicians have been aware that various types of cancer show a predictable pattern of metastatic dissemination — one type spreading primarily to the brain, another to the lung, yet others to the liver or bone. This seeding into varied sites can be in part simply the result of proximity or of mechanical and rheological factors such as the force, velocity, and volume of blood flow; the site of arrest of a twig in a stream is influenced by these same physical elements. However, these considerations alone do not fully explain the pattern of distribution of various tumors in the body.

A burst of investigative work in the last decade has demonstrated, through many imaginative experimental approaches, that some tumor cells have a predilection for colonizing certain organs of the body and that the interactions between the circulating tumor cell and the host organ overrides proximity and mechanical forces and are the primary determinants of tumor cell arrest, extravasation, survival, angiogenesis, and growth in a given site.[1-14]

The following five aspects of metastasis comprise the principal interactions between the host organ and the blood-borne metastatic cell: (1) attachment to the endothelium, (2) extravasation to the abluminal side of the endothelium, (3) survival in the organ microenvironment, (4) establishment of a blood supply, and (5) growth in the new site. It is the first of these that shall be discussed in this chapter, that is to say, the attachment of circulating tumor cells to the endothelium of a specific organ site. Other components of the tumor cell-host interaction, each of which is complex, are discussed in Chapters 12 to 17.

II. DEVELOPMENTAL PERSPECTIVES

The endothelium lines the lumen of all blood vessels and represents the total cellular makeup of the small capillaries in which tumor cell arrest occurs.[15-20] Until the recent past, it was generally assumed that the endothelium was a monolithic layer, and thus, it was difficult to conceptualize a differential interaction between tumor cells and endothelial cells of different capillary beds. His,[21] in 1868, proposed that all blood vessels arose from preexisting blood vessels, which grew centripetally to vascularize each new organ as it developed during embryogenesis. His exhaustive treatise describes in detail the gradual emergence of blood vessels in the yolk sac, their penetration into the embryo, and their subsequent gradual extension as the embryo elongates and undergoes organogenesis. His's view, which has prevailed to the present, was consistent with the assumption that endothelial cells were a homogeneous entity. Scientists, accepting this argument, elected to use the aorta, pulmonary artery and vein, or, in the case of humans, the umbilical vein, as a source of endothelial cells because of the greater accessibility of these vessels, the ease with which their endothelial cells could be isolated, and the large number of cells which they could yield. Hundreds of publications dealing with the behavior of endothelial cells *in vitro,* their response to growth factors, and their interactions with various cells such as leukocytes and muscle cells have appeared in the literature, and the conclusions drawn have been based on the tacit assumption of endothelial cell homogeneity.

Arguing against His's theory were the experimental embryologists of the 1920s who viewed capillary development as distinct from the development of large blood vessels.[22-28] Morphological observations as well as some experimental studies suggested that the endothelial cells comprising the microvasculature arose from within each organ during ontogeny. Even these investigators, however, did not propose that a diverse origin should necessarily mean that endothelial cells vary from organ to organ.

In recent years, the arguments have been reviewed by new experimental studies using avian embryos. The question of endothelial cell origin was studied using chimeric embryos in which chick embryonic rudiments were grafted into quail embryos or prevascularized quail tissue was transplanted into chick embryos.[29-32] The source of endothelial cells then could be determined by using antibodies generated against quail-specific endothelial cells to detect quail-derived cells wherever they might ultimately be located. The dominant pattern of vascularization indeed was found to confirm His's view: endothelial cells move as a coherent group, penetrating organ rudiments such as the limb or kidney as these organs grow and differentiate.[29,31,33] Histological preparations of chick rudiments grafted into quail embryos confirmed that the blood vessels of these grafted chick organs were of quail origin. Yet Noden,[32] by careful analysis of serial sections of chick embryos grafted with quail tissue from prevascularized embryos, also discovered that there were single quail endothelial cells, far removed from the original quail graft site, that were incorporated into various organ rudiments to participate in the *in situ* differentiation of blood vessels whose endothelium was primarily of chick origin. Thus, as is so often a case between divergent hypotheses, both views of vasculogenesis have been confirmed: vessels arise from preexisting vessels *and* from individual cells that differentiate *in situ.*

It does not necessarily follow that site-specific differentiation of endothelial cells depends on an intrinsic origin of the precursor cells that develop into blood vessels.[28,34] Thus, even though it has been clearly demonstrated that the blood vessels found in the cerebral hemispheres migrate into the developing brain from the outside, the vessels acquire brain-specific properties including, for example, the establishment of a mature blood-brain barrier[35] and the synthesis of gamma glutamyl synthetase.[36,37]

III. ORGAN-SPECIFIC ADHESION OF TUMOR CELLS TO THE ENDOTHELIUM

H.S.N. Greene, following many years of studying tumor transplants in ectopic sites, proposed that tumor cells metastasize following an initial adhesion to the endothelial cell surface, i.e., on the luminal side of microvascular endothelial cells.[38] Some years later, Woodruff and her colleagues demonstrated adhesion of lymphocytes to endothelial cells, specifically to the endothelial cells comprising the high endothelial venules.[39-41] These studies employed the technique of overlaying test cells onto sectioned frozen tissue samples — a technique that was subsequently employed by Zetter and his associates[42-44] and by Brodt[45] and others in their analysis of lung specific tumor cell metastasis (see below).

Experimental studies using tumor transplants or tumor cells injected into the arterial or venous system confirmed that different tumors had different predilections for establishing metastases in one or in another location.[5,6,46-48] These studies, however, did not focus specifically on a single component of the metastatic process and thus could not distinguish selective adhesion from other factors in determining the fate of metastatic tumor cells: entry into the bloodstream (for tumor transplants), arrest, penetration of the endothelium, angiogenesis, or growth.

Kahan used *in vitro* adhesion assays to demonstrate that tumor cells exhibited preferential adhesion to organ explants from their predicted site of metastasis.[49,50] Thus, teratoma cells with a known predilection for metastasizing to the ovary showed preferential adhesion to explants of whole mouse ovary. However, these studies were not designed to distinguish between particular ovarian cell types.

One of the earliest experimental observations of organ specificity of microvascular endothelial cells was the detection of brain-specific antigens on mouse brain-derived capillary endothelial cells.[28,51,52] These cells were found to express both Thy 1 and other brain-associated antigens as detected by monoclonal antibodies. The studies were significant in two ways: (1) mouse brain endothelial cells were antigenically different from other endothelial cells and (2) mouse brain endothelial cells expressed some antigens that were also present on nonendothelial cells from brain.

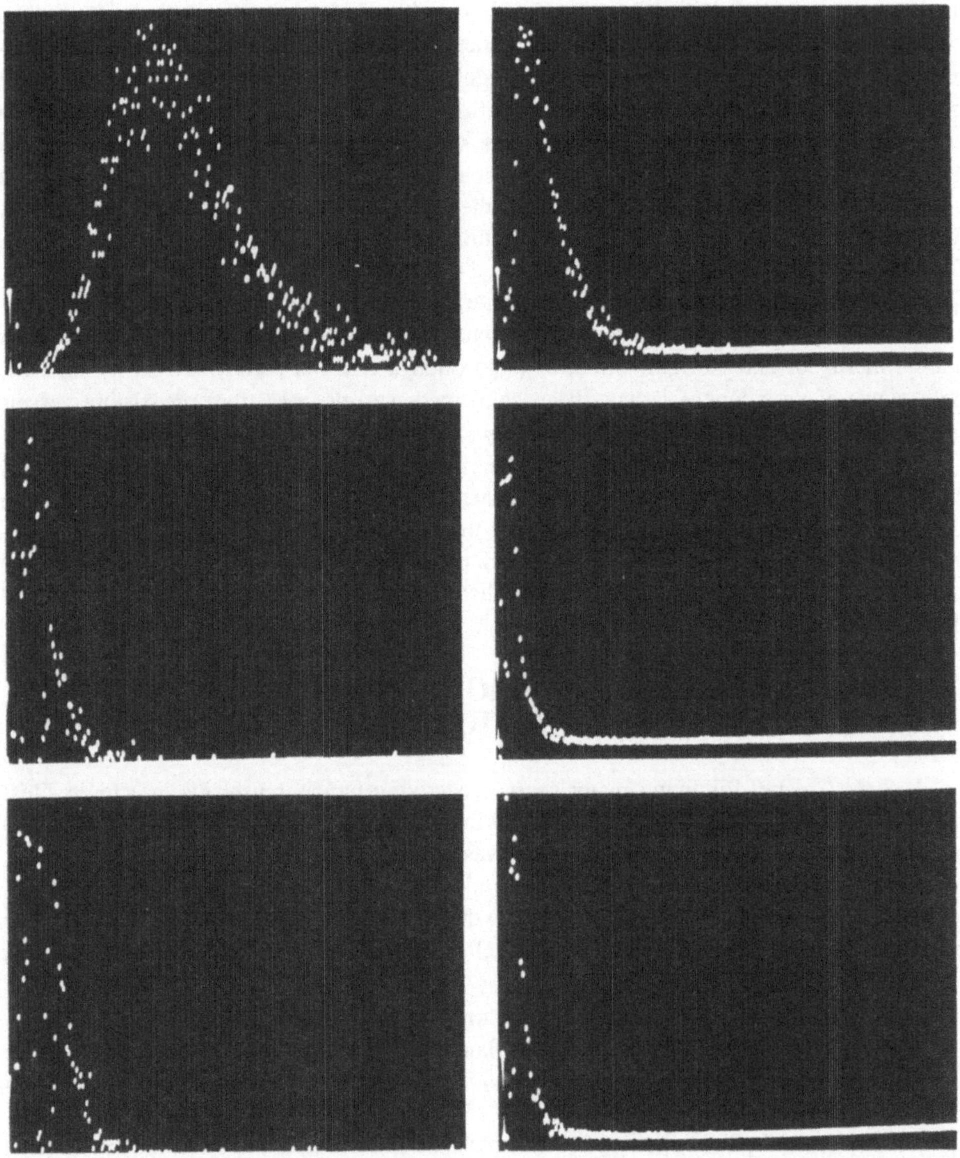

FIGURE 1. Flow cytometric analysis of antibody binding to mouse brain endothelial cells (left: MBE-1) and mouse ovary endothelial cells (right: MOE). Top panel: α-MBE P5E3 (positive by ELISA tests and immunohistology); Middle panel: α-MBE P5C3 (negative isotype control); Bottom panel: second-antibody only. (From Auerbach, R., Alby, L., Morissey, L. W., Tu, M., and Joseph, J., *Microvasc. Res.*, 29, 401, 1985. With permission.)

Similar findings were reported for other microvascular endothelial cells. For example, endothelial cells from mouse ovaries expressed some ovary-specific antigens that were common between them and ovary-derived fibroblasts, but they did not express on either endothelial or nonendothelial cells from other organs.[51] Similarly, lung endothelial cells shared some antigens with lung fibroblasts (Figure 1).

These new findings concerning organ-specific cell surface heterogeneity of endothelial cells prompted our re-examination of selective metastasis from this perspective, i.e., as a function of tumor cell/endothelial cell interaction. Our first experiments were carried out using two mouse tumors: the OTT6050 teratoma and the GL26 glioma.[53] The teratoma cell

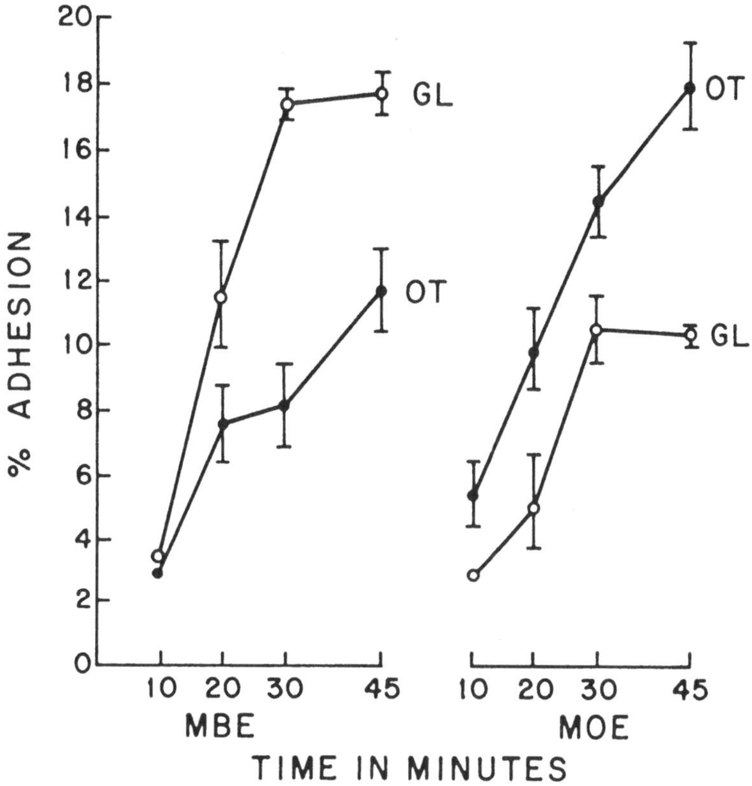

FIGURE 2. Comparison of glioma (GL) and ovarian teratocarcinoma (OT) cell adhesion to MBE and MOE endothelial cells derived from mouse brain (P16) or mouse ovary (P15) microvessels (1 of 13 experiments; three samples per data point). Cultures were agitated at room temperature at a rotational speed of 100 rpm. (From Alby, L. and Auerbach, R., *Proc. Natl. Acad. Sci. U.S.A.*, 81, 5739, 1984. With permission.)

line routinely metastasized to the ovary, following either intraperitoneal or intravenous injection. The GL26 glioma showed affinity for neural tissues. As already described above, we had isolated murine endothelial cells from brain and ovary during the course of our studies on organ-specific antigens.[51] We now use these same cell lines to examine the question of preferential adhesion of tumor cells to endothelial cells of a specific organ. Monolayers of mouse brain or ovary endothelial cells were grown to confluence. GL26 and OTT6050 tumor cells were radiolabelled by overnight incubation with ^{3}H-thymidine. Labelled tumor cells were then added to the endothelial cell monolayers and permitted to adhere for varying periods of time under constant agitation to reduce nonspecific adhesion. Following washing, adherent cell numbers were determined on the basis of retained radioactivity. The results were clear-cut: glioma cells preferred brain endothelium while teratoma cells adhered preferentially to ovary-derived endothelial cells. (Figure 2).

Subsequent studies were carried out using different tumors and different monolayer substrates.[54] Among the tumors tested, in addition to the original glioma and teratoma lines, were rat hepatoma cells, as well as various murine tumors including a bladder tumor, a hemangioendothelioma, a sarcoma, a lymphoma, a mastocytoma, and a mammary carcinoma. Hepatoma cells adhered preferentially to liver-derived endothelium, glioma cells to brain-derived endothelium, teratomas to endothelial cells obtained from the ovary, and mammary tumor cells to lymphatic endothelium. Some tumors such as the S180 sarcoma showed no selectivity, and some, like the MBT-2 bladder tumor line, were so self-adherent that they could not be distributed evenly on the monolayer, while others such as a murine endothelioma cell line unexpectedly adhered best to 3T3 fibroblasts. (Figures 3 and 4).

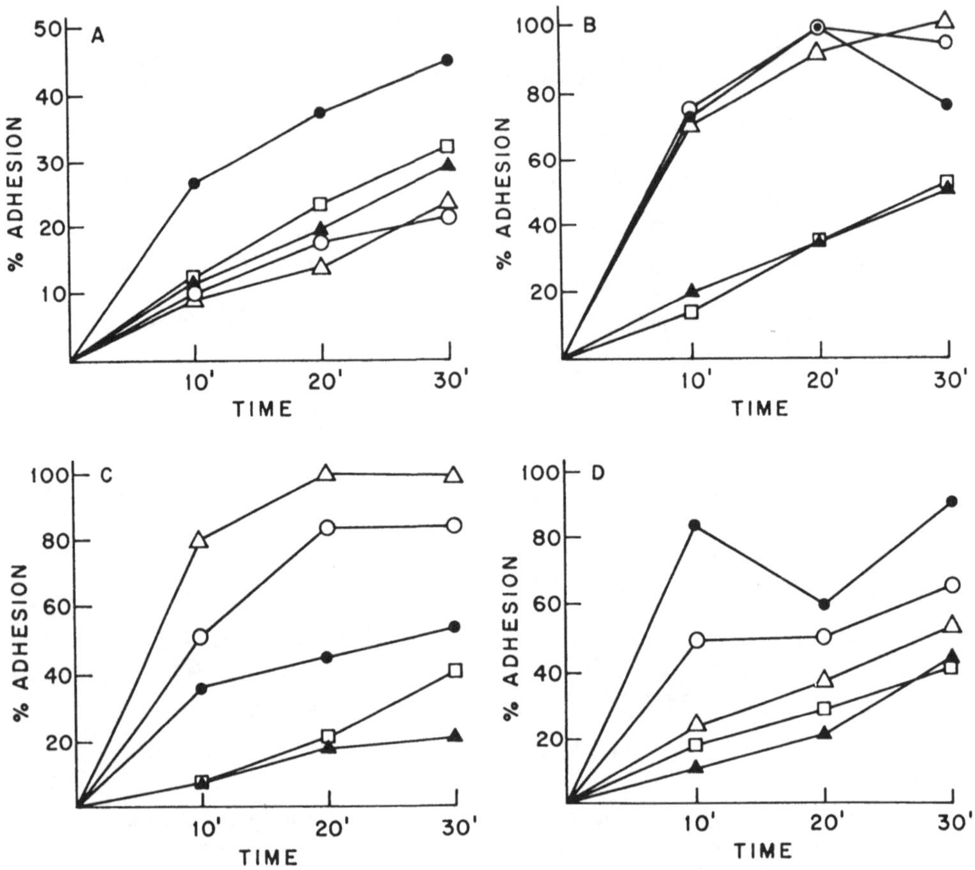

FIGURE 3. Adhesion of different mouse tumors (A = endothelioma; B = S180 sarcoma; C = teratoma; D = MBT-2 bladder tumor) to different murine confluent culture monolayers: (△) lung endothelium; (○) 3T3 fibroblasts; (●) liver; (□) thoracic duct lymphatic endothelium; (▲) brain endothelium. (From Auerbach, R., Lu, W. C., Pardon, E., Gumkowski, F., Kaminska, G., and Kaminski, M., *Cancer Res.*, 47, 1492, 1987. With permission.)

Several other laboratories also have observed organ-specific adhesion of tumor cells to endothelial cells. Experiments documenting the strong preference of hepatoma cells for adhesion to hepatic endothelium were most convincing.[13,55] The classic studies of the B16 melanoma sublines[56,57] have been extended to measurement of adhesion to endothelium, and to some extent, also have exhibited organ-specific selective adhesion.[5,6,46,47] In a recent study of lymphoma variants, a lung-selective subline adhered preferentially to pulmonary vascular endothelial cells while another variant that manifested preferential metastasis to the liver adhered preferentially to liver-derived microvascular endothelium.[58] Mizrachi et al. observed specific adhesion between pheochromocytoma cells and adrenal medullary endothelial cells in co-culture.[59] A striking organ preference of lung tumor cells for lung endothelium was also demonstrated by documenting selective adhesion of these tumor cells to the endothelium present in frozen lung sections.[42-44]

IV. ADHESION-MEDIATING MOLECULES

Several recent experiments have used functional assays to help identify particular moieties important in the adhesion between tumors and endothelial cells (see also Chapters 9 and 10). Among the most intriguing was the finding of Pauli and Lee that "neutral" endothelial cells acquired specificity by being cultured on extracellular matrix components released from

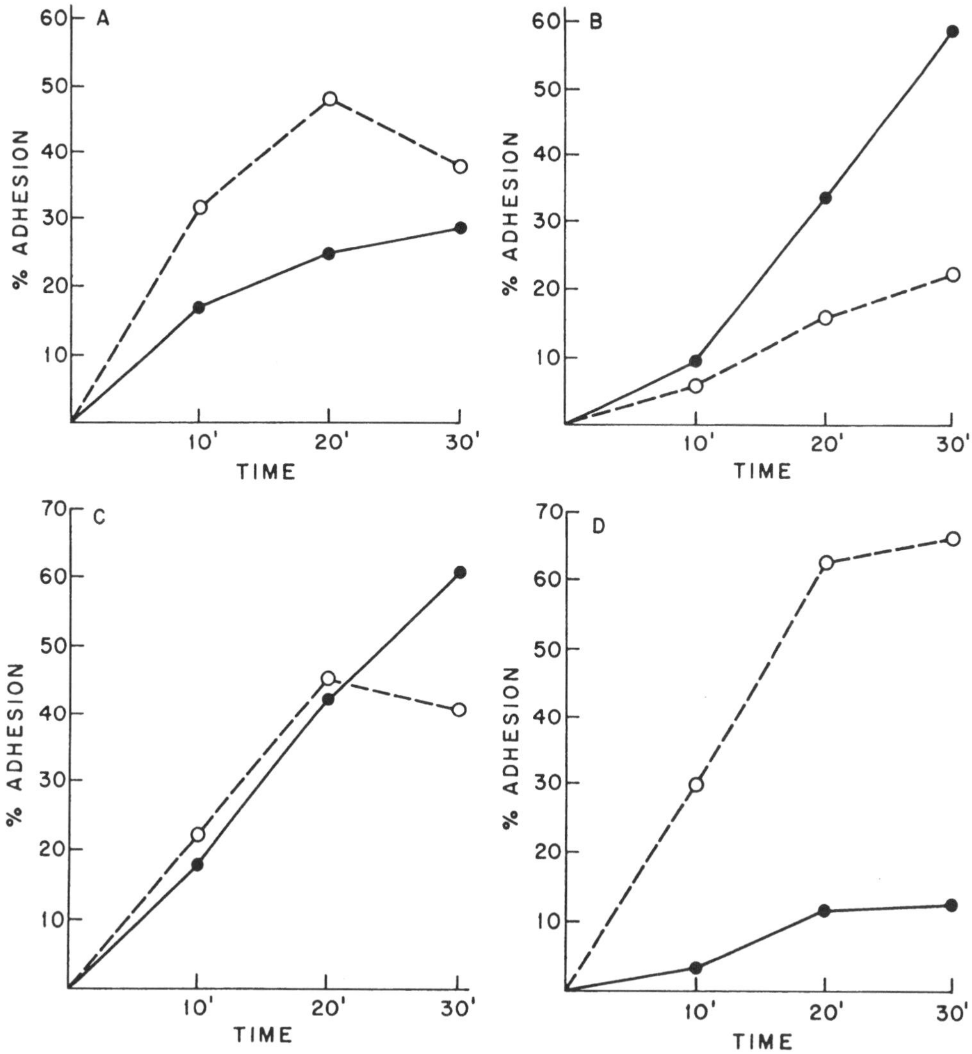

FIGURE 4. Adhesion of rat hepatoma H7777 (○) and mouse GL26 glioma (●) cells to mouse-derived cell cultures. (A = liver endothelium; B = brain endothelium; C = thoracic duct lymphatic endothelium; D = 3T3 fibroblasts. (From Auerbach, R., Lu, W. C., Pardon, E., Gumkowski, F., Kaminska, G., and Kaminski, M., *Cancer Res.*, 47, 1492, 1987. With permission.)

specific endothelial cells.[60] These studies increased the likelihood that the earlier work of Nicolson and his colleagues,[47] which emphasized the dominant role of the subendothelial matrix, might reflect the same molecules.

A more general adhesion-mediating substance has been identified by Zetter and his group.[42] As already mentioned, Netland and Zetter demonstrated selective adhesion between lung tumor cells and lung endothelial cells, but they now have convincing evidence that elastin plays a role and that tumor cells adhering to the lung bear elastin receptors on their cell surface.

Recently, a large number of investigations have been directed at determining the molecular basis for selective adhesion between tumors and the endothelium. The literature dealing with specific adhesion molecules is vast and will not be reviewed here. The reader is referred to several recent, excellent reviews.[61-63] Most important, both experimentally and conceptually, is the identification of vascular addressins, a term used to describe those specific adhesion molecules that appear, at first glance, to be particularly or exclusively involved in the adhesion to the endothelium of various circulating cells, including not only tumor cells but neutrophils, eosinophils, and other leukocytes.[64,65] A separate literature is developing that deals with lectin-binding sites on both tumors and endothelial cells,[42,55] and research in this area becomes all the more relevant in the light of the demonstration that a lectin-like domain has been identified on the family of adhesion molecules that includes the vascular addressins.[61,66]

V. IMMUNE SURVEILLANCE OF TUMORS: ROLE OF THE ENDOTHELIUM

An intriguing and original finding was made in our laboratory by Kaminski who studied the effectiveness of natural killer (NK) cells on different tumor cell lines.[67] Arguing that tumor cells are generally not present in the circulation for long but rather adhere to endothelium, he designed experiments to test the ability of tumor cells to be lysed *in vitro* by splenic NK cells when the tumor cells were adherent to cell monolayers.[3] The studies initially showed that a substrate of cells, whether fibroblasts or endothelial cells, afforded significant protection of the tumor cells from lysis by NK-mediated immune surveillance methods (Figure 5). Further investigation demonstrated that the protective effect was directly proportional to the extent of cell adhesion, from which followed that specific adhesion to endothelial cells would be a most effective method for tumor cells to survive NK-mediated lysis (Figure 6). Experiments verified this concept: since glioma cells adhered most effectively to brain endothelial cells, it was these that afforded the greatest protection.[68]

The protective effect of endothelial cells could be modified in various ways. For example, treatment of endothelial cell monolayers with glutaraldehyde reduced adhesion and simultaneously increased tumor cell sensitivity to NK cell-mediated lysis. More subtle effects were also demonstrated: pretreatment of endothelial cells with ultraviolet light reduced their ability to promote adhesion, although the effects were not cytotoxic.[72] In line with previous findings, there was a concomitant decrease in the protection that these treated endothelial cells could provide for tumor cells plated on these irradiated monolayers.

Studies to date indicate that the role of the endothelium in protecting tumor cells is not limited to NK-mediated cytotoxicity. Its role is more general, since tumor cells, on adhering to endothelial cells, are also a less susceptible target for antibody-mediated cytotoxicity.[73] Although selective adhesion also may play a role here, the studies of ADCC-mediated tumor cell destruction have not directly addressed the question of cell adhesion.

VI. ENDOTHELIAL CELL CYTOKINES AND GROWTH FACTORS

A relatively new area of investigation that has a potential impact on tumor cell/endothelial cell interactions is the role played by various cytokines produced by endothelial cells. In the last several years, a variety of studies have led to the demonstration that there are numerous factors produced by endothelial cells. One of the earliest was Hybridoma Growth Factor, which since has been found to be identical to IL-6.[69] Included in the list are several vasoconstrictive and vasodilation-inducing factors, prostaglandins, IL-1, IL-8, and IL-9, as well as a number of less well-defined growth promoting factors.

These cell products are traditionally considered nonspecific in that they have broad regulatory functions. Not generally examined, however, are two questions of specificity: (1) Are these factors selectively produced by *different* endothelial cells? and (2) Do endothelial cells also produce *specific* factors that may modulate tumor cell behavior? Moreover, with respect to the latter, are the specific factors produced by endothelial cells themselves separable either by organ site or by their selective action on particular tumor types?

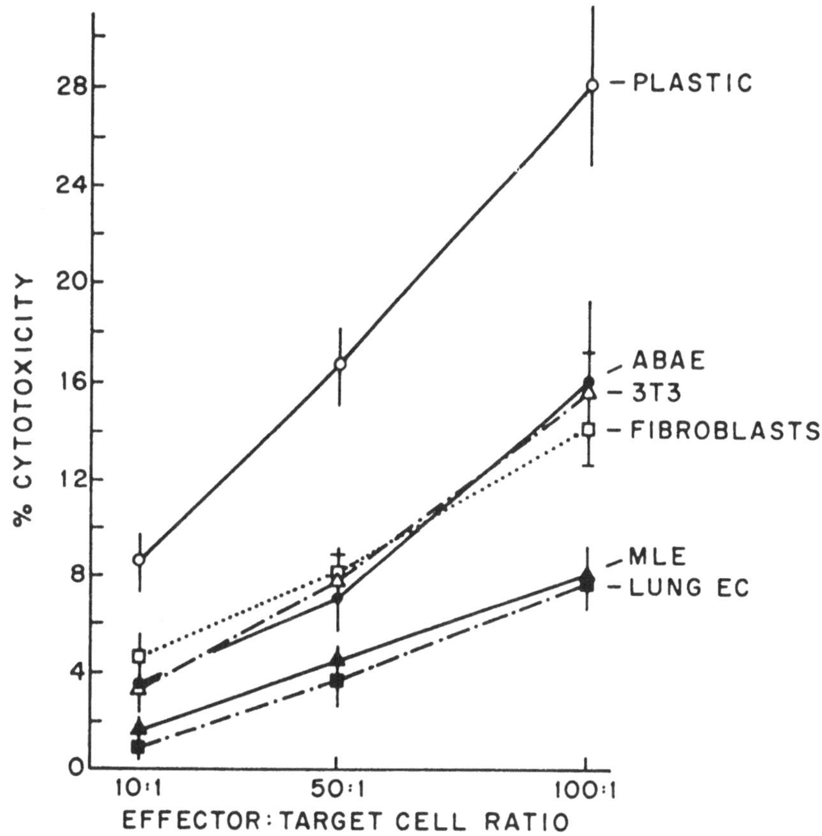

FIGURE 5. Cytotoxicity of mouse splenocytes against YAC-1 tumor cells on different cell monolayers. Data from 6 separate experiments; n = 3 for each data point for each experiment. Results are expressed as mean percentage release of ^{51}chromium ± SEM. ▲ = mouse thoracic duct; ■ = mouse lung endothelial cells; □ = mouse lung fibroblasts; △ = 3T3 cells; ● = adult bovine aortic endothelial cells; ○ = control wells without cell substrata. (From Kaminiski, M. and Auerbach, R., *Int. J. Cancer,* 41, 847, 1988. With permission.)

There is a long history of using organ-specific conditioned medium to promote organ-specific differentiation and growth. Most of the literature is difficult to interpret because of the complex media and conditions under which cells were grown or under which the media were assayed. But almost invariably, the conventional wisdom that has led to the adoption of certain techniques, such as using organ-specific conditioned medium, has a valid, even though not firmly established, basis. Our current molecular tools permit us to determine both the validity and the basis for organ-specific growth factors.

VII. CONCLUDING COMMENTS

Throughout its long history, experimental embryology has emphasized the processes of cell interactions and tissue interactions as fundamental to diversity and morphogenesis. This emphasis was applied to tumor biology in the 1940s and 1950s, where it provided an intellectual framework for such concepts as induction and promotion of tumors, two-stage carcinogenesis, and the phenomenon of tumor progression. Although the concepts were valid, they focused on questions which were not then readily amenable to experimentation. These approaches, important to tumor biology in earlier days, have a new validity and

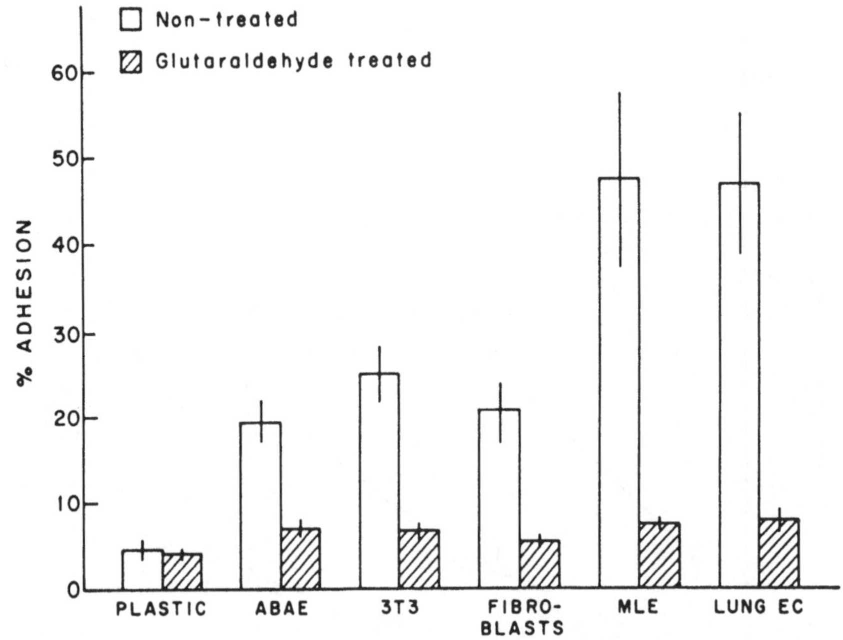

FIGURE 6. Adhesion of YAC-1 cells to different monolayers. Adhesion data (wells without splenocytes, 4 hr incubation, ^{51}chromium retention assay); details in "Material and Methods" for the standard monolayers as well as for monolayers pretreated with glutaraldehyde are shown. Data from 6 separate experiments; n = 3 for each data point. □ = untreated monolayers; ▨ = glutaraldehyde-treated monolayers. (From Kaminski, M. and Auerbach, R., *Int. J. Cancer,* 41, 847, 1988. With permission.)

urgency when viewed in the context of the remarkable progress made at the molecular and genetic levels. We are once again asking these complex, fundamental questions in tumor biology and endothelial cell biology: What tissues modulate expression of specific cell surface receptors? What factors are produced in response to cell or tissue interactions? What products do tumor cells release that influence endothelial cells? What products do endothelial cells secrete that either influence tumor cells directly or alter the likelihood of their transit out of the circulation?

Endothelial cells represent a heterogenous cell type, manifesting organ and site-specific differences[28,51,70,71] (Table 1). They possess the capacity to engage, variably, in a multitude of cell functions, many of which influence the behavior of those tumor cells with which they come into contact. On the other hand, the complex nature of tumor cells themselves also must be recognized. Tumor cells, too, represent an array of dissimilar cell types. They vary in their basic histotypic differentiation, in the products they synthesize or release, and in the particular set of oncogenes they harbor and express. They show complex patterns of metastatic preference. They vary in their ability to induce angiogenesis. They differ in their immunogenicity and in the type of immune response that they can evoke. All of these properties of tumor cells have an impact on their interactions with vascular endothelial cells.

As we gain a greater understanding of the individual molecules that regulate specific events such as cell adhesion, it will be particularly important not to equate the identification of such molecules with an understanding of the overall processes that underlie cell interactions. Each newly identified moiety will, however, provide more insight into the complex processes underlying these interactions, so that in time, the aggregate information can lead to a better comprehension of the events that regulate the interface between endothelial cells and the tumor cells with which they come into contact.

TABLE 1
Lectin-Binding Properties of Different Endothelial Cells

Cell	PBS	Con-A	DBA	PNA	RCAI	SBA	UEAI	WGA
Lung								
%[a]		94.6	1.6	16.3	97.0	21.1	0	97.7
Mean[b]	58.6	120.7	57.2	70.6	129.9	75.2	53.6	130.2
MBE								
%		98.7	1.1	98.6	90.7	35.6	0	98.5
Mean	53.5	124.4	54.5	122.3	91.3	70.3	50.9	131.9
MLyE								
%		97.2	0.3	37.7	98.0	77.5	0.4	97.7
Mean	58.5	125.2	62.3	77.5	121.9	86.7	60.1	137.5
ABAE								
%		97.7	0	6.3	98.3	82.5	0	97.6
Mean	60.1	118.1	56.8	67.7	128.3	88.5	52.4	141.3
E'oma								
%		97.6	0	0.5	98.2	64.1	0	95.9
Mean	62.6	115.6	59.9	66.4	137.6	89.2	55.0	146.6
Liver								
%		98.4	3.7	92.6	97.8	31.3	0.5	98.4
Mean	56.9	124.9	58.3	89.9	139.0	71.1	56.2	132.6
Mixed liver								
%		95.0	11.5	29.7	92.8	17.0	3.5	94.9
Mean	61.3	109.8	63.6	70.6	123.8	65.1	58.0	128.8
Fibroblasts								
%		98.4	7.8	18.5	94.1	73.5	0	98.8
Mean	55.1	114.5	57.7	62.0	127.1	86.8	51.1	146.1

Note: PBS = Phosphate-buffed saline; Con-A = concanavalin A; DBA = Dolichos biflorus agglutinin; PNA = peanut agglutinin; RCAI = *Ricinus communis* agglutinin; SBA = soybean agglutinin; UEAI = *Ulex europaeus* agglutinin; WGA = wheat germ agglutinin; MBE = mouse brain endothelium; MLyE = mouse lymphatic endothelium; ABAE = adult bovine aortic endothelium; E'oma = endothelioma.

[a] Percentage corrected for PBS control values (PBS = 0%).
[b] Mean channel value. Log amplification: 36 channels = 1 decade increase in fluorescence.

REFERENCES

1. **Auerbach, R.,** Patterns of tumor metastasis: organ selectivity in the spread of cancer cells, *Lab. Invest.,* 58, 361, 1988.
2. **Fidler, I. J.,** Origin and biology of cancer metastasis, *Cytometry,* 10, 673, 1989.
3. **Killion, J. J. and Fidler, I. J.,** The biology of tumor metastasis, *Semin. Oncol.* 16, 106, 1989.
4. **Weiss, L.,** *Principles of Metastasis,* Academic Press, Orlando, FL., 1985.
5. **Nicolson, G. L.,** Organ specificity of tumor metastasis role of preferential adhesion, invasion and growth of malignant cells at specific secondary sites, *Cancer Metast. Rev.,* 7, 143, 1988.
6. **Nicolson, G. L.,** Cancer metastasis: organ colonization and the cell surface properties of malignant cells, *Biochim. Biophys. Acta,* 695, 113, 1982.
7. **Roos, E. and Dingemans, K. P.,** Mechanisms of metastasis, *Biochim. Biophys. Acta,* 560, 135, 1979.
8. **Schirrmacher, V.,** Cancer metastasis, *Adv. Cancer Res.,* 43, 1, 1985.
9. **Hart, I. R.,** Seed and soil revisited. Mechanisms of site specific metastasis, *Cancer Metast. Rev.,* 1, 5, 1982.
10. **Tarin, D.,** Clinical and experimental studies on the biology of metastasis, *Biochim. Biophys. Acta,* 780, 227, 1985.

11. **Weiss, L., Orr, F. W., and Honn, K. V.,** Interactions between cancer cells and the microvasculature: a rate-regulator for metastasis, *Clin. Exp. Metastasis,* 7, 127, 1989.
12. **Nicolson, G. L.,** Cancer metastasis: tumor cell and host organ properties important in metastasis to specific secondary sites, *Biochim. Biophys. Acta,* 948, 175, 1988.
13. **Schirrmacher, V.,** Mechanisms of metastatic spread to liver, *Recent Results Cancer Res.,* 100, 23, 1986.
14. **Murphy, P., Alexander, P., Senior, P. V., Fleming, J., Kirkham, N., and Taylor, I.,** Mechanisms of organ selective tumor growth by bloodborne cancer cells, *Br. J. Cancer,* 57, 19, 1988.
15. **Ryan, U., Ed.,** *Endothelial Cells,* Vol. 3, CRC Press, Boca Raton, FL, 1989.
16. **Jaffe, E. A.,** *The Biology of Endothelial Cells,* Martinus Nijhoff, The Hague, 1983.
17. **Simionescu, N. and Simionescu, M.,** *Endothelial Cell Biology in Health and Disease,* Plenum Press, New York, 1988, 1.
18. **Simionescu, N. and Simionescu, M.,** *Endothelial Cell Dysfunction,* Plenum Press, New York, 1991.
19. **Feinberg, R. and Shearer, G.,** *Development of the Vascular System,* S. Karger, New York, 1991.
20. **Shepro, D.,** Endothelial cells, inflammatory edema and the microvascular barrier: comments by a "free radical", *Microvasc. Res.,* 35, 247, 1988.
21. **His, W.,** *Untersuchungen ueber die erste Anlage des Wirbelthierleibes,* FCW Vogel, Leipzig, 1868.
22. **McClure, C.,** The endothelial problem, *Anat. Rec.,* 22, 219, 1921.
23. **Reagan, P. R.,** Vascularization phenomena in fragments of embryonic bodies completely isolated from yolksac blastoderm, *Anat. Rec.,* 9, 329, 1916.
24. **Sabin, F. R.,** Studies on the origin of blood vessels and of red blood corpuscles as seen in the living blastoderm of chicks during the second day of incubation, *Contr. Embryol. Carnegie Inst.,* 9, 213, 1920.
25. **Clark, E. R. and Clark, E. L.,** Observations on changes in blood vascular endothelium in the living animal, *Amer. J. Anat.,* 57, 385, 1935.
26. **Jolly, J.,** Recherches sur la formation du systeme vasculaire de l'embryon, *Arch. d'Anat. Microsc.,* 35, 295, 1939.
27. **Wagner, R. C.,** Endothelial cell embryology and growth, *Adv. Microcirc.,* 9, 45, 1980.
28. **Auerbach, R. and Joseph, J.,** Cell surface markers on endothelial cells: a developmental perspective, in *The Biology of Endothelial Cells,* Jaffe, E. A., Ed., Martinus Nijhoff, The Hague, 1983, 393.
29. **Peault, B., Coltey, M., and Le Douarin, N. M.,** Ontogenic emergence of a quail leukocyte/endothelium cell surface antigen, *Cell Differ.,* 23, 165, 1988.
30. **Pardanaud, L., Yassine, F., and Dieterlen-Lievre, F.,** Relationship between vasculogenesis, angiogenesis and haemopoiesis during avian ontogeny, *Development,* 105, 473, 1989.
31. **Labastie, M. C., Poole, T. J., Peault, B. M., and Le Douarin, N. M.,** MB1, a quail leukocyte-endothelium antigen: partial characterization of the cell surface and secreted forms in cultured endothelial cells, *Proc. Natl. Acad. Sci. U.S.A.,* 83, 9016, 1986.
32. **Noden, D. M.,** Embryonic origins and assembly of blood vessels, *Am. Rev. Respir. Dis.,* 140, 1097, 1989.
33. **Sariola, H., Ekblom, P., Lehtonen, E., and Saxen, L.,** Differentiation and vascularization of the metanephric kidney grafted on the chorioallantoic membrane, *Dev. Biol.,* 96, 427, 1983.
34. **Risau, W., Sariola, H., Zerwes, H. G., Sasse, J., Ekblom, P., Kemler, R., and Doetschman, T.,** Vasculogenesis and angiogenesis in embryonic-stem-cell derived embryoid bodies, *Development,* 102, 471, 1988.
35. **Risau, W. and Wolburg, H.,** Development of the blood-brain barrier, *Trends Neurosci.,* 13, 174, 1990.
36. **Cancilla, P. A. and DeBault, L. E.,** Neutral amino acid transport properties of cerebral endothelial cells *in vitro, J. Neuropathol. Exp. Neurol.,* 42, 191, 1983.
37. **Meresse, S., Dehouck, M. P., Delorme, P., Bensaid, M., Tauber, J. P., Delbart, C., Fruchart, J. C., and Cecchelli, R.,** Bovine brain endothelial cells express tight junctions and monoamine oxidase activity in long-term culture, *J. Neurochem.,* 53, 1363, 1989.
38. **Greene, H. S. N. and Harvey, E. K.,** The relationship between the dissemination of tumor cells and the distribution of metastases, *Cancer Res.,* 24, 799, 1964.
39. **Clarke, L. M. and Chin, Y. H.,** Specific cell-adhesion mechanisms determining migration pathways of recirculating lymphocytes, *Annu. Rev. Immunol.,* 5, 201, 1987.
40. **Chin, Y. H., Rasmussen, R. A., Woodruff, J. J., and Easton, T. G.,** A monoclonal anti-HEBFPP antibody with specificity for lymphocyte surface molecules mediating adhesion to Peyer's patch high endothelium of the rat, *J. Immunol.,* 136, 2556, 1986.
41. **Woodruff, J. J. and Kuttner, B. J.,** Adherence of lymphocytes to the high endothelium of lymph nodes *in vitro, Ciba Found. Symp.,* 71, 243, 1980.
42. **Zetter, B. R.,** The cellular basis of site-specific tumor metastasis, *New Engl. J. Med.,* 322, 605, 1990.
43. **Netland, P. A. and Zetter, B. R.,** Organ-specific adhesion of metastatic tumor cells *in vitro, Science,* 224, 1113, 1984.
44. **Netland, P. A. and Zetter, B. R.,** Metastatic potential of B16 melanoma cells after *in vitro* selection for organ-specific adherence, *J. Cell Biol.,* 101, 720, 1985.

45. **Brodt, P.**, Tumor cell adhesion to frozen lymph node sections — an *in vitro* correlate of lymphatic metastasis, *Clin. Exp. Metastasis,* 7, 135, 1989.
46. **Nicolson, G. L. and Winkelhake, J. L.**, Organ specificity of blood-borne tumour metastasis determined by cell adhesion?, *Nature,* 255, 230, 1975.
47. **Kramer, R. H., Vogel, K. G., and Nicolson, G. L.**, Tumor cell interactions with vascular endothelial cells and their extracellular matrix, *Prog. Clin. Biol. Res.*, 89, 333, 1982.
48. **Nicolson, G. L.**, Metastatic tumor cell attachment and invasion assay utilizing vascular endothelial cell monolayers, *J. Histochem. Cytochem.*, 30, 214, 1982.
49. **Kahan, B.**, Experimental metastasis of mouse embryonal carcinoma cell lines to specific locations, *Cancer Res.*, 47, 6315, 1987.
50. **Kahan, B.**, Ovarian localization of embryonal teratocarcinoma cells derived from female germ cells, *Somatic Cell Genet.*, 5, 763, 1979.
51. **Auerbach, R., Alby, L., Morrissey, L. W., Tu, M., and Joseph, J.**, Expression of organ-specific antigens on capillary endothelial cells, *Microvasc. Res.*, 29, 401, 1985.
52. **Auerbach, R.**, Cell surface antigens and differentiation, *Prog. Clin. Biol. Res.*, 149, 3, 1984.
53. **Alby, L. and Auerbach, R.**, Differential adhesion of tumor cells to capillary endothelial cells *in vitro, Proc. Natl. Acad. Sci. U.S.A.*, 81, 5739, 1984.
54. **Auerbach, R., Lu, W. C., Pardon, E., Gumkowski, F., Kaminska, G., and Kaminski, M.**, Specificity of adhesion between murine tumor cells and capillary endothelium: an *in vitro* correlate of preferential metastasis *in vivo, Cancer Res.*, 47, 1492, 1987.
55. **Schirrmacher, V., Uhlenbruck, G., and Pulverer, G.**, Inhibition of liver tumor cell colonization in two animal tumor models by lectin blocking with D-galactose or arabinogalactan, *Clin. Exp. Metastasis,* 6, 115, 1988.
56. **Fidler, I. J.**, Selection of successive tumor lines for metastasis, *Nature,* 242, 148, 1973.
57. **Hart, I. R. and Fidler, I. J.**, Role of organ selectivity in the determination of metastatic patterns of B16 melanoma, *Cancer Res.*, 40, 2281, 1980.
58. **Doerr, R., Zvibel, I., Chiuten, D., D'Olimpo, J., and Reid, L. M.**, Clonal growth of tumors on tissue-specific biomatrices and correlation with organ site specificity of metastases, *Cancer Res.*, 49, 384, 1989.
59. **Mizrachi, Y., Lelkes, P. I., Ornberg, R. L., Goping, G., and Pollard, H. B.**, Specific adhesion between pheochromocytoma (PC12) cells and adrenal medullary endothelial cells in co-culture, *Cell Tissue Res.*, 256, 365, 1989.
60. **Pauli, B. M. and Lee, C.-L.**, Organ preference of metastasis: the role of organ-specific modulated endothelial cells, *Lab. Invest.*, 58, 379, 1988.
61. **Patarroyo, M. and Makgoba, M. W.**, Leukocyte adhesion to cells. Molecular basis, physiological relevance, and abnormalities, *Scand. J. Immunol.*, 30, 129, 1989.
62. **Rutishauser, U. and Jessell, T. M.**, Cell adhesion molecules in vertebrate neural development, *Physiol. Rev.*, 68, 819, 1988.
63. **Pabst, R. and Binns, R. M.**, Heterogeneity of lymphocyte homing physiology: several mechanisms operate in the control of migration to lymphoid and non-lymphoid organs *in vivo, Immunol. Rev.*, 108, 83, 1989.
64. **Streeter, P. R., Berg, E. L., Rouse, B. T. N., Bargatze, R. F., and Butcher, E. C.**, A tissue-specific endothelial cell molecule involved in lymphocyte homing, *Nature,* 331, 41, 1988.
65. **Berg, E. L., Goldstein, L. A., Jutila, M. A., Nakache, M., Picker, L. J., Streeter, P. R., Wu, N. W., Zhou, D., and Butcher, E. C.**, Homing receptors and vascular addressins: cell adhesion molecules that direct lymphocyte traffic, *Immunol. Rev.*, 108, 5, 1989.
66. **Yednock, T. A. and Rosen, S. D.**, Lymphocyte homing, *Adv. Immunol.*, 44, 313, 1989.
67. **Kaminski, M. and Auerbach, R.**, Tumor cells are protected from NK-cell-mediated lysis by adhesion to endothelial cells, *Int. J. Cancer,* 41, 847, 1988.
68. **Rozental, J., Kaminska, G. M., and Kaminski, M. J.**, Cultured brain endothelium inhibits the cytocidal action of natural killer cells on glioma, *J. Neurooncol.*, 7, 65, 1989.
69. **Pober, J. and Cotran, R. S.**, Cytokines and endothelial cell biology, *Physiol. Rev.*, 70, 427, 1990.
70. **Zetter, B. R.**, Endothelial heterogeneity: influence of vessel size, organ localization and species specificity on the properties of cultured endothelial cells, in *Endothelial Cells,* Vol. 2, Ryan, U. S., Ed., CRC Press, Boca Raton, FL, 1989, 63.
71. **Gumkowski, F., Kaminska, G., Kaminski, M., Morrissey, L. W., and Auerbach, R.**, Heterogeneity of mouse vascular endothelium. *In vitro* studies of lymphatic, large blood vessel and microvascular endothelial cells, *Blood Vessels,* 24, 11, 1987.
72. **Auerbach, R.**, unpublished observations.
73. **Auerbach, R.**, unpublished observations.

Chapter 12

SELECTIVE INVOLVEMENT OF A SPECIFIC SINUSOIDAL DOMAIN IN HEPATIC METASTASIS

Emilio Barberá-Guillem and Fernando Vidal-Vanaclocha

TABLE OF CONTENTS

I. INTERACTION OF TUMOR CELLS WITH HEPATIC TISSUE

In order for liver metastasis to occur, tumor cells reaching the organ through the hepatic artery or the portal vein must travel from the portal venules (PV) to the central venules or terminal hepatic venules (THV) and through a microvascular bed in the form of a sinusoidal network. In the liver, the sinusoids form recurring structures of capillary pathways arranged between leaflets of parenchymal cells (Figure 1). They basically appear in bundles of microvessels measuring 5 to 7 μm in diameter and are arranged in a theoretically radial pattern following into the THV, which are tributaries of the hepatic veins.[1] The true arrangement of the sinusoids, however, is not strictly radial. Some sinusoids follow a circumferential route in the areas furthest from the THV and run along the area between two adjacent PV. The specific region occupied by these specially arranged sinusoids is, in the liver of certain animals such as the pig, the area occupied by a septum of connective tissue. These sinusoids are thus called septal sinusoids in order to distinguish them from the radial sinusoids, which are the ones that finally flow into the THV.[2,3] The branched network of PV and hepatic arteries, together with the abundant, repetitive sinusoidal network and THV flowing into the hepatic veins, constitute the extensive labyrinth of the hepatic microvasculature[3,4] through which the tumor cells circulate, stop, and establish interactions with different types of liver cells and extracellular matrix molecules.

In the Kiernan space, the terminal branches of PV and arterioles are surrounded by the extracellular matrix of the connective tissue and have a continuous endothelial lining.[1] PVs measure more than 30 μm in diameter, while the terminal arterioles measure between 10 and 50 μm. The veins are connected to the sinusoids via orifices measuring 5 μm in diameter.[3,4] Somewhere along this complex microvascular route, tumor cells may adhere — alone or in groups — to the walls of the different microvascular segments, but they do not reduce their diameters in order to continue on their way, except at the exits from the PV to the sinusoids and in the final stretches of the arterioles. At these points, the tumor cells can become physically trapped and forced to change shape in order to continue onward.

The medium surrounding the cells in the PV is comprised of incoming blood from the spleen and mesentery that has yet to be processed by the liver. In the branches of the hepatic arteries, however, the oxygen content of the medium is higher, corresponding to levels in the arterial bloodstream.[3,5]

Once inside the sinusoids, the cancer cell must travel through a winding pathway that changes in diameter before finally reaching the THV. The average diameter of this pathway is 5 to 7 μm, i.e., narrower than the average diameter of the cancer cells.[6,7] Here then, the cells must reduce their diameters by altering their shape in order to proceed. The sinusoidal walls are lined with fenestrated endothelial cells[8,9] (Figure 2), which in turn are covered with a blood cell surface interface of special glycoproteins comprising their glycocalix.[10] Sinusoids branch out and anastomose with other neighboring sinusoids, organizing a true labyrinth (Figure 3).[3,5] It often happens that the sinusoidal pathway becomes almost completely obstructed by the cell body or cytoplasmic prolongations of the hepatic resident macrophages, i.e., the Kupffer cells[11] (Figure 4). Also found in the sinusoidal lumen are the Pit cells[12] (asialo GM-1 positive cells) and various subpopulations of lymphoid cells.[13,14] As the blood travels through the sinusoid from the portal or septal zones to the central zone, it gradually changes composition. The concentrations of oxygen, metabolic substrates, hormones, etc. increase or decrease according to the distance from the PV or THV.[5] All these resident cells and microenvironmental conditions in the sinusoid are possible candidate elements for tumor-host cell interactions, which would affect the fate of tumor cells passing through.

Outside the endothelial cells is the Disse space,[9] in which are found a number of extracellular matrix molecules (fibronectin, entactin, laminin, collagen IV, and some cell-

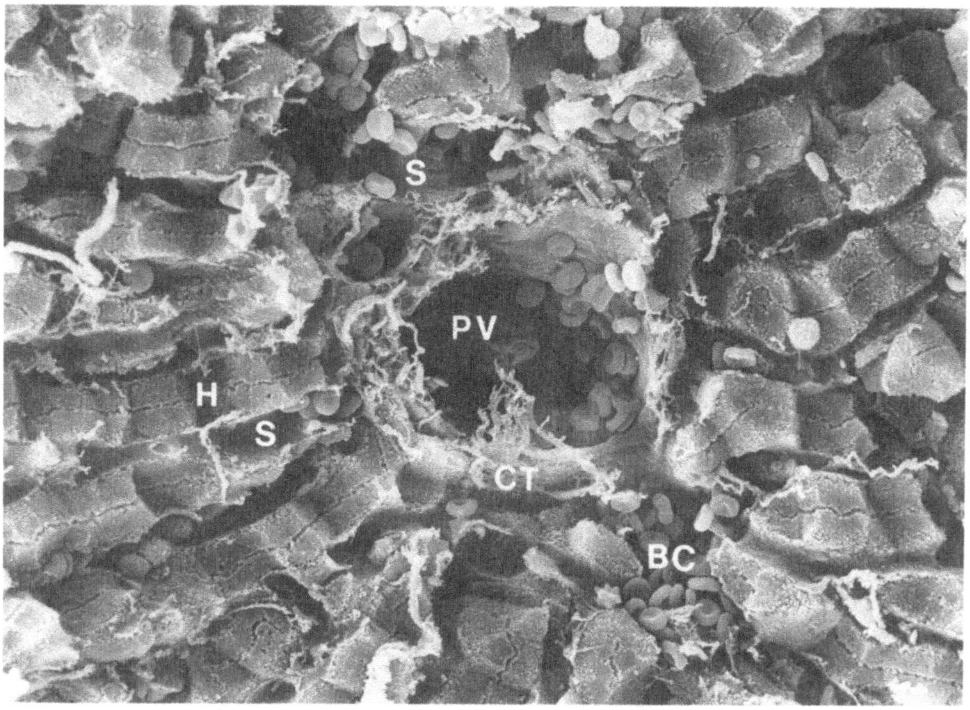

FIGURE 1. Scanning electron micrograph (SEM) of a portal venule (PV) area and its surrounding tissue. Radial periportal sinusoids (S); hepatocyte leaflets (H); blood-cells (BC) in the sinusoidal lumen; connective tissue (CT). × 462.

associated proteoglycans) that never finally form a true basal lamina.[15] Here, we find plasma filtered through the endothelial fenestrae and Ito or fat-storing cells.[14] On the other side of the Disse space are the hepatocytes with their microvilli (Figure 2). Finally, the end of the sinusoidal pathway is reached with a sudden emptying into a THV (average diameter of 45 μm).[4] From this point on, the tumor cell travels through larger and larger veins whose walls are lined with a continuous endothelium resting on a thin extracellular basal lamina. In these segments, the blood medium is similar to that in the final stretch of the sinusoid.

II. HEPATIC FUNCTIONAL ZONES AND THEIR MICROVASCULAR IMPLICATIONS

The parenchyma of the liver tissue is functionally and regionally heterogeneous. For example, in the area around the PV, the hepatocytes develop certain preferential and sometimes exclusive functions revealed by the marked activity of various enzymes, whereas in the area around the THV, the enzymatic activities engaged in by the hepatocytes are quite different.[16,17,18] Consequently, Rappaport[5] proposed the existence of microcirculatory acini in which the following functional zones could be identified: zone 1, corresponding to the periportal and septal areas; zone 3, corresponding to the pericentral or centrilobular area; and zone 2, the border area between these two end zones (Figure 5). These zones are easily distinguished using histochemical and immuno-histochemical techniques. For example, there are certain enzymes such as succinate-dehydrogenase (SDH) that are not distributed homogeneously along the strings of hepatocytes running from zones 1 to 3. SDH activity actually decreases as we move from the area closest to the PV towards the area next to the THV, and thus there is a more or less smooth transition between zones 1 and 3 (Figure 6).

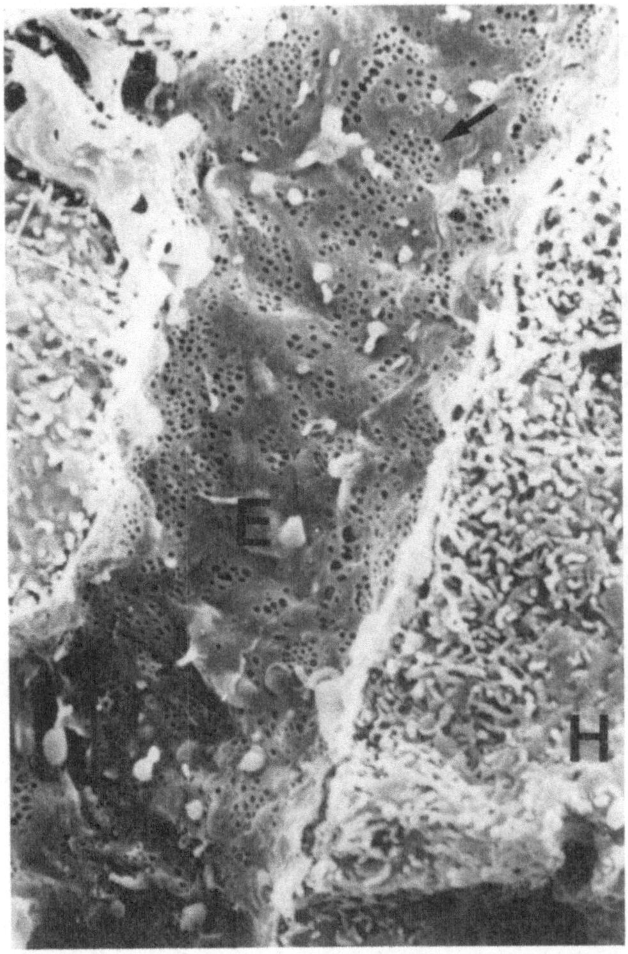

FIGURE 2. Frontal view of the hepatic sinusoidal wall (SEM). Capillary lining consists of endothelial cells (E) with flattened processes perforated by small fenestrae (arrow) of about 0.1 μm in size. H = hepatocytes. × 4400.

A few years ago,[8] we showed that the sinusoidal endothelium of zone 1 is clearly distinct from that of zone 3. In zone 1, the endothelial cells are less porous than in zone 3, suggesting less communication between the sinusoidal lumen and the Disse space in zone 1. In developing livers from the fetal to the adult stage, this zonal differentiation of the endothelial cells lining the sinusoids precedes the zonal differentiation of the hepatocytes.[20,21] What is more, the wall of the zone 3 sinusoidal endothelium facilitates the intravasation of hemopoietic cells by creating large-sized endothelial fenestrae that are present even after birth.[20,22] The endothelial cells of zones 1 and 3 can be distinguished by their specific lectin-binding patterns produced by the different carbohydrate residue compositions of their surface glycoproteins (Table 1).[23] Zone 1 endothelial cells have a higher concentration of *N*-acetyl-neuraminic acid, galactose, and *N*-acetyl-glucosamine, while mannose and glucose concentrations are more evenly distributed in all the endothelial cells lining the sinusoidal wall; *N*-acetyl-galactosamine and fucose molecules are absent. In a detailed quantitative study on wheat germ agglutinin (WGA) surface binding, we showed that the zone 1 endothelial cells have six times more binding sites for this lectin than the zone 3 endothelial cells (Figure 7). This quality is maintained following separation by enzyme digestion of liver tissue, thus

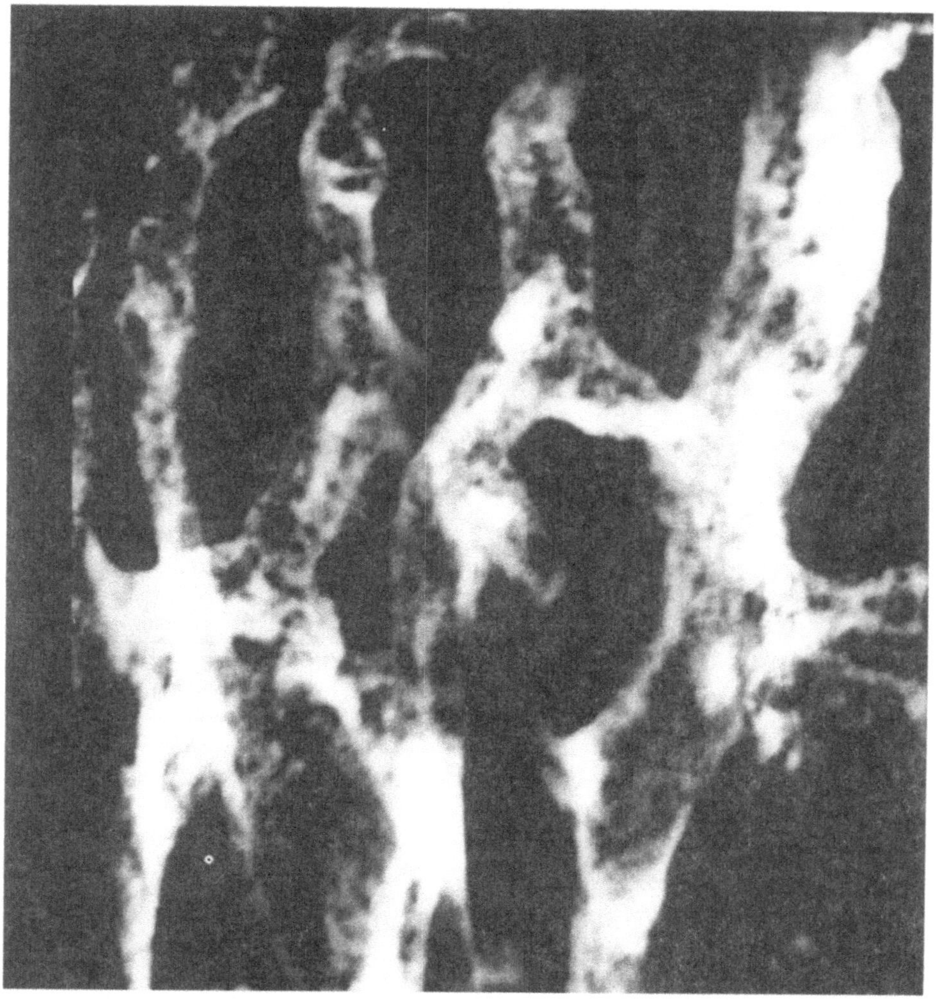

FIGURE 3. High-resolution confocal microscopic image of the sinusoidal segments located in the periportal area (acinar zone 1) of liver tissue.

making it possible to separate the two endothelial cell populations *in vitro* (Figure 8). An additional distinction between the endothelial cells of zones 1 and 3 is that the sinusoidal endothelial cells of zone 1 are able to take up latex beads perfused through the portal vein[24] or administered to endothelial cells *in vitro,*[25] in a greater degree than those of zone 3.[26]

The Kupffer cells are another heterogeneous sinusoidal cell population with zone-related differences. In physiological conditions, they are somewhat more frequent in zone 1, where phagocytosis is greater, as measured by counting their uptake of tracer particles.[11] Moreover, when a hepatic metastasis is forming, the Kupffer cells interact with the tumor cells[27] and respond with significant dynamic changes in numerical density, acinar distribution, and phagocytic capacity.[7,28]

Zone 1 sinusoids have been described as more winding and anastomotic than the straighter, less anastomotic zone 3 sinusoids.[3,5] Following perfusion of fluorochrome-conjugated lectins, confocal microscopy can be used to show that in zone 1, there is indeed a tree of twisted varicose sinusoids lined with endothelial cells, having high concentrations of WGA-binding sites on their surface. In zone 3, the sinusoids are more cylindrical in shape, more parallel, and lined with low WGA-affinity endothelial cells (Figure 9).

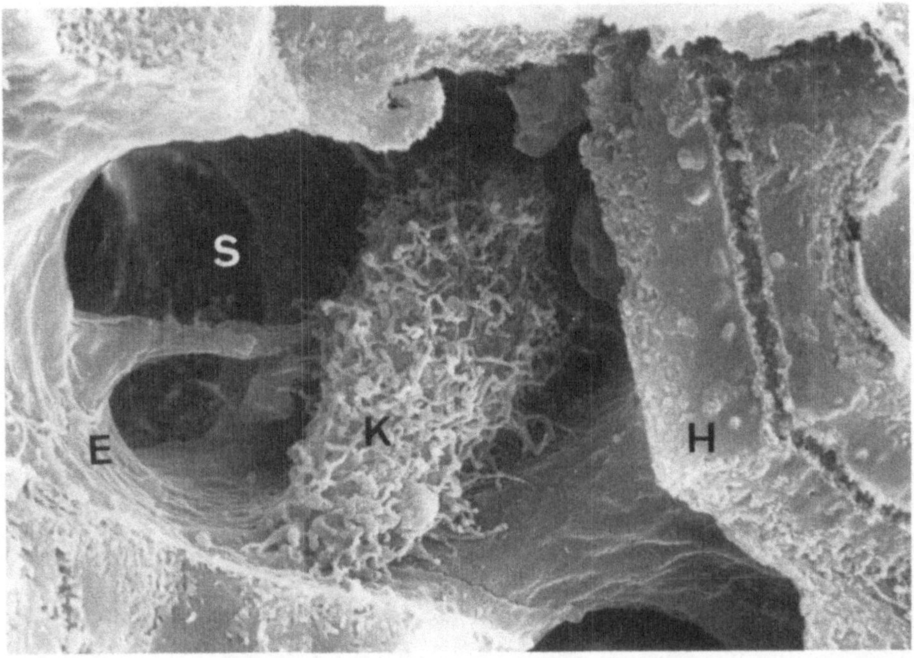

FIGURE 4. Scanning electron micrograph of a liver sinusoid. A large Kupffer cell (K) within the sinusoidal lumen (S) showing an irregular surface with folds, ruffles, and microvilli. H = hepatocyte; E = sinusoidal endothelium. × 3500.

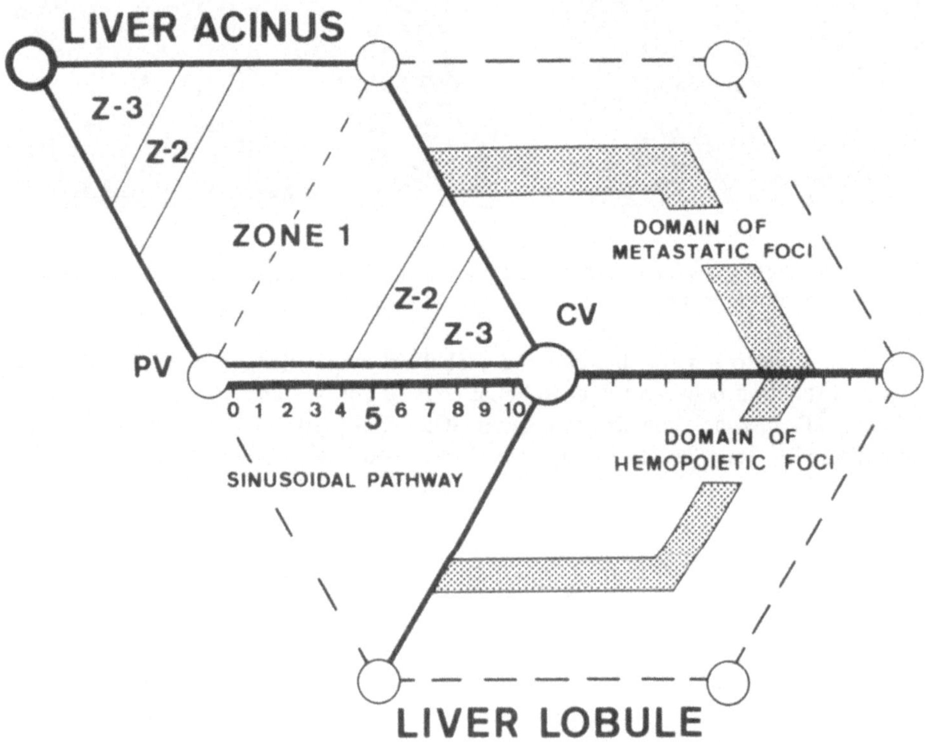

FIGURE 5. Diagrammatic representation of acinar and lobular models of liver tissue organization and the specific distribution domains (dotted areas) of both hematopoietic colonies from PHZ-treated mice and all the metastatic foci, regardless of the tumor cell type or its vascular delivery route. The calculated average position on the theoretical sinusoidal pathway going from the portal vein (PV) to the central vein (CV) was 3.3 (range: 2.8—3.8) for hematopoietic foci and 3.1 (range: 2.4—4.0) for metastatic foci.

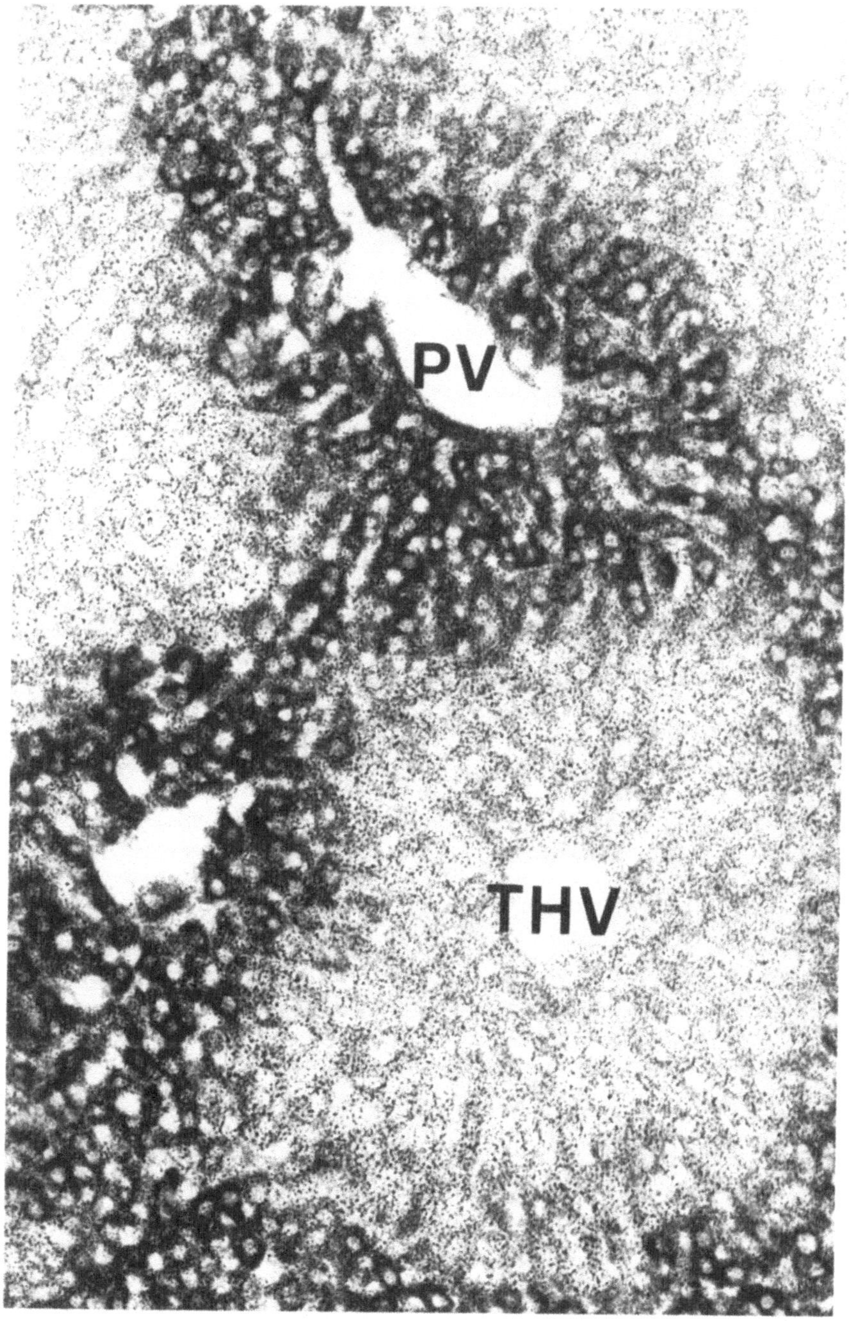

FIGURE 6. Liver tissue section obtained following a succinate-dehydrogenase (SDH) histochemical reaction. Highly-stained parenchymal areas are identified as periportal and septal (acinar zone 1) hepatocytes; low-stained areas correspond to perivenous (acinar zone 3) hepatocytes. PV = portal venule; THV = terminal hepatic venule.

TABLE 1
Assessment of the Lectin-Binding Pattern of Different Microvascular Segments

Labeling pattern groups	Hepatic section incubation						Intraportal liver perfusion					
		Microvascular segment						Microvascular segment				
	Lectin	PV	CV	PS	SS	CS	Lectin	PV	CV	PS	SS	CS
I	CON-A[b]	2	2	2	2	2	CON-A[b]	2	2	2	2	2
	RCA60	2	2	2	2	2						
II	WGA[b]	3	1	3	3	1	WGA[b]	3	0	3	3	0
							RCA60	3	0	3	2	0
	PHA-E[b]	3	2	2	2	1	PHA-E[b]	3	2	2	2	0
	ECA	3	2	3	3	1	ECA	2	0	2	2	0
	LOA	3	2	3	1	0						
	PSA	2	2	2	0	0	PSA	2	0	2	2	0
	BSI-A4	3	1	3	1	1						
	WA	2	1	2	1	0						
III	MPA	0	0	2	2	0	LOA	1	1	3	3	0
							PHA-P	1	1	3	3	0
IV	DBA,SBA,WFA,SJA,CAA,HAA,PNA,BPA, UEA-I,LTA						DBA,WA,SBA,WFA,SJA,MPA,CAA, HAA,PNA,BPA,UEA-I,LTA					

Note: I: equal binding in all segments; II: different affinities depending on acinar zone; III: preferential binding to the sinusoidal network; IV: negative binding to the hepatic microvasculature. Results are expressed as intensity of fluorescence microscopy labeling (0: negative; 1: low; 2: moderate; 3: intense).

Concanavalin A (CON-A); Pisum sativum (PSA); Lathyrus odoratus (LOA); Wheat germ agglutinin (WGA); Dolichos biflorus (DBA); Vicia villosa (WA); Soybean (SBA); Wisteria floribunda (WFA); Sophora japonica (SJA); Maclura pomifera (MPA); Caragana arborescens (CAA); Griffonia simplicifolia ($BSI\text{-}A_4$); Helix aspersa (HAA); Peanut (PNA); Bauhinia purpurea (BPA); Ricinus communis toxin (RCA_{60}); Ulex europaeus (UEA-I); tetragonolobus purpureus (LTA); erythrina cristagalli (ECA); phaseolus vulgaris (PHA-P and PHA-E).

[a] From liver tissue labeled by *in situ* intraportal perfusion or *in vitro* incubation of cryostat sections with different FITC-lectins.

[b] Concordant lectins when comparing their lectin-binding patterns obtained by the incubation or perfusion procedures.

Zones 1 and 3 can be easily distinguished in hepatic sections, but zone 2 remains poorly defined. Using immunohistochemical analysis for revealing the presence of carbamoyl-phosphate synthetase, it has been shown that staining is most intense in the hepatocytes around PV and decreases towards THV.[29] This way of distinguishing the tissue heterogeneity is sufficient to identify tissue position qualitatively. Moreover, it has proved possible to demonstrate that for certain enzymes such as glucose-6-phosphatase and lactate dehydrogenase, there is a gradual decrease in activity along the radial lines going from the PV and septa to the THV.[30,31] Although these straight lines drawn from the PV to the THV are not the true pathways of the sinusoids, it is legitimate to use them as the theoretical pathway of the radial sinusoids. We use an enzymatic histochemical reaction to reveal SDH activity, followed by microspectrophotometric measurement of the intensity of the activity along the lines drawn from the PV to the THV (Figure 10). This enables us to estimate on a scale of 0 to 10, the relative position between the two vessels of any point of the parenchyma by measuring the intensity of the SDH activity and interpolating it in the function.[19] This method affords precise measurement of the relative position along the PV-THV pathway of the

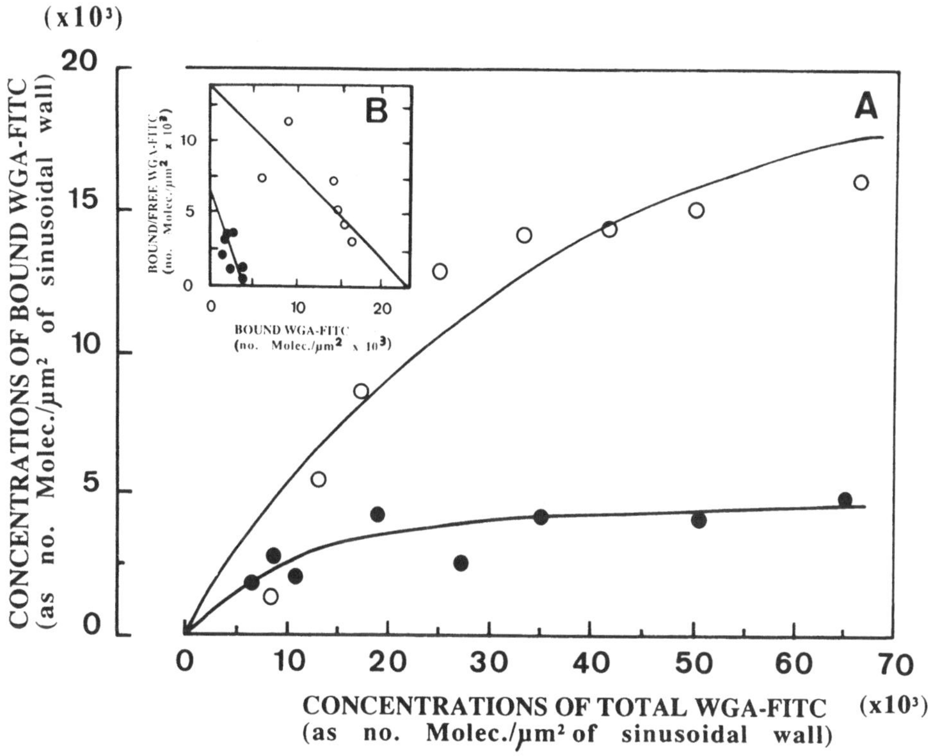

FIGURE 7. Comparison of specific binding of various concentrations of FITC-WGA lectin to the acinar zone 1 (○) and 3 (●) sinusoidal segments of liver tissue as resolved by *in situ* cytofluorimetry. Values express concentrations ± SD of bound FITC-WGA (as number of molecules/µm² in the sinusoidal wall). A = saturation curves of WGA-binding sites in zone 1 and zone 3 sinusoidal walls; B = Scatchard plot of the data from A. The WGA-binding site concentration, calculated from the intercept of the abscissa, indicates 22.5 × 10³ molecules/µm² for zone 1 sinusoids and 4.32 × 10³ molecules/µm² for zone 3 sinusoids.

normal and metastic tumor cells[32] and of the hemopoietic foci[33,34] without being affected by the distorted image of the hepatic lobules.

III. ARRIVAL, ARREST, AND CLEARANCE OF TUMOR CELLS IN THE HEPATIC MICROVASCULATURE

Most experiments done to examine the arrest of tumor cells in organs have been based on the introduction of radiolabeled cells. The results obtained demonstrate the number of cells retained in each organ and clearance times. It has generally been concluded that tumor cells tend to lodge in the first organ they reach following injection (arterial, venous, or lymphatic) and that later disappearance from the organ occurs at a very poorly defined rate.[6-8,35] Other studies using injection of fluorochrome-labeled tumor cells, followed by microscopic examination of the cells' progress, have produced different data on their retention and clearance in the liver.[6,39,40] In some studies, hepatic metastasis has been associated with the invasion of the connective tissue of the portal spaces. The tumor cells reaching the liver through the portal vein are arrested mostly in the sinusoidal stretch closest to the portal vein.[41,42] This arrest occurs even in sinusoids whose diameter is much greater than that of the tumor cells, due to a possible tumor cell-endothelial cell contact mechanism in which neither platelets nor leukocytes are involved.[6] Certain types of tumor cells have been described as establishing contact with and projecting cytoplasmic processes through the endothelial cells, even passing through to the Disse space.[42] Most studies coincide in observing

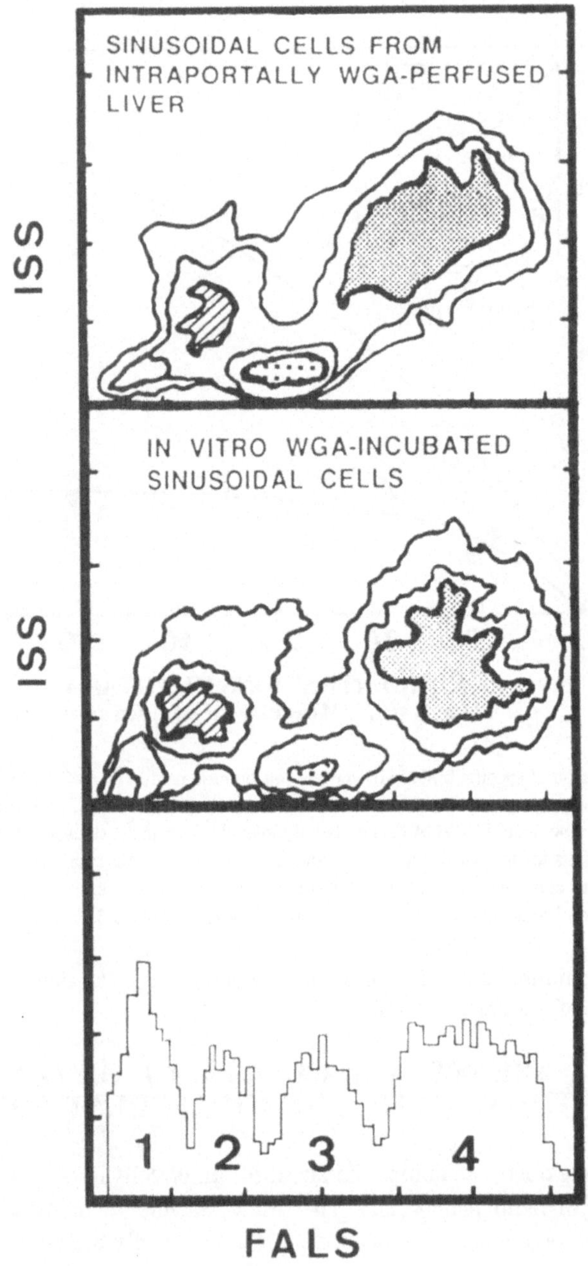

FIGURE 8. Flow cytometric analysis of isolated liver sinusoidal cells. Two-parameter slice plots of the forward (FALS) vs. the integrated side (ISS) light scatter of sinusoidal cell populations obtained from intraportally FITC-WGA-perfused livers and from non-WGA perfused livers *in vitro* incubated with FITC-WGA. FALS distribution of identified sinusoidal cell types: 1 = lymphoid and large vessel endothelial cells; 2 = type I sinusoidal endothelial cell; 3 = type II sinusoidal endothelial cell; and 4 = Kupffer cells.

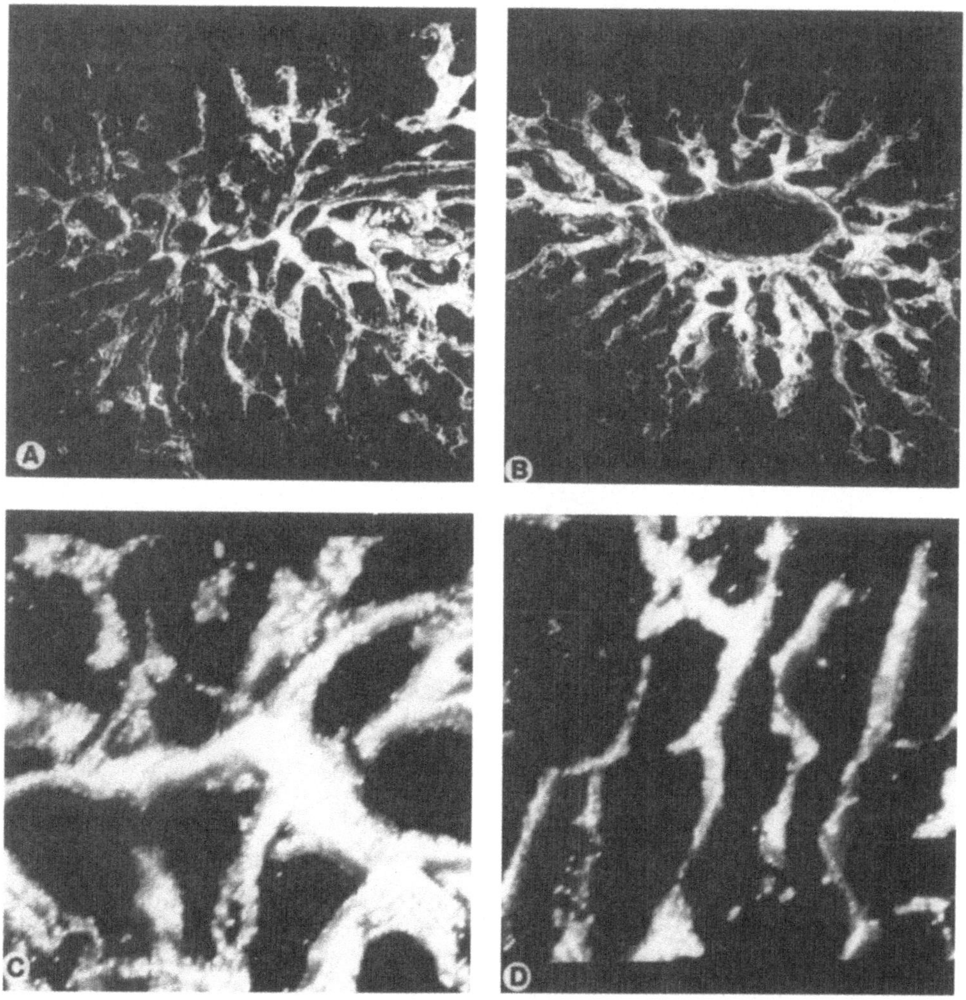

FIGURE 9. Confocal microscopic images of the liver microvasculature: (A) terminal portal venules and its surrounding sinusoidal network and (B) terminal hepatic venule and their converging sinusoidal segments. High-resolution images of (C) interconnecting sinusoidal segments in the acinar zone 1 and of (D) most parallel sinusoidal segments in the acinar zone 3.

that tumor cells do not stop in the large and medium-sized vessels, except when they form thrombi. Instead, their arrest occurs individually in the sinusoids.[6,41,42] Some studies have reported observations on injected cells as late as 30 d following injection.[39] But the cells that remain are so few and the methods for labeling them so fragile that it is difficult to carry out quantitative studies.

Bromodeoxy-uridine (BrdUrd)-labeled injected cells may be detected by means of MoAb against BrdUrd sequences — no matter where they are located in the liver[32] (Figure 11). Using this technique, it has been shown that large numbers of tumor cells become trapped in the liver following injection and that most of these cells are destroyed during the first hour[43] (Table 2). In addition, the number of cells destroyed during this first period depends on the type of tumor. A small number of cells stay in the liver where they remain for at least 72 h, although according to a mathematical simulation calculation, it appears likely that they could remain there for more than 20 d if they do not proliferate.[43]

Another detailed study on the position of tumor cells arrested in the liver showed that

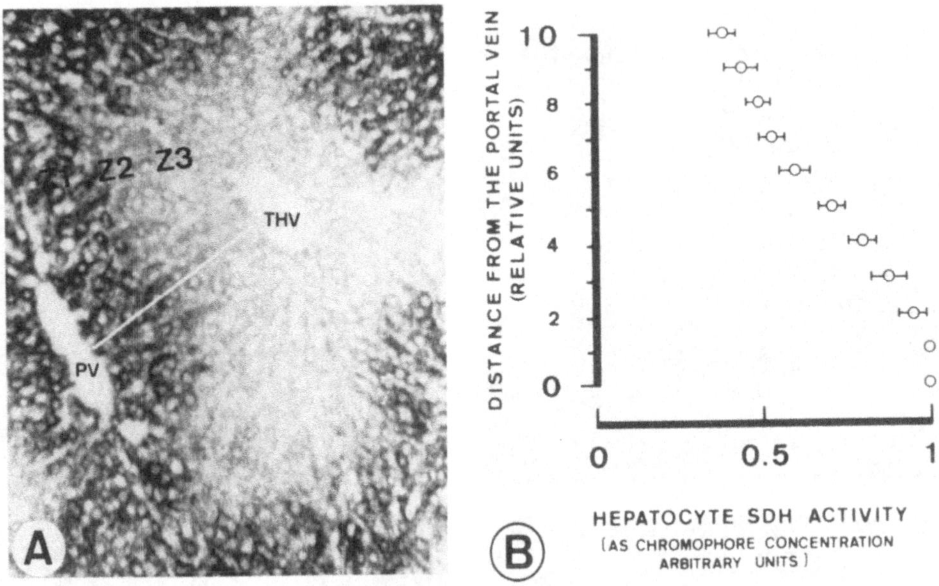

FIGURE 10. (A): Digitalized image of a liver tissue field following a SDH histochemical reaction. Zones of the liver acinus as described by Rappaport:[5] Zone 1 (Z1), zone 2 (Z2), and zone 3 (Z3). For microspectrophotometric measurement of chromophore concentration in the cytoplasm of hepatocytes, imaginary lines that run from the portal (PV) to the terminal hepatic venules (THV) are drawn. (B): Acinar gradient curve of hepatocyte SDH activity calculated from recording of this enzyme activity on the imaginary lines drawn from the PV-to-THV distance and its correlation with the position on the sinusoidal pathway from the PV to the THV.

these cells are retained along the entire sinusoidal pathway, although their number is greater in the stretch near the PV. Using the same simulation study mentioned earlier, it was possible to demonstrate that the time the tumor cells remain in zone 1 is approximately six times higher than that in the sinusoidal segments near the centrilobular vessels. Stated in another way, tumor cells abandon zone 3 sinusoids six times more quickly than zone 1. This then helps to explain the apparent concentration of tumor cells in zone 1 and the reason why most of the relations between tumor cells and the cells in the hepatic environment occur in zone 1[43] (Table 2).

The greater retention of tumor cells in zone 1 can be explained in various ways: (a) by the higher degree of anastomosis in this area of the sinusoids,[3,5] (b) by the greater presence of Kupffer cells, which might act as sinusoidal sphincters,[3,11,12,44] (c) by the lower pressure and sinusoidal flow in this stretch,[5,45] and (d) by the existence of a specific type of endothelial cell whose surface has a much higher concentration of carbohydrate residues, giving the zone greater adhesiveness.[25] And of course, the opposite reasons can be used to justify the swifter passage of the tumor cells through the sinusoids in zone 3.

The participation of endothelial cells in the longer retention of tumor cells in zone 1 can be substantiated through numerous studies showing that tumor cell-endothelial cell adhesion[46-49] depends on certain molecules that not only give the endothelial lining in each organ its particular characteristics,[50,51] but also, in reactive states, increase the adhesiveness of the endothelium for tumor cells under the influence of molecules such as IL-1.[52] This hypothesis is rendered more plausible by the fact that various experiments have related metastatic organ affinity to the type of endothelial cell in the target organ.[48,51] It is in fact possible to establish a hypothetical relation between the special type of endothelial cell occupying the sinusoidal segments in zone 1[25] and the arrest of tumor cells. This phenomenon is theoretically comparable to the homing of lymphocytes in the postcapillary venules of the

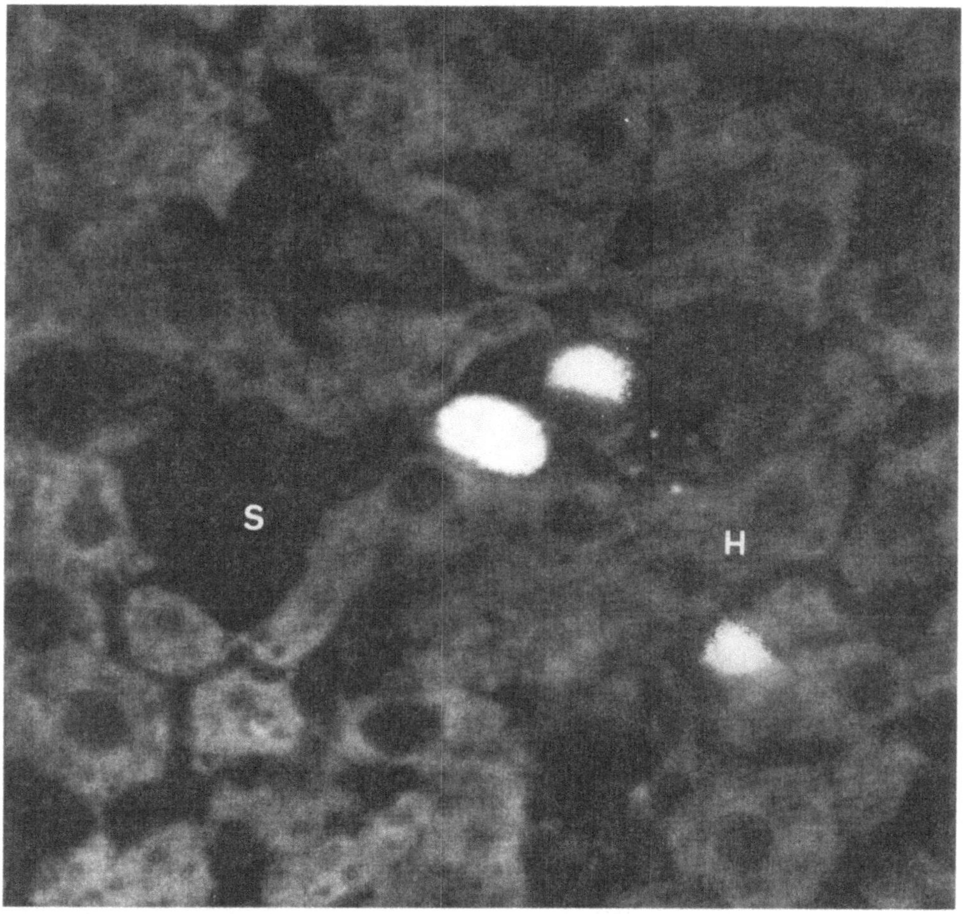

FIGURE 11. Confocal microscopic image showing an isolated tumor cell (highly fluorescent cell) arrested within the sinusoidal lumen (S) of the hepatic microvasculature from an intrasplenically tumor cell-injected mouse, which was sacrified 2 h later. The arrested tumor cell closely contacts the endothelial cells that are lining the sinusoidal wall between the hepatocytes (H).

lymph node.[53,54] Further strengthening of the hypothesis comes from the fact that in the liver, the sinusoidal zone where the largest number of tumor cells stop,[32,43] is also the place where hemopoietic colony-forming cells stop and proliferate,[33,34] thus, sharing the same physical space with the metastatic cells (Figure 5).

The large number of tumor cells destroyed on their journey through the sinusoids succumb mostly in the zone 1 sinusoidal segments. The destruction of tumor cells in the sinusoidal pathway may be conditioned by three factors commonly recognized as responsible for metastatic inefficiency: (1) the mechanical effect of having to pass through vessels measuring 5 μm,[54] (2) the aggression on the part of Kupffer,[27] and (3) the Pit cells in the liver.[13,55] Using BrdUrd-labeled tumor cells, we have shown that Kupffer cells retain nuclear fragments of the tumor cells during the first 6 h postinoculation[43] (Figure 12). This observation indicates either the participation of Kupffer cells in eliminating cancer cells or in endocytosing their fragments. But the fact that the mass destruction of tumor cells occurs in the first hour suggests a mechanism involving superoxide anions[56] and/or mechanical destruction[54] as the most probable, albeit nonspecific, mechanism of cancer cell destruction. Our results also suggest the participation of T-lymphocytes, Pit and/or Kupffer cells in the elimination of tumor cells since the cyclosporin A-induced inhibition on host cell responsiveness correlates with the increase in the seeding of tumor cells in the liver.[57]

TABLE 2
Assessment of the Initial Intrahepatic Arrest of Intrasplenically-Injected BrdUrd-Labeled B16F10 Tumor Cells and Their Intra-Acinar Distribution[a]

		Intra-acinar distribution	
Time post-injection	Total no.[b](%)[c]	Zone 1[b,c](%)[d]	Zone 3[b,c](%)[d]
5 min	5.12 ± 2.13 (100%)	5.12 (100%)	0 (0%)
30 min	2.68 ± 0.81 (52.3%)	2.63 (98.2%)	0.05 (1.6%)
1 h	0.56 ± 0.12 (10.9%)	0.49 (88.7%)	0.07 (11.9%)
2 h	0.36 ± 0.13 (7.0%)	0.33 (93.9%)	0.03 (6.1%)
6 h	0.41 ± 0.10 (8.0%)	0.39 (95.3%)	0.02 (4.6%)
24 h	0.18 ± 0.00 (3.5%)	0.15 (85.2%)	0.03 (15.2%)

[a] According to the two major microcirculatory domains of the sinusoidal network.
[b] As the number of arrested tumor cells per mm^2 of liver tissue (10 μ thick).
[c] Percentage of the total number of arrested cells.
[d] All the values were statistically significant ($p < 0.01$) between the partial cell arrests in zone 1 vs. zone 3.

In experiments involving the collection of cancer cells from the hepatic vein as they are injected through the portal vein, we have shown that virtually none pass directly through the liver.[13] Thus, the cells which, according to other experiments, appeared capable of metastasizing other organs beyond the liver must come from previous hepatic metastases.[58] No clear answer has been given as to how the tumor cells trapped for 60 h in the hepatic sinusoids manage to remain alive. They are most probably cells that are especially adapted to the conditions of the organ[59,60] or that have certain particular functional properties such as endowment with the adhesion molecules, enabling them to remain anchored to the endothelium or to its subendothelial matrix.[61,62,63]

Cancer cells undergoing DNA synthesis may be detected by injecting animals with BrdUrd and using fluorescence-conjugated anti-BrdUrd MoAb on histological sections taken from organs where the cells have lodged. Using this method, we have shown that during the first 50 to 60 h following injection and the arrest of the tumor cells in the sinusoids, none undergo synthesis.[43] It is only after the first 60 h that the onset of a nearly synchronous replication of all the arrested tumor cells occur. This DNA replication takes place mostly in zone 1, although it is also possible to find some tumor cells undergoing DNA-synthesis in the zone 3 sinusoidal segments between 80 and 90 h post-injection.[43] This period of silence and the synchronous activation of the cancer cells may well indicate that the organ must either produce cell growth-regulating humoral factors or alternate some very strict selection of a subpopulation of tumor cells, whose distinguishing feature is that they are undergoing a specific phase of the cell cycle at the moment of arrest. In this regard, the factors inducing synthesis could originate in the sinusoidal cells themselves.[64] For example, melanoma B16 tumor cells are activated by IL-2,[65] and other experiments indicate a possible relationship between cancer cell and sinusoidal cell activation.

When spleen cells are delivered to the liver following intrasplenic injection of medium, they are retained in the sinusoids, and proliferation of these intrasinusoidal cells occurs after 60 h. Although it is difficult to distinguish those proliferating cells that come from the spleen between those that come from the liver, the important point in the present context is that they all begin proliferating simultaneously at 60 h, thus, coinciding with the proliferation

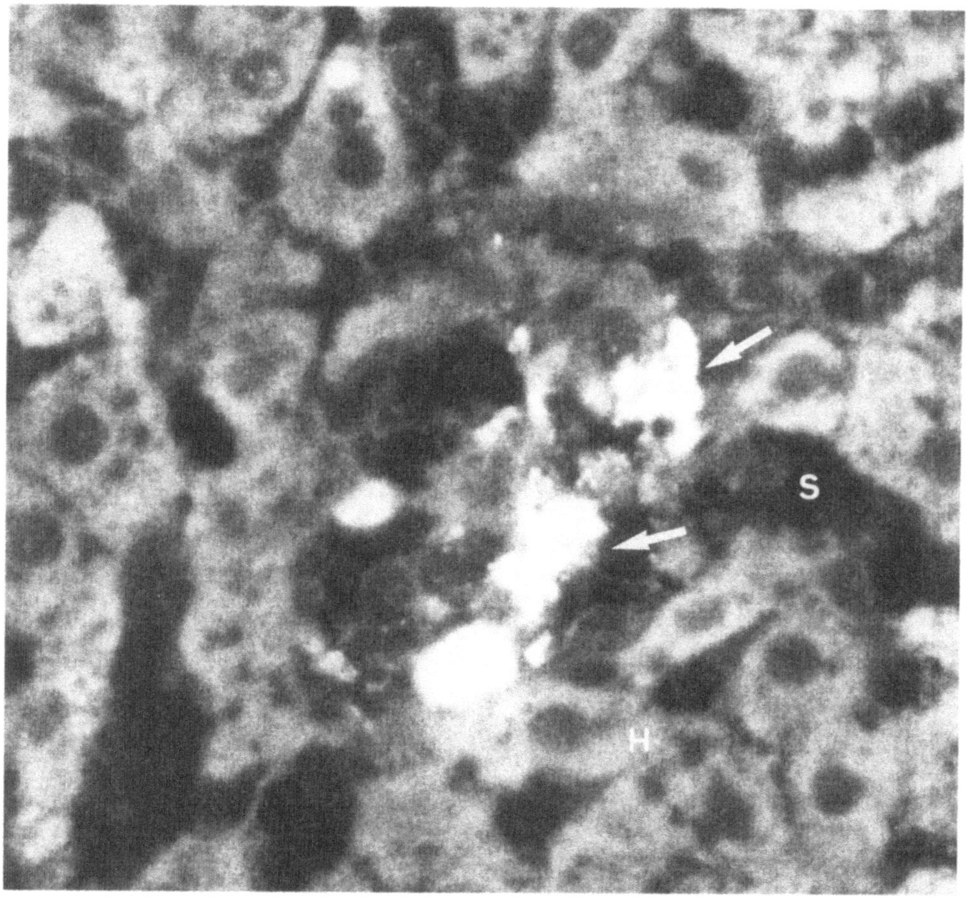

FIGURE 12. Confocal microscopic image showing the intrasinusoidal tumor cell destruction 6 h postinjection of BrdUrd-labeled tumor cells (highly fluorescent cells). Fragments of labeled tumor cell nuclei (arrows) are taken up by Kupffer cells. S = sinusoidal lumen; H = hepatocytes.

of cancer cells (Figure 13). The proliferation of intrasinusoidal cancer cells follows the same patterns, regardless of the type of tumor (melanoma B16, Lewis lung carcinoma, M5076 reticulosarcoma). This, together with the fact that arrest and proliferation occur synchronously, lead us to think that there are noncancer cell-specific mechanisms participating in the regulation of hepatic metastasis.[33,34]

IV. SPECIFIC LOCATION OF HEPATIC METASTASIS

Nearly all observations coincide in locating the site of hepatic metastasis as near the vessels,[7,32,41] especially those of the portal zone.[62] The most detailed studies on the early development of metastasis have demonstrated that metastatic foci in the liver develop as intrasinusoidal strings of cells, whose location in the sinusoid becomes impossible to pinpoint as the colony spreads and adopts its characteristic structure.[36] Detailed studies of incipient metastatic microfoci (colonies of 10 to 20 cells) revealed that hepatic metastasis originates inside the sinusoids with the lodging of cancer cells in the second quarter of the radial sinusoidal pathway going from the PV to the THV.[32,34] This position has been confirmed for various experimental tumors with metastatic affinity for the liver such as reticulum cell sarcoma M5076 in the mouse or rhabdomyosarcoma S4MH in the rat, as well as tumor lines, such as B16 melanoma and 3LL carcinoma that do not spontaneously develop liver

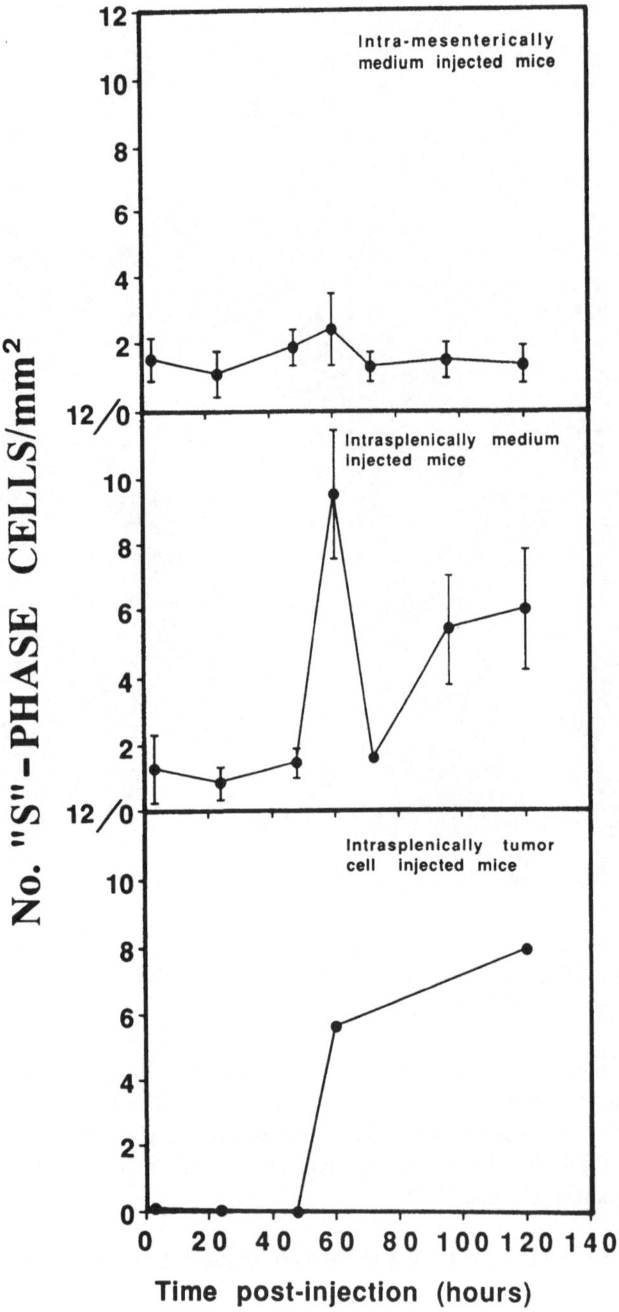

FIGURE 13. Assessment of the S-phase cell population in the liver sinusoidal compartment of normal and tumor cell injected mice. Following the intra-mesenteric vein injection of a balanced salt solution, the normal rate of sinusoidal S-phase cells was determined. The intrasplenic injection of the same solution allows to obtain the number of S-phase cells in hepatic sinusoids containing delivered splenic cells. Following the intrasplenic injection of tumor cells, the temporal profile of S-phase activation in the tumor cell population arrested in liver sinusoids was determined.

TABLE 3
Hepatocyte SDH-Activity Around Hepatic Tumors and Phenylhydrazine-Induced Hematopoietic Foci and Relative Positions of Foci (D.F.P.V.) Within the Liver Acini of C57BL/6 Mice

Hepatic foci	Average SDH activity[a]	D.F.P.V.[b] Average value	Range
B16 melanoma (F1)	0.80 ± 0.18	3.97	(3.48—4.49)
B16 melanoma (F10)	0.89 ± 0.23	2.86	(2.44—3.39)
LLC (Parent)	0.88 ± 0.19	3.00	(2.56—3.53)
LLC (MH10)	0.85 ± 0.21	3.39	(2.91—3.92)
RMS (S4MH)	0.90 ± 0.19	2.73	(2.31—3.23)
M5076 reticulum cell sarcoma metastasis (s.c. injection)	0.86 ± 0.22	3.00	(2.50—3.50)
M5076 reticulum cell sarcoma metastasis (i.s. injection)	0.84 ± 0.21	3.50	(3.00—4.00)
PHZ-induced hematopoietic foci	0.83 ± 0.24	3.30	(2.80—3.80)

[a] Succinate dehydrogenase activity is expressed as Relative Optical Density Units (R.O.D.U.).
[b] D.F.P.V. express the Distance From the Portal Vein, which was obtained by interpolating the peri-focal, average hepatocyte SDH-activity values.

TABLE 4
Hepatocyte Succinate Dehydrogenase (SDH) Activity Around B16F10 Micrometastatic Foci and Their Relative Position Within the Liver Acini of Treated Mice

Tumor cell type	Average SDH activity[a]	D.F.P.V.[b] Average value	Range
Control mice	0.89 ± 0.23	2.87	(2.44—3.39)
Partially hepatectomized	0.88 ± 0.24	3.00	(2.56—3.53)
17αEE-treated	0.80 ± 0.19	3.97	(3.48—4.49)
CCl_4-treated	0.81 ± 0.20	3.86	(3.37—4.38)

[a] SDH activity is expressed as Relative Optical Density Units (R.O.D.U.) ± S.D. The number of samples per experimental group was higher than 100.
[b] D.F.P.V. express the Distance From the Portal Vein, which was obtained by interpolating peri-metastatic hepatocyte average SDH-activity values in the corresponding equation.

metastases, but that only produce colonies experimentally following cell injection through the portal vein[32,34] (Table 3). The location of all metastases has proved to be so stable that even in experiments altering the zonal organization of the liver, the position remains the same. Specifically, changing the speed of flow and intrasinusoidal pressure through partial hepatectomy, dilating the sinusoidal diameter in the periportal segments by more than 10 μm by administering high doses of 17-α-ethynyl-estradiol, enriching the subendothelial laminina in zone 3 sinusoidal segments with severe intoxication of carbon tetrachloride, and depleting zone 1 of Kupffer cells causing them to concentrate in zone 3 through carbon tetrachloride intoxication were all unable to alter the arrest and proliferation site of the metastatic foci[32] (Table 4).

The organ affinity described repetitively for over a hundred years[66] now has been related to the topology of endothelial cells specific to each organ[46,47,48] and associated with the specific regional distribution of liver tissue metastases.[32] Indeed, although some tumor cells do proliferate in zone 3 of the sinusoids, no metastases ever appear in this zone. Metastasis

TABLE 5
Assessment of Hepatic Colonization from Intrasplenic B16F10 Melanoma, Lewis Lung Carcinoma, or M5076 Reticulum Cell Sarcoma Cells in Phenylhydrazine-Treated and Control Mice

Experimental groups	Metastasis density (No. foci/mm^3)	Metastasis area (μm^2)	Metastasis volume (as % liver volume)	Focal growth index[a] (mm^3/d)
B16 melanoma/controls	15.43 ± 6.81	4843 ± 456	11.93 ± 6.28	1.28 ± 0.71
B16 melanoma/phenylhydrazine-treated	18.62 ± 7.54	22140 ± 1153[b]	25.60 ± 12.60[b]	4.00 ± 0.8[b]
3LL/controls	2.73 ± 1.27	1980 ± 259	0.37 ± 0.27	0.15 ± 0.08
3LL/phenylhydrazine-treated	3.45 ± 0.83	5366 ± 977[b]	0.77 ± 0.21[b]	0.36 ± 0.1[b]
M5076 reticulum cell sarcoma/controls	29.74 ± 8.83	3750 ± 280	0.46 ± 0.16	0.21 ± 0.14
M5076 reticulum cell sarcoma/phenylhydrazine-treated	67.08 ± 21.44[b]	2782 ± 151[b]	0.59 ± 0.3	0.11 ± 0.02

Note: Data are expressed as mean values ± S.D. in at least ten mice per experimental group (five liver sections per mouse).

[a] Focal growth index: $\frac{\text{Metastasis volume/Metastasis density}}{\text{Days after cancer cell injection}}$

[b] Statistically significant ($p<0.05$) differences between PHZ-treated and control mice.

always occupies a position in the second quarter of the hepatic sinusoidal pathway; this position does not change with alteration of the hemodynamics of the hepatic acinus, the distribution of Kupffer cells, or the diameter of the sinusoidal lumen. By default, this suggests that the intrahepatic distribution of metastases is related to the characteristics of the endothelial cells in zone 1.[32]

The proliferation-induction property of zone 1 of the sinusoids has been observed not only with metastatic foci, but also with hemopoietic foci (Figure 5).[33,34] When hemopoietic and metastatic activity occur simultaneously in the liver tissue, interaction between the two proliferative processes has been demonstrated following tumor cell inoculation in phenylhydrazine-treated mice. In these cases, while hemopoietic colony proliferation is occurring in zone 1, metastases grow in the same site, although more quickly than in controls lacking hemopoietic production[34] (Table 5).

In summary, the liver is an organ having marked zonal differences related to its microvascular structure.[5,16,17] Sinusoidal cells having different functional phenotypes co-exist and interrelate with each other since they share common hormonal, metabolic, and immunological processes.[67] More specifically, within the hepatic sinusoid, there are two clearly defined zones that can be distinguished morphologically,[19] although the more important distinction is the different types of endothelial cells lining their walls,[25,68] together with the subsets of other sinusoidal cells they contain.[11-14,67] That is, in zone 1, we find the necessary circumstances, enabling colony-forming cells to initiate hemopoietic cell proliferation in the case of the arrest of blood-progenitor cells[33] or proliferation of cancer cells in the case of metastatic cell implantation.[32] We conclude that the characteristics of zone 1, which favor hepatic metastasis, also could represent more general regulatory mechanisms involved in physiological cell proliferation in this segment of the hepatic sinusoid and therefore, would not be specific for the process of metastasis.[34]

REFERENCES

1. **Wisse, E., De Wilde, A., and De Zanger, R.,** Perfusion fixation of human and rat liver tissue for light and electron microscopy: a review and assessment of existing methods with special emphasis on sinusoidal cells and microcirculation, in *Science of Biological Specimen Preparation,* SEM, AMF O'Hare, Chicago, 1984, 31.
2. **Teutsch, H.,** Regionality of glucose-6-phosphate hydrolysis in the liver lobule of the rat: metabolic heterogeneity of "portal" and "septal" sinusoids, *Hepatology,* 8, 311, 1988.
3. **McCuskey, R. S.,** The hepatic microvascular system: microcirculation, in *The Alimentary Tract,* Koo, A., Lam, S. K., and Smaje, L. H., Eds., World Scientific Publishing, Singapore, 1983, 57.
4. **Campra, J. L. and Reynolds, T. B.,** The hepatic circulation, in *The Liver: Biology and Pathobiology,* Arias, I., Popper, H., Schachter, D., and Shafritz, D. A., Eds., Raven Press, New York, 1982, chap. 37.
5. **Rappaport, A. M.,** The microcirculatory unit, *Microvasc. Res.,* 6, 212, 1973.
6. **Bagge, U., Skolnik, G., and Ericson, L. E.,** The arrest of circulating tumor cells in the liver microcirculation, *J. Cancer Res. Clin. Oncol.,* 105, 134, 1983.
7. **Vidal-Vanaclocha, F., Alonso-Varona, A., Ayala, R., and Barberá-Guillem, E.,** Functional variations in liver tissue during the implantation process of metastatic tumor cells, *Virchows Arch. A. Pathol. Anat.,* 416, 189, 1990.
8. **Vidal-Vanaclocha, F. and Barberá-Guillem, E.,** Fenestration patterns in endothelial cells of rat liver sinusoids, *J. Ultrastruct. Res.,* 90, 115, 1985.
9. **Wisse, E., De Zanger, R. B., Charels, K., Van Der Smissen, P., and McCuskey, R. S.,** The liver sieve: considerations concerning the structure and function of endothelial fenestrae, the sinusoidal wall and the space of Disse, *Hepatology,* 5, 683, 1985.
10. **Ghitescu, L. and Fixman, A.,** Surface charge distribution on the endothelial cell of liver sinusoids, *J. Cell Biol.,* 99, 639, 1984.
11. **Wake, K., Decker, K., Kirn, A., Knook, D. L., McCuskey, R. S., Bouwens, L., and Wisse, E.,** Cell biology and kinetics of Kupffer cells in the liver, *Int. Rev. Cytol.,* 118, 173, 1989.
12. **Bouwens, L., Baeckeland, M., De Zanger, R., and Wisse, E.,** Quantitation, tissue distribution and proliferation kinetics of Kupffer cells in normal rat liver, *Hepatology,* 6, 718, 1986.
13. **Geerts, A., Bouwens, L., and Wisse, E.,** Ultrastructure and function of hepatic fat-storing and Pit cells, *J. Electron Microsc. Tech.,* 14, 247, 1990.
14. **Freudenberg, N., Schalk, J., Galanos, C., Katschinski, T., Datz, O., Pein, U., and Freduedenberg, M. A.,** Identification and percentage frequency of isolated non-parenchymal liver cells (NPLC) in the mouse, *Virchows Arch. B. Cell Pathol.,* 57, 109, 1989.
15. **Bissel, D. M., Friedman, S. L., Maher, J. J., and Roll, F. J.,** Connective tissue biology and hepatic fibrosis, *Hepatology,* 11, 488, 1990.
16. **Gumucico, J. J.,** Hepatocyte heterogeneity: the coming of age from the description of a biological curiosity to a partial understanding of its physiological meaning and regulation, *Hepatology,* 9, 154, 1989.
17. **Jungermann, K.,** Metabolic zonation of liver parenchyma, *Semin. Liver Dis.,* 8, 329, 1988.
18. **Lamers, W. H., Hilberts, A., Furt, E., Smith, J., Jonges, G. N., van Noorden, C. J. F., Janzen, J. W. G., Charles, R., and Moorman, A. F. M.,** Hepatic enzyme zonation: a reevaluation of the concept of the liver acinus, *Hepatology,* 10, 72, 1989.
19. **Barberá-Guillem, E., Alonso-Varona, A., Boyano, M. D., and Vidal-Vanaclocha, F.,** Estimating anatomical-functional position coordinates in liver tissue, *Anat. Rec.,* 228, 267, 1990.
20. **Barberá-Guillem, E., Arrue, J. M., Ballesteros, J., and Vidal-Vanaclocha, F.,** Structural changes in endothelial cells of developing rat liver in the transition from fetal to postnatal life, *J. Ultrastruct. Res.,* 97, 197, 1986.
21. **Barberá-Guillem, E. and Vidal-Vanaclocha, F.,** Structural and functional interrelationships between hepatocytes and sinusoidal endothelium in the maturing process of rat liver, in *Progress in Developmental Biology,* Part A, Slavkin, H. C., Ed., Alan R. Liss, New York, 1986, 325.
22. **Barberá-Guillem, E., Ayala, R., and Vidal-Vanaclocha, F.,** Coincident position of large endothelial fenestrae and residual hemopoietic colonies in the centrilobular domain of postnatal rat liver acini, in *Cells of the Hepatic Sinusoid,* Vol. 2, Wisse, E., Knook, D. L., and Decker, K., Eds., Kupffer Cell Foundation, Rijswijk, 1989, 423.
23. **Dan, C. and Wake, K.,** Modes of endocytosis of latex particles in sinusoidal endothelial and Kupffer cells of normal and perfused rat liver, *Exp. Cell Res.,* 158, 75, 1985.
24. **Steffan, A. M., Gendrault, J.-L., McCuskey, R. S., McCuskey, P. A., and Kirn, A.,** Phagocytosis, an unrecognized property of murine endothelial liver cells, *Hepatology,* 6, 830, 1986.
25. **Barberá-Guillem, E., Rocha, M. A., Alvarez, A., and Vidal-Vanaclocha, F.,** Differences in the lectin-binding patterns of periportal and perivenous endothelial domains in the liver sinusoids, *Hepatology,* in press.

26. **Rocha, M. A.,** Identification of two different functional subsets of endothelial cells in the sinusoids of mouse liver, Doctoral thesis, University of the Basque Country, Leioa, Vizcaya, Spain, 1990.
27. **Philips, N. C.,** Kupffer cells and liver metastasis, *Cancer Metastasis Rev.*, 8, 231, 1989.
28. **Barberá-Guillem, E., Alonso-Varona, A., and Vidal-Vanaclocha, F.,** Acinar re-distribution of Kupffer cells concomitant to the implantation and focal growth in rat liver of metastatic rhabdemyosarcoma cells, in *Cells of the Hepatic Sinusoid,* Vol. 2, Wisse, E., Knook, D. L., and Decker, K., Eds., Kupffer Cell Foundation, Rijswijk, 1989, 421.
29. **Moorman, A. F. M., Vermeulen, J. L. M., Charles, R., and Lamers, W. H.,** Localization of ammonia-metabolizing enzymes in human liver: ontogenesis of heterogeneity, *Hepatology,* 9, 387, 1989.
30. **Hildebrand, R. and Schleicher, A.,** Image analysis of histochemical demonstration of glucose-6-phosphatase activity in rat liver, *Histochemistry,* 86, 181, 1986.
31. **Ebert, S., Hildebrand, R., and Haubitz, I.,** Sinusoidal profiles of lactate dehydrogenase activity in rat liver, *Histochemistry,* 87, 371, 1987.
32. **Barberá-Guillem, E., Alonso-Varona, A., and Vidal-Vanaclocha, F.,** Selective implantation and growth in rats and mice of experimental liver metastasis in acinar zone one, *Cancer Res.*, 49, 4003, 1989.
33. **Barberá-Guillem, E., Ayala, R., and Vidal-Vanaclocha, F.,** Differential location of hemopoietic colonies within liver acini of postnatal and phenylhydrazine-treated adult mice, *Hepatology,* 9, 29, 1989.
34. **Barberá-Guillem, E., Alonso-Varona, A., Ayala, R., Boyano, M. D., and Vidal-Vanaclocha, F.,** Coincident implantation, growth and interaction sites within the liver of cancer and reactive hematopoietic cells, *Int. J. Cancer,* 46, 267, 1990.
35. **Fidler, I. J.,** Metastasis: quantitative analysis of distribution and fate of tumor emboli labeled with 125-I-5iodo-2'deoxyuridine, *J. Natl. Cancer Inst.*, 45, 773, 1970.
36. **Hart, I. R., Talmadge, J. E., and Fidler, I. J.,** Metastatic behavior of a murine reticulum cell sarcoma exhibiting organ-specific growth, *Cancer Res.*, 41, 1281, 1981.
37. **Weiss, L., Ward, P. M., Harlos, J. P., and Holmes, J. C.,** Target organ patterns of tumors in mice following the arterial dissemination of B16 melanoma cells, *Int. J. Cancer,* 33, 825, 1984.
38. **Orr, F. W., Adamson, I. Y. R., and Young, L.,** Promotion of pulmonary metastasis in mice by bleomycin-induced endothelial injury, *Cancer Res.*, 46, 891, 1986.
39. **Potter, K. M., Juacaba, S. F., Price, J. E., and Tarin, D.,** Observations on organ distribution of fluorescein-labelled tumour cells released intravascularly, *Invasion Metastasis,* 3, 221, 1983.
40. **Blomqvist, G., Skolnik, G., Braide, M., Bjursten, L. M., Blixt, A., and Baggue, U.,** Differences in lodgement of tumour cells in muscle and liver, *Clin. Exp. Metastasis,* 6, 285, 1988.
41. **Roos, E., Dingemans, K. P., Van de Pavert, I. V., and Van den Bergh-Weerman, M. A.,** Mammary carcinoma cells in mouse liver: infiltration of liver tissue and interaction with Kupffer cells, *Br. J. Cancer,* 38, 74, 1978.
42. **Dingemans, K. P.,** Invasion of liver tissue by blood-borne mammary carcinoma cells, *J. Natl. Cancer Inst.*, 53, 1813, 1974.
43. **Smith-Zubiaga, I.,** Arrival, arrest and clearance of tumor cells in the mouse liver microvasculature, Doctoral thesis, University of the Basque Country, Leioa, Vizcaya, Spain, 1991.
44. **Wisse, E. and McCuskey, R. S.,** On the interaction of blood cells with the sinusoidal wall as observed by *in vivo* microscopy of rat liver, in *Cells of the Hepatic Sinusoid,* Vol. 1, Kirn, A., Knook, D. L., and Wisse, E., Eds., Kupffer Cell Foundation, Rijswijk, 1986, 477.
45. **Henriksen, J. H. and Niels, A. L.,** Pressure profile in liver sinusoids. A model of localization of sinusoidal resistance in the normal and cirrhotic liver, *Liver,* 8, 88, 1988.
46. **Pauli, B. U. and Lee, C. L.,** Organ preference of metastasis. The role of organ-specifically modulated endothelial cells, *Lab. Invest.*, 58, 379, 1988.
47. **Netland, P. A. and Zetter, B. R.,** Tumor-cell interactions with blood vessels during cancer metastasis, in *Fundamental Aspects of Cancer,* Goldfarb, R. H., Ed., Kluwer Academic Publishers, Dordrecht, The Netherlands, 1989, 84.
48. **Auerbach, R., Pardon, L. W. C., Gumkowski, F., Kaminska, G., and Kaminski, M.,** Specificity of adhesion between murine tumor cells and capillary endothelium: an *in vitro* correlate of preferential metastasis *in vivo, Cancer Res.*, 47, 1492, 1987.
49. **Azzarelli, B., Easterling, K., and Norton, J. A.,** Leukemic cell-endothelial cell interactions in leukemic cell dissemination, *Lab. Invest.*, 60, 45, 1989.
50. **Gumkowski, F., Kaminska, G., Kaminski, M., Morrisey, L. W., and Auerbach, R.,** Heterogeneity of mouse vascular endothelium. *In vitro* studies of lymphatic, large blood vessel and microvascular endothelial cells, 24 11, 1987.
51. **Belloni, P. N. and Tressler, R. J.,** Microvascular endothelial cell heterogeneity: interactions with leukocytes and tumor cells, *Cancer Metastasis Rev.*, 8, 353, 1990.
52. **Dejana, E., Bertocchi, F., Bortolami, M. C., Regonesi, A., Tonta, A., Breviario, F., and Giavazzi, R.,** Interleukin 1 promotes tumor cell adhesion to cultured human endothelial cells, *J. Clin. Invest.*, 82, 1466, 1988.

53. **Geoffroy, J. S. and Rosen, S. D.,** Demonstration that a lectin-like receptor (gp90 mel) directly mediates adhesion of lymphocytes to high endothelial venules of lymph nodes, *J. Cell Biol.*, 109, 2463, 1989.
54. **Weiss, L. and Schmid-Schoenbein, G. W.,** Biomechanical interactions of cancer cells with the microvasculature during metastasis, *Cell Biophys.*, 14, 187, 1989.
55. **Cohen, S. A., Tzung, S. P., Doerr, R. J., and Goldrosen, M. H.,** Role of asialo-GM1 positive liver cells from athymic nude or polyinosinic-polycytidylic acid-treated mice in suppressing colon-derived experimental hepatic metastasis, *Cancer Res.*, 50, 1834, 1990.
56. **Glaves, D.,** Intravascular death of disseminated cancer cells mediated by superoxide anion, *Invasion Metastasis*, 6, 101, 1986.
57. **Barberá-Guillem, E., Cañavate, M. L., Lopez de Tejada, I., and Vidal-Vanaclocha, F.,** Influence of host defenses on the hepatic colonization of B16F10 melanoma cells, *Clin. Exp. Metastasis*, 2, 153, 1988.
58. **Weiss, L., Ward, P. M., Harlos, J. P., and Holmes, J. C.,** Target organ patterns of tumors in mice following the arterial dissemination of B16 melanoma cells, *Int. J. Cancer*, 33, 825, 1984.
59. **Barberá-Guillem, E., Barceló, J. R., Urcelay, B., Alonso-Varona, A. I., and Vidal-Vanaclocha, E.,** Noncorrelation between implantation and growth of tumor cells for their final metastatic efficiency, *Invasion Metastasis*, 8, 266, 1988.
60. **Brodt, P.,** Characterization of two highly metastatic variants of the Lewis lung carcinoma with different organ specificities, *Cancer Res.*, 46, 2422, 1986.
61. **Netland, P. A. and Zetter, B. R.,** Organ-specific adhesion of metastatic tumor cells *in vitro*, *Science*, 224, 1113, 1984.
62. **Bresalier, R. S., Rockwell, R. W., Dahiya, R., Duh, C. Y., and Kim, Y. S.,** Cell surface sialoprotein alterations in metastatic murine colon cancer cell lines selected in an animal model for colon cancer metastasis, *Cancer Res.*, 50, 1299, 1990.
63. **Chung, D. C., Zetter, B. R., and Brodt, P.,** Lewis lung carcinoma variants with differing metastatic specificities adhere preferentially to different defined extracellular matrix molecules, *Invasion Metastasis*, 8, 103, 1988.
64. **Rosenbaum, J., Mavier, P., Preaux, A. M., and Dhumeaux, D.,** Demonstration of a basic fibroblast growth factor-like molecule in mouse hepatic endothelial cells, *Biochem. Biophys. Res. Commun.*, 164, 1099, 1989.
65. **Barberá-Guillem, E., Cañavate, M. L., García de Galdeano, A., Boyano, M. D.,** Interleukin-2 responsiveness of B16 melanoma cells, unpublished results.
66. **Paget, S.,** The distribution of secondary growths in cancer of the breast, *Lancet*, 1, 571, 1889.
67. **Wisse, E., Geerts, A., Bouwens, L., van Bossuyt, H., Vanderkerken, K., and van Goethem, F.,** Cells of the hepatic sinusoid *anno* 1988, in *Cells of the Hepatic Sinusoid*, Vol. 2, Wisse, E., Knook, D. L., and Decker, K., Eds., Kupffer Cell Foundation, Rijswijk, 1989, 1.
68. **Morin, O., Patry, P., and Lafleur, L.,** Heterogeneity of endothelial cells of adult rat liver as resolved by sedimentation velocity and flow cytometry, *J. Cell Physiol.*, 119, 327, 1984.

Chapter 13

THE MORPHOLOGY OF CANCER CELL ARREST AND EXTRAVASATION

John D. Crissman, Robert F. Cerra, and Fuzlul Sarkar

TABLE OF CONTENTS

I. INTRODUCTION

Mechanisms or steps in the metastasis of cancer have been heavily investigated during the past decade. Unfortunately, tumor metastases still account for the majority of significant clinical morbidity and mortality. Most metastasis evolve via lymphatic or blood vasculature, and this mechanism will be the focus of this review. The multiple steps involved in the dissemination of a malignant tumor include numerous and diverse interactions between the tumor cell and the microenvironment of the host organ. In general, for a successful metastatic focus to be formed, a tumor cell must invade the host stroma of the primary tumor and the tissue surrounding the neoplasm, penetrate into the blood or lymphatic circulation (intravasation), escape immune surveillance and mechanical trauma while in the circulation, and undergo successful arrest by interacting with endothelial cells. The latter is usually widened by induction of platelet aggregation and/or fibrin production. Subsequent retraction of the endothelium follows, allowing attachment of the arrested tumor cells to the extracellular matrix and finally, proliferation of the attached cells along the extracellular matrix and displacing the endothelial cells within the vasculature (Figure 1). The last steps involve penetration of the extracellular matrix, presumably through the excretion of proteolytic enzymes. Continued tumor cell proliferation after extravasation ultimately requires tumor-induced angiogenesis to provide nutrients for continued growth. This review will focus on the extravasation portion of the metastatic cascade and will examine in detail what happens to the tumor cell, beginning with the initial arrest of circulating tumor cells and ending with the penetration of the extracellular matrix (completion of extravasation).

Several animal models have evolved to investigate the extravasation process. Most utilize an "experimental" metastasis model in which the initial steps of the metastatic cascade, including tumor invasion, intravasation, and immune and mechanical trauma of circulating cells, are bypassed. In such experiments, a suspension of single cells derived from either a cell culture line or a dissociated solid tumor are injected either into a vein (usually the tail vein) or an artery of the animal. This model has been termed experimental metastasis to differentiate it from spontaneous occurring metastasis that transverse all steps in the metastatic cascade from "primary" tumor growth and invasion to successful extravasation. The experimental model often uses cells derived from culture that may or may not have the same capacity for arrest and extravasation as cells derived from primary tumors. Cell surface changes appear to vary with the culture phase (i.e., exponential growth phase vs. confluence, etc.), and this represents a potential source of biologic variation in the experimental metastasis model, which needs to be recognized. In addition, single cells derived from dissociated solid tumors are sensitive to the method of disaggregation. Enzymatic dissociation has the ability to alter surface molecules, which in turn may alter tumor cell-endothelial cell interactions during circulating tumor cell arrest. Thus, the source and preparation of the cell suspension either from cell culture or solid tumors remains a critical step (variable) in the development and definition of an experimental metastasis model (Table 1).

The major advantage of the experimental metastasis model is the ability to identify the various steps involved in arrest and extravasation, assuring definition of each step by sampling organs at various time intervals following the tumor cell injection. Observation of the multiple extravasation steps can be documented beginning at time intervals as short as 30 s. Since a large bolus of tumor cells is introduced into the circulation, adequate observations of the subsequent steps can be made. Conversely, spontaneous metastases models (discussed below) result in a significant, yet relatively small number of cells entering the circulation over a predictable, but wide span of time.

A "spontaneous" metastatic model also has been used in some studies in which a tumor is permitted to grow, usually in the flank of an animal, and days to weeks later, the animal is sacrificed. This more closely approximates a true, or physiologic, metastatic process since

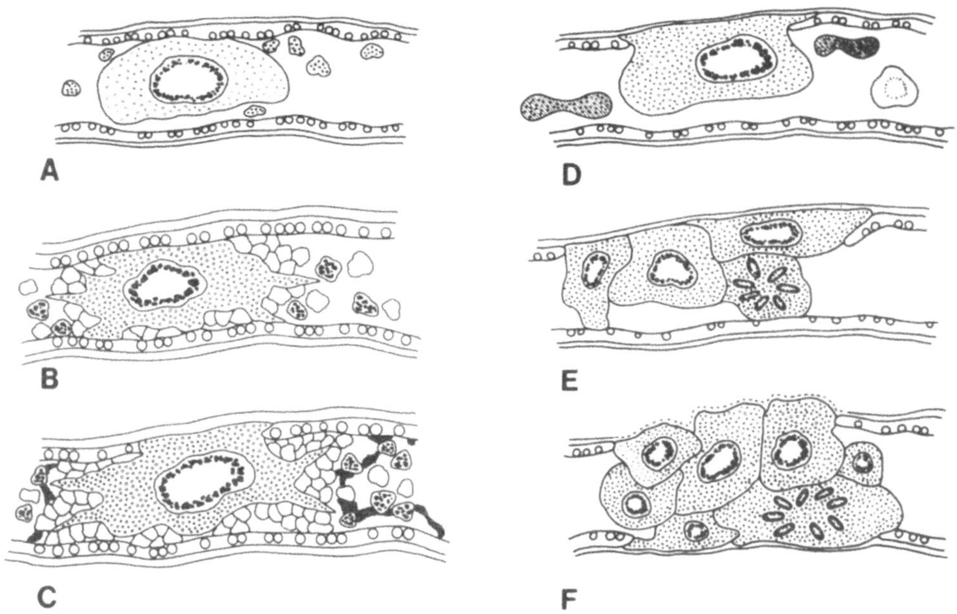

FIGURE 1. Schematic for the events involved in the arrest and extravasation of circulating tumor cells. A: The initial arrest involves interaction of the cell membrane (? adhesive molecules) of the tumor cell and the endothelium; B: Platelet activation with early thrombus formation; C: Platelet activation with continued thrombus development and alteration in the tumor cell with "pseudopodia"; D: Retraction of endothelial cells, adherence of the tumor cell to capillary basal lamina, and dissolution of the thrombus. Re-establishment of the circulation. E: Proliferation of tumor cells along the capillary basal lamina; F: Dissolution of capillary basal lamina by proliferating tumor cells and "extravasation".

it includes the multiple steps in the initial phases of the metastatic cascade, including intravasation. In addition, it is more physiologic in the sense that the cells successful in intravasation may or may not have the capacity for arrest and extravasation. This is in contrast to injection of a large bolus of cells (experimental model) in which the organ that the cells encounter may greatly affect the efficiency of forming tumor colonies. However, it is nearly impossible to document carefully steps in the metastatic cascade, including arrest and extravasation with the spontaneous model, due to the variable time course of producing sufficient circulating tumor cells to allow for accurate assessment of the steps involved in the complex metastatic cascade.

When tumor cells are injected via the tail vein, the cells first encounter the lung capillary filter which, for most cell lines, results in the successful development of pulmonary tumor colonies or "metastatic" foci. However, some cell lines do not form lung colonies after tail vein injection, but the circulating tumor cells pass through the pulmonary vascular bed and successfully arrest, survive, and proliferate in specific organs. This experimental observation supports the concept of organ selection or "homing" of some tumors. Our laboratory has noted that there is a transient "hold up" of circulating cells in the pulmonary bed, usually lasting from 2 to 10 min with secondary peaks of cell concentrations in other organs, especially in organs developing tumor colonies. This observation documents the ability of circulating tumor cells to pass through capillary beds and re-arrest in secondary organs, resulting often in successful extravasation. the two prevailing theories regarding the distribution of metastases include the mechanical theory,[1] which hypothesizes that optimum metastasis occurs in the first organ capillary bed the tumor cells are exposed to or "trapped in". The second explanation for patterns of metastases is the "seed and soil" hypothesis,[2] which represents the explanation for organ specific distribution of metastasis and is explained

TABLE 1
Comparison of Capillary Extravasation in Experimental Metastatic Models

0	30 min	3 h	6 h	12 h	24 h	48 h	Ref.
Arrest thrombi formation		Thrombi dissolution		Thrombi formation	Proliferation; penetration of endothelium		3
Arrest thrombi formation	Decrease number of platelets		Endothelial breaching		Proliferation; extravascularization		4
Arrest thrombi formation		Retraction; attachment			Thrombi dissolution; proliferation; dissolution of basement membrane		5, 6
Arrest thrombi formation			Retraction of endothelial cells	Covering of tumor cells by endothelium	Dissolution of basement membrane	Interstitial localization	11
Arrest thrombi formation		Thrombi dissolution		Adhesion to endothelial lining	Penetration of cell layer	Perivascular growth	24
Arrest thrombi formation	Thrombi dissolution; endothelial defects; attachment to basement membrane		Proliferation in lumen; endothelium penetration		Proliferation in subendothelial space		25
Thrombi formation; thrombi enlargement	Thrombi enlargement; thrombi dissolution		Penetration of endothelium (retraction); penetration of basement membrane		Dissolution of basement membrane		48

by the interactions between host organ endothelial cell properties where tail vein injection is the most common site of innoculation and circulating tumor cells. Other routes of cell delivery include injection of tumor cells into the spleen, portal vein of the liver, aortic arch, and other vascular sites and are used to test for patterns of metastases based on mechanical trapping or specific tumor cells-endothelial cell interactions in other organs. Each of these routes of tumor cell inoculation of the experiment models have their own advantages and disadvantages, and the details are beyond the extended scope of this review.

II. HOMOTYPIC VS. HETEROTYPIC AGGREGATES

Many tumors invading stroma and penetrating into vascular lumens may actually proliferate within the lymphatic and blood capillaries. This is consistent with the common observation of large homotypic aggregates of intravascular tumor cells adjacent to a primary carcinoma common in tumors of breast and colon. These cohesive aggregates are released into the lymphatic or blood vasculature as microemboli and result in mechanical trapping within the microvascular screen of the first organ encountered. This is the most likely explanation for the common clinical course of liver metastasis in colon adenocarcinoma and characteristic patterns of invasion noted in other types of cancer. Heterotypic aggregates of tumor cells and other cellular elements such as platelets, polymorphonuclear leukocytes, and lymphocytes remain a theoretical possibility, but have not been consistently described in either animal models or observed in human cancers. In contrast, we and others have observed platelet activation, and aggregation commonly occurs after initial tumor cell arrest. A description of some of these changes will be discussed in greater detail.

III. METASTATIC CASCADE, ARREST, AND EXTRAVASATION

Extravasation can be broken down into six general stages (diagrammatically shown in Figure 1). These consist of (1) circulating tumor cell arrest with endothelial-tumor cell interactions, (2) platelet activation/thrombi formation and development of tumor cytoplasmic protrusions into platelet thrombus, (3) endothelial cell retraction/basement membrane exposure and apposition by the tumor cell, (4) thrombi dissolution, (5) intravascular tumor cell proliferation, and (6) penetration of the basement membrane and invasion/proliferation of the host organ's stroma.

IV. ARREST OF THE TUMOR CELL

The initial step of extravasation is the arrest of a circulating tumor cell within the microvasculature of the target organ. This stage is characterized by intimate contact between a single tumor cell and the capillary endothelium. Wood[3] was one of the first to demonstrate tumor cell arrest. Using microcinematography techniques of blood flow through an ear of a rabbit, he observed intravenously injected rabbit V2 carcinoma cells adhering to the capillary endothelium. Jones et al.,[4] using a Walker 256 rat model, observed single tumor cells with occasional homotypic aggregates of up to six cells, arresting within 2 min after i.v. inoculation of the cells. More extensive electron microscopy studies by Crissman et al.[5,6] of three morphologically distinct murine cell lines also reported single tumor cells adhering to the capillary endothelium.

Although some early studies[7-9] have suggested that heterotypic aggregates consisting of platelets and tumor cells may be involved in cell arrest, it is more likely that thrombi formation plays a role later in the extravasation cascade. The reported tumor emboli in several of these studies were observed only at a much later time and, as discussed in greater detail in the following section, platelet activation and thrombi formation follow within 2 min of the initial arrest of a tumor cell. Therefore, in the capillaries, these emboli may result from platelet activation following the initial arrest of circulating tumor cells.

The initial arrest of tumor cells in the arterioles, however, may involve different mechanisms. Baserga and Saffiotti[9] have observed freely floating platelet/tumor cell emboli in the arterioles. Chew and Wallace[10] also have found tumor cells associated with platelets in the arterioles as early as 30 s post-injection of the cells. More recently, Lapis et al.[11] have compared extravasation in both the capillary and arterioles and have suggested that different mechanisms may be involved. In terms of initial attachment, they suggest that the thrombi composed of tumor cells, platelets, and fibrin form prior to attachment. This heterotypic cellular aggregate may result in mechanical trapping of the tumor cell embolus, which is a different sequence than single tumor cells attaching to endothelium. Homotypic tumor cell aggregates most likely arrest due to mechanical trapping, especially when the aggregates are cohesive with intracellular attachments or the desmosomes are sufficiently developed to withstand the shear forces exerted by the pulsatile blood flow in arterioles. Homotypic aggregates may occur in the experimental metastases model when incomplete dissaggregation occurs or when cells re-attach to each other during cell concentration prior to injection. In human tumors, intravascular growth of tumor cells after intravasation is a potential source of homotypic cell emboli. The mechanism by which a circulating tumor cell attaches to the capillary endothelium appears to involve an interaction between both the endothelial and the tumor cell surfaces. This remains the only plausible explanation for the numerous observations of the arrest of circulating single cells. Single tumor cells are $\sim$ 25 μm in diameter and, even though shown to be highly deformable,[12,13] may still physically lodge in the smaller diameter capillary. Experimental evidence has demonstrated that, for some tumor cell lines, these cells will momentarily arrest in the first capillary bed encountered and that they either pass through the capillary bed or are destroyed by hemodynamic shear forces. After passing through the initial capillary bed, the cells may form tumor colonies in other organ systems or be destroyed in the hostile environment of the circulation. Clearly, interaction between circulating tumor cells and endothelial cell surfaces initiate the events leading to extravasation. Evidence exists to suggest that an organ-specific recognition event may occur in many tumor lines. Nicholson and Winkelhake[14] have shown, *in vitro,* that specific adhesive interactions occur between murine tumor cells that colonize liver or lung specifically and cells derived from dissociated liver or lung, respectively. Pauli and Lee[15] also have developed an *in vitro* model of organ-specific tumor cell- endothelial cell interactions and demonstrated a correlation between metastatic phenotype *in vivo* with the ability to attach to endothelium *in vitro*. Morphologically, once the tumor cell contacts the endothelium, they maintain a smooth area of contact.[5,6,16] However, platelet aggregation on the luminal side of the tumor cell results in irregular cytoplasmic protrusions into the platelet aggregate.[17]

V. PLATELET ACTIVATION

The involvement of platelets is the second critical step of extravasation. As evidenced by shape change and degranulation, platelet activation is observed within 2 min of the initial tumor cell attachment to the endothelial cell and, although there has been some debate as to whether this thrombus forms prior to or following tumor cell attachment to a capillary endothelial cell, it clearly occurs after the tumor cell has arrested.[3-6,11,24,25] Wood[3] was the first to visualize the platelet activation following the initial arrest. Subsequent electron microscopy observations have shown the progressive nature of platelet aggregation adjacent to the arrested tumor cells. The tumor cells then develop cell extensions that project into the platelet thrombi and are presumably induced by the activated platelets.[17]

Platelet activation may play several roles in assuring tumor cell survival and colony formation. First, the attached platelets have been suggested to serve as protection of the arrested tumor cell from recognition and/or attack by the immune system.[26] Second, the association of the tumor cell with the endothelium is a relatively weak bond, and thrombi formation may serve to enhance this attachment by mechanical protection of the tenuously attached tumor cell from the stresses secondary to continued blood flow.[27,28] Grossi et al.[29] and Chopra et al.[30] have recently identified a cell surface glycoprotein, which is immunologically related to, or identical with, the GpIIb/IIIa complex. This complex is a member of the integrin family and may serve as a mediator of tumor cell-endothelial cell adhesion and platelet attachment. As demonstrated by Grossi et al.,[31] the expression of the GpIIb/IIIa protein is enhanced by a lipoxygenase metabolite of arachidonic acid, 12(S)-hydroxyeicosatetraenoic acid (12-HETE). The 12-HETE molecule is generated during platelet aggregation. Therefore, as platelets become actively attached to a tumor cell, 12-HETE is released, stimulating an increase in GpIIb/IIIa appearance on the cell surface, which results in additional platelet activation.

Fibrin formation parallels the platelet activation, but whether it is a critical component of the metastatic cascade is debatable. Early observations showed what appeared to be fibrin in the tumor-platelet emboli, and it was assumed to play an important role in thrombi stabilization.[3,32,33] Others, however, have reported little to no fibrin present in the emboli. Chew and Wallace,[10] in the Walker 256 carcinoma model, found only immunohistochemical staining unpolymerized fibrin with small amounts of stable fibrin developing after 5 min. Crissman et al.,[5,6] Machado,[34] and Jones[4] have identified occasional fibrin deposits at the periphery of the platelet thrombi that were visible by light microscopy. The fibrin deposition, however, was a transient event that usually disappeared within 1 h.

VI. ENDOTHELIAL CELL RETRACTION

The third step of the extravasation process begins approximately 4 h following arrest and is characterized by endothelial cell retraction with subsequent attachment of the tumor cell to the subendothelial cell basement membrane. By 24 h post-injection, all the arrested cells are in contact with the basement membrane. The primary site of penetration of the endothelial layer occurs at the intracellular junctions with little to no degradation of the endothelial cell layer by direct action of the tumor cell. Chew et al.[10] have observed similar retraction when tumor cells were applied to an opened capillary with an intact endothelial lining. Kinjo[25] has reported that, with the AH130 rat ascites tumor model, cells were associated with the basement membrane at sites of large endothelial cell defects. Similar observations by Crissman[5,6] also found that with increasing time, a marked thinning of the endothelial cell cytoplasm occurred, resulting in the eventual exposure of the subendothelial matrix. Degenerative changes in the endothelial layer were not observed. In some instances, the invasion of the endothelium by a tumor cell in diapedesis has been found;[3,35] tumor cell cytoplasmic processes were found to protrude between the endothelial cells and to contact the underlying basement membrane. The exact mechanism of tumor cell displacement of endothelial cells is not clear. Whether a single or multiple mechanism is operational has not been clarified. Nevertheless, tumor cell (or platelet)-induced endothelial cell retraction and/or active displacement by tumor cell migration remain the likely mechanisms.

The mechanism of endothelial cell disruption is not a simple event. Machado et al.[34] have suggested that the pressure from the growing tumor emboli results in mechanical disruption of the endothelial layer. More recently, other investigators have proposed that molecular factors, possibly secreted by the tumor cell, induce endothelial cell retraction. Kramer and Nicolson[36] and Kramer et al.,[37] using *in vitro* models, have demonstrated endothelial cell retraction induced by an adherent monolayer of tumor cells. Honn et al.[38] have shown that 12-HETE (discussed above), but not the related isomers 12(R)-, 5(s), or 15(s)-HETE, causes a reversible endothelial cell retraction.

VII. THROMBI DISSOLUTION

Following attachment by the tumor cell to the subendothelial matrix, the platelet-tumor thrombus dissolves and marks the fourth stage of extravasation. The establishment of contact with the subendothelial matrix apparently secures the attachment of the tumor cell. Warren et al.[39] and Winkelhake et al.[40] have suggested that the initial adhesion to the endothelium (Stage 1) is a weak association stabilized by the development of the tumor-platelet thrombi (Stage 2). As the tumor cell develops more stable contacts, the thrombus dissipates, and normal blood flow is re-established. The tumor cells no longer activate the platelets, as evidenced by circulating inactivated platelets.[5] In addition, little interaction with polymorphonuclear leukocytes (PMNs), lymphocytes, and monocytes is observed and can be attributed to a downregulation of the cell surface receptors for these molecules. Clearly, the tumor cell related or initiated events are no longer operational, and the cell appears to move to the next set of obstacles in the metastatic cascade.

VIII. SUBENDOTHELIAL MATRIX ATTACHMENT

The fifth stage of extravasation is characterized by the tumor cell attachment to the subendothelial basement membrane and the cell's subsequent proliferation. Some of the earliest evidence of a receptor-mediated cell arrest came from the work of Terranova et al.[18] and Vollmers et al.[19] They were able to block metastasis by injecting fragments of laminin, a cell-binding protein, along with the tumor cells. This phenomenon was abrogated by inclusion of antilaminin antibodies. More recently, Languino et al.[20] have shown that endothelial cells contain an integrin, a heterodimeric protein involved in cell adhesion,[21,22] as a laminin receptor, and Yannariello-Brown et al.[23] have identified a $M_r \sim 69,000$ protein that interacts with laminin. However, whether laminin present on the tumor cell surface influences the initial arrest or induces endothelial retraction (discussed below) remains unclear.

Proliferation of the tumor cell begins after establishment of contact with the matrix. Mitotic figures have been observed[3-6,25] within 4 h of contact with the matrix. The proliferating cells maintain the attachment to the matrix and induce further displacement of endothelial cells. This proliferative response may be induced by molecules present within the basement membrane. Such factors have been shown to play a role in embryological development and are known to regulate various cellular functions.

IX. DISSOLUTION OF BASEMENT MEMBRANE

The final step of extravasation involves dissolution of the basement membrane and penetration into the extravascular spaces. This stage begins as early as 3 d[5,6] after initial arrest and can proceed for up to 8 d. The penetration of the subendothelial basement membrane by the tumor cells proceeds potentially by two mechanisms. Cells have been reported to overcome the matrix barrier by a diapedesis-like mechanism.[3,8] The cells' pseudopodia, in contact with the matrix, digests a small hole in the matrix and extends the pseudopod through this hole. Cytoplasmic streaming then follows until the entire cell is present in the interstitial space. Tumor cell locomotion plays a critical role in this process.

Alternatively, tumor cells also have been observed to induce dissolution of the basement membrane prior to migration into the interstitial space. Crissman et al.[5,6] found that single cells did not penetrate the matrix, but observed that multi-focal dissolution of the matrix occurred as the mass of intravascular tumor cells continued to proliferate and expand. The subendothelial basement membrane in contact with the proliferating tumor nodule became irregular, indistinct, and eventually dissolved, which resulted in contact by the tumor cell with the extravascular collagen fibers.

Proteolytic enzymes either secreted[41,42] or activated[43,44] by the tumor cell are necessary for basement membrane penetration. Collagenase, a protease that digests the basement membrane collagen IV molecule, has been shown to play a role in metastasis.[43] Sloane and Honn[41] have demonstrated a correlation between the ability of a tumor cell to secrete Cathepsin B and tumor colony formation in murine lungs, while Cathepsin D has been shown to be implicated in human breast cancer metastasis.[49]

The digested matrix material may then act to influence the tumor cell during the latter stages of the metastatic cascade. Several investigators have reported the endogenous chemotactic substances are present in the host organ[45] or are contained within the extracellular matrix[46] and may be released during proteolytic breakdown, thus inducing further invasion. Saksela and Rifkin[47] have found the endogenous bFGF (basic Fibroblast Growth Factor) is associated with heparin sulfate proteoglycan and released from basement membrane due to the action of plasmin.

X. CONCLUSIONS

As a result of numerous investigators' efforts, an understanding of the extravasation process is beginning to emerge. A single circulating tumor cell attaches to the capillary endothelium primarily via a cell surface interaction. Platelet activation follows, resulting in a more secure attachment and protection from the immune system. this also may induce other factors (e.g., 12-HETE) that cause an upregulation in tumor cell surface adhesion receptor and retraction of the subendothelial basement membrane. The tumor cell then attaches to the exposed subendothelial matrix, at which time platelets no longer associate with the cell, presumably by downregulation of the tumor cell surface receptors. The firmly attached tumor cell may then secrete or activate proteolytic enzymes to digest the basement membrane to permit invasion into the extravascular space.

REFERENCES

1. **Weiss, L.,** A critical overview of the metastatic process, in *Mechanisms of Cancer Metastasis,* Honn, K. V., Powers, W. E., Sloane, B. F., Eds., Martinus Nijhoff, Boston, 1986, 23.
2. **Crissman, J. D.:** Metastases from metastasis: clinical relevance in human cancer, in *Cancer Growth and Progressions,* Goldfarb, R. H., Ed., Kluwer Academic Publishing, Norwell, MA., 1989, 156.
3. **Wood, S.,** Pathogenesis of metastasis formation observed *in vivo* in the rabbit ear chamber, *Arch. Pathol.,* 66, 550, 1958.
4. **Jones, D. S., Wallace, A. C., Fraser, E. E.,** Sequence of events in experimental metastases of Walker 256 tumor: light, immunofluorescent, and electron microscopic observations, *J. Natl. Cancer Inst.,* 46, 493, 1971.
5. **Crissman, J. D., Hatfield, J., Schaldenbrand, J., Sloane, B. F., Honn, K. V.,** Arrest and extravasation of B16 amelanotic melanoma in murine lungs, *Lab. Invest.,* 53, 470, 1985.
6. **Crissman, J. D., Hatfield, J. S., Menter, D. G., Sloane, B., Honn, K. V.,** Morphological study of the interaction of intravascular tumor cells with endothelial cells and subendothelial matrix, *Cancer Res.,* 48, 4065, 1988.
7. **Warren, S. and Gates, O.,** The fate of intravenously injected tumor cells, *Am. J. Cancer,* 27, 485, 1936.
8. **Ludatscher, R. M., Luse, S. A., Suntzeff, V.,** An electron microscopic study of pulmonary tumor emboli from transplantable Morris hepatoma 5123, *Cancer Res.,* 27, 1939, 1967.
9. **Baserga, R., Saffiotti, R.,** Experimental studies on histogenesis of blood-borne metastases, *Arch. Pathol.,* 59, 26, 1955.
10. **Chew, E. C. and Wallace, A. C.,** Demonstration of fibrin in early stages of experimental metastasis, *Cancer Res.,* 36, 1904, 1976.
11. **Lapis, K., Paku, S., and Liotta, L. A.,** Endothelialization of embolized tumor cells during metastasis formation, *Clin. Exp. Metastasis,* 6, 73, 1988.

12. **Zeidman, I.,** The fate of circulating tumors, cells. I. Passage of cells through capillaries, *Cancer Res.,* 21, 38, 1961.
13. **Sato, H. and Suzuki, M.,** Deformability and viability of tumor cells by transcapillary passage, with reference to organ affinity of metastasis in cancer, in *Fundamental Aspects of Cancer,* Weiss, L., Ed., North Holland, Amsterdam, 1976, 311.
14. **Nicolson, G. L. and Winkelhake, J.,** Organ specificity of blood-borne tumor metastasis determined by cell adhesion? *Nature,* 255, 230, 1975.
15. **Pauli, B. V. and Lee, C. L.,** Organ preference metastasis. Role of organ-specifically modulated endothelial cells, *Lab. Invest.* 58, 379, 1988.
16. **Kawaguchi, T., Tobai, S., and Nakamura, K.,** Extravascular migration of tumor cells in the brain: an electron microscopic study, *Invasion and Metastasis,* 2, 40, 1982.
17. **Menter, D. G., Hatfield, J. S., Harkins, C., Sloane, B. F., Taylor, J. D., Crissman, J. D., and Honn, K. V.,** Tumor cell-platelet interactions *in vitro* and their relationship to *in vivo* arrest of hematogenously circulating tumor cells, *Clin. Exp. Metastasis,* 5, 65, 1987.
18. **Terranova, V. P., Hujanen, E. S., and Martin, G. R.,** Basement membrane and the invasive activity of metastatic tumor cells, *J. Natl. Cancer Inst.,* 77, 311, 1986.
19. **Vollmers, H. P., Imhof, B. A., Braum, S., Waller, C. A., Schirrmacher, V., and Birchmejer, W.,** Monoclonal antibodies which prevent experimental lung metastasis, *FEBS Lett.,* 172, 17, 1984.
20. **Languino, L. R., Gehlsen, K. R., Wayner, E., Carter, W. G., Engnall, E., and Ruoslahti, E.,** Endothelial cells use B_1 integrin as a laminin receptor, *J. Cell Biol.,* 109, 2455, 1989.
21. **Hynes, R. O.,** Integrins: a family of cell surface receptors, *Cell,* 48, 549, 1987.
22. **Ruoslahti, E. and Pierschbacher, M. D.,** New perspective in cell adhesion: RGD and integrins, *Science,* 238, 491, 1987.
23. **Yannariello-Brown, J., Wewer, U., Liotta, L., and Madri, J. A.,** Distribution of a 69-kD laminin-binding protein in aortic and microvascular endothelial cells: modulation during cell attachment, spreading and migration, *J. Cell Biol.,* 106, 1773, 1988.
24. **Sindelar, W. F., Tralka, T. S., and Ketchan, A. S.,** Electron microscopic observations on formation of pulmonary metastases, *J. Surg. Res.,* 18, 137, 1975.
25. **Kinjo, M.,** Lodgement and extravasation of tumor cells in blood-borne metastasis: an electron microscopic study, *Br. J. Cancer,* 38, 293, 1978.
26. **Tobgo, A., Tanaka, N. G., and Ogawa, M.,** Platelet aggregating activities of metastasizing tumor cells, *Invasion Metastasis,* 6, 58, 1986.
27. **Menter, D. G., Sloane, B. F., Steinert, B. W., Onoda, J., Craig, R., Harkins, C., Taylor, J. D., and Honn, K. V.,** Platelet enhancement of tumor cell adhesion to subendothelial matrix: role of platelet cytoskeleton and platelet membrane, *J. Natl. Cancer Inst.,* 79, 1077, 1987.
28. **Menter, D. G., Steinert, B. W., Sloane, B. F., Gundlach, N., O'Gara, C. Y., Marnett, L. J., Diglio, C., Walz, D., Taylor, J. D., and Honn, K. V.,** Role of platelet membrane in enhancement of tumor cell adhesion to endothelial cell extramurally matrix, *Cancer Res.,* 47, 6751, 1987.
29. **Grossi, I. M., Hatfield, J. S., Fitzgerald, L. A., Newcombe, M., Taylor, J. D., and Honn, K.,** Role of tumor cell glycoproteins immunologically related to glycoprotein Ib and IIb/IIIa in tumor cell-platelet and tumor cell-matrix interactions, *FASEBJ,* 2, 2385, 1988.
30. **Chopra, H., Hatfield, J. S., Chang, Y. S., Grossi, I. M., Fitzgerald, L. A., O'Gara, C. Y., Marnett, L. J., Diglio, C. A., Taylor, J. D., and Honn, K. V.,** Role of tumor cell cytoskeleton and membrane glycoprotein IRGpIIb/IIIa in platelet adhesion to tumor cell membrane and tumor cell-induced platelet aggregation, *Cancer Res.,* 48, 3787, 1988.
31. **Grossi, I. M., Fitzgerald, L. A., Umbargar, L. A., Nelson, K. K., Diglio, C. A., Taylor, J. D., and Honn, K. V.,** Bidirectional control of membrane expression and/or activation of the tumor cell IRGpIIb/IIIa receptor and tumor cell adhesion by lipoxygenase products of arachidonic acid and linoleic acid, *Cancer Res.,* 49, 1029, 1989.
32. **Gastpar, J.,** Coagulation processes in tumor dissemination, in *Metastatic Tumor Growth,* Grundemann, E., Ed., Gustav Fischer Verlag, New York, 1980, 321.
33. **Dvorak, H. F., Dvorak, A. M., Munseau, E. J., Wiber, J., Churchhill, W. H.,** Fibrin gel investment associates with line 1 and line 10 solid tumor growth, angiogenesis, and fibroplasia in guinea pigs. Role of cellular immunity, myofibroblasts, microvascular damage and infarction of line 1 tumor regression, *J. Natl. Cancer Inst.,* 62, 1459, 1979.
34. **Machado, E. A., Gerard, D. A. Mitchell, J. R., Lozzio, B. B., and Lozzio, C. B.,** Arrest and extravasation of neoplastic cells. An electron microscopy study of serial sections of sequestial stages, *Virchows Arch. A: Pathol. Anat.,* 396, 73, 1982.
35. **Ludatscher, R. M., Luse, S. A., and Suntzeff, V.,** An electron microscopic study of pulmonary tumor emboli from transplantable Morris hepatoma 5123, *Cancer Res.,* 27, 1939, 1967.
36. **Kramer, R. H. and Nicolson, G. L.,** Interaction of tumor cells with vascular endothelial cell monolayers: a model for metastatic invasion, *Proc. Natl. Acad. Sci. U.S.A.,* 76, 5704, 1979.

37. **Kramer, R. H., Gonzalez, R., and Nicolson, G. L.,** Metastatic tumor cells adhere preferentially to the extramurally matrix underlying vascular endothelial cells, *Int. J. Cancer,* 26, 639, 1980.
38. **Honn, K. V., Grossi, I. M., Diglio, C. A., Wojtukiewicz, M., and Taylor, J. D.,** Enhances tumor cell adhesion to the subendothelial matrix resulting from 12(s)-HETE-induced endothelial cell retraction, *FASEBJ,* 3, 2285, 1989.
39. **Warren, B. A. and Vales, O.,** The adhesion of thromboplastic tumor emboli to vessel walls *in vivo, Br. J. Exp. Pathol.,* 53, 301, 1972.
40. **Winkelhake, J. L. and Nicolson, G. L.,** Determination of adhesive properties of variant metastatic melanoma cells to BALB/3T3 cells and their virus-transformed derivatives by a monolayer attachment assay, *J. Natl. Cancer Inst.,* 56, 285, 1976.
41. **Sloane, B. F. and Honn, K. V.,** Cysteine proteinases and metastasis, *Cancer Metastasis Rev.,* 3, 249, 1984.
42. **Terranova, V. P., Hujanen, E. S., and Martin, G. R.,** Basement membrane and the invasive activity of metastatic tumor cells, *J. Natl. Cancer Inst.,* 77, 311, 1986.
43. **Liotta, L. A., Thorgeirsson, V. P., and Garbisa, S.,** Role of collagenases in tumor cell invasion, *Cancer Metastasis Rev.,* 1, 277, 1982.
44. **Vlodavsky, F., Ariau, Y., Atzmon, R., and Fuks, Z.,** Tumor cell attachment to the vascular endothelium and subsequent degradation of the subendothelial extramurally matrix, *Exp. Cell Res.,* 140, 149, 1982.
45. **Hujanen, E. S. and Terranova, V. P.,** Migration of tumor cells to organ-derived chemoattractants, *Cancer Res.,* 45, 3517, 1985.
46. **Cerra, R. F. and Nathanson, S. D.,** Organ specific chemotactic factors present in lung extramurally matrix, *J. Surg. Res.,* 46, 422, 1989.
47. **Saksela, O. and Rifkin, D. B.,** Release of basic fibroblast growth factor-heparin sulfate complexes from endothelial cells by plasminogen activator-mediators proteolytic activity, *J. Cell Biol.,* 110, 767, 1990.
48. **Paku, S., Pawelet, N., Spiess, E., Avlenbacher, P., Werling, H.-O., and Knierm, M.,** Ultrastructural analysis of experimentally induced invasion in the rat lung by tumor cells metastasizing lymphatically, *AntiCancer Res.,* 6, 957, 1986.
49. **Tandon, A. K., Clark, G. M., Chamness, G. C., Chirgwin, J. M., and McGuire, M. L.,** Cathepsin D and prognosis in the breast cancer, *N. Engl. J. Med.,* 322, 297, 1990.

Chapter 14

FATTY ACID METABOLISM AND CANCER CELL-ENDOTHELIAL CELL INTERACTIONS

Michael R. Buchanan, Maria C. Bertomeu, and Thomas A. Haas

TABLE OF CONTENTS

I. INTRODUCTION

Epidemiological studies of both Western and Eastern societies suggest that dietary fat intake and subsequent body fat content significantly influence the incidence of cancer.[1-6] For example, Carroll and Khor[3,4] found a significant correlation between both total fat and animal fat intake and the incidence of breast, colon, and prostate cancer. Other studies suggest that the lower incidence in mortality in breast, prostate, and colon cancers, as seen, for example, in the Japanese compared to the Western populations, is related, in part, to a lower ingestion of dietary fats. Interestingly, in post-World War II Japan, the caloric intake of total fats of the Japanese averaged 10% as compared to 40% in the Americans. However, by 1980, the caloric intake of dietary fats by the Japanese had increased to 25%, yet over the same period, the caloric intake of dietary fats by the North Americans remained the same.[5] The increase in Japanese dietary fat-related caloric intake from 1945 to 1980 was parallelled by an increase in mortality rates for both breast and colon cancer, while the mortality rates remained constant in U.S. Similar relationships between dietary fat ingestion and the incidence of cancer have been reported for northern and southern Italians. In southern Italy, where more starch and less fat are consumed, the prevalence of cancer is markedly less than that seen in northern Italy where less starch and more fat are consumed.[6]

A more in-depth examination of the fatty acid composition of these various diets suggests that consumption of specific poly- and monounsaturated fatty acids affords a protective effect against cancer, whereas other polyunsaturated and saturated fatty acids increase its incidence.

Thus, there is an abundance of evidence to suggest that dietary fats play an important role in either enhancing or inhibiting the onset and/or progression of metastasis. Undoubtedly, fatty acid metabolism may alter cancer cell function at the various stages of metastasis, including initial tumor growth, invasion, extravasation, and secondary metastasis. In this chapter, we will focus predominately on those specific mechanisms in vascular endothelial cells and in cancer cells that influence one of the steps, namely, cancer cell attachment to the endothelium, and we will discuss how these mechanisms may be altered by changes in dietary fat intake. First, we will review the basic pathways, which result in the synthesis of cyclo-oxygenase and lipoxygenase derived fatty acid metabolites. We will then review the evidence concerning the manner by which these metabolites are thought to regulate the surface properties of the vascular endothelium and/or the cancer cells, thereby affecting subsequent cancer cell-endothelial cell interactions and subsequent metastasis. Finally, we will examine how diet may modulate these processes.

II. CYCLO-OXYGENASE METABOLISM OF ARACHIDONIC ACID IN ENDOTHELIAL CELLS

It is interesting to note that while the fatty acid composition of the vessel wall, in particular the endothelium, is complex,[7,8] most investigators have focussed their attention solely on the role of the 20 carbon fatty acid, *arachidonic acid,* and its metabolism via the *cyclo-oxygenase* pathway in *stimulated* endothelial cells.

Numerous biological stimuli such as thrombin, endotoxin, and a variety of cytokines have been shown to induce the synthesis by and subsequent release of prostacyclin (i.e., prostaglandin I_2 or PGI_2) from endothelial cells,[9-16] presumably by activating endothelial cell plasma membrane phospholipases (Figure 1).

PGI_2 is synthesized via the cyclo-oxygenase pathway following the liberation of a free arachidonic acid from the endothelial cell membrane phospholipids.[15-17] Free arachidonic acid is metabolized by cyclo-oxygenase in the presence of molecular oxygen (Figure 1). One oxygen molecule is inserted into the C_9 position of arachidonic acid, and a second oxygen molecule is inserted at C_{11} (Figure 2). This compound rapidly isomerizes, resulting

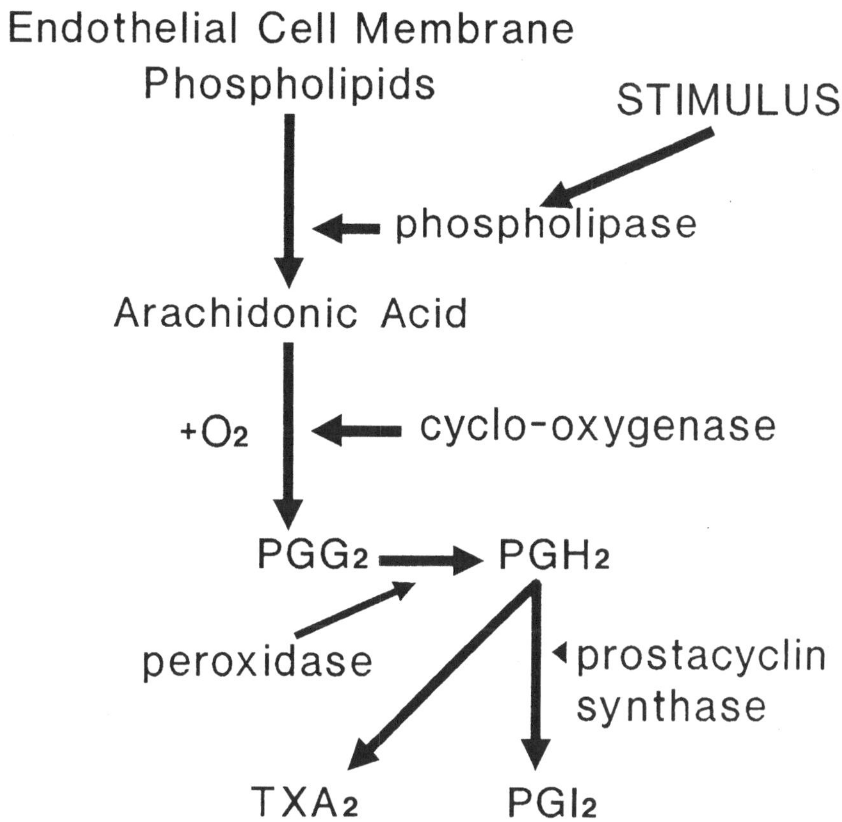

FIGURE 1. Synthesis of PGI_2 and TxA_2 via the cyclo-oxygenase pathway.

in a ring closure between C_8 and C_{12} and forming an oxygen bridge between C_9 and C_{11} (Figure 2). A third oxygen molecule is then inserted at C_{15}, completing the formation of the 15-hydroperoxy endoperoxide or PGG_2 (Figure 2).[17] PGG_2 is then rapidly hydrolysed into PGH_2,[17] which is labile and is subsequently metabolized into a variety of eicosanoids. In endothelial cells, PGH_2 is metabolized by prostaglandin synthase into prostacyclin or PGI_2. PGI_2 is thought to be the principle cyclo-oxygenase-derived fatty acid metabolite produced by endothelial cells,[9,10] although some studies suggest that endothelial cells may also synthesize small amounts of thromboxane A_2 or TxA_2.[19,20] The significance of the latter observations is not clear since TxA_2 is only produced by endothelial cells in culture.[19,20] Other studies suggest that the apparent synthesis of TxA_2 by endothelial cells is, in fact, due to contaminating fibroblasts in the cell culture preparation.[21]

PGI_2 is best recognized as a potent inhibitor of platelet aggregation and a potent vasodilator of the vessel wall.[9,10] PGI_2 is thought to inhibit platelet aggregation by activating platelet adenylate cyclase, thereby, elevating cyclic adenosine monophosphate (cAMP) and rendering platelets less responsive to untoward stimuli. The activation of adenylate cyclase by PGI_2 is thought to be mediated through a PGI_2 receptor and to be common to a variety of cells.[23-26] This effect is opposite to that initiated by the platelet-derived cyclo-oxygenase arachidonic acid metabolite, TxA_2.[18] Consequently, it was postulated that the relative amounts of TxA_2 and PGI_2 play important opposing roles in the regulation of platelet endothelial cell interactions following blood cell and vessel wall injury.[25] Since platelets are thought to play an important role in cancer cell activation and subsequent extravasation,[27-29] endothelial cell-derived PGI_2 influences on platelet function may also result in secondary effects on cancer cell-vessel wall interactions. Endothelial cell-derived PGI_2 also may have direct effects on

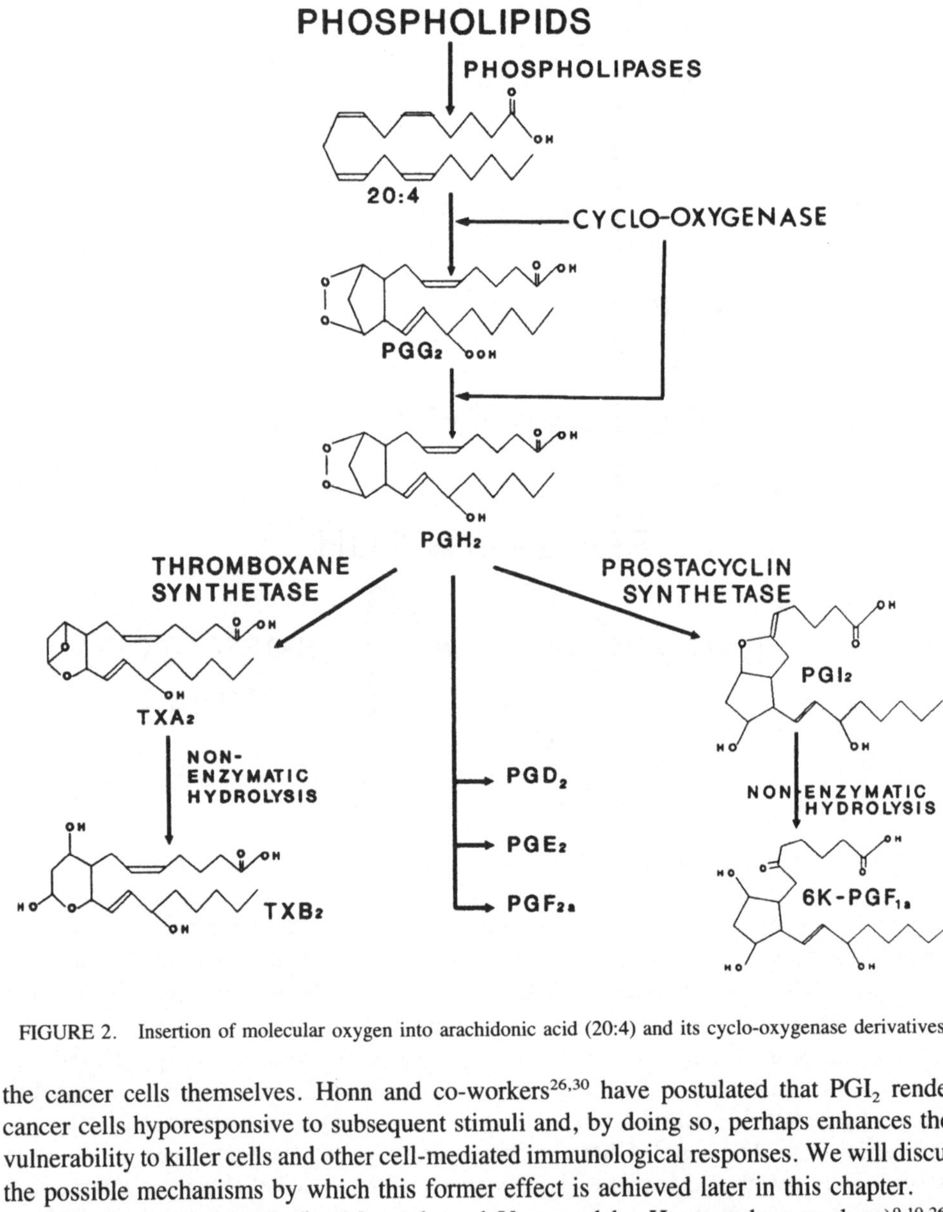

FIGURE 2. Insertion of molecular oxygen into arachidonic acid (20:4) and its cyclo-oxygenase derivatives.

the cancer cells themselves. Honn and co-workers[26,30] have postulated that PGI_2 renders cancer cells hyporesponsive to subsequent stimuli and, by doing so, perhaps enhances their vulnerability to killer cells and other cell-mediated immunological responses. We will discuss the possible mechanisms by which this former effect is achieved later in this chapter.

The above hypotheses (by Moncada and Vane and by Honn and co-workers)[9,10,26,30] assume that PGI_2 per se is the most important "antiplatelet" and "antimetastatic" prostanoid to regulate cell responsiveness. It should be recognized, however, that PGI_2 has an exceedingly short biological half-life, $\approx$ 30 s,[10,25] and its inhibition is not accompanied by enhanced thrombosis or by enhanced metastasis *in vivo*.[31,32] Thus, from the perspective of a PGI_2-induced inhibition of platelet effects (involved in either thrombus formation or cancer cell-vessel wall interactions) or from the perspective of a PGI_2-induced direct inhibition of cancer cell function, these effects are likely to be transient at best. Ideally, a more stable form of PGI_2 synthesized at a time of insult, i.e., during platelet-cancer cell-endothelial cell interactions, might be better able to influence these pathophysiological events and, hence, be more biologically relevant.

One possible candidate in this regard is 6-keto-PGE_1, a prostanoid that has received less attention than PGI_2, but undoubtedly has potent biologic effects. Mehta et al.[33,34] found that circulating blood cells generate PGI_2-like activity. At the same time, Wong et al.[35,36] and

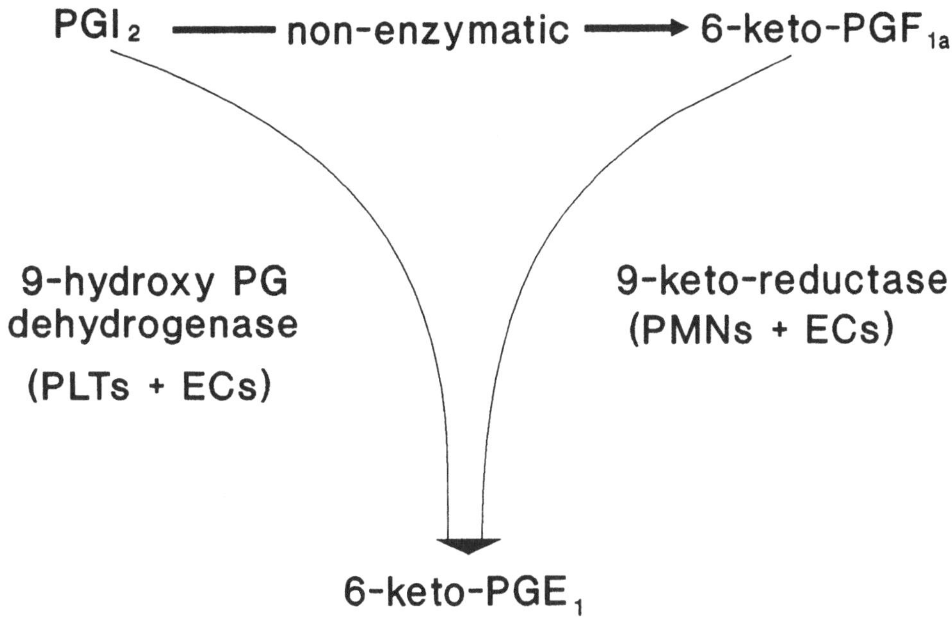

FIGURE 3. Metabolism of 6-keto-PGE_1 by the platelet (PLT) and leukocyte (PMN) enzymes, 9-hydroxy prostaglandin (PG) dehydrogenase and 9-keto-reductase. Activation of both enzymes requires a cofactor derived from endothelial cells.

Chang et al.[37] found that both leukocytes and platelets had the biochemical machinery to convert PGI_2, its stable, or the inactive end-product, 6-keto-$PGF_{1\alpha}$ into 6-keto-PGE_1, namely, by the platelet-derived 9-hydroxy-prostaglandin dehydroxygenase or by the leukocyte-derived 9-keto reductase (Figure 3). The significance of these observations is that 6-keto-PGE_1 is as stable as 6-keto-$PGF_{1\alpha}$, but at least as equipotent as PGI_2.[36,38] The potent effect of 6-keto-PGE_1, like PGI_2, is achieved by stimulating adenylate cyclase, thereby increasing cAMP.[36,39] Thus, 6-keto-PGE_1 inhibits platelet aggregation and antagonizes the proaggregatory effect of TXA_2.[36,38,39] More recent studies performed in our laboratory provide evidence that the *in vivo* synthesis of 6-keto-PGE_1 occurs only during dynamic blood cell-vessel wall interactions following injury or insult. Thus, we demonstrated that both activated leukocytes and platelets can convert PGI_2 or 6-keto-$PGF_{1\alpha}$ into 6-keto-PGE_1.[40,41] More importantly, activation of the enzymes in both platelets and leukocytes requires the presence of the endothelium. Neither platelets alone nor leukocytes alone are able to synthesize 6-keto-PGE_1.[40,41] Therefore, our data raise the possibility that (1) PGI_2 is converted into a more potent and more stable product, 6-keto-PGE_1, during blood/vessel wall insult or injury, and (2) the synthesis of 6-keto-PGE_1 requires an enzyme or co-factor derived from pertubated or injured endothelial cells. At present, the identity of this co-factor is unknown.

In summary, endothelial cells, in response to stimulation or injury, metabolize arachidonic acid via the cyclo-oxygenase pathway into the prostanoid, PGI_2. Since PGI_2 synthesis is a product of *in vivo* cell stimulation, it is also expected that the very unstable PGI_2 and its breakdown product, 6-keto-$PGF_{1\alpha}$ are then converted into the more stable yet equipotent metabolite, 6-keto-PGE_1, by blood cells also involved in the response to injury or insult, e.g., platelets, leukocytes, and/or cancer cells interacting at the site of endothelial cell damage. Endothelial cells contribute to this latter process by providing a co-factor which appears to ''turn on'' the leukocyte and platelet enzymes necessary for 6-keto-PGE_1 conversion. It is not yet known whether cancer cells are also capable of converting PGI_2 or 6-keto-$PGF_{1\alpha}$ into 6-keto-PGE_1 when they interact with endothelial cells. Our current suspicion is that they cannot, since the generation of such a potent and stable 6-keto-PGE_1 prostanoid

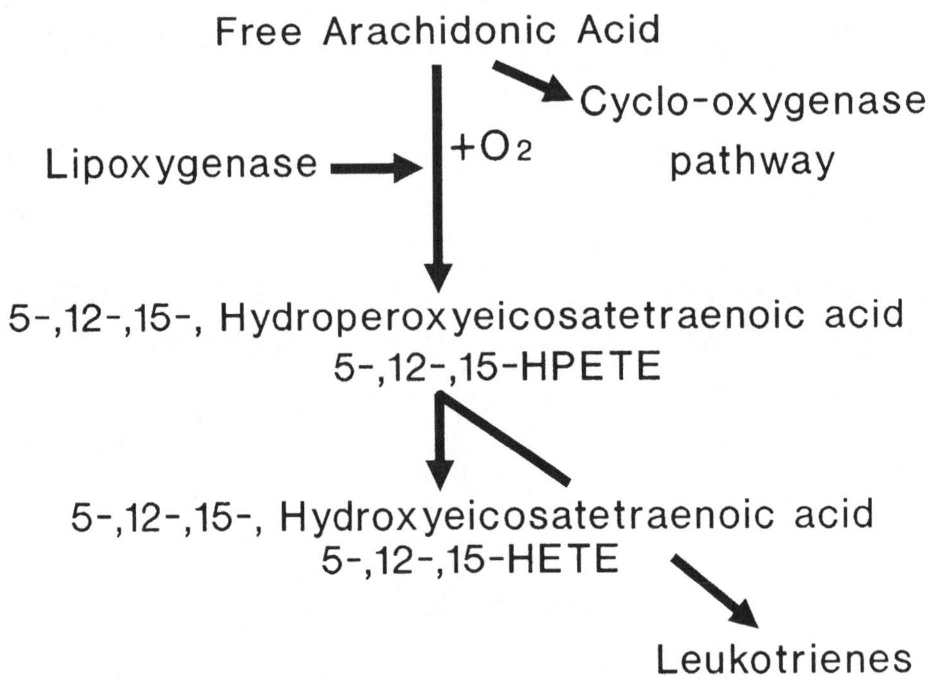

FIGURE 4. Arachidonic acid metabolism via the lipoxygenase pathway.

can impede the cancer cell-endothelial cell interactions, thereby, impairing the metastatic potential of the cancer cells.

III. LIPOXYGENASE METABOLISM OF ARACHIDONIC ACID

When blood cells are stimulated, free arachidonic acid is also metabolized by a second enzyme, lipoxygenase, which is located within the cytosol of cells (e.g., in platelets and leukocytes).[15,17,42] Lipoxygenase, in the presence of molecular oxygen, converts arachidonic acid into the unstable hydroperoxy-eicosatetraenoic acid (HPETE), which is then hydrolysed by a cytosolic-associated peroxidase into hydroxyeicosatetraenoic acid or HETE (Figure 4). The position of the first double bond in the HETE structure, e.g., 5-HETE and 12-HETE, is dependant upon the cell-specific enzyme, i.e., 5-lipoxygenase in leukocytes[17] and 12-lipoxygenase in platelets.[42]

Ten years ago, it was thought that there was no lipoxygenase pathway in the vascular wall cells. The evidence to support that conclusion was based upon the evidence that there were no lipoxygenase metabolites released from vascular wall cells following stimulation or injury *in vitro*. However, studies by Greenwald et al.[43] suggested that a lipoxygenase pathway did exist in the vessel wall since a 12-HETE-like substance was isolated from intact aortic segments. More detailed studies by us and other investigators using *in vitro* cell culture systems demonstrated that not only vascular endothelial cells, but also smooth muscle cells and fibroblasts could metabolize *exogenous* arachidonic acid into a HETE-like metabolite.[44-46] However, in these conditions, the HETE produced had its first double bond in the 15 position (15-HETE) and not in the 12 position.[41,44,45] These observations indicated that the endothelial cell lipoxygenase metabolite was 15-HETE, not 12-HETE, and that the lipoxygenase enzyme in endothelial cells was the omega—6-lipoxygenase, therefore, distinctly different from the lipoxygenase enzymes found in leukocytes (which synthesize 5-HETE) and platelets (which synthesize 12-HETE). It should be emphasized, however, that while these observations confirmed the existence of a lipoxygenase pathway in vascular wall cells, they did not provide any evidence that synthesis of 15-HETE by endothelial cells was biologically relevant. In fact, there is no evidence to demonstrate that any 15-HETE derived from their *endogenous* arachidonic acid stores is produced by endothelial cells.[41]

In summary, endothelial cells are capable of metabolizing arachidonic acid into two major metabolites, PGI_2, via the cyclo-oxygenase pathway and, 15-HETE, via the lipoxygenase pathway. However, it should be noted that both freshly isolated vascular tissue and cultured endothelial cells synthesize only PGI_2 from their endogenous arachidonic acid stores only after *stimulation* and only under the conditions when these cells are in isolation. Under more pathophysical conditions *in vivo* involving vessel or blood cell injury and subsequent blood cell-vessel wall interactions, we believe that PGI_2 is likely to be converted into a more stable metabolite, 6-keto-PGE_1. Finally, there is no evidence to suggest that cultured endothelial cells and intact human vessel walls are capable of synthesizing 15-HETE from endogenous arachidonic acid.[12,40,47]

This latter point was perplexing to us since we had found in earlier studies that various lipoxygenase inhibitors had specific effects on platelet-endothelial cell interactions *in vitro* and thrombus formation *in vivo,* and these effects were achieved independent of a platelet effect.[48-51] This prompted us to hypothesize that vessel wall biocompatibility with circulating blood cells under "resting" or homeostatic conditions was regulated, in part, by an active lipoxygenase pathway in endothelial cells, but apparently independent of arachidonic acid metabolism per se.[52] Since we were unable to detect any lipoxygenase metabolites in the ambient surroundings, we were prompted to look inside the cells.

IV. LIPOXYGENASE METABOLISM OF LINOLEIC ACID

A number of subsequent studies confirmed that endothelial cells were indeed metabolically active under basal conditions, and this activity involved the lipoxygenase pathway.[52-55] In particular, Denning et al.[53] first demonstrated that triglycerides were rapidly turned over in the unstimulated endothelial cell. Then we found that linoleic acid was continuously released from this cytosolic triglyceride pool and metabolized *intracellulary* by the endothelial cell enzyme, 15-lipoxygenase, into the monohydroxide, 13-hydroxyoctadecadienoic acid or 13-HODE (Figure 5).[52,54,55]

We found that 13-HODE was retained intracellularly and *was not released* into the ambient surroundings,[52,54,55,56] like PGI_2. Furthermore, when endothelial cells were stimulated, 13-HODE synthesis rapidly decreased, such as following stimulation by thrombin, endotoxin, or a number of cytokines.[46,52,56] It should also be noted that following stimulation, 13-HODE *was not released* from the endothelial cells.[46,52,54-57]

The level of intracellular 13-HODE in vascular endothelial cells can be elevated by increasing the resting levels of intracellular cAMP both *in vitro* and *in vivo*.[50,52,55,56] This effect appears to be associated with an increase in linoleic acid turnover in the triglyceride pool, thereby providing more substrate for the lipoxygenase enzyme.[55] We should, perhaps, remind the reader at this time that PGI_2, 6-keto-PGE_1, and some other prostanoids increase intracellular cAMP. The obvious implications, therefore, are that all of these prostanoids are capable of increasing intracellular levels of 13-HODE by elevating cAMP.

It should be noted that other investigators have suggested that endothelial cells metabolize linoleic acid into 13-HODE and 9-HODE via the cyclo-oxygenase pathway and following stimulation.[58] However, it should be emphasized that these observations are based upon the addition of industrial concentrations of *exogenous* linoleic acid, an 18 carbon chain fatty acid. Fatty acid substrates with 18 carbons and 2 double bonds are poor substrates for the cyclo-oxygenase enzyme. As a consequence, supra physiological concentrations of the exogenous linoleic acid are needed to generate 13- and 9-HODE via the cyclo-oxygenase

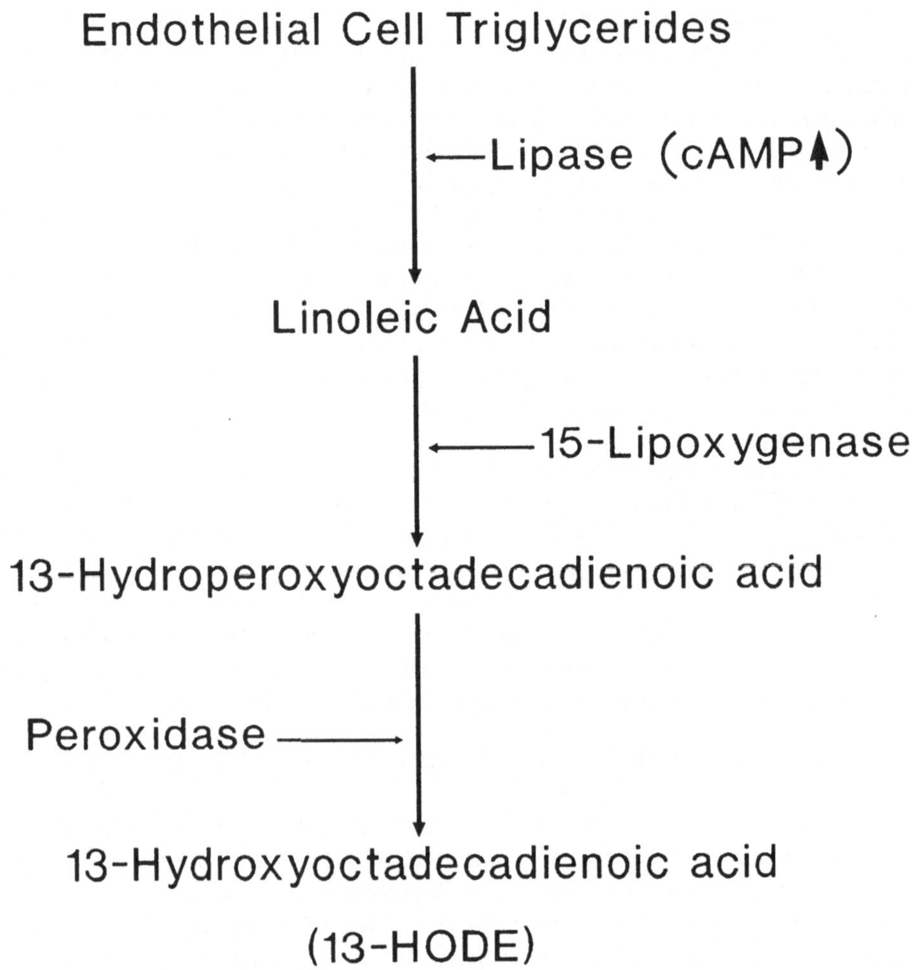

FIGURE 5. Synthesis of 13-HODE-from linoleic acid in endothelial cells under basal conditions.

pathway. Whether such supra-concentrations of free extracellular linoleic acid can be achieved in the plasma in a more biological relevant setting *in vivo* is unknown. If so, it may have some interesting implications concerning metabolism of linoleic acid via the cyclo-oxygenase pathway in endothelial cells, or in any other cell, and subsequent effects in cancer cell-endothelial cell interaction. On the other hand, cyclo-oxygenase metabolism of 9- and 13-HODE may be simply an artefact *in vitro* due to the artificial conditions, particularly since the investigators who demonstrated the synthesis of 9- and 13-HODE from exogenous linoleic acid provide no evidence either *in vitro* or *ex vivo* that 9- and 13-HODE also can be synthesized via the cyclo-oxygenase pathway from endogenous stores of linoleic acid.

V. ARACHIDONIC AND LINOLEIC ACID METABOLISM BY CANCER CELLS

Metabolism of arachidonic acid and linoleic acid in cancer cells also proceeds via the cyclo-oxygenase and lipoxygenase pathways.[52,56,59-64] Under basal conditions, linoleic acid and arachidonic acid are metabolized intracellularly into the lipoxygenase-derived 13-HODE and 15-HETE metabolites, which are retained within the cancer cells.[52,56] This suggests that there is a 15-lipoxygenase species in different cancer cells like in the endothelial cells.

Furthermore, the ratio of 13-HODE:15-HETE within cancer cells varies markedly among cancer cell derived from different origins.[56] Whether the synthesis of these two metabolites reflects differences in available substrates (more linoleic acid and less arachidonic acid in some and the opposite in other) or reflects differences in the distribution of the lipoxygenase enzyme within the cell is not known, but it is strikingly obvious that these differences are reflected by significant differences in cancer cell metastatic potential.[65]

When cancer cells are stimulated, arachidonic acid metabolism via both the cyclo-oxygenase and lipoxygenase pathway predominate. A number of investigators have demonstrated that a variety of cancer cells, e.g., those obtained from squamous cell carcinoma, adenocarcinoma, small cell carcinoma, and mixed cell carcinoma, as well as other metastatic tumors, synthesize uniquely different profiles of prostaglandins, including PGE_1, PGE_2, $PGF_{2\alpha}$, and TxA_2.[59-64] The biological relevance of the different prostanoid profiles in these cells is unclear. Bennett et al.[62] and Rolland et al.[63] found that prostaglandin production in human breast cancer was markedly elevated. They suggested, therefore, that the elevated prostaglandin production was a marker of high metastatic potential for neoplastic cells. In contrast, Fulton[61] and Vergate et al.[64] found the opposite and suggested that increased production of prostanoids was a marker of good prognosis. The explanation for these discrepancies is unclear, but without an inclusion of the profile of the other fatty acid metabolites, derived not only from the cyclo-oxygenase pathway, but also from the lipoxygenase pathway, our understanding of the delicate balance of fatty acid metabolism as it relates to the metastatic processes is obscured. At the end of this chapter, we will integrate these two pathways and propose an explanation for the discrepancy.

VI. INFLUENCE OF FATTY ACID METABOLITES ON ENDOTHELIAL AND CANCER CELL ADHESION MOLECULE EXPRESSION

A number of recent studies suggest that the intracellular levels of 13-HODE in endothelial cells and the intracellular ratio of 13-HODE:15-HETE in cancer cells contribute to the regulation of adhesion molecule expression on their extracellular surfaces.[46,52,54,56,57] When 13-HODE synthesis is increased in the resting endothelial cell, i.e., by adding exogenous db-cAMP or by growing the cells in the presence of a phosphodiesterase inhibitor, dipyridamole, there is a corresponding dose-related decrease in the ability of untreated cancer cells to adhere to an endothelial cell surface.[56] In contrast, when endothelial cells are stimulated with cytokines such as interleukin 1, tumor necrosis factor, or the synthetic peptide, fMLP, endothelial cell 13-HODE synthesis decreases and cancer cell endothelial cell adhesion increases.[56,57,65]

Similar observations have been seen when manipulating cancer cell fatty acid metabolism.[56,65] For example, when cancer cells are grown in the presence of the phosphodiesterase inhibitor, cancer cell cAMP levels also increase. The increase in cAMP is parallelled by a dose-related increase in intracellular 13-HODE synthesis and by a decrease in the ability of the cancer cells to adhere to the untreated endothelial cells. Interestingly, the decrease in 13-HODE synthesis in cancer cells following stimulation is associated with an increase in 15-HETE synthesis. It should be noted that under these conditions, there was no detectable 13-HODE or 15-HETE released into the ambient surroundings.

Thus, studies using a variety of human and murine cancer cell lines indicate that the ratio of 13-HODE:15-HETE in cancer cells correlates significantly with their adhesive ability; the more the 13-HODE and the less the 15-HETE, the less adhesive is the cancer cell under resting conditions. Following stimulation, 13-HODE synthesis decreases, and there are corresponding increases in 15-HETE synthesis and in the ability of cancer cells to adhere.[56,65]

The rapid development in molecular biologic techniques has lead to the identification

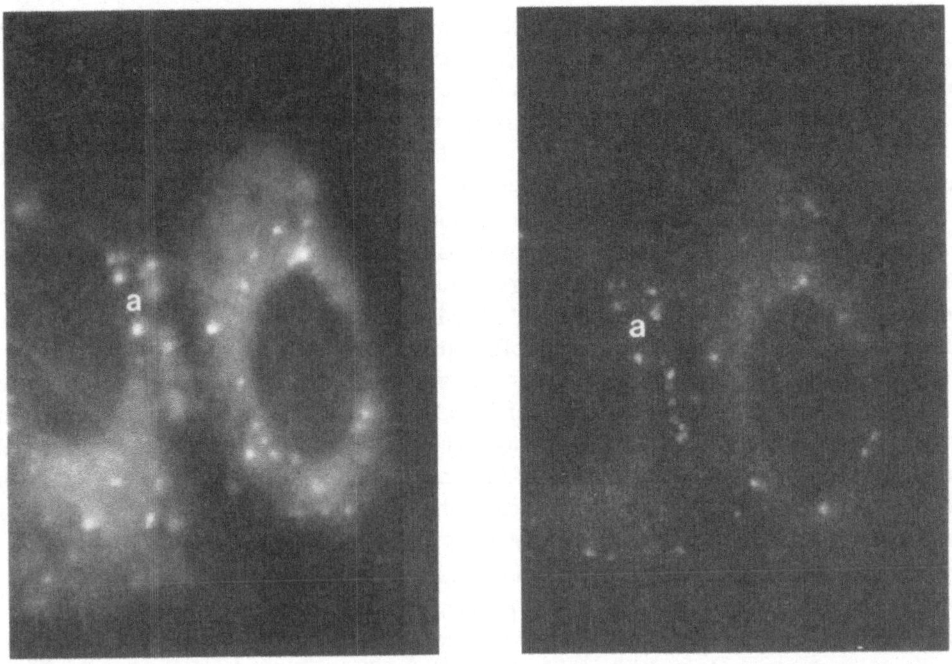

FIGURE 6. Colocalization of 13-HODE (left) and the vitronectin receptor, VnR (right), inside nonadhesive endothelial cells. For example, the pattern of histoimmunofluorescence around (a) of endothelial cells expressed to the fluorescein tagged 13-HODE antibody is identical to the pattern of histoimmunofluorescence around (a) of the same endothelial cells exposed to the rhodamine red tagged VnR antibody.

of a host of adhesion receptors on various cell surfaces. This is elegantly reviewed in detail by Kramer et al. in Chapter 10. Little, however, is known about the biochemical regulators inside the cells, which influence the expression of these adhesion molecules on the external surface of the cells. Honn et al. (Chapter 7) described how following stimulation, cancer cells express a glycoprotein IIb/IIIa-like molecule on their surface. The expression of this molecule and other RGD-recognizing integrins is coincidental with enhanced cancer cell adhesion,[66–68] and their expression is coincidental with a decrease in 13-HODE.[56,65,69] We raised the possibility that the expression of these adhesion molecules, in cancer cells and endothelial cells, was regulated by 13-HODE, thereby influencing cancer cell/endothelial cell adhesion.[52,70]

One possible mechanism by which 13-HODE could achieve this effect was to physically influence the conformational expression of the integrin on the cell surface, and hence, influence its ability to recognize its specific adhesion ligands. Consistent with this possibility, earlier studies by Conforti et al.[71] demonstrated that by changing the phospholipids associated with the vitronectin receptor, they could alter the ability of the vitronectin receptor to recognize its various ligands, including von Willebrand factor, fibronectin, and vitronectin. Recently, we found that interleukin 1 stimulated both endothelial cell expression and *de novo* synthesis of the vitronectin receptor on the apical surface of endothelial cells.[66] Therefore, we performed studies to determine whether a physical relationship existed between 13-HODE and the vitronectin receptor in unstimulated and interleukin 1-stimulated endothelial cells. We were unable to detect any 13-HODE or vitronectin receptor on the apical surface of unstimulated endothelial cells, i.e., nonadhesive endothelial cells. However, we were able to colocalize both 13-HODE and the vitronectin receptor within the same nonadhesive endothelial cells (Figure 6). [Earlier studies by our laboratory confirmed that 13-HODE was located in specific vesicles immediately below but adjacent to the plasma mem-

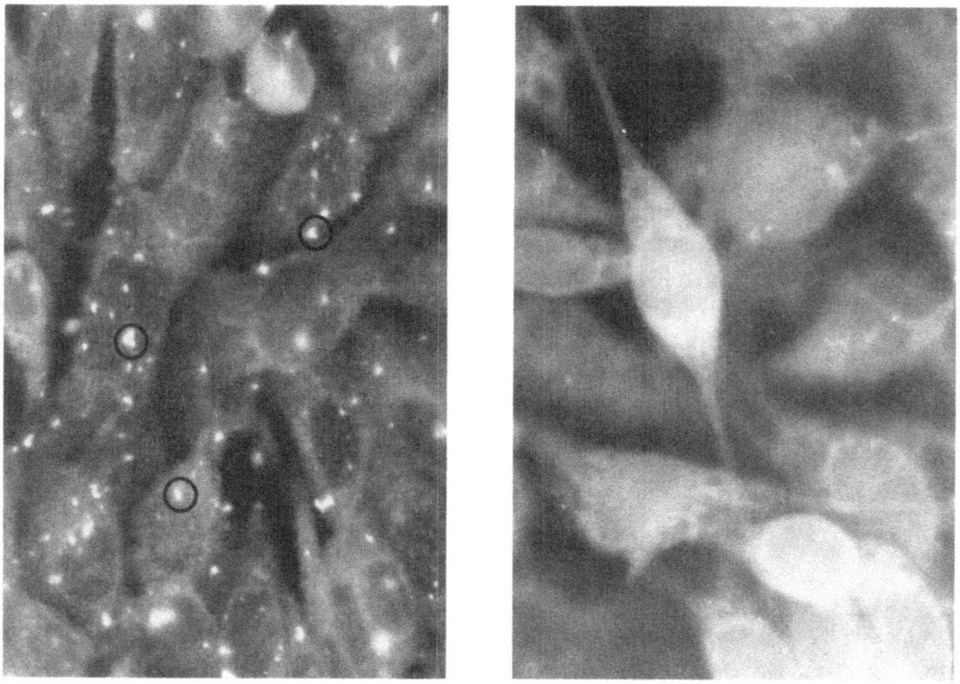

FIGURE 7. Histoimmunofluorescent localization of 13-HODE in nonmetastatic (left) and metastatic cancer cells (right). The nonmetastatic cells contained more 13-HODE than the metastatic cells as highlighted by the circles. × 320.

brane within the cytosol of the endothelial cells[72]]. When endothelial cells were stimulated, the vitronectin receptor and the 13-HODE dissociated, and the vitronectin receptor was detected on the apical surface of the cells, i.e., at a time when the endothelial cells had become adhesive.

These observations provided the first evidence that 13-HODE acted as a downregulator of adhesion molecule expression on endothelial cells. Consistent with this possibility, Singer et al.[73] found that the laminin and fibronectin receptors were also located in specific vesicles or ''adhesomes'' in other cells under resting condition. Upon stimulation, these adhesion molecules were also transferred to the cell surface.

Similar results have been obtained when examining the relationship between the amount of 13-HODE in cancer cells and their abilities to adhere to endothelial cells, their underlying basement membrane, and their abilities to metastasize. Thus, Bastida et al.[56,57] found a significant inverse relationship between the ability of cancer cells to produce 13-HODE and their ability to adhere to various surfaces. The more the 13-HODE were in the human- and murine-derived cancer cells, the less adhesive the cells were. Furthermore, upon stimulation of any of these cells, 13-HODE synthesis decreased, and the ability of the cancer cells to adhere to any surface increased.[56,57] To make matters more complicated, however, as the 13-HODE levels decreased, the intracellular levels of 15-HETE increased. Bertomeu et al.[65,69] found a similar relationship *in vivo*. Thus, cancer cells with more metastatic potential produced less 13-HODE than cancer cells with minimal metastatic potential. Moreover, by selectively inhibiting vessel wall/13-HODE synthesis, the metastatic potential was increased.

Finally, studies currently ongoing in our laboratory confirm that nonmetastatic cells contain significantly more 13-HODE than metastatic cells; these are measured both by high performance chromatography[56,57,65,69] and by histoimmunofluorescence (Figure 7).

In other studies, Grossi et al.[68] found that exogenous 13-HODE blocked the expression of adhesion molecules on a variety of cancer cells and that the expression of the adhesion receptor was enhanced by exogenous 12-HETE.

All of these observations have lead us to conclude that lipoxygenase metabolites derived from arachidonic acid and linoleic acid act as intracellular regulators to influence integrin expression and subsequent cell adhesivity from the perspective of both the endothelial cell surface and the cancer cell surface.[70]

It also should be recognized that a number of investigators have reported that other receptors on cancer cells such as the EGF receptor (required for cell growth[74]) are more ubiquitous on metastatic cells.[75,76] Whether or not one of these lipoxygenase metabolites (13-HODE or 15-HETE) influences the expression of this particular receptor is presently unknown. However, this may be a possibility, particularly since Gleeson et al.[77] have reported that the expression of the EGF receptor on cervical squamous carcinoma cells and their subsequent growth can be altered by changing the composition of the fatty acid cell membrane.

VII. 13-HODE AND PGI_2 SYNTHESIS AND CANCER CELL/ ENDOTHELIAL CELL ADHESION

A number of investigators have proposed that PGI_2 plays an important role in metastasis, presumably by influencing cancer cell function.[26,30,59-64] However, there is no consensus of how these prostanoids achieve these anti- or pro-metastatic effects. We would like to propose a possible mechanism by which PGI_2 influences metastasis, which might resolve some of these apparent inconsistencies (see Section II). First, we must remind the reader that when cancer cell adhesion to endothelial cells is *enhanced* following endothelial injury or stimulation, the enhanced cancer cell adhesion occurs at a time when endothelial cell PGI_2 synthesis is increased.[52,55-57,78-80] Since PGI_2 is purported to be antimetastatic, these observations would appear at first glance to be totally inconsistent. In another study, we found that the levels of both PGI_2 and 6-keto PGE_1 increased during *symptomatic episodes* in a patient with primary thrombocythemia, i.e., at a time when the patient was suffering a transient ischemia attack or during intravascular cell-cell interactions.[38] We postulated that the increased production of both metabolites reflected a response to injury; however, at that time, we had no idea by which mechanism. Given our more recent observations, namely that (1) 13-HODE appears to downregulate integrin expression,[56,57,81,82] (2) 13-HODE synthesis can be upregulated by elevating cAMP,[55,56] and (3) PGI_2 and its more stable end-product 6-keto PGE_1 elevate cAMP, we propose the following model: when cAMP levels are normally high, i.e., in healthy unstimulated cells, there is a continuous turnover of triglycerides that results in the liberation of free linoleic acid (Figure 7). Free linoleic acid, in turn, is continuously metabolized by the lipoxygenase enzyme into 13-HODE. The newly synthesized 13-HODE complexes with adhesion receptors, for example, with the vitronectin receptor in endothelial cells and retains the receptor in specific vesicles inside the cell, i.e., 13-HODE prevents its expression on the apical surface (Figure 8). However, when the cells are stimulated, cAMP levels dramatically drop, and triglyceride turnover decreases. This reduces the liberation of linoleic acid and hence provides less substrate for the synthesis of 13-HODE. As a consequence, the remaining 13-HODE and the vitronectin dissociate, allowing the vitronectin receptor to relocate to the plasma cell membrane phospholipids. As a consequence the receptor undergoes a conformational change and renders the apical surface more adhesive.

We also recognize that following cell stimulation, the decrease in cAMP is parallelled by an activation of the membrane-associated phospholipases, which facilitate the liberation of arachidonic acid.[15-18] As a consequence, PGI_2 is synthesized via the cyclo-oxygenase pathway. PGI_2 can act either directly, or by being further metabolized into 6-keto-PGE_1, as

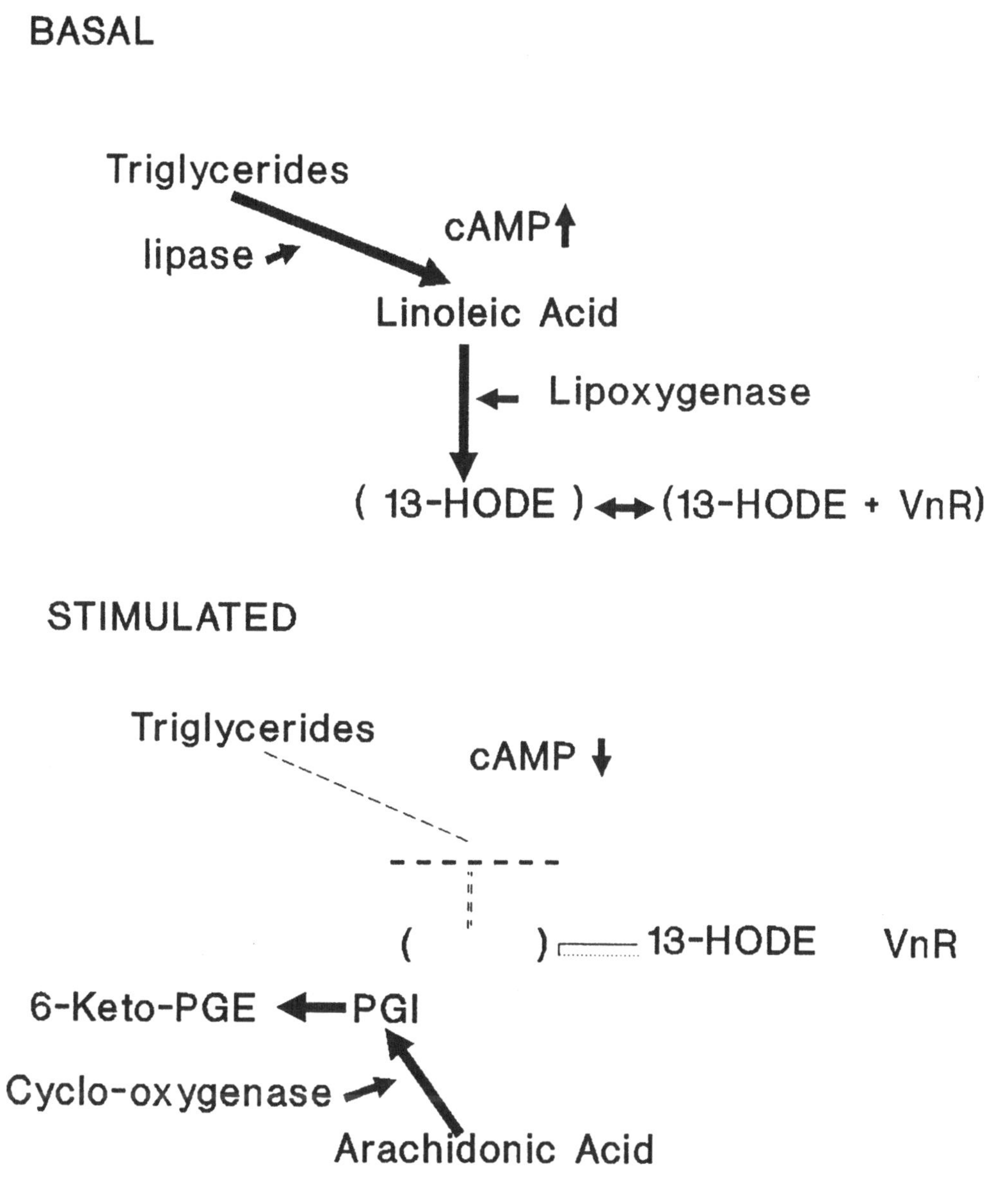

FIGURE 8. Proposed model for the regulation of vitronectin receptor in vascular endothelial cells. VnR = vitronectin receptor.

a negative feedback mechanism to elevate the cAMP levels, and reverse the adhesive process by facilitating 13-HODE synthesis. This would downregulate adhesion receptor expression and return the endothelial cell apical surface to its original nonadhesive state.

A number of dietary studies, both clinical and in experimental animals, as well as *in vitro* cell culture experiments, support this possibility as a basic model for the regulation of adhesion molecule expression and subsequent cell-cell interactions involved in metastasis both in endothelial and cancer cells.

VIII. INFLUENCES OF DIET ON LIPOXYGENASE FATTY ACID METABOLISM: POSSIBLE RELEVANCE IN METASTASIS

As indicated earlier in this chapter, differences in dietary fat intake have been associated with differences in the incidence of cancer in various populations.[1-6] The ingestion of high

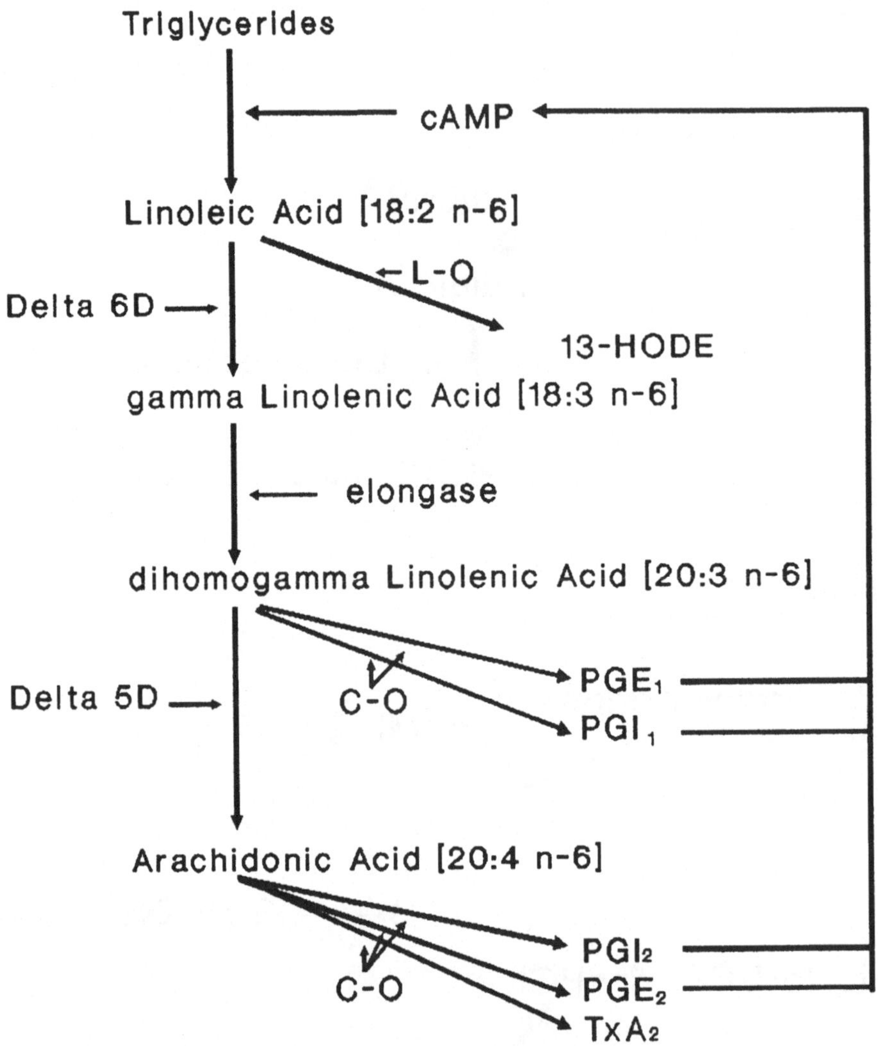

FIGURE 9. Metabolism of dietary essential fatty acids. Delta-5D and Delta-6D represent the desaturase enzymes creating double bonds at the 5 and 6 carbon positions. n-6 indicates the position of the first C-atom involved in a double bond determined from the terminal methyl group.

cholesterol diets and saturated fats are associated with an increased incidence of metastasis, whereas the ingestion of vegetable fats containing both linoleic acid and γ-linolenic acid is associated with a decreased incidence of metastasis. A number of hypothesis have been postulated to explain these effects. We will focus on one of these, but before doing so, we will first briefly review the metabolism of dietary fats.

Saturated fatty acids are synthesized in the body from the precursor, acetyl-Co-A.[82] However, polyunsaturated fatty acids, such as linoleic acid and α-linolenic acid, and their derivatives (e.g., arachidonic acid and eicosapentenoic acid) cannot be synthesized. These polyunsaturated fatty acids, therefore, are considered as "essential fatty acids" since they must be obtained directly from the diet. When linoleic acid is absorbed from the diet, it is metabolized by a number of desaturase and elongation steps, which eventually results in the formation of arachidonic acid (Figure 9). Approximately 1% of the linoleic acid liberated from the triglycerides stores is metabolized into 13-HODE. The remaining linoleic acid is desaturated and elongated into a sequential series of fatty acids, including dihomo-γ-linolenic acid, which precedes the formation of arachidonic acid (Figure 9). It should also be recognized that dihomo-γ-linolenic acid can be metabolized by the *cyclo-oxygenase pathway* into the prostanoid, PGE_1 (in cancer cells) or PGI_1 (in endothelial cells). Both metabolites are as effective as PGI_2 and 6-keto-PGE_1 in stimulating adenylate cyclase, thereby, elevating cAMP. It appears possible, therefore, that both of these prostanoids can act as a negative feedback mediator to enhance triglyceride turnover, liberation of linoleic acid, and 13-HODE synthesis following cell-cell interaction.

Booyens et al.[83-85] investigated the inhibitory effects of evening primrose (which contains high concentrations of both linoleic and γ-linolenic acid) on cancer cell growth and survival and found that the evening primrose decreased cancer cell growth *in vitro*. Van der Merwe found that there was a prolonged survival of patients with terminal cancer who ingested a dietary supplement of evening primrose.[86] Their explanation for these potentially antimetastatic effects was similar to the hypothesis proposed by Horrobin,[87] who said that cancer could be reversed by increasing the intracellular cAMP levels of malignant cells and that this effect was achieved by influencing the metabolism of essential fatty acids. In particular, when γ-linolenic is elongated to dihomo-γ-linolenic acid, dihomo-γ-linolenic acid can be metabolized to prostaglandin E_1 by the cyclo-oxygenase pathway. Prostaglandin E_1 (PGE_1) is as potent as PGI_2 in elevating cAMP and, presumably, renders cancer cells less "metastically abnormal". Other investigators have suggested that cancer cells with a high proliferative capacity often have a parallelled lowering of cAMP levels as compared to their parent cell line.[88-90] However, these investigations were not clear concerning the mechanism by which high cAMP levels rendered the cancer cells less metastatic.

Given that cancer cell proliferation requires cancer cell adhesion to a substrate, the most recent data suggest a possible explanation. Increasing the substrate, dihomo-γ-linolenic acid provides for an increased synthesis of PGE_1, which in turn increases 13-HODE synthesis by elevating cAMP. As a result, the cancer cells become less adhesive, cannot attach to the vessel wall surface, and escape into the extravascular tissue. Instead, they remain suspended in the circulating blood and are more vulnerable to killer cell-mediated defense mechanisms. Results from other studies are consistent with that possibility. Fujiwara et al.[91,92] found that exogenous γ-linolenic acid altered the membrane fatty acid composition of two human neuroblastoma cells, resulting in their dysfunction and subsequent death. Burns and Spector[93] demonstrated that cancer cells harvested from animals fed a linoleic acid-rich diet were more susceptible to chemotherapy and cell death. Linoleic acid is the substrate for both 13-HODE (via the cyclo-oxygenase pathway) and dihomo-γ-linolenic acid (via the desaturase/elongation process) (Figure 9). The growth of human breast carcinoma cells grown in athymic mice pretreated with evening primrose is also decreased.[2]

Other investigators raised the possibility that these fatty acids mediated a direct cytotoxic effect associated with the generation of free radicals. Thus, Das et al.[94] demonstrated that human breast adenocarcinoma cells exposed to essential fatty acids *in vitro* result in the generation of free radicals associated with elevated levels of lipid peroxidases and superoxide anion formation, all of which lead to cancer cell death. They based their conclusion on the observation that when vitamin E, an antioxidant that scavenges free radicals, was added back, the effect of the dietary fats on cancer cell death was minimized. However, most oxygen radicals *in vivo* are rapidly scavenged, and the possibility of such a cytotoxic effect occurring *in vivo* is very unlikely.

Other evidence suggest that delta-6-desaturase activity is lower in cancer cells than in their normal cell counterpart.[87] If so, this would reduce the elongation of linoleic acid to dihomo-γ-linolenic and arachidonic acids. At first glance, this may appear to be beneficial since it would suggest that synthesis of 13-HODE would be enhanced and 15-HETE synthesis would be decreased. However, this is unlikely to be the case. Excess accumulation of any of a number of unsaturated fatty acid, such as linoleic acid, suppresses hepatic fatty acid synthetase and decreases fatty acid release.[95] Consistent with that observation, we found that vessel wall/13-HODE synthesis was higher in animals that were fed a diet containing a lower amount of linoleic acid in combination with γ-linolenic acid, (43 and 16 molar percent, respectively) than in animals that were fed a diet containing higher amounts of linoleic acid (59 molar percent) and no γ-linolenic acid.[65,96]

Such selective effects of these essential fatty acids on subsequent metabolic activity also may explain the apparent inconsistencies associated with the prometastatic and antimetastatic potential of linoleic acid. For example, Hubbard et al.[97] found dose-related increases in metastasis of mammary tumors injected into the inguinal mammary fat pad of mice that were fed increasing amounts of linoleic acid. Interestingly, there was no difference in prostanoid synthesis by any of the cancer cells obtained from the different treatment groups, yet the author concluded that prostanoids played an important role in the enhanced metastatic effect since indomethacin, a reversible cyclo-oxygenase inhibitor, blocked the linoleate-induced metastasis. The authors did not consider, however, that inhibition of the cyclo-oxygenase pathway results in an enhanced production of lipoxygenase-derived metabolites, including 13-HODE (from linoleic acid) and 5-, 12- and/or 15-HETE (from arachidonic acid).[15,17,41,42,46,48,49,54] An alternative explanation for their results is that the high linoleic acid in the absence of γ-linolenic acid (which is elongated to dihomo-γ-linolenic acid) resulted in a shut-down of lipases, reducing the amount of linoleic acid liberated from the triyglycerides. This effect may be reversed by enhancing lipoxygenase activity or prostanoid production. Consistent with the latter possibility, when similar experiments were performed, feeding animals a dietary mixture containing both linoleic and γ-linolenic acid, metastasis was *inhibited* in a dose-related manner.[65,98,99]

IX. CONCLUDING REMARKS

Epidemiological studies and experimental studies performed both *in vivo* and *in vitro* provide an abundance of data which suggest that fatty acid metabolism plays an important role in cancer cell-endothelial cell interactions and subsequent metastasis. These studies have lead to a number of hypotheses to explain the modulating influence of fatty acid metabolites on metastasis. For the most part, however, our attention has been focussed on those metabolites derived from the essential fatty acid and arachidonic acid via the cyclo-oxygenase pathway. However, it is difficult to ignore the overwhelming evidence that the incidence of cancer and metastasis is lower in those populations that ingest a high amount of vegetable diets or dietary supplements containing both linoleic and γ-linolenic acid. Albeit incomplete, the recent studies in the last five years, which examine the one series of prostaglandins and the lipoxygenase metabolites derived both from linoleic and arachidonic acids, have added to our understanding of how these dietary fats may influence cancer. From the perspective of cancer cell-endothelial cell interactions, the data supports the hypothesis that a delicate balance in the synthesis of prostanoids (which upregulate cAMP activity) and the subsequent synthesis of 13-HODE from linoleic acid and the HETEs from arachidonic acid influence cancer cell/tumor cell adhesion moiety expression and subsequent interactions. 13-HODE appears to downregulate adhesion, and the arachidonic acid metabolites appear to upregulate adhesion. Prostanoids derived from dihomo-γ-linolenic acid and arachidonic acid enhance cAMP. However, other eicosanoids such as thromboxane A_2 and PGE_2 derived from arachidonic acid regulate other pathways in cancer cells and circulating blood cells, which may antagonize this effect. Hence, metabolism of dihomo-γ-linolenic acid by the cyclo-oxygenase pathway may better circumvent some of these unwanted responses and complete a better circuit to maintain this delicate homeostatic mechanism.

ACKNOWLEDGMENTS

The studies referred to from our laboratory were supported by a number of grants obtained from the Ontario Heart and Stroke Foundation, the Medical Research Council of Canada, and Merck-Frosst Canada.

REFERENCES

1. **Armstrong, B. and Doll, R.**, Environmental factors and cancer incidence and mortality in different countries, with special reference to dietary practices, *Int. J. Cancer,* 15, 617, 1975.
2. **Pritchard, G. A., Jones, D. L., and Mansel, R. E.**, Lipids in breast carcinogenesis, *Br. J. Surg.*, 76, 1069, 1989.
3. **Carroll, K. K. and Khor, H. T.**, Effects of dietary fat and dose level of 7,12-dimethylbenz-(α) anthracene on mammary tumour incidence in rats, *Cancer Res.*, 30, 2260, 1970.
4. **Carroll, K. K. and Khor, H. T.**, Dietary fat in relation to tumorigenesis, *Prog. Biochem. Pharmacol.*, 10, 308, 1975.
5. **Wynder, E. L. and Hiyama, T.**, Comparative epidemiology of cancer in the United States and Japan: preventive implications, *Gann Monogr. Cancer Res.*, 33, 183, 1987.
6. **La Vecchia, C., Harris, R., and Wynder, E. L.**, Comparative epidemiology of cancer between the United States and Italy, *Cancer Res.*, 48, 7285, 1988.
7. **Funk, C. D. and Powell, W. S.**, Metabolism of linoleic acid by prostaglandin endoperoxide synthase from adult fetal blood vessels, *Biochim. Biophys. Acta,* 754, 57, 1983.
8. **Lagarde, M., Sicard, B., Guichardant, M., Felisi, O., and Dechavanne, M.**, Fatty acid composition in native and cultured human endothelial, *In Vitro,* 20, 33, 1984.
9. **Moncada, S., Herman, A. G., Higgs, E. A., and Vane, J. R.**, Differential formation of prostacyclin (PGX or PGI) by layers of the arterial wall. An explanation for the anti-thrombotic properties of vascular endothelium, *Thromb. Res.*, 11, 323, 1977.
10. **Moncada, S., Gryglewski, R., Bunting, S., and Vane, J. R.**, An enzyme isolated from arteries transforms prostaglandin endoperoxides to an unstable substance that inhibits platelets aggregation, *Nature,* 263, 663, 1976.
11. **Dejana, E., Balconi, G., Castellarnau, C. D., Barbieri, B., Vergara-Dauden, M., and Gaetano, G. D.**, Prostacyclin production by human endothelial and bovine smooth muscle cells in culture, *Biochim. Biophys. Acta,* 750, 261, 1983.
12. **Buchanan, M. R., Crozier, G. L., and Haas, T. A.**, Fatty acid metabolism and the vasculature endothelial cell, *Haemostasis,* 18, 360, 1988.
13. **Dejana, E., Breviario, F., Erroi, A., Bussolino, F., Mussoni, L., Gramse, M., Pintucci, G., Casali, B., Dinarello, C. A., Van Damme, J., Jr., Mantovani, A.**, Modulation of endothelial cell function by different molecular species of interleukin 1, *Blood,* 69, 695, 1987.
14. **Buchanan, M. R.**, Uncontrolled PGI_2 production by whole vessel wall segments due to thrombin generation *in vivo* and its prevention by heparin, *Thromb. Res.*, 16, 551, 1979.
15. **Hamberg, M., Svensson, J., and Samuelsson,B.**, Prostaglandin endoperoxides, a new concept concerning the mode of action and release of prostaglandins, *Proc. Natl. Acad. Sci. U.S.A.*, 71, 3824, 1974.
16. **Warso, M. A. and Lands, W. E. M.**, Lipid peroxidation in relation to prostacyclin and thromboxane physiology and pathophysiology, *Br. Med. Bull.*, 39, 277, 1983.
17. **Marcus, A. J.**, Transcellular metabolism of eicosanoids, *Prog. Hemost. Thromb.*, 8, 127, 1986.
18. **Hamberg, M., Svensson, J., and Wakabayashi, T.**, Isolation and structure of two prostaglandin endoperoxides that cause platelet aggregation, *Proc. Natl. Acad. Sci. U.S.A.*, 71, 345, 1974.
19. **Ingerman-Wolenski, C., Silver, M. I., Smith, J. B., and Macarack, E.**, Bovine endothelial cells in culture produce thromboxane as well as prostacyclin, *J. Clin. Invest.*, 67, 1292, 1981.
20. **Weksler, B. B., Marcus, A. J., and Jaffe, E. A.**, Synthesis of prostaglandin I2 (prostacyclin) by cultured human and bovine endothelial cells, *Proc. Natl. Acad. Sci. U.S.A.*, 74, 3922, 1977.
21. **Ali, A. E., Barret, J. C., and Eling, T. E.**, Prostaglandin and thromboxane production by fibroblasts and vascular endothelial cells, *Prostaglandins,* 20, 667, 1988.
22. **Gorman, R. R., Bunting, S., and Miller, D. V.**, Modulation of human platelet adenylate cyclase by prostacyclin (PGX), *Prostaglandins,* 13, 377, 1977.

23. **Hajjar, D. P., Weksler, B. B., Falcone, D. J., Hefton, J. M., Tack-Goldman, K., and Minick, C. R.,** Prostacyclin modulates cholesteryl ester hydrolytic activity by its effects on cyclic adenosine monophosphate in rabbit aortic smooth muscle cell, *J. Clin. Invest.*, 70, 479, 1982.
24. **Pohlman, T., Yates, J., Needleman, P., and Klahr, S.,** Effects of prostacyclin on short-circuit current and water flow in the food urinary bladder, *Am. J. Physiol.*, 244, 270, 1983.
25. **Moncada, S. and Vane, J. R.,** Arachidonic acid metabolites and the interactions between platelets and blood-vessel walls, *N. Engl. J. Med.*, 300, 1142, 1979.
26. **Honn, K. V. and Marnett, L. J.,** Prostaglandin, thromboxane, and leukotriene biosynthesis: target for antitumor and antimetastatic agents, in *Novel Approaches to Cancer Therapy*, Honn, K. V. and Marnett, L. J., Eds., Academic Press, New York, 1984, 128.
27. **Karpatkin, S. and Pearlstein, E.,** Role of platelets in tumor cell metastases, *Ann. Intern. Med.*, 95, 636, 1981.
28. **Gasic, G., Gasic, T., Stewart, C. C.,** Anti-metastatic effects associated with platelet reduction, *Proc. Natl. Acad. Sci. U.S.A.*, 61, 46, 1968.
29. **Hildgard, P.,** Blood platelets and experimental metastasis, in *Platelets a Multidisciplinary Approach*, de Gaetano, G., Ed., Raven Press, New York, 1978, 107.
30. **Honn, K. V. and Dunn, J. R.,** Nafazatrom (Bay g 6575) inhibition of tumor cell lipoxygenase activity and cellular proliferation, *FEBS Lett.*, 139, 65, 1982.
31. **Buchanan, M. R. and Hirsch, J.,** Effect of aspirin on hemostasis and thrombosis, *N. Engl. Reg. Allergy Proc.*, 7, 6, 1986.
32. **Karpatkin, S., Ambrogio, C., and Pearlstein, E.,** Lack of effect of *in vivo* prostacyclin on the development of pulmonary metastasis in mice following intravenous injection of CT26 colon carcinoma, Lewis lung carcinoma or B16 amelanotic melanoma cells, *Cancer Res.*, 44, 3880, 1984.
33. **Mehta, J., Mehta, P., Lawson, D. L., Ostrowski, N., and Brigmon, L.,** Influence of selective thromboxane synthetase blocker CGS-13080 on thromboxane and prostacyclin biosynthesis in whole blood: evidence for synthesis of prostacyclin by leukocytes from platelet-derived endoperoxides, *J. Lab. Clin. Med.*, 106, 246, 1985.
34. **Mehta, P., Mehta, J., Lawson, D., and Patel, S.,** Ethanol stimulates prostacyclin biosynthesis by human neutrophils and potentiates anti-platelet aggregatory effects of prostacyclin, *Thromb. Res.*, 48, 653, 1987.
35. **Wong, P. Y. K., Lee, W. H., Chao, P. H. W., Reiss, R. F., and McGiff, J. C.,** Metabolism of prostacyclin by 9-hydroxy-prostaglandin dehydrogenase in human platelets, *J. Biol. Chem.*, 255, 9021, 1980.
36. **Wong, P. Y. K., McGiff, J. C., Sun, F. F., and Lee, W. H.,** 6-ketoprostaglandin E inhibits the aggregation of human platelets, *Eur. J. Pharmacol.*, 60, 245, 1979.
37. **Chang, D. G. B. and Tai, H. H.,** A radioimmunoassay for 6-ketoprostaglandin E_1, *Prost. Leuk. Med.*, 8, 11, 1982.
38. **Gibson, B. E. S., Buchanan, M. R., Barr, R. D., White, J. G.,** Primary thrombocythaemia in childhood: symptomatic episodes and their relationship to thromboxane A2, 6-keto-PGE_1 and 12-hydroxyeicosatetraenoic acid production: a case report, *Prost. Leuk. Med.*, 26, 221, 1987.
39. **Adaikan, P. G., Tai, M. Y., Lau, L. C., Karim, S. M. M., and Kottegoda, S. R.,** A comparison of some pharmacological actions of prostaglandin E1, 6-OXO-PGE1 and PGI2, *Prostaglandins*, 27, 505, 1984.
40. **Buchanan, M. R.,** Inhibition of thrombosis by leukocytes: role of endogenous fatty acid metabolites, in *Fondation Sanofi Thrombose pour La Recherche*, Choay, H., Ed., Choay Foundation, Paris, 1989, 14.
41. **Buchanan, M. R., Nakamura, K., Haas, T. A., and Hullin, F.,** Endothelium blood cell interactions: role of fatty acid metabolism, in *Biology of Icosanoids*, Lagarde, M., Ed., Colloque INSERUM, Paris, 1987, 247.
42. **Lagarde, M., Croset, M., Authi, K. S., and Crawford, N.,** Subcellular localization and some properties of lipoxygenase activity in human blood platelets, *Biochem. J.*, 222, 495, 1984.
43. **Greenwald, J. E., Bianchine, J. R., and Wong, L. K.,** The production of the arachidonate metabolite HETE in vascular tissue, *Nature*, 281, 588, 1979.
44. **Hopkins, N. K., Oglesby, T. D., Bundy, G. L., and Gorman, R. R.,** Biosynthesis and metabolism of 15-hydroperoxy-5,8,11,13-eicosatetraenoic acid by human umbilical vein endothelial cells, *J. Biol. Chem.*, 259, 14048, 1984.
45. **Kuhn, H., Ponicke, K., Halle, W., Wiesner, R., Schewe, T., and Forster, W.,** Metabolism of (1-14C) — arachidonic acid by cultured calf aortic endothelial cells: evidence for the presence of a lipoxygenase pathway, *Prost. Leuk. Med.*, 17, 291, 1985.
46. **Buchanan, M. R., Butt, R. W., Magas, Z., Van Ryn, J., Hirsh, J., and Nazir, D. J.,** Endothelial cells produce a lipoxygenase derived chemorepellent which influences platelet/endothelial cell interactions: effects of aspirin and salicylate, *Thromb. Haemost.*, 53, 306, 1985.
47. **Brister, S. J., Haas, T. A., Bertomeu, M. C., Austin, J., Buchanan, M. R.,** 13-HODE synthesis in internal mammary arteries and saphenous veins: implications in cardiovascular surgery, in *Advances in Prostaglandin and Thromboxane Leukotriene Research*, Samuelson, B., Ramwell, P. W., Paoletti, R., Folco, G., Gramstrom, E., Eds., Raven Press, New York, 1990, 21.

48. **Buchanan, M. R., Blajchman, M., and Hirsh, J.**, Inhibition of arterial thrombosis and platelet function by nafazatrom, *Thromb. Res.*, 28, 157, 1982.
49. **Buchanan, M. R. and Hirsh, J.**, Effect of aspirin and salicylate on platelet-vessel wall interactions in rabbit, *Arteriosclerosis*, 4, 403, 1984.
50. **Weber, E., Haas, T. A., Muller, T. H., Eisert, W. G., Hirsh, J., Richardson, M., and Buchanan, M. R.**, Relationship between vessel wall 13-HODE synthesis and vessel wall thrombogenecity following injury: influence of salicylate and dipyridamole treatment, *Thromb. Res.*, 57, 383, 1990.
51. **Kelton, J. G., Hirsh, J., Carter, C. J., and Buchanan, M. R.**, Thrombogenic effect of high-dose aspirin in rabbits, *J. Clin. Invest.*, 62, 892, 1978.
52. **Buchanan, M. R. and Bastida, E.**, The role of 13-HODE and HETE's in vessel wall/circulating blood cell interactions, *Agents Actions*, 3, 337, 1987.
53. **Denning, G. M., Figard, P. H., Kaduce, T. L., and Spector, A. A.**, Role of triglycerides in endothelial cell arachidonic acid metabolism, *J. Lipid Res.*, 24, 993, 1983.
54. **Buchanan, M. R., Haas, T. A., Lagarde, M., and Guichardant, M.**, 13-Hydroxyoctadecadienoic acid is the vessel wall chemorepellent factor, LOX, *J. Biol. Chem.*, 260, 16056, 1985.
55. **Haas, T. A., Bertomeu, M. C., Bastida, E., and Buchanan, M. R.**, Cyclic AMP regulation of endothelial cell triacylglycerol turnover, 13-hydroxyoctadecadienoic acid (13-HODE) synthesis and endothelial cell thrombogenecity, *Biochim. Biophys. Acta*, 1051, 174, 1990.
56. **Bastida, E., Bertomeu, M. C., Haas, T. A., Almirall, L., Lauri, D., Orr, F. W., and Buchanan, M. R.**, Regulation of tumor cell adhesion by intracellular 13-HODE: 15-HETE ratio, *J. Lipid Med.*, 2, 281, 1990.
57. **Bastida, E., Almirall, L., Ordinas, A., Buchanan, M. R., Bertomeu, M. C., and Haas, T. A.**, Effects of antiplatelet drugs and cytokines on endothelial cell 13-HODE synthesis and tumor cell/endothelial cell adhesion, *Thromb. Haemost.*, 62, 443, 1989.
58. **Kaduce, T. L., Figard, P. H., Leifur, R., and Spector, A. A.**, Formation of 9-hydroxyoctadecadienoic acid from linoleic acid in endothelial cells, *J. Biol. Chem.*, 264, 6823, 1989.
59. **McLemore, T. L., Hubbard, W. C., Litterst, C. L., Liu, M. C., Miller, S., McMahon, N. A., Eggleston, J. C., and Boyd, M. R.**, Profiles of prostaglandin biosynthesis in normal lung and tumor tissue from lung cancer patients, *Cancer Res.*, 48, 3140, 1988.
60. **Lau, S. S., McMahon, J. B., McMenamin, M. G., Schuller, H. M., and Boyd, M. R.**, Metabolism of arachidonic acid in human lung cancer cell lines, *Cancer Res.*, 47, 3757, 1987.
61. **Fulton, A. M.**, The role of eicosanoids in tumor metastasis, *Prost. Leuk. Essen. Fatty Acids*, 34, 229, 1988.
62. **Bennett, A., Charler, E. M., McDonald, A. M., Simpson, J. S., Stamford, I. F., and Zebro, T.**, Prostaglandins and breast cancer, *Lancet*, 2, 624, 1977.
63. **Rolland, P. H., Martin, P. M., Jacquemier, J., Rolland, A. M., and Toga, M.**, Prostaglandins in human breast cancer: evidence suggesting that an elevated prostaglandin production is a marker of high metastatic potential for neoplastic cells, *J. Natl. Cancer Inst.*, 64, 1061, 1980.
64. **Vergate, I. B., Laekeman, G. M., Keersmakers, G. H., Uyllenbroeck, F. L., Vanderheyden, J. S., Abbertyn, G. P., Haensch, C. F., De Roy, G. J., and Herman, A. F.**, Prostaglandin $F_{2\alpha}$ in benign and malignant breast tumors, *Br. J. Cancer*, 51, 827, 1985.
65. **Bertomeu, M. C., Crozier, G. L., and Buchanan, M. R.**, Differential effects of dietary fats on primary tumor growth and secondary metastasis, Proc. 7th Int. Conf. Prostaglandins Related Compounds, Florence, May 28 to June 1, 1990, 277.
66. **Lafrenie, R. M., Podor, T. J., Buchanan, M. R., and Orr, F. W.**, Interleukin-1α induced vitronectin receptor expression and tumor cell endothelial cell adhesion, *FASEB*, 4, A1134, 1990.
67. **Cheresh, D. A., Smith, J. W., Cooper, H. M., and Quaranta, V.**, A novel vitronectin receptor integrin (alpha v beta x) is responsible for distinct adhesive properties of carcinoma cells, *Cell*, 57, 59, 1989.
68. **Grossi, I. M., Fitzgerald, L. A., Umbarger, L. A., Nelson, K. K., Diglio, C. A., Taylor, J. D., and Honn, K. V.**, Bidirectional control of membranes expression and/or activation of tumor cell IRGpIIb/IIIa receptor and tumor cell adhesion by lipoxygenase products of arachidonic acid and linoleic acid, *Cancer Res.*, 49, 1029, 1989.
69. **Bertomeu, M. C., Whybourne, K., Orr, F. W., and Buchanan, M. R.**, Influence of interleukin 1 on 13-HODE synthesis, integrin expression and B16 melanoma cell metastasis *in vivo*, in Proc. 1st Intl. Conf. Eicosanoids Bioactive Lipids in Cancer and Radiation Injury, Detroit, 1989, IIB-2.
70. **Buchanan, M. R., Bertomeu, M. C., and Bastida, E.**, Fatty acid metabolism and cell/cell interactions, *Agents Actions*, 29, 16, 1990.
71. **Conforti, G., Zanetti, A., Pasquali-Ronchetti, I., Quaglino, D., Jr., Neyroz, P., and Dejana, E.**, Modulation of vitronectin receptor binding by membrane lipid composition, *J. Biol. Chem.*, 265, 4011, 1990.
72. **Aznar-Salatti, J., Bastida, E., Buchanan, M. R., Castillo, R., Ordinas, A., and Escolar, G.**, Differential localization of von Willebrand factor, fibronectin and 13-HODE in human endothelial cell culture, *Histochemistry*, 93, 507, 1990.

73. **Singer, I. I., Scott, S., Kawka, D. W, and Kazazis, D. M.,** Adhesomes: specific granules containing receptors for laminin, C_3bi/fibrinogen, fibronectin, and vitronectin in human polymorphonuclear leukocytes and monocytes, *J. Cell Biol.*, 109, 3169, 1989.
74. **Gullick, W. I. and Waterfirld, M. D.,** Experimental growth factor and its receptor, in *Molecular Biology of Receptors*, Strosberg, A. D., Ed., Ellis Howard, Chichester, 1987, 15.
75. **Kudlow, J. E., Cheung, C.-Y. M., and Bjorge, T. D.,** Epidemial growth factor stimulates the synthesis of its own receptor in a human breast cancer cell line, *J. Biol. Chem.*, 261, 4134, 1986.
76. **Sainburg, J. R. C., Faindern, J. R., Needham, G. K., Malcolm, A. J., and Haries, A. L.,** Epidermal growth factor receptor status as a predictor of early recurrence and death from breast cancer, *Lancet*, 1398, 1987.
77. **Gleeson, R. P., Ayub, M., Wright, J. T., Wood, C. B., Habib, N. A., Soutter, S. P., Sullivan, M. H. F., and White, J. O.,** Fatty acid control of growth of human cervical and endometrial cancer cells, *Br. J. Cancer*, 61, 500, 1990.
78. **Haas, T. A., Bastida, E., Nakamura, K., Hullin, F., Almirall, L., and Buchanan, M. R.,** Binding of 13-HODE, 5-, 12- and 15-HETE to endothelial cells and subsequent platelet, neutrophil and tumor cell adhesion, *Biochem. Biophys. Acta*, 961, 153, 1988.
79. **Buchanan, M. R. and Bastida, E.,** Endothelial and underlying membrane reactivity with platelets, leukocytes and tumor cells: regulation by the lipoxygenase-derived fatty acid metabolites, 13-HODE and HETEs, *Med. Hypothesis*, 27, 317, 1988.
80. **Buchanan, M. R., Bertomeu, M. C., Haas, T. A., Gallo, S., and Eltringham-Smith, L.,** Endothelial Cell 13-HODE synthesis and tumor cell endothelial cell adhesion, in *Advances in Prostaglandin Thromboxane and Leukotriene Research*, Samuelson, B., Ramwell, P. W., Paoletti, R., Folco, G., Gramstrom, E., Eds., Raven Press, New York, 1990, 21.
81. **Buchanan, M. R., Bertomeu, M. C., Brister, S. J., Lafrenie, R. M., Haas, T. A., Orr, F. W., and Bastida, E.,** Vessel wall 13-HODE synthesis, vitronectin expression and metastasis: *in vitro* and *in vivo* studies, Proc. 7th Int. Conf. Prostaglandins Related Compounds, Florence, May 28 to June 1, 1990, 214.
82. **Sprecher, H. and James, A. T.,** Biosynthesis of long-chain fatty acids in mammalian systems, in *Geometrial and Positional Fatty Acids Isomers*, Em Keu, E. A. and Dutton, H. J., Eds., American Oil Chemist's Society, Washington, D.C., 1979, 303.
83. **Booyens, J., Dippenaar, N., Fabbri, D., Engelbrecht, P., and Katzeff, I. E.,** The effect of gamma-linolenic acid on the growth of human osteogenic sarcoma and esophageal carcinoma cells in culture, *S. Afr. Med. J.*, 65, 204, 1984.
84. **Booyens, J., Dippenaar, N., Fabbri, D., Engelbrecht, P., Louwrens, C. C., and Katzeff, I. E.,** Some effects of linoleic acid and gamma-linolenic acid on the proliferation of human hepatoma cells in culture, *S. Afr. Med. J.*, 65, 607, 1984.
85. **Dippenaar, N., Booyens, J., Fabbri, D., and Katzeff, I. E.,** The reversibility of cancer: evidence that malignancy in melanoma cells is gamma-linolenic acid deficiency-dependent, *S. Afr. Med. J.*, 62, 505, 1982.
86. **van der Merwe, C. F.,** Evening primrose oil in cancer treatment. Follow-up of an ongoing pilot open clinical trial, Proc. 7th Int. Conf. Prostaglandins Related Compounds, Florence, May 28 to June 1, 1990, 279.
87. **Horrobin, D. F.,** The reversibility of cancer: the relevance of cyclic AMP, calcium, essential fatty acids and prostaglandins E_1, *Med. Hypothesis*, 6, 469, 1980.
88. **Hsie, A. W., Jones, C., and Puck, T. T.,** Further changes in differentiation state accompanying the conversion of Chinese hamster cells to fibroblast HC form by dibutyryl adenosine cyclic monophosphate and hormones, *Proc. Nat. Acad. Sci. U.S.A.*, 68, 1648, 1971.
89. **Puck, T. T.,** Cyclic AMP, the microtubule/microfilament system and cancer, *Proc. Nat. Acad. Sci. U.S.A.*, 74, 4491, 1977.
90. **Pastan, I., Willingham, M., Carchman, R., et al.,** Cyclic AMP metabolism in normal and transformed fibroblast, in *The Role of Cyclic Nucleotids in Carcinogenesis*, Schultz, J. and Gratzner, H. G., Eds., Academic Press, New York, 1973, 44.
91. **Fujiwara, F., Todo, S., and Imashuku, S.,** Fatty acid modification of cultured neuroblastoma cells by gamma linolenic acid relevant to its antitumor effect, *Prost. Leuk. Med.*, 30, 37, 1987.
92. **Fujiwara, F., Todo, S., and Imashuku, S.,** Antitumor effect of gamma-linolenic acid on cultured human neuroblastoma cells, *Prost. Leuk. Med.*, 23, 311, 1986.
93. **Burns, C. P. and Spector, A. A.,** Membrane fatty acid modification in tumor cells: a potential therapeutic adjunct, *Lipids*, 22, 178, 1987.
94. **Das, U. N., Huang, Y. S., Begin, M. E., Ells, G., and Horrobin, D. F.,** Uptake and distribution of CIS-unsaturated fatty acid and their effects of free radical generation in normal and tumor cells *in vitro*, *J. Free Rad. Biol. Med.*, 3, 9, 1987.
95. **Kandutsch, A. A. and Hancock, R. L.,** Regulation of the rate of sterol synthesis and the level of beta-hydroxy-beta-methylglutaryl coenzyme A reductase activity in mouse liver and hepatomas, *Cancer Res.*, 31, 1396, 1971.

96. **Bertomeu, M. C., Crozier, G. L., Haas, T. A., Fleith, M., and Buchanan, M. R.,** Selective effects of dietary fats on vascular 13-HODE synthesis and platelet/vessel wall interactions. *Thromb. Res.*, 59, 819, 1990.
97. **Hubbard, N. E., Chapkin, R. S., and Erickson, K. L.,** Inhibition of growth and linoleate-enhanced metastasis of a transplantable mouse mammary tumor indomethacin, *Cancer Lett.*, 43, 111, 1988.
98. **Sobajima, T., Tamiya-Koizumi, K., Ishihara, H., and Kojima, K.,** Effects of fatty acid modification of ascites' tumor cells on pulmonary metastasis in rat, *Jpn. J. Cancer Res.*, 77, 657, 1986.
99. **Robinson, K. M. and Botha, J. H.,** Effects of gamma-linolenic acid, dihomo-gamma-linolenic acid and ethanol on cultured human mammary carcinoma cells, *Prost. Leuk. Med.*, 20, 209, 1985.

Chapter 15

THE INFLUENCE OF ENDOTHELIAL INJURY AND INFLAMMATORY PROCESSES ON METASTASIS

F. William Orr

TABLE OF CONTENTS

I. INTRODUCTION

The bloodstream is the main route for the transport of cancer cells from primary tumors to the distant sites where they proliferate to form metastatic tumors. At the same time, the circulatory pathways do not constitute ideal environments for the growth and survival of these cells. Indeed, as pointed out by Weiss (Chapter 9), many cancer cells are destroyed during the hematogenous phase of metastasis. Thus, the microvasculature can be regarded as a major regulator of cancer metastasis.[1,2] Since endothelial cells and their basement membranes are the main barriers to entry and exit of cancer cells to and from the bloodstream, it has been postulated that damage to these structures might occur during metastasis. If superimposed on the metastatic process, vessel wall injury would facilitate cancer dissemination by removing the barrier between the circulation and the extravascular tissue. Indeed, morphologic studies of metastasis (described by Crissman in Chapter 13) and functional studies (reviewed by Terranova in Chapter 2) have indicated that injury to basement membranes is a major feature of the transvascular passage of cancer cells.

The microvasculature, especially the endothelium, is susceptible to damage from irradiation, drugs and environmental toxins, intravascular leukocytes, and ischemia-reperfusion. Cells of the pulmonary microvasculature, situated in an organ that is a frequent site for metastatic tumor growth, are particularly vulnerable to such injuries. In this chapter, I will review major points of evidence that endothelial damage can promote cancer metastasis, and I will discuss some of the pathophysiologic mechanisms that relate to this evidence.

II. EVIDENCE THAT ENDOTHELIAL CELL INJURY PROMOTES METASTASIS

A. PHYSICIAL TRAUMA

There is a large number of literature concerning the formation of metastatic tumors at sites of tissue trauma such as fractures, needle tracts, and surgical wounds;[3-7] this has been reviewed recently.[8] Since some of these metastatic sites were far from the primary tumor, the phenomenon cannot be explained entirely on the basis of direct local spread of tumor cells. Early observations led to experimental studies that demonstrated enhanced localization of intravascular radiolabeled cancer cells at sites of trauma, suggesting a regional mechanism.[9] However, in other experiments, the induction of distant metastases suggested activation of one or more systemic processes such as changes in vessel wall adhesiveness, blood coagulation, and/or platelet activation.[7,10,11]

B. IRRADIATION

Endothelium and vessel walls are susceptible to injury by irradiation. The responses of endothelial cells *in vitro* and *in vivo* are characterized by altered prostaglandin metabolism, incorporation of ^{3}H-thymidine, permeability changes, increased adhesiveness for leukocytes and platelets, lysis, and detachment of cells from the substrate.[12] These are of potential importance in metastasis. Clinical evidence showing that irradiation might facilitate tumor spread was suggested by increased formation of metastatic tumors in the skin and lung of breast cancer patients after radiotherapy.[13] Further, the proportion of breast cancer patients whose treatment failures presented as distant metastases was greater after irradiation.[14]

Irradiation of *primary* tumors can lead to an increase in metastatic frequency of some experimental and human cancers, e.g., veruccous carcinoma of the larynx.[15] While this might be due to an effect on the cancer cell,[16] there is also evidence that damage to the supporting connective tissue of the tumor, the so-called "tumor bed effect", can facilitate metastasis while resulting in decreased growth of the primary tumor.[17] This has been postulated to result from increased permeability of the irradiated vessels,[18,19] tumor necrosis,[17] or a growth-promoting effect on the metastatic cancer cells.[20]

It also has been established that irradiation of *metastatic* target organs (usually the lungs or liver) prior to giving animals an intravenous injection of cancer cells results in greatly increased number of target organ metastases.[21,22] Other studies have shown that prophylactic irradiation increases the incidence of spontaneous pulmonary metastases from a canine osteosarcoma.[23] The effects in experimental studies are likely to be local as they can be prevented in one lung if that lung is shielded from the X-ray.[21,24] They are dependent upon radiation dose and the interval between radiation and tumor cell injection;[21,22,24] maximum enhancement occurred when cancer cells were injected at times of greatest injury (judged histologically).[21,24] The phenomenon of post-radiation enhancement could be correlated with increased retention of cancer cells in irradiated lungs[22,25,26] and was speculated to relate to increased penetration of tumor cells through damaged endothelial cells[25] or to increased tumor growth.[24] The experimental design in these studies indicated that the effect was unlikely to be due to generalized immunosuppression.[22,24]

C. CHEMOTHERAPEUTIC DRUGS AND TOXINS

Noting the studies in which irradiation of rodent lungs had enhanced the development of pulmonary metastases by intravenously injected cancer cells, van Putten et al. demonstrated that treatment of mice with several commonly employed cytostatic drugs increased the metastastasis of a nonimmunogenic murine osteosarcoma after intravenous injection of cancer cells.[27] The magnitude of the increase in numbers of lung nodules was variable from drug to drug, but treatment with cyclophosphamide, in particular, amplified pulmonary metastasis by as much as 1000-fold. These authors provided evidence that the promoting effect of the drugs was not related to immunosuppression and suggested injury to an unidentified host target cell as the mechanism for increased lung metastasis.

These observations have been corroborated in models of spontaneous metastasis[28,29] and metastasis of intravenously-injected cancer cells.[30-32] Some additional findings are noteworthy. Moore and Dixon[28] reported greater amplification of lung metastasis when cyclophosphamide treatment was coupled with irradiation. Carmel and Brown,[30] Steel and Adams,[31] and Gasic et al.,[32] found that metastatic enhancement was optimized if drug treatment was given 2 to 4 d *before* the injection of tumor cells. Histologic studies by Steel and Adams on the lungs of cyclophosphamide-treated, nontumor-bearing mice showed evidence of acute pulmonary injury with congestion, edema, and hyperplasia of cellular elements. Indeed, the peak of metastatic enhancement was noted to coincide with the period of acute injury.[31] Poupon et al.[29] found that pretreatment or treatment of tumor-bearing rats with the nitrosourea, CZT, resulted in enhanced spontaneous metastasis of a transplantable rhabdomysarcoma. These workers were unable to demonstrate that drug treatment altered the subsequent metastatic potential of surviving tumor cells, suggesting that the promotion of metastasis was due to an effect of the drug on the host rather than on the cancer cell. Gasic et al.[32] were able to block the drug effect by simultaneous treatment of animals with leech salivary gland extract. The latter, which inhibits platelet aggregation and acts as an inhibitor of proteolytic enzymes, decreased the retention of radiolabeled cancer cells in the lung after intravenous injection, but this effect did not appear to be related to an effect on NK cell activity or to a cytotoxic effect of leech extract on cancer cells.[32] While Carmel and Brown failed to alter the metastatic pattern by anticoagulants, their results also suggested that an immunosuppressive mechanism was unlikely to be operant.[30] They, Gasic et al.[32] and Poupon et al.,[29] speculated that cytotoxic drugs might facilitate metastasis by inducing damage to the pulmonary microvasculature, but this mechanism was not examined directly.

Based on these observations, we and others have sought more direct evidence for relationships between pulmonary endothelial injury and the promotion of metastasis. This has been accomplished by taking advantage of *in vivo* models where there is a predictable sequence of lung endothelial injury and repair after exposure of animals to cytotoxic drugs or hyperoxia (Table 1).

TABLE 1
Effects of Acute Pulmonary Microvascular Injury and Repair on the Metastasis of Experimental Cancer Cell Lines

Treatment	Tumor line/species	Interval[a]	Index of injury	Effect on metastasis 24 h[b]	Effect on metastasis 14 d[c]	Ref.
Bleomycin (120 mg/kg single i.v. injection)	Fibrosarcoma/C57bl/6 mouse					
	Test	5 d	0.43[d]	10.9	6.4	36,37
	Test	10 d	0.36	4.2	4.2	
	Test	21 d	0.19	0.5	0.4	
	Saline control	5 d	0.18	1.8	0.9	
Hyperoxic atmosphere (90% oxygen for 4 d)	Fibrosarcoma/C57bl/6 mouse					
	Test	0	0.85[d]	47.0	12.6	46
	Air control	0	0.08	1.6	2.2	
Monocrotaline pyrrole (60 mg/kg single i.v. injection)	Walker carcinosarcoma/Wistar rat					
	Test	10 d	0.45[d]	6.6	39.4	39
	Saline control	—	0.09	2.7	3.1	
Cobra venom factor (5 units single i.v. injection)	Walker carcinosarcoma/Sprague-Dawley rat					
	Test	Simult	368[e]	10.2	5.2	48
	Control	Simult	13	4.2	1.0	
	Fibrosarcoma/C57BL/6 mouse					
	Test	Simult	12.3[f]	4.5	5.5	64
	Control	Simult	0.2	1.4	0.5	

[a] Microvascular injury was assessed, and cancer cells were injected i.v. at various times after administration of the treatment. "0" indicates that cells were administered immediately following cessation of the treatment. "Simult" indicates simultaneous administration of cancer cells and the toxic agent.
[b] % of ^{125}IUDr-labeled cancer cells in lungs 24 h after i.v. injection.
[c] % of host lung occupied by metastatic cancer 14 d after i.v. cancer cells.
[d] Protein levels in bronchoalveolar lavage fluids (mg/ml).
[e] dpm ^{125}I-albumin/mg dry lung 30 min after leukocyte activation.
[f] μg intravenously-injected Evans blue/mg dry lung.

1. Bleomycin

Bleomycin, a glycopeptide-derived antibiotic, is used as a chemotherapeutic agent in many cancer treatment protocols. The drug binds to DNA in the form of an iron-bleomycin complex, which reacts with molecular oxygen to produce reactive oxygen species, including superoxide anion and hydroxyl radical. This leads to DNA fragmentation by the oxygenation of deoxyribose and to the generation of free bases as well as to the peroxidation of cell membrane lipids.[33,34] While this action accounts for the beneficial effects of the drug as an anticancer drug, it also relates to the side effects of bleomycin on the lung, including the production of pulmonary fibrosis. Following a single intravenous injection, the initiating event in pulmonary damage is injury to the endothelium followed by a well characterized sequence of events, including endothelial regeneration, focal epithelial injury, and pulmonary fibrosis.[35] To look for a relationship between this injury-repair sequence and metastasis, C57BL/6 mice were given a single i.v. injection of bleomycin (120 mg/kg). Five days later,

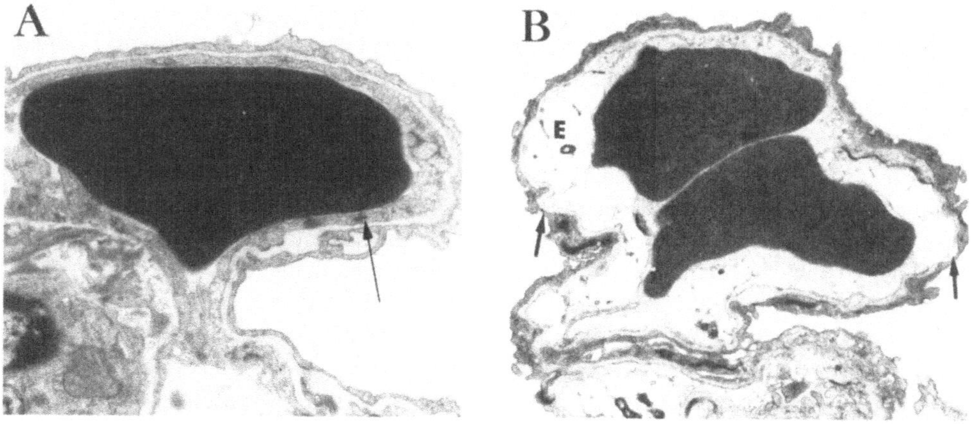

FIGURE 1. A: Ultrastructure of a normal murine pulmonary capillary. The air-blood barrier consists of a thin Type 1 epithelial cell separated by a continuous basement membrane from a thin endothelial lining (arrow). × 11,840. B: 5 d after bleomycin. The endothelial lining (E) is swollen and disrupted. In some places, the cells have become separated from the underlying basement membrane (arrows). × 7,770.

endothelial injury was detected by bronchoalveolar lavage with an increase in total bronchoalveolar lavage (BAL) protein as well as leakage of previously-injected intravenous ^{125}I-albumin into the BAL fluids. Electron microscopy of the pulmonary capillaries demonstrated edema of the endothelial cells as well as the areas of denuded basement membrane (Figure 1). When radiolabeled fibrosarcoma cells were injected during this period, the percentage of cells retained in the bleomycin-injured lungs, liver, and kidney after 24 h increased 2 to 8 times that seen in controls. The bleomycin-treated animals also developed a greater number of metastases after 14 d.[36] However, if cancer cells were injected after endothelial repair, the number of cancer cells that localized in the lung and the number of subsequent metastatic tumors was the same as in control animals, even though there was pulmonary fibrosis.[37] Thus, in this model, there was a direct correlation between the alteration in endothelial integrity after bleomycin and the effect on metastasis.

2. Pyrrolizidine Alkaloids

Monocrotaline is a pyrrolizidine alkaloid present in the seeds and leaves of the leguminous plant *Crotalaria spectabilis*. Rats given a single subcutaneous injection of monocrotaline develop a severe, well-studied, chronic hypertensive pulmonary disease associated with an initial period of endothelial injury.[38] Vincic et al. have studied the effect of monocrotaline-induced lung injury on the retention and metastasis of intravenously injected Walker 256 cells in the lung and the effect of this injury on spontaneous metastasis in animals with intramuscular tumor transplants.[39] Female Wistar rats were given a single subcutaneous injection of monocrotaline (60 mg/kg). The degree of lung injury was assessed by morphology, bronchoalveolar lavage, and determination of right ventricular hypertrophy. The effect of monocrotaline on metastasis was followed by measurement of cell localization after intravenous injection and by quantitative histology. There was a direct correlation between the severity of lung injury and measurements of metastasis after i.v. cell injection. When r^2 was computed, these data suggested that 64 to 98% of cancer cell retention and 46 to 83% of subsequent tumor burden could be related directly to indices of lung injury. Monocrotaline also altered the rate of spontaneous metastasis of cells from a solid intramuscular tumor transplant. There was a 4.6-fold increase in lung tumor burden in monocrotaline-treated animals compared to controls.

3. Environmental Pollutants

Exposure of animals to nitrogen dioxide[40-42] or ozone,[43] common components of urban smog, has been reported to promote the blood-borne metastasis of experimental tumors. In an atmosphere with ambient or near-ambient levels of NO_2, mice developed microthrombi in their lung capillaries with endothelial blisters and cell loss by electron microscopic examination.[42] These lesions correlated with an increased incidence in the metastasis of B16 melanoma cells after intravenous injection. Increased pulmonary capillary permeability with endothelial injury, suppression of host immunity, or altered clotting mechanisms were suggested as possible explanations for the increased metastatic rate.[40,42]

Exposure of mice to atmospheric ozone for 1 to 14 d before intravenous injection of a murine fibrosarcoma resulted in enhanced lung metastasis. The magnitude of the effect varied with the duration of ozone exposure and concentration.[43] In this study, the mechanisms were not examined, but it was suggested that ozone could interfere with natural resistance, promote platelet aggregation (by inhibiting lung prostacyclin synthesis), induce endothelial swelling, or decrease host antiprotease activity (to facilitate host tissue destruction by cancer cell proteases).

4. Hyperoxia

Exposure to high concentrations of oxygen can also lead to vessel wall injury in pulmonary capillaries. This can be identified by electron microscopy as swelling and retraction of microcapillary endothelial cells and can be quantified by measuring the leakage of protein into bronchoalveolar lavage fluids. Potential mediators of this injury are oxygen radicals, proteases, or metabolites of arachidonic acid.[44] Since periods of maximum injury are associated with the adherence of neutrophils to damaged endothelium, the release of proteases and reactive oxygen species from these cells also may be involved.[45] Using established models of hyperoxic injury, C57BL/6 mice were exposed to an atmosphere of 90% oxygen for a period of 2 to 4 d. After intravenous injection, more radiolabeled cancer cells were retained in the lungs of animals that had been exposed to hyperoxia than in the lungs of control animals. By electron microscopy, tumor cells were seen at sites of denuded basement membrane, which was often associated with platelet-fibrin thrombi or with sequestered neutrophils. Two weeks later, more metastases were found in animals exposed to 90% oxygen. The effect of hyperoxic injury on metastasis was abrogated if the vessels were allowed to repair before injecting the cancer cells intravenously.[46] These experiments demonstrated a direct relationship between the degree of pulmonary endothelial damage and the effect on metastatic tumor growth ($r = 0.90$).

D. LOCALIZED AND SYSTEMIC INFLAMMATORY REACTIONS

The microvasculature is a major effector of acute inflammatory reactions, regulating permeability responses and the egress of leukocytes. At the same time, oxygen radicals and proteases released by activated leukocytes during inflammation can be toxic to the endothelium and basement membrane.[45,47] Given the foregoing evidence that endothelial damage can promote metastasis, it would seem reasonable to expect that inflammatory reactions also could have an influence on the metastatic fate of circulating cancer cells.

1. Neutrophil-Mediated Injury

Leukocytes account for a significant proportion of circulating host cells and are able to interact with intravenous cancer cells, forming heterotypic aggregates.[48-50] While there is evidence that intravascular homotypic aggregation of cancer cells promotes metastasis,[51] the effect of interactions between cancer cells and leukocytes are more controversial (see Chapter 6 by Glaves).

On the one hand, it appears that leukocytes can promote metastasis. The early studies by Wood suggested that rabbit VX2 carcinoma cells leave the microvasculature through defects caused by leukocytes.[52] In humans, leukocytosis has been associated with poor prognosis for some solid tumors with increased metastatic burden.[53] In experimental systems, intravenous injection of cancer cells into animals with granulocytosis,[54] injection of preformed leukocyte-tumor aggregates,[49] infusion of neutrophils with tumor cells,[55] or injection of cancer cells into animals with localized inflammatory processes[56,57] has resulted in greater retention of cancer cells in target organs and/or more metastatic tumors. These results have been explained on the basis of several mechanisms, including embolic localization of heterotypic aggregates,[49] elevated levels of heparanase and type IV collagenolytic activity in the leukocytes of rats with highly metastatic tumors,[55] the generation of localized chemoattractants for cancer cells,[56] release of neutrophil-derived growth factors,[57] and stimulation of the invasive or metastatic potentials of the cancer cells by leukocytes.[58]

Contradictory results have been obtained by others, in particular Glaves, who has provided evidence that neutrophil-derived superoxide anion can release trapped intravascular tumor cells from arrest sites in target organs[59,60] and Jones et al.,[61] who have identified the heterogeneous effects of leukocytes, possibly related to the activation state of leukocytes and/or the differential sensitivity of different cancer cells to the cytolytic effects of activated neutrophils.

Activated neutrophils damage endothelial cells *in vitro* primarily by releasing proteolytic enzymes and free radicals.[62,63] To test the possibility that neutrophil-mediated pulmonary endothelial injury could promote the metastasis of circulating cancer cells, neutrophils were activated by the intravenous injection of cobra venom factor. In both rats[48] and mice,[64] this resulted in complement activation and neutropenia with sequestration of neutrophils in the lung. Damage to the endothelium was confirmed by electron microscopic examination and by increased vasopermeability. In CoF-treated rats, increased vasopermeability was measured by leakage of ^{125}I-albumin from the circulation into lung tissue. This was detected within 5 min after CoF injection and increased to maximum values within 30 min. In mice, there was a 60-fold increase in the amount of intravascular Evans blue retained in the lungs after cobra venom treatment. Aggregates of neutrophils and tumor cells were observed within pulmonary capillaries 2 h after injecting cancer cells i.v. in CoF-treated animals (Figure 2). Twenty-four hours after intravenous injection, there were more tumor cells in the lungs of CoF-treated animals than in controls. In CoF-treated rats, there was a 2- to 3-fold increase in the retention of radiolabelled Walker 256 carcinosarcoma cells. In mice, the simultaneous injection of CoF and radiolabelled fibrosarcoma cells resulted in a 3- to 4-fold increase in the retention of tumor cells. Pretreatment of animals with antineutrophil antiserum reduced tumor cell localization by 55 to 96%. While animals pretreated with catalase demonstrated a 70 to 85% reduction in tumor cell localization following the simultaneous injection of tumor cells and CoF, pretreatment with superoxide dismutase had no effect, suggesting involvement of H_2O_2. There was a direct correlation between the localization of cancer cells at 24 h and the formation of metastasis at 14 d. In CoF-treated rats, morphometric examination and histologic sections of lung demonstrated a 5-fold increase in the percentage of lung involved with tumor. In CoF-treated mice, there was a 3 to 20-fold increase in the number of metastatic pleural tumor nodules and a 4- to 10-fold increase in the area of lung involved with metastatic tumor. In the mouse, endothelial damage and its effect on metastasis were shown to be dependent upon the C5-component of serum complement and upon the intact function of circulating neutrophils.

II. MECHANISTIC CONSIDERATIONS

A. ENDOTHELIAL RETRACTION

Studies on experimental metastasis have demonstrated initial attachment of cancer cells to endothelial surfaces at junction points between adjacent endothelial cells, followed by

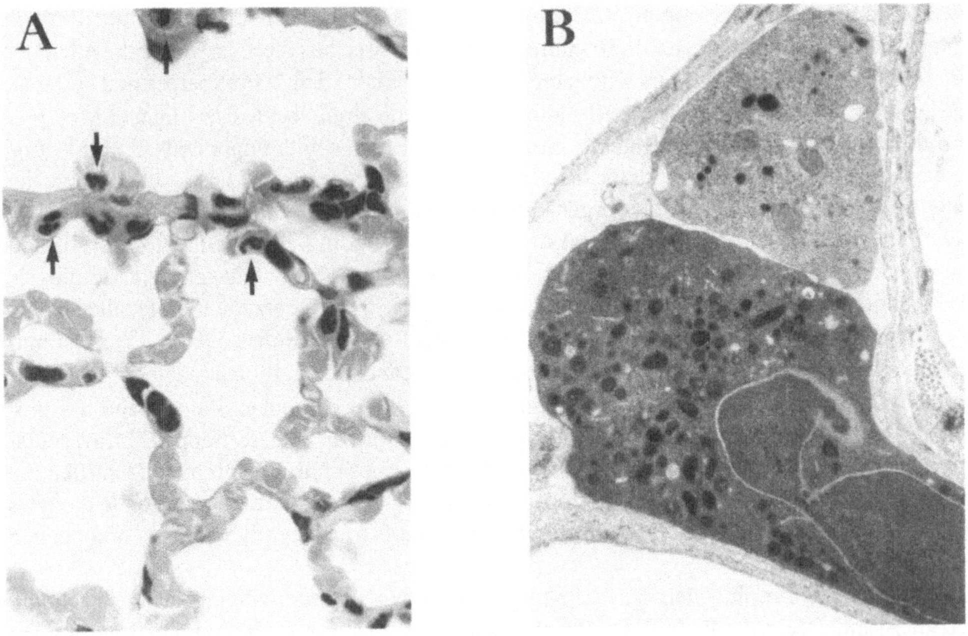

FIGURE 2. A: Histologic section of rat lung 30 min after an intravenous injection of 5 units cobra venom factor. Neutrophil accumulation in the lung microvasculature is shown by the arrows. × 260. B: Two hours after injecting Walker 256 carcinosarcoma cells and cobra venom factor, heterotypic aggregates of neutrophils and cancer cells are found in the pulmonary vessels. × 3,250

endothelial retraction and by adhesion of cancer cells to the underlying basement membrane.[65,66] *In vitro* endothelial retraction also is seen at points of interaction with cancer cells, and there is substantial evidence that cancer cells adhere more readily to the underlying basement membranes than to the endothelium.[67-70] Thus, it has been postulated that retraction of the endothelium, leading to exposure of the more adhesive basement membrane substrate, could upregulate the metastatic process. Direct evidence for this suggestion has been provided by Nicholson's and Custead's experiments in which commonly employed chemotherapeutic agents at concentrations relevant to clinical practice induced retraction of cultured endothelial monolayers, exposure of the basement membrane, and adhesion of platelets and cancer cells to the exposed matrix.[71] *In vivo* retraction of endothelial cells also has been observed by Orr et al. in mice treated with bleomycin[36] or hyperoxia.[46] Reversible endothelial retraction may be initiated by the release of 12-lipoxygenase metabolites of arachidonic acid from activated platelets and/or tumor cells at sites of cancer cell attachment to the vessel wall. This mechanism has been related to enhanced adhesion of cancer cells to endothelial basement membranes in culture.[72] However, it may be that retraction alone is insufficient to promote metastasis *in vivo* since it has been demonstrated that the local or systemic infusion of vasopermeability factors (which presumably induce endothelial retraction) does not change the metastatic behavior of cancer cells injected into the circulation.[73,74] Further, as stated above, Milas et al. found little evidence that increased permeability after irradiation could account for increased metastasis.[17] Thus, agents that induce endothelial retraction coincident with upregulation of metastasis may act through other mechanisms in addition to those responsible for endothelial retraction, and some form of vessel wall injury may be necessary.

B. EXPRESSION OF ADHESION MOLECULES

The arrest and survival of cancer cells within the microvasculature appear to be mandatory for hematogenous metastasis. As pointed out by Weiss (Chapter 9), mechanical arrest is important in initiating the attachment of circulating cells to the vessel wall. It is possible that mechanical factors contribute to the enhanced retention of circulating cancer cells after hyperoxic or bleomycin-induced injury where there is endothelial swelling with reduction in the luminal diameter of small vessels.[36,46] However, the subsequent retention of cells at arrest points is likely to depend upon their fixation to adhesion molecules on the endothelial surface and (following retraction) the basement membrane. As pointed out in recent reviews of this subject, there are organ-specific differences in endothelial surfaces[75-77] and correlations between the adhesion of cancer cells to endothelial monolayers and their malignancy *in vivo*.[68,78] There is evidence for involvement of many adhesive proteins and their receptors[77] (see Chapter 10 by Kramer).

Activation of endothelial cells by stimulants such as interleukin-1, tumor necrosis factor, platelet activating factor, thrombin, and interferon (all cytokines potentially involved in the inflammatory process) is followed by increased expression and/or synthesis of adhesion molecules that are able to mediate enhanced attachment of neutrophils, monocytes, and lymphocytes to endothelial surface and their subsequent penetration of endothelial monolayers.[79-82] This *in vivo* phenomenon has been seen to occur at sites of inflammation and is thought to account for localized attachment of inflammatory cells at these sites.[83]

Recent evidence indicates that the expression of similar surface adhesion molecules may be relevant to the metastatic process. It has been confirmed by several groups that pretreatment of human endothelial cell monolayers with inflammatory cytokines leads to an increased adhesion of various cancer cells to the monolayers.[84-86] The nature of the induced adhesion molecule(s) is currently under investigation. Work in this laboratory by Lauri et al. has shown that the effects are time-dependent, reaching a plateau after 4 to 6 h, and are dependent upon protein synthesis. Adhesion is not blocked by antibodies to fibronectin, to glycoprotein IIb/IIIa, or to endothelial adhesion molecules for leukocytes (ICAM, LFA).[87] However, cancer cell attachment could be blocked by the peptide GRGDS, which is consistent with the involvement of a member of the integrin adhesion molecule family.[88,89] It is notable that competition by RGD-containing peptides was not observed in the experiments reported by Rice et al.[86,90] More recently, Lafrenie et al. have provided evidence that enhanced adhesion can be related to expression of the vitronectin receptor on perturbed endothelial monolayers.[91]

These observations appear to be relevant *in vivo*. Treatment of nude mice with interleukin-1α 4 h before intravenous injection of radiolabeled A549 human lung carcinoma cells induced a five-fold enhancement of cancer cell retention in the lungs after 24 h.[87] In other studies, Bertomeu et al. found that IL-1α pretreatment of C57BL/6 mice enhanced the subsequent pulmonary retention of B16 melanoma cells after intravenous injection with increased development of metastatic nodules at 14 d. This effect could be blocked by injecting GRGDS peptides at the same time as the cancer cells, inferring involvement of the vitronectin receptor or another integrin-related molecule.[92] The experiments may provide an additional explanation for the localization of metastatic tumors at sites of inflammation[56,57,93] and suggest that metastatic mechanisms can be regulated in an analogous manner to the acute inflammatory response.

C. CHEMOTACTIC MECHANISMS

The metastatic phenotypes of many cancer cells, such as motility and enzyme release, are susceptible to regulation by factors in the external environment, including connective tissue matrix molecules and humoral mediators. There is compelling evidence that chemoattractants can promote the retention of circulation cancer cells in target organs and the subsequent development of local metastatic tumors.

Recognizing parallels between metastasis and the inflammation, Hayashi et al. were the first to isolate a factor that was chemotactic for tumor cells and that induced the local formation of metastatic nodules when injected into the dermis of mice with intravascular tumor cells.[73,94] Generation of this factor and a related peptide appeared to be dependent upon interaction of a tissue protein with a protease released from cancer cells and normal cells by a process analogous to the *in vivo* generation of a previously described leukocyte chemoattractant.[95]

1. Inflammatory Chemoattractants for Cancer Cells

Subsequently, it was demonstrated by Romualdez, Ward, and others, that a portion of the fifth component of serum complement (C5) is chemotactic for cancer cells and can be generated *in vitro* by partial digestion of C5 or C5a with a number of proteolytic enzymes, including leukocyte-derived neutral proteases.[96,97] Because C5 and/or C5a and lysosomal hydrolyses are likely to be found at sites of acute inflammation, Orr et al. predicted that inflammatory exudates would provide an appropriate environment for the generation of the C5-derived chemotactic factor for cancer cells *in vivo.* It was subsequently shown that this chemoattractant can be detected in experimental and naturally occurring inflammatory exudates[98,99] and that after injecting rat 256 Walker carcinosarcoma cells intravenously, more mesenteric metastases formed in animals with peritonitis or in animals given intraperitoneal injections of chemoattractant than in control animals.[98] Because the lung is a frequent site of inflammation and metastatic tumors, Orr et al. then looked for tumor cell chemotactic factors in alveolar inflammatory exudates and examined the effect of inflammation on the localization and metastasis of a circulation syngeneic fibrosarcoma in C57BL/6 mice. Pneumonitis was induced by intratracheal injection of 1 mg carbon suspension and quantified by serial bronchoalveolar lavage. In the Boyden chamber assay, the cancer cells demonstrated chemotactic responses to factors in the lavage fluids from animals with inflamed lungs, and the magnitude of the chemotactic response correlated directly with the intensity of the inflammatory process. When radiolabelled cancer cells were injected intravenously during periods of active pneumonitis, there was a 3- to 5-fold increase in retention of these cells after 24 h and a 2- to 5-fold increase in the numbers of detectable metastases in the lungs after 1 to 3 weeks.[56] These data provide evidence to support the hypothesis that inflammatory processes facilitate the metastatic cascade through the generation of chemoattractant molecules at the sites of inflammation.

2. Endothelial-Derived Chemoattractants

Activated or perturbed endothelial cells produce increased amounts of prostacyclin, platelet activating factor, growth factors, tissue factor like procoagulant activity, and interleukins.[100,101] Recently, enhanced gene expression and synthesis of chemotactic factors for monocytes and neutrophils have been described following cytokine-mediated activation.[102,103] Lipoxygenase-derived lipid chemoattractants for neutrophils are also released from endothelial cell cultures following irradiation.[12] Since interleukin-1 had been reported to be a potent chemoattractant for human neutrophils, T-lymphocytes, and nonleukocytic cells,[104,105] we proposed that this cytokine also could influence tumor cell motility. Initially, we determined that recombinant human Il-1α and Il-1β can stimulate dose-dependent, random, and directed migration of human tumor cell populations in the Boyden chamber assay. We then found that the conditioned media from human endothelial cell monolayer cultures contain a chemoattractant for neoplastic cells. This chemotactic activity is greatest in the media of cultures that have been stimulated 4 h previously with bacterial lipopolysaccharide or the synthetic peptide FMLP. The generation of this chemoattractant activity correlates directly with the expression of intracellular mRNA for interleukin-1 and with the presence of interleukin-1 growth factor activity in the conditioned media. The tumor cell chemotactic activity in these media was lost after they had been incubated with anti-Il-1.[106] On the basis of these experiments, we speculate that the production of IL-1 or expression of tumor cell adhesion sites by endothelial cells at sites of inflammation could modulate the behavior of cancer cells within the circulation. Since activation of the endothelium is likely to take place at sites of inflammation, we postulate that this mechanism provides another possible explanation for the effect of inflammatory processes on cancer metastasis.

D. GROWTH FACTOR PRODUCTION

It has been suggested by van den Brenk that inflammatory process could promote metastasis through the local generation of growth factors,[57] although in some experiments, a search for these was unsuccessful.[107] These data do not rule out the existence of local or microvascular-derived growth factor activities. On the contrary, in some cases, intravascular growth of trapped cancer cells seems to provide a means for their subsequent exit from the circulation by mechanical rupture.[66] Cancer cells are frequently sequestered by platelets and fibrin thrombi at sites of arrest. Platelet-derived growth factor and platelet-derived TGFβ in these foci also could act as growth promoting or motility promoting factors.[108,109] Activated or injured endothelial cells have been shown to produce growth factors (βFGF, PDGF, GMCSF)[110-113] that might contribute to cancer cell growth at sites of tumor arrest. The influence of coagulation and platelet factors is discussed in detail in Chapters 7 and 8.

E. ENDOTHELIAL INJURY BY CANCER CELLS

Walker 256 carcinosarcoma cells have been used extensively as an experimental model for cancer metastasis in the rat. These cells are similar to leukocytes in that they carry specific receptors for the peptide, *N*-formyl-Met-Leu-Phe, and phorbol esters. Leukocytes and W256 cells respond to these ligands by chemotaxis, increased adhesiveness, and cell swelling.[114,115] Since leukocytes respond to fMLP by secreting proteolytic enzymes and by generating oxygen-derived free radicals that can cause endothelial injury, we postulated that W256 cells would similarly produce oxygen-derived free radicals upon fMLP addition and that this response could damage endothelial cell monolayers *in vitro*. As an assay for free radical production by W256 cells, we employed chemiluminescence amplified in the presence of luminol as well as the reduction of acetylated ferricytochrome c.[116] In both cases, there was a dose-dependent response. Low levels of background chemiluminescence also were observed in the absence of fMLP. The chemiluminescence response of W256 cells was inhibited by 50% upon the addition of either superoxide dismutase (1 mg/ml) or catalase (1,000 units/ml), inferring production of O_2 and H_2O_2. In addition, mannitol (5 m*M*), a known scavenger of hydroxyl radicals, inhibited W256-promoted chemiluminescence by 66%. Under anaerobic conditions, the chemiluminescence response of fMLP-activated W256 cells was greatly diminished. To examine the possibility that W256-generated free radicals could damage endothelium, we prelabeled endothelial monolayers with ^{3}H-2-deoxyglucose and added activated or unactivated W256 cells to the endothelial cultures. When fMLP-activated W256 cells were incubated with prelabeled endothelial cell monolayers, there was a 27% increase in the specific release of isotope after a 90 min incubation. A small but significant increase in ^{3}H-2-deoxyglucose also was observed in the absence of fMLP. Catalase (1,000 units/ml) inhibited tumor cell-induced release of isotope by 84% while superoxide dismutase at a concentration of 1 mg/ml had no effect, suggesting that H_2O_2 is the main effector of cell damage. We found that contact between the cancer cell and endothelial target is needed for damage since the supernatant of activated tumor cells failed to promote the release of ^{3}H-2-deoxyglucose from endothelial cell monolayers. The requirement for contact also was shown by preincubating W256 cells with I μ*M* cytochalasin B prior to their incubation with labelled endothelium. Although there was a threefold increase in chemiluminescence in the presence of cytochalasin B, there was a decreased release of isotope from labeled endothelium, and scanning electron micrographs demonstrated 60 to 80% fewer adherent W256 cells on the endothelial monolayer.[117] More recent experiments indicate that W256 cancer cell-mediated free radical damage to endothelium is dependent upon adhesion between the effector and target via the vitronectin receptor.[118]

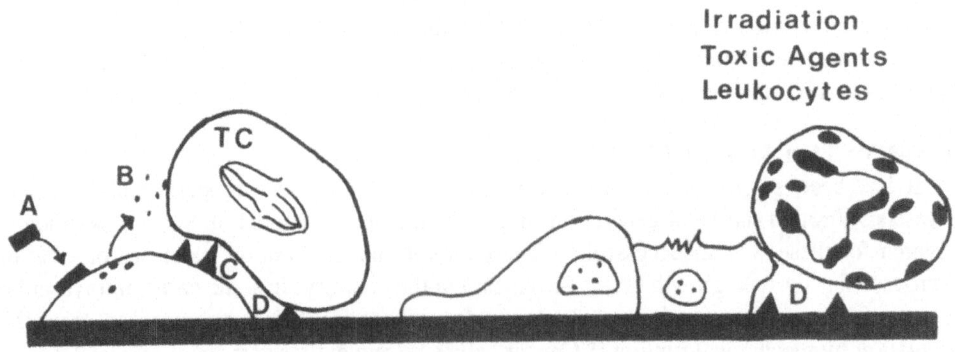

FIGURE 3. Mechanisms by which endothelial perturbation and injury can influence the rate of cancer metastasis. Endothelial cells are subject to activation by circulating humoral mediators, e.g., endotoxins or interleukin-1(A), which result in the synthesis and/or release of humoral chemoattractants or growth factors (B) and/or the expression of cell surface adhesion molecules (C). Other adhesion molecules may be expressed constitutively on the endothelial cells and the basement membrane. Exposure of the latter could occur if endothelial cells retract actively in response to perturbation or sublethal injury (D). Endothelial injury can result from irradiation, the action of drugs and environmental toxins, or free radicals and proteases released from activated host leukocytes and from some tumor cells (TC).

It is not known if these observations apply to the behavior of other cancer cell types. However, there is evidence that platelets, as well as leukocytes, can be activated to produce free radicals and to induce endothelial injury.[119,120] This may be a means by which interactions between platelets and cancer cells could facilitate the transvascular passage of circulating cancer cells.

F. MECHANISMS UNRELATED TO MICROVASCULAR INJURY

Treatment of tumor-bearing mice with ketamine, halothane, thiopental sodium, and N_2O can promote metastasis and, in the case of halothane and ketamine, the effect has been correlated with a decrease in natural killer cell activity.[121] Many recent studies have placed emphasis on the ability of chemotherapies to alter the metastatic phenotype of (target) cancer cells. Thus, by inducing genetic mutation, amplifying genes relevant to metastasis, or altering gene expression, drug treatment may select for or promote the growth of more malignant tumor subpopulations.[122-125] This subject has been reviewed recently by McMillan and Hart.[126]

III. CONCLUSION

Cancer cells frequently disseminate via the bloodstream where the endothelium acts as a barrier between the circulating tumor cells and the extravascular tissue. Environmental factors, inflammatory reactions, host cells, and tumor cells can cause microvascular damage, and there is evidence that these injuries can promote the metastasis of intravascular tumor cells. The endothelium is also a potential regulator of metastasis by virtue of its ability to express adhesion molecules and to secrete chemoattractants or growth factors. Figure 3 briefly summarizes these concepts, most of which are based on evidence from *in vitro* studies. The significance of these phenomena *in vivo* is not fully known and is an area worthy of additional study.

ACKNOWLEDGMENTS

The author's work, cited in this review, is supported by grants from the National Cancer Institute of Canada and the Medical Research Council of Canada.

REFERENCES

1. **Weiss, L., Orr, F. W., and Honn, K. V.,** Interactions between cancer cells and the microvasculature: a rate-regulator for metastasis, *Clin. Exp. Metastasis,* 7, 127, 1989.
2. **Blood, C. H. and Zetter, B. R.,** Tumor interactions with the vasculature: angiogenesis and tumor metastasis, *Biochim. Biophys. Acta Rev. Cancer,* 1032, 89, 1990.
3. **Rate, W. R. and Solin, L. J.,** Mediastinoscopy incision site metastasis: implications for radiotherapeutic treatment, *Cancer,* 63, 68, 1989.
4. **Jewell, W. R. and Romadahl, M. M.,** Recurrent malignant disease in operative wounds not due to surgical implantation from the resected tumor, *Surgery,* 58, 806, 1965.
5. **Black, J. W.,** The localisation of metastatic Brown-Pearce carcinoma in granulation tissue, *Br. J. Cancer,* 18, 143, 1964.
6. **Ewing, J.,** Modern attitude toward traumatic cancer, *Arch. Pathol.,* 19, 690, 1935.
7. **Alexander, J. W. and Altemeier, W. A.,** Susceptibility of injured tissues to hematogenous metastases: an experimental study, *Ann. Surg.,* 159, 933, 1964.
8. **Weiss, L.,** Some effects of mechanical trauma on the development of primary cancers and their metastases, *J. Forensic Sci.,* 35, 614, 1990.
9. **Fisher, B., Fisher, E. R., and Fuduska, N.,** Trauma and the localization of tumor cells, *Cancer,* 20, 23, 1967.
10. **Agostino, D. and Cliffton, E. E.,** Trauma as a cause of localization of blood-borne metastases: preventive effect of heparin and fibrinolysin, *Ann. Surg.,* 161, 97, 1965.
11. **Skolnik, G., Ivarsson, L., and Bagge, U.,** The influence of antiserotonin treatment with ketanserin on the pulmonary lodgement of circulating tumour cells in normal and traumatized rats, *Eur. J. Cancer,* 19, 843, 1983.
12. **Eldor, A., Vlodavsky, I., Fuks, Z., Matzner, Y., and Rubin, D. B.,** Arachidonic metabolism and radiation toxicity in cultures of vascular endothelial cells, *Prost. Leuk. Essen. Fatty Acids,* 36, 251, 1989.
13. **Dao, T. L. and Kovaric, J.,** Incidence of pulmonary and skin metastasis in women with breast cancer who received postoperative irradiation, *Surgery,* 52, 203, 1962.
14. **Fisher, B., Slack, N. H., Cavanaugh, P. J., Gardner, B., and Ravdin, R. G.,** Postoperative radiotherapy in the treatment of breast cancer: results of the NSABP clinical trial, *Ann. Surg.,* 172, 711, 1970.
15. **Edstrom, S., Johansson, S. L., Lindstrom, J., and Sandin, I.,** Verrucous squamous cell carcinoma of the larynx: evidence for increased metastatic potential after irradiation, *Otolaryngol. Head Neck Surg.,* 97, 381, 1987.
16. **Milas, L., Iwakawa, M., and Hunter, N.,** Enhancement of lung colony formation by admixing irradiated with viable tumor cells: dependence on host status, *Clin. Exp. Metastasis,* 5, 213, 1987.
17. **Milas, L., Hirata, H., Hunter, N., and Peters, L. J.,** Effect of radiation-induced injury of tumor bed stroma on metastatic spread of murine sarcomas and carcinomas, *Cancer Res.,* 48, 2116, 1988.
18. **van den Brenk, H. A. S., Crowe, M. D., and Stone, M. G.,** Reactions of the tumor bed to lethally irradiated tumor cells and the Revesz effect, *Br. J. Cancer,* 36, 94, 1977.
19. **Rappaport, D. S. and Brown, J. M.,** Influence of localized preinoculation irradiation of the foot on lymphatic metastasis from a primary tumor growing in the foot, *Radiat. Res.,* 78, 108, 1979.
20. **Fisher, B., Saffer, E. A., and Deutsch, M.,** Influence of irradiation of a primary tumor on the labeling index and estrogen receptor index in a distant tumor focus, *Int. J. Radiat. Oncol. Biol. Phys. [G97],* 12, 879, 1986.
21. **Dao, T. L. and Yogo, H.,** Enhancement of pulmonary metastases by x-irradiation in rats bearing mammary cancer, *Cancer,* 29, 2020, 1967.
22. **Withers, H. R. and Milas, L.,** Influence of preirradiation of lung on development of artificial pulmonary metastases of fibrosarcoma in mice, *Cancer Res.,* 33, 1931, 1973.
23. **Owen, L. N. and Bostock, D. E.,** Treatment of canine osteosarcoma, *Vet. Rec.,* 92, 212, 1973.
24. **Thompson, S. C.,** Tumour colony growth in the irradiated mouse lung, *Br. J. Cancer,* 30, 337, 1974.
25. **Brown, J. M.,** The effect of lung irradiation on the incidence of pulmonary metastases in mice, *Br. J. Radiol.,* 46, 613, 1973.
26. **Peters, L. J., Mason, K., McBride, W. H., and Patt, Y. Z.,** Enhancement of lung colony-forming efficiency by local thoracic irradiation: interpretation of labeled cell studies, *Radiology,* 126, 499, 1978.
27. **van Putten, L. M., Kram, L. K. J., van Dierendonck, H. H. C., Smink, T., and Fuzy, M.,** Enhancement by drugs of metastatic lung nodule formation after intravenous tumour cell injection, *Int. J. Cancer,* 15, 588, 1975.
28. **Moore, J. V. and Dixon, B.,** Metastasis of a transplantable mammary tumour in rats treated with cyclophosphamide and/or irradiation, *Br. J. Cancer,* 36, 221, 1977.
29. **Poupon, M. F., Pauwels, C., Jasmin, C., Antoine, E., Lascaux, V., and Rosa, B.,** Amplified pulmonary metastases of a rat rhabdomyosarcoma in response to nitrosourea treatment, *Cancer Treat. Rep. [CNM],* 68, 749, 1984.

30. **Carmel, R. J. and Brown, J. M.**, The effect of cyclophosphamide and other drugs on the incidence of pulmonary metastases in mice, *Cancer Res.*, 37, 145, 1977.
31. **Steel, G. G. and Adams, K.**, Enhancement by cytotoxic agents of artificial pulmonary metastasis, *Br. J. Cancer*, 36, 653, 1977.
32. **Gasic, G. J., Iwakawa, A., Gasic, T. B., Viner, E. D., and Milas, L.**, Leech salivary gland extract from haementeria officinalis, a potent inhibitor of cyclophosphamide- and radiation-induced artificial metastasis enhancement, *Cancer Res.*, 44, 567, 1984.
33. **Hecht, S. M.**, DNA strand scission by activated bleomycin group antibiotics, *Fed. Proc.*, 45, 2784, 1986.
34. **Twentyman, P. R.**, Bleomycin-mode of action with particular reference to the cell cycle, *Pharmacol. Ther.*, 23, 417, 1984.
35. **Adamson, I. Y. R.**, Drug-induced pulmonary fibrosis, *Environ. Health Perspect.*, 55, 25, 1984.
36. **Orr, F. W., Adamson, I. Y. R., and Young, L.**, Promotion of pulmonary metastasis in mice by bleomycin-induced endothelial injury, *Cancer Res.*, 46, 891, 1986.
37. **Adamson, I. Y. R., Orr, F. W., and Young, L.**, Effects of injury and repair of the pulmonary endothelium on lung metastasis after bleomycin, *J. Pathol.*, 150, 279, 1986.
38. **Kay, J. M., Keane, P. M., and Suyama, K. L.**, Pulmonary hypertension induced in rats by monocrotaline and chronic hypoxia is reduced by p-chlorophenylalanine, *Respiration*, 47, 48, 1985.
39. **Vincic, L., Orr, F. W., Warner, D. J. A., Suyama, K. L., and Kay, J. M.**, Enhanced cancer metastasis after monocrotaline-induced lung injury, *Toxicol. Appl. Pharm.*, 100, 259, 1989.
40. **Richters, A. and Kuraitis, K.**, Inhalation of NO2 and blood borne cancer cell spread to the lungs, *Arch. Environ. Health*, 36, 36, 1981.
41. **Richters, A. and Richters, V.**, A new relationship between air pollutant inhalation and cancer, *Arch. Environ. Health*, 38, 69, 1983.
42. **Richters, A. and Richters, V.**, Nitrogen dioxide (NO2) inhalation, formation of microthrombi in lungs and cancer metastasis, *J. Environ. Pathol. Toxicol. Oncol.*, 9(1), 45, 1989.
43. **Kobayashi, T., Todoroki, T., and Sato, H.**, Enhancement of pulmonary metastasis of murine fibrosarcoma NR-FS by ozone exposure, *J. Toxicol. Env. Health*, 20, 135, 1987.
44. **Hageman, J. R., Babler, S., Lee, S. C., Cobb, M., Pachman, L. M., Smith, L. J., and Hunt, C. E.**, The early involvement of pulmonary prostaglandins in hyperoxic lung injury, *Prost. Leuk. Med.*, 25, 105, 1986.
45. **Ginsburg, I., Gibbs, D. F., Schuger, L., Johnson, K. J., Ryan, U. S., Ward, P. A., and Varani, J.**, Vascular endothelial cell killing by combinations of membrane-active agents and hydrogen peroxide, *Free Rad. Biol. Med.*, 7, 369, 1989.
46. **Adamson, I. Y. R., Young, L., and Orr, F. W.**, Tumor metastasis after hyperoxic injury and repair of the pulmonary endothelium, *Lab. Invest.*, 57, 71, 1987.
47. **Weiss, S. J., Curnutte, J. T., and Regiani, S.**, Neutrophil-mediated solubilization of the subendothelial matrix: oxidative and nonoxidative mechanisms of proteolysis used by normal and chronic granulomatous disease phagocytes, *J. Immunol.*, 136(2), 636, 1986.
48. **Orr, F. W. and Warner, D. J. A.**, Effects of neutrophil-mediated pulmonary endothelial injury on the localization and metastasis of circulating Walker carcinosarcoma cells, *Invasion Metastasis*, 7, 183, 1987.
49. **Starkey, R., Liggitt, H. D., Jones, W., and Hosick, H. L.**, Influence of migratory blood cells on the attachment of tumour cells to vascular endothelium, *Int. J. Cancer*, 34, 535, 1984.
50. **Orr, F. W. and Mokashi, S.**, Effect of leukocyte activation on the formation of heterotypic tumour-cell aggregates *in vitro*, *Int. J. Cancer*, 35, 101, 1985.
51. **Liotta, L. A., Kleinerman, J., and Saidel, G. M.**, The significance of hematogenous tumor cell clups in the metastatic process, *Cancer Res.*, 36, 889, 1976.
52. **Wood, S.**, Pathogenesis of metastasis formation observed *in vivo* in the rabbit ear chamber, *Arch. Pathol.*, 66, 550, 1958.
53. **Shoenfeld, Y., Tal, A., Berliner, S., and Pinkhas, J.**, Leukocytosis in non-hematological malignancies — a possible tumour-associated marker, *J. Cancer Res. Clin. Oncol.*, 111, 54, 1986.
54. **Ishikawa, M., Koga, Y., Hosokawa, M., and Kobayashi, H.**, Augmentation of B16 melanoma lung colony formation in C57BL/6 mice having marked granulocytosis, *Int. J. Cancer*, 37, 919, 1986.
55. **Aeed, P. A., Nakajima, M., and Welch, D. R.**, The role of polymorphonuclear leukocytes (PMN) on the growth and metastatic potential of 13762NF mammary adenocarcinoma cells, *Int. J. Cancer*, 42, 748, 1988.
56. **Orr, F. W., Adamson, I. Y. R., and Young, L.**, Pulmonary inflammation generates chemotactic activity for tumor cells and promotes lung metastasis, *Am. Rev. Respir. Dis.*, 131, 607, 1985.
57. **van den Brenk, H. A. S., Stone, M., Kelly, H., Orton, C., and Sharpington, C.**, Promotion of growth of tumour cells in acutely inflamed tissues, *Br. J. Cancer*, 30, 246, 1974.
58. **Welch, D. R., Schissel, D. J., Howrey, R. P., and Aeed, P. A.**, Tumor-elected polymorphonuclear cells, in contrast to "normal" circulating polymorphonuclear cells, stimulate invasive and metastatic potentials of rat mammary adenocarcinoma cells, *Proc. Natl. Acad. Sci. U.S.A.*, 86, 5859, 1989.

59. **Glaves, D.**, Role of polymorphonuclear leukocytes in the pulmonary clearance of arrested cancer cells, *Invasion Metastasis*, 3, 160, 1983.
60. **Glaves, D.**, Intravascular death of disseminated cancer cells mediated by superoxide anion, *Invasion Metastasis*, 6, 101, 1986.
61. **Jones, C. L., Nelson, K. K., Hatfield, J. S., Honn, K. V., and Onoda, J. M.**, Regulation of metastasis by polymorphonuclear neutrophils, *Proc. Am. Assoc. Cancer Res.*, 29, 62, 1988.(Abstr.)
62. **Henson, P. M. and Johnston, R. B.**, Tissue injury in inflammation: oxidants, proteinases, and cationic proteins, *J. Clin. Invest.*, 79, 669, 1987.
63. **Ward, P. A. and Varani, J.**, Mechanisms of neutrophil-mediated killing of endothelial cells, *J. Leukocyte Biol.*, 48, 97, 1990.
64. **Orr, F. W. and Warner, D. J. A.**, Effects of systemic complement activation and neutrophil-mediated pulmonary injury on the retention and metastasis of circulating cancer cells in mouse lungs, *Lab. Invest.*, 62, 331, 1990.
65. **Crissman, J. D., Hatfield, J., Schaldenbrand, M., Sloane, B. F., and Honn, K. V.**, Arrest and extravasation of B16 amelanotic melanoma in murine lungs. A light and electron microscopic study, *Lab. Invest.*, 53, 470, 1985.
66. **Crissman, J. D., Hatfield, J. S., Menter, D. G., Sloane, B., and Honn, K. V.**, Morphological study of the interaction of intravascular tumor cells with endothelial cells and subendothelial matrix, *Cancer Res.*, 48, 4065, 1988.
67. **Kramer, R. H., Gonzales, R., and Nicolson, G. L.**, Metastatic tumor cells adhere preferentially to the extracellular matrix underlying vascular endothelial cells, *Int. J. Cancer*, 26, 639, 1980.
68. **Nicolson, G. L.**, Metastatic tumor cell attachment and invasion assay utilizing vascular endothelial cell monolayers, *J. Histochem. Cytochem.*, 30, 214, 1982.
69. **Vlodavsky, I., Atzmon, A. R., and Fuks, Z.**, Tumor cell attachment to the vascular endothelium and subsequent degradation of the subendothelial extracellular matrix, *Exp. Cell Res.*, 140, 149, 1982.
70. **Boxberger, H.-J., Paweletz, N., Spiess, E., and Kriehuber, R.**, An *in vitro* model study of BSp73 rat tumour cell invasion into endothelial monolayer, *Anticancer Res.*, 9, 1777, 1989.
71. **Nicolson, G. L. and Custead, S. E.**, Effects of chemotherapeutic drugs on platelet and metastatic tumor cell-endothelial cell interactions as a model for assessing vascular endothelial integrity, *Cancer Res.*, 45, 331, 1985.
72. **Honn, K. V., Grossi, I. M., Diglio, C. A., Wojtukiewicz, M., and Taylor, J. D.**, Enhanced tumor cell adhesion to the subendothelial matrix resulting from 12(S)-HETE-induced endothelial cell retraction, *FASEB J.*, 3, 2285, 1989.
73. **Ozaki, T., Yoshida, K., Ushijima, K., and Hayashi, H.**, Studies on the mechanisms of invasion in cancer. II. *In vivo* effects of a factor chemotactic for cancer cells, *Int. J. Cancer*, 7, 93, 1971.
74. **Lam, W. C., Delikatny, J., Orr, F. W., Wass, J., Varani, J., and Ward, P. A.**, The chemotactic response of tumor cells: a model for cancer metastasis, *Am. J. Pathol.*, 104, 69, 1981.
75. **Nicolson, G. L.**, Organ specificity of tumor metastasis: role of preferential adhesion, invasion and growth of malignant cells at specific secondary sites, *Cancer Metast. Rev.*, 7, 143, 1988.
76. **Auerbach, R., Alby, L., Morrissey, W., Tu, M., and Joseph, J.**, Expression of organ-specific antigens on capillary endothelial cells, *Microvasc. Res.*, 29, 401, 1985.
77. **Belloni, P. N. and Tressler, R. J.**, Microvascular endothelial cell heterogeneity: interactions with leukocytes and tumor cells, *Cancer Metast. Rev.*, 8, 353, 1990.
78. **Alby, L. and Auerbach, R.**, Differential adhesion of tumor cells to capillary endothelial cells *in vitro*, *Proc. Natl. Acad. Sci. U.S.A.*, 81, 5739, 1984.
79. **Renkonen, R., Mattila, P., Turunen, J.-P., and Häyry, P.**, Lymphocyte binding to and penetration through vascular endothelium is stimulated by platelet-activating factor, *Scand. J. Immunol.*, 30, 673, 1989.
80. **Furie, M. B. and McHugh, D. D.**, Migration of neutrophils across endothelial monolayers is stimulated by treatment of the monolayers with interleukin-1 or tumor necrosis factor-α, *J. Immunol.*, 143, 3309, 1989.
81. **Bevilacqua, M. P., Pober, J. S., Wheeler, M. E., Cotran, R. S., and Gimbrone, M. A., Jr.**, Interleukin-1 acts on cultured human vascular endothelium to increase the adhesion of polymorphonuclear leukocytes, monocytes, and related leukocyte cell lines, *J. Clin. Invest.*, 76, 2003, 1985.
82. **Cavender, D., Saegusa, Y., and Ziff, M.**, Stimulation of endothelial cell binding of lymphocytes by tumor necrosis factor, *J. Immunol.*, 139, 1855, 1987.
83. **Cotran, R. S., Gimbrone, M. A., Jr., Bevilacqua, M. P., Mendrick, D. L., and Pober, J. S.**, Induction and detection of a human endothelial activation antigen *in vivo*, *J. Exp. Med.*, 164, 661, 1986.
84. **Lauri, D., Bertomeu, M.-C., Orr, F. W., Bastida, E., Sauder, D. N., and Buchanan, M. R.**, Differential effects of interleukin-1 and fMLP on chemotaxis and human endothelium adhesivity for A549 tumor cells, *Lab. Invest.*, 60, 161, 1989.
85. **Dejana, E., Bertocchi, F., Bortolami, M. C., Fegonesi, A., Tonta, A., Brevario, F., and Giavazzi, R.**, Interleukin-1 promotes tumor cell adhesion to cultured human endothelial cells, *J. Clin. Invest.*, 82, 1466, 1988.

86. **Rice, G. E., Gimbrone, M. A., Jr., and Bevilacqua, M. P.,** Tumor cell-endothelial interactions. Increased adhesion of human melanoma cells to activated vascular endothelium, *Am. J. Pathol.*, 133, 204, 1988.
87. **Lauri, D., Bertomeu, M.-C., Orr, F. W., Bastida, E., Sauder, D. N., and Buchanan, M. R.,** Interleukin-1 increases tumor cell adhesion to endothelial cells through an RGD-dependent mechanism: *in vitro* and *in vivo* studies, *Clin. Exp. Metast.*, 8, 27, 1990.
88. **Hynes, R. O., Marcantonio, E. E., Stepp, M. A., Urry, L. A., and Yee, G. H.,** Integrin heterodimer and receptor complexity in avian and mammalian cells, *J. Cell Biol.*, 109, 409, 1989.
89. **Van Mourik, J. A., Von dem Borne, A. E. G. K., and Giltay, J. G.,** Pathophysiological significance of integrin expression by vascular endothelial cells, *Biochem. Pharmacol.*, 246, 1303, 1989.
90. **Rice, G. E. and Bevilacqua, M. P.,** An inducible endothelial cell surface glycoprotein mediated melanoma adhesion, *Science*, 246, 19203, 1989.
91. **Lafrenie, R. M., Podor, T. J., Buchanan, M. R., and Orr, F. W.,** Adhesion of A549 adenocarcinoma cells to interleukin-1alpha stimulated endothelial cells is partially mediated by the vitronectin receptor, 1990, (unpublished).
92. **Bertomeu, M. C., Whybourne, K., Gallo, S., Haas, T. A., Orr, F. W., Bastida, E., and Buchanan, M. R.,** Increased integrin expression on the endothelium and its effects on cancer metastasis following interleukin 1 stimulation: *in vitro* and *in vivo* studies with human and mouse tissue, 1990, (unpublished).
93. **DerHagopain, R. P., Sugarbaker, E. V., and Ketcham, A.,** Inflammatory oncotaxis, *JAMA*, 240, 374, 1978.
94. **Hayashi, H., Yoshida, K., Ozaki, T., and Ushijima, K.,** Chemotactic factor associated with invasion of cancer cells, *Nature*, 226, 1174, 1970.
95. **Koono, M., Katsuya, H., and Hayashi, H.,** Studies on the mechanisms of invasion in cancer. IV. A factor associated with release of neutral protease of tumor cell, *Int. J. Cancer*, 13, 334, 1974.
96. **Romualdez, A. G., Jr. and Ward, P. A.,** A unique complement derived chemotactic factor for tumor cells, *Proc. Natl. Acad. Sci. U.S.A.*, 72, 4128, 1975.
97. **Orr, W., Varani, J., Kreutzer, D. L., Senior, R. M., and Ward, P. A.,** Digestion of the fifth component of complement by human leukocyte enzymes: sequential generation of chemotactic activities for leukocytes and for tumor cells, *Am. J. Pathol.*, 94, 75, 1979.
98. **Orr, F. W., Mokashi, S., and Delikatny, J.,** Generation of a complement-derived factor for tumor cells in experimentally induced peritoneal exudates and its effect on the local metastasis of circulating tumor cells, *Am. J. Pathol.*, 108, 112, 1982.
99. **Orr, F. W., Delikatny, E. J., Mokashi, S., Krepart, G. V., and Stiver, H. G.,** Detection of a complement-derived chemotactic factor for tumor cells in human inflammatory and neoplastic effusions, *Am. J. Pathol.*, 110, 41, 1983.
100. **Pober, J. S.,** Cytokine-mediated activation of vascular endothelium: physiology and pathology, *Am. J. Pathol.*, 133, 426, 1988.
101. **Pober, J. S. and Cotran, R. S.,** Cytokines and endothelial cell biology, *Physiol. Rev.*, 70, 427, 1990.
102. **Rollins, B. J., Yoshimura, T., Leonard, E. J., and Pober, J. S.,** Cytokine-activated human endothelial cells synthesize and secrete a monocyte chemoattractant, MCP-1/JE, *Am. J. Pathol.*, 136, 1229, 1990.
103. **Sica, A., Matsushima, K., Van Damme, J., Wang, J. M., Polentarutti, N., Dejana, E., Colotta, F., and Mantovani, A.,** IL-1 transcriptionally activates the neutrophil chemotactic factor/IL-8 gene in endothelial cells, *Immunology*, 69, 548, 1990.
104. **Sauder, D. N., Monick, M. M., and Hunninghake, G. W.,** Epidermal cell thymocyte activating factor (ETAF) is a potent T-cell chemoattractant, *J. Invest. Dermatol.*, 85, 431, 1985.
105. **Sauder, D. N., Orr, F. W., Matic, S., Stesko, D., Parker, K. P., and Kilian, P. L.,** Human interleukin-1-alpha is chemotactic for normal human keratinocytes, *Immunol. Lett.*, 22, 123, 1989.
106. **Orr, F. W., Buchanan, M. R., Tron, V. A., Guy, D., Lauri, D., and Sauder, D. N.,** Chemotactic activity of endothelial cell-derived interleukin-1 for human tumor cells, *Cancer Res.*, 48, 6758, 1988.
107. **Orr, F. W., Lam, W.-C., Delikatny, E. J., Mokashi, S., and Varani, J.,** Localization of intravenously injected tumor cells in the rat mesentery after intraperitoneal administration of chemotactic stimuli, *Invasion Metastasis*, 1, 239, 1981.
108. **Orr, F. W., Millar-Book, W., and Singh, G.,** Chemotactic activity of bone and platelet-derived TGF-beta for bone-metastasizing rat Walker 256 carcinosarcoma cells, *Invasion Metastasis*, 10, 241, 1990.
109. **Millar-Book, W., Orr, F. W., and Singh, G.,** *In vitro* effects of bone and platelet-derived transforming growth factor-beta on the growth of Walker 256 carcinosarcoma cells, *Clin. Exp. Metastasis*, 8, 503, 1990.
110. **Gajdusek, C. M. and Carbon, S.,** Injury-induced release of basic fibroblast growth factor from bovine aortic endothelium, *J. Cell. Physiol.*, 139, 570, 1989.
111. **Sieff, C. A., Tsai, S., and Faller, D. V.,** Interleukin-1 induces cultured human endothelial cell production of granulocyte-macrophage colony stimulating factor, *J. Clin. Invest.*, 79, 48, 1987.
112. **McNeil, P. L., Muthukrishnan, L., Warder, E., and D'Amore, P. A.,** Growth factors are released by mechanically wounded endothelial cells, *J. Cell Biol.*, 109, 811, 1989.

113. **Witte, L., Fuks, Z., Haimovitz-Friedman, A., Vlodavsky, I., Goodman, D. S., and Eldor, A.,** Effects of irradiation on the release of growth factors from cultured bovine, porcine, and human endothelial cells, *Cancer Res.*, 49, 5066, 1989.
114. **Wass, J. A., Varani, J., and Ward, P. A.,** Size increase induced in Walker ascites cells by chemotactic factors, *Cancer Lett.*, 9, 313, 1980.
115. **Varani, J. and Fantone, J. C.,** Phorbol myristate acetate-induced adherence of Walker 256 carcinosarcoma cells, *Cancer Res.*, 42, 190, 1982.
116. **Leroyer, V., Werner, L., Shaughnessy, S., Goddard, G. J., and Orr, F. W.,** Chemiluminescence and oxygen radical generation by Walker carcinosarcoma cells following chemotactic stimulation, *Cancer Res.*, 47, 4771, 1987.
117. **Shaughnessy, S. G., Buchanan, M. R., Turple, S., Richardson, M., and Orr, F. W.,** Walker carcinosarcoma cells damage endothelial cells by the generation of reactive oxygen species, *Am. J. Pathol.*, 34, 787, 1989.
118. **Shaughnessy, S. G., Lafrenie, R. M., Buchanan, M. R. Podor, T. J., and Orr, F. W.,** Endothelial cell damage by Walker carcinosarcoma cells is dependent upon tumor cell adhesion, *Clin. Exp. Metast.*, 8, 60, 1990. (Abstr.)
119. **Joseph, M., Capron, A., Tsicopoulos, A., Ameisen, J. C., Martinot, J. B., and Tonnel, A. B.,** Platelet activation by IgE and aspirin, *Agents Actions*, 21 (Suppl.), 169, 1987.
120. **Larsen, T., Sorensen, M. B., Olsen, R., and Jorgensen, L.,** Effect of scavengers of active oxygen species and pretreatment with acetyl-salicylic acid on the injury to cultured endothelial cells by thrombin-stimulated platelets, *In Vitro Cell. Dev. Biol.*, 25, 276, 1989.
121. **Katzav, S., Shapiro, J., Segal, S., and Feldman, M.,** General anesthesia during excision of a mouse tumor accelerates postsurgical growth of metastases by suppression of natural killer cell activity, *Isr. J. Med. Sci.*, 22, 339, 1986.
122. **Takenaga, K.,** Modification of the metastatic potential of tumor cells by drugs, *Cancer Metast. Rev.*, 5, 67, 1986.
123. **Cillo, C., Ling, V., and Hill, R. P.,** Drug resistance in KHT fibrosarcoma cell lines with different metastatic ability, *Int. J. Cancer*, 43, 107, 1989.
124. **McMillan, T. J. and Hart, I. R.,** Enhanced experimental metastatic capacity of a murine melanoma following pre-treatment with anticancer drugs, *Clin. Exp. Metast.*, 4, 285, 1986.
125. **Kerbel, R. S. and Davies, A. J. S.,** Facilitation of tumour progression by cancer therapy, *Lancet*, 2, 977, 1982.
126. **McMillan, T. J. and Hart, I. R.,** Can cancer chemotherapy enhance the malignant behaviour of tumours, *Cancer Metast. Rev.*, 6, 503, 1987.

Chapter 16

THE ROLE OF VASCULARIZATION IN TUMOR METASTASIS

Marsha A. Moses

TABLE OF CONTENTS

I. INTRODUCTION

Tumor growth to approximately 1 mm^3 in size can be accomplished in the absence of vascularization since all of the essential nutrients and waste products are capable of diffusing across this distance. However, once a tumor has reached this threshold level of growth, vascularization is essential if there is to be additional (exponential) tumor growth and progression into the final stages of tumor metastasis, secondary tumor growth. This chapter is designed to focus on the role of angiogenesis, the process of new capillary formation, in the metastatic process. Following a brief history of angiogenesis as it relates to tumor growth and metastasis, this section will review current information on the control of neovascularization by a number of key regulators including the positive (angiogenesis stimulators) and negative (angiogenesis inhibitors) modulators of vascular growth as well as other less direct yet nonetheless effective regulatory factors.

II. TUMORS ARE ANGIOGENESIS-DEPENDENT

For years, most researchers, while noting the extensive capillary proliferation associated with tumors, viewed this neovascularization response as one secondary to tumor metabolism or necrosis.[1] However, the compelling work of Algire and co-workers suggested that the continuous growth of a tumor was virtually dependent on its vascularization.[2] Gimbrone, Folkman and their co-workers reported that tumors implanted into a perfused organ grew to a limit of 2 mm in diameter in the absence of a vascular supply, yet when removed from this system and reimplanted into animals, those tumors grew into large tumor masses. Upon histological analysis, it was observed that the tumors obtained from the *in vitro* system were avascular, whereas the reimplanted tumors were highly vascularized.[3] Another study on tumors implanted into the anterior chamber resulted in two important conclusions: first, that vascularization is an absolute requirement for successful solid tumor growth and second, that the degree of vascularization is a critical determinant in the ultimate size of the tumor.[4] These conclusions led, in turn, to the hypothesis that ''anti-angiogenesis'' strategies might ultimately lead to control of solid tumor growth.[5,6]

In vitro work also has supported the concept of the angiogenesis dependence of solid tumors. *In vitro* studies of the prevascular state demonstrated that only dormant tumors could be obtained under *in vitro* conditions at this avascular stage in tumor growth.[7] Additionally, Tannock and colleagues showed that capillary blood vessels were surrounded by tumor cells in a cylindrical manner with a radius equal to the diffusion distance of oxygen (150 to 200 μm). It was also observed that the further the distance between tumor cells and the nearest capillary, the lower the level of tumor cell DNA synthesis.[8,9]

These observations regarding tumor angiogenesis were extended by the work of Ausprunk and co-workers who demonstrated that tumor vessels were dependent on the continuous presence of a stimulus for their continued growth. Using the chick chorioallantoic membrane assay (CAM), they demonstrated that the removal of an angiogenic stimulus resulted in total regression of the blood vessels originally induced by that stimulus.[10]

The angiogenic capacity of tumors was first demonstrated by Greenblatt and Shubik who reported that even if a tumor was separated from the host vasculature by a Millipore filter (0.45 μm), it could still elicit new blood vessel growth, suggesting that vascularization was induced via a diffusible, tumor-derived angiogenesis factor.[11] In the early 1970s, isolation of the first angiogenic factor from rat tumor extracts was reported[12] followed by the isolation of an angiogenic factor from the conditioned media of transformed cells[13] and the subsequent isolation of other tumor-derived angiogenesis factors from various sources.[14-19] Purification and identification of the active component in these angiogenic extracts remained a formidable task.

III. THE ANGIOGENIC PROCESS

The purification of tumor-derived angiogenesis factors was severely limited by the lack of appropriate bioassays. A number of *in vivo* angiogenesis assays had been developed and were routinely used (rabbit corneal pocket, chick CAM, rat dorsal air sac, and rabbit ear chamber; see Reference 20 for further review), however, these assays were extremely time consuming and expensive, and they required large amounts of precious test material. The cloning of capillary endothelial cells[21] ushered in a period of rapid progress in the study of neovascularization. As an understanding of the biology of angiogenesis developed, *in vitro* assays were established, which could both qualitatively and quantitatively measure the cellular and biochemical components of angiogenesis in a more rapid and reproducible fashion.

It is now established that the phenomenon of tumor angiogenesis occurs via the "sprouting" of new capillaries from the preexisting microvasculature as described originally by Ausprunk and Folkman.[22] Enzymatic degradation of the basement membrane of the parent microvessel is followed by capillary endothelial cell (EC) migration (in response to an angiogenic stimulus) towards the tumor. The migrating EC align themselves to form a new sprout. Trailing EC proliferate, thereby, increasing the immature sprout length. Subsequently, the process of lumen formation occurs in which two hollow sprouts join to form vascular loops. Pericytes and basement membrane components surround the immature capillaries, completing the formation of the mature capillary bed.[23]

With the knowledge of the sequence of events required for neovascularization, the development and use of the *in vitro* assays focused on these key components of the angiogenic process: the degradation of basement membrane,[24] the migration,[25] the proliferation of capillary EC,[26,27] and the formation of three dimensional capillary tubes.[28] With the advent of these *in vitro* assay systems and the cloning of capillary endothelial cells for use in these studies, the purification and characterization of a number of angiogenesis factors, from both normal and tumor sources, were greatly facilitated.

IV. STIMULATORS OF ANGIOGENESIS

A number of different molecules have been shown to be angiogenic either by virtue of stimulating neovascularization *in vivo* and/or by their ability to stimulate capillary EC proliferation, migration, and/or capillary formation. Many of these factors have pleiotropic effects on blood vessel formation as will be evident in a discussion of these factors below. This topic has been extensively reviewed elsewhere[29-31] and will be briefly covered in this chapter. A summary of these angiogenesis stimulators is presented in Table 1.

TABLE 1
Angiogenesis Stimulators

Factor	EC Proliferation	EC Migration	Angiogenesis
FGF	+	+	+
Angiogenin	0	0	+
VEGF/VPF	+	+	+
TGF-β	−	−	+
PD-ECGF	+	+	+
TGF-α	+	+	+
Angiotropin	0	+	+
TNF-α	−	+	+

Note: + = stimulates; 0 = does not stimulate; − = inhibits.

A. ANGIOGENIC FACTORS

1. Fibroblast Growth Factors (FGF)

One family of angiogenic molecules, the FGFs, was found to possess an extremely strong affinity for the glycosaminoglycan heparin.[32-36] This observation greatly facilitated the purification of FGFs via the use of heparin affinity chromatography. The prototypes of this factor are basic (bFGF) and acidic (aFGF) FGF. The biochemical characterization of FGF is extensive. bFGF, a cationic (pI 9.6) 18 kDa polypeptide, recently has been shown to exist in higher molecular weight forms as well. aFGF, also an 18 kDa polypeptide, is anionic (pI 5) and has been shown to have a 53% absolute sequence similarity to bFGF. Both proteins share the characteristics of heat lability and stability to sulfhydryl reducing agents.[37-42] Both are mitogenic for vascular ECs, smooth muscle cells, and connective tissue cells, and they also have been shown to stimulate neural differentiation in PC12 cells[43,44] and to promote neuronal survival.[45] FGF is also chemotactic for EC, stimulates their production of collagenase and plasminogen activator, induces capillary-like tube formation *in vitro,* and has been shown to be a potent stimulator of angiogenesis *in vivo* in both the CAM and corneal pocket bioassays[24,46-48] (Figure 1). Tissue surveys reveal that bFGF appears to be ubiquitous. It has been isolated from tumors, skeletal, neural, and reproductive tissue, numerous organs, and white blood cells. aFGF has been predominantly found in neural tissues, including hypothalamus, brain, eye, and retina, and it also has been isolated from bone.[29]

As noted earlier, FGF is a potent mitogen for endothelial cells. These cells also possess receptors for FGF, bind FGF, and synthesize significant amounts of this factor.[49-52] Neither acidic nor basic FGF is secreted, but have been demonstrated to be cell-associated and "stored" in the extracellular matrix.[53,54] It has been suggested that the activity of extracellular matrix degrading enzymes might release the mitogenic molecules associated with the basement membranes, thereby, making these stimulators available.[55] An alternate hypothesis suggests that the lysis of cells of ischemic or damaged tissue could release cellular FGF, making it available to the immediate microenvironment. This theory is particularly intriguing when applied to the ischemic tissue of a necrotic tumor center.[56]

Of particular relevance to the study of tumor growth and metastases is the identification of oncogenes encoding for heparin-binding proteins. These proteins share 40 to 50% homology to bFGF and aFGF, but differ in that they possess signal peptides and are secreted proteins.[29] These include int-2[57] and the hst[58,59] oncogenes as well as the K-fgf,[60] which was isolated from a Kaposi's tumor and is identical to hst, FGF-5[60] and kFGF, (keratinocyte fibroblast growth factor), a specific epithelial cell mitogen.[61] Unlike their normal counterparts, the FGF-like oncogenes have been isolated predominantly from tumor and embryonic tissue rather than from adult tissue.[62,63]

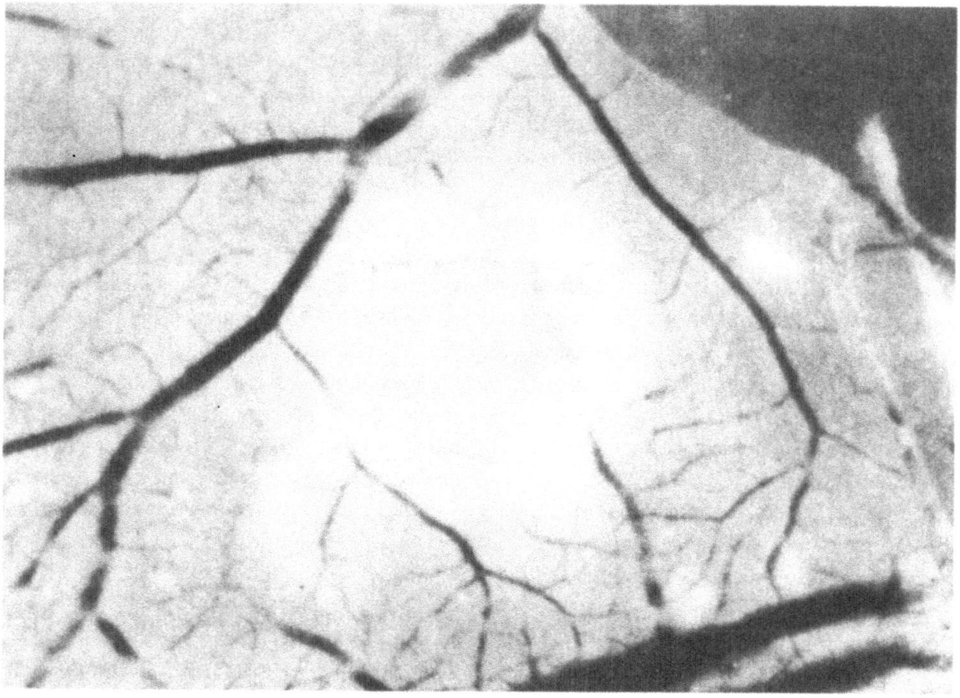

A

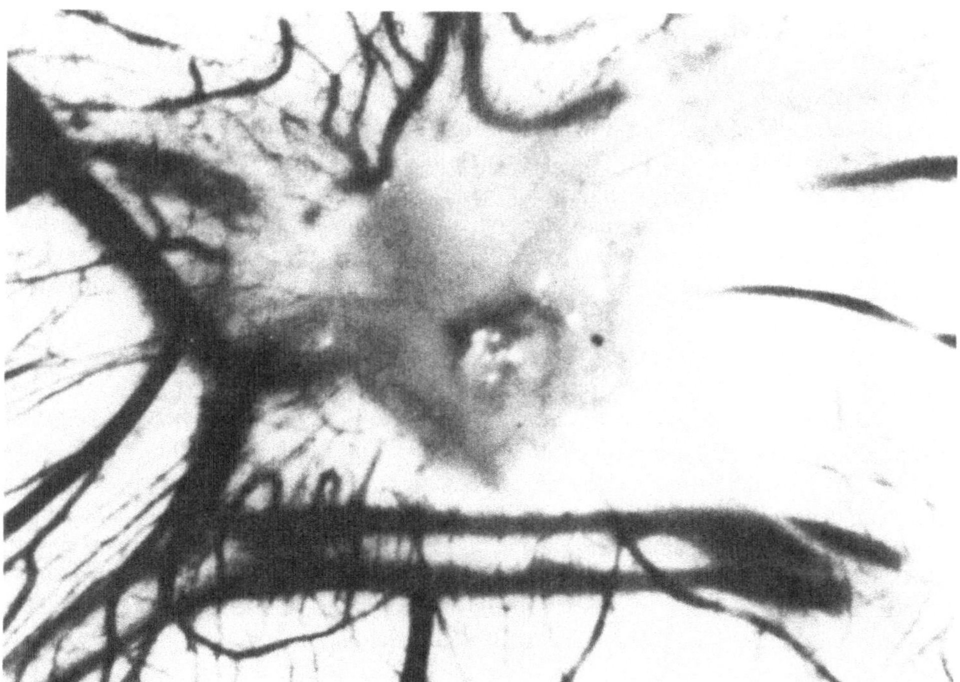

B

FIGURE 1. Stimulation of angiogenesis on the chorioallantoic membrane caused by chondrosarcoma-derived growth factor. Normal (A) and stimulated (B). (From Shing, Y., Folkman, J., Haudenschild, C., Lund, D., Crum, R., and Klagsbrun, M., *J. Cell Biochem.*, 29, 275, 1985. With permission.)

2. Angiogenin

Angiogenin is a single chain (14.1 kDa) cationic protein (pI 9.5), which is a stimulator of angiogenesis *in vivo*. However, this molecule does not appear to exert any effect on endothelial cell migration or proliferation; it does, however, activate endothelial cell phospholipase C.[64] A secreted protein, angiogenin was isolated from the conditioned medium of a number of tumor cell lines such as lung carcinoma and hepatoma cells as well as from normal cell lines including WI-38 and lymphocytes[65] and also has been found in human plasma.[66]

Analysis of the nucleotide sequence of angiogenin reveals a 35% absolute sequence homology between this molecule and pancreatic RNase A.[67] It is interesting to note that although angiogenin is angiogenic, pancreatic RNase is not, and the ribonucleolytic activity of angiogenin is weak relative to RNase. However, it has been shown that the ribonucleolytic activity and angiogenic activity of angiogenin are related.[68] Messenger RNA studies have demonstrated that angiogenesis is primarily made in adult rat liver[69] with lower amounts synthesized in the developing fetus. This suggests that angiogenin gene expression does not temporally relate to vascular development since, in the rat, vascular development is highest in the developing fetus and lowest in the adult. The role of angiogenin in the process of neovascularization remains unknown.

3. Vascular Permeability Factor/Vascular Endothelial Growth Factor (VEGF/VPF)

Recently, several laboratories have independently isolated a non-heparin-binding growth factor specific for vascular endothelial cells.[70-72] This vascular endothelial growth factor (VEGF) is similar to a vascular permeability factor (VPF), also recently purified with the exception that a 24 amino acid insert present in VPF is absent in VEGF.[73]

These mitogens are cationic (pI 8.5) highly glycosylated dimers (46 to 48 kDa) composed of 2 to 24 kDa subunits. They are stable to low pH and heat, but are labile to treatment by sulfhydryl reducing agents. VEGF/VPF demonstrates a 21 to 24% nucleotide homology with platelet-derived growth factor (PDGF) A and B chains and conservation of the cysteine residues determined in both PDGF chains. Unlike VEGF/VPF, which appear to be highly specific for endothelial cells, PDGF is a smooth muscle cell mitogen.[74]

Unlike FGF, VEGF/VPF is secreted into the conditioned media of many cell types such as rat glioma cells[72] and bovine pituitary follicular cells[70] as well as tumor cells such as mouse sarcoma 180 cells[71] and NB41 neuroblastoma cells[75] among others. These mitogens are angiogenic *in vivo* and unlike other angiogenic stimuli, VPF possesses the somewhat unique characteristic of increasing the fluid permeability from blood vessels.[73]

4. Platelet-Derived Endothelial Cell Growth Factor (PD-ECGF)

A nonheparin-binding endothelial cell growth factor, PD-ECGF, was first isolated from platelets,[76] but has since been shown to be produced by human foreskin fibroblasts as well as tumor cell lines such as human squamous carcinoma cells and anaplastic thyroid carcinoma cells. An intracellular protein that, like FGF, is not secreted, PD-ECGF is an acidic, single chain polypeptide with a molecular weight of 45,000, which is stable to reduction with sulfhydryl reducing agents, but labile to heat and acid treatment. This endothelial cell mitogen also has been shown to be chemotactic for bovine aortic endothelial cells and is a potent stimulator of angiogenesis *in vivo*. Whether this mitogen plays a role in tumor angiogenesis is yet to be determined, however, it is worth noting that tumors derived from tumor cells transfected with PD-ECGF and grown in nude mice were extremely vascular relative to control tumors.[76,77]

5. Transforming Growth Factor Beta (TGF-β)

First isolated from tumor cells, TGF-β has since been found in bone, cartilage, kidney, placenta, and platelets.[78,79] It is a homodimeric polypeptide with a molecular weight of 25 kDa.[80] This factor is secreted in a biologically latent form that can be activated by heat, proteases, or acid treatment.[80,81] TGF-β is a potent angiogenesis stimulator *in vivo* despite the fact that it is not mitogenic for endothelial cells (in fact it is an inhibitor of capillary EC proliferation as discussed below).[82] It is suggested that TGF-β's ability to stimulate angiogenesis may be a function of its chemotactic ability for monocytes and other accessory cells that may, in turn, release EC mitogens.[83]

6. Transforming Growth Factor Alpha (TGF-α)

This factor was originally isolated from transformed fibroblasts and has since been found in a number of tumor cells as well as macrophages.[84,85] It is a 5.5 kDa polypeptide that shares 40% homology with epidermal growth factor (EGF) and binds to the EGF receptor.[86,87] TGF-α is considered to be a secreted protein by virtue of the fact that it is released by proteolytic cleavage from an 18 kDa transmembrane protein precursor. TGF-α significantly stimulates EC proliferation, whereas EGF is primarily an epithelial cell mitogen. TGF-α has been shown to be capable of transforming normal cells into cells with a transformed phenotype. TGF-α and EGF are both angiogenic *in vivo,* although EGF is less potent.[88]

7. Angiotropin

Isolated from the conditioned medium of peripheral blood monocytes, angiotropin is a copper-containing polyribonucleoprotein of 4.5 kDa. This factor is highly angiogenic *in vivo* and stimulates EC chemokinesis, but not their proliferation *in vitro*. It is also able to potentiate capillary tube formation *in vitro* and has been suggested to have a role in stimulating the neovascularization required for wound healing.[89]

8. Tumor Necrosis Factor Alpha (TNF-α)

Produced predominantly by activated macrophages and tumor cells, TNF-α, also known as cachectin, was first identified as causing solid tumor necrosis regression.[90] It is also cytotoxic for some tumor cells. TNF-α is an anionic 17 kDa polypeptide that is 28% homologous with a lymphotoxin, TNF-β.[91] Interestingly, TNF-α's effect on angiogenesis is very similar to that of TGF-β. Both factors inhibit EC proliferation and stimulate capillary tube formation *in vitro* as well as angiogenesis *in vivo*.[92] TNF-α also has been shown to stimulate granulocyte-macrophage colony-stimulating factors (GM-CSF) synthesis, interleukin synthesis, and ICAM-1 induction and may, through these effects, indirectly effect the response of ECs.[93,94]

B. LOW MOLECULAR WEIGHT ANGIOGENIC FACTORS

A number of other nonpeptide factors have been shown to be angiogenic. These include prostaglandins E_1 and E_2, which are angiogenic *in vivo* and, although they do not directly effect EC proliferation or migration, are thought to modulate angiogenesis indirectly by attracting macrophages and other cells to a site where they produce angiogenesis stimulators.[95,96]

Monobutyrin (1-butyryl-glycerol) has been purified from adipocytes and demonstrated to be a potent stimulant of angiogenesis *in vivo* and endothelial cell migration, but not proliferation *in vitro*.[97]

Nicotinamide, purified from Walker 256 carcinoma cells, has been reported to stimulate angiogenesis *in vivo,* but its mechanism of action remains unknown.[98] The vasodilators adenosine diphosphate and adenosine also have been shown to be angiogenic *in vivo*.[99,100]

Finally, it should be noted that a group of undefined low molecular weight angiogenesis factors has been reported from retina, serum, tumors, synovial fluid, and other sources. Until purification and characterization of these molecules have been achieved, their roles in the angiogenic process remain unclear.[29]

It is obvious from the review of the angiogenesis stimulators presented above that there must be significant variability in the mechanism(s) by which these factors stimulate neovascularization. Some factors directly stimulate EC proliferation and migration, some stimulate only one of these events, and some do neither. Some factors exert their influence by affecting the differentiation of endothelial cells or by affecting the endothelium. Other angiogenic factors appear to work indirectly by attracting accessory cells, which then can directly affect the angiogenic process. Still other agents may act by releasing growth factors stored in the extracellular matrix (ECM). Inasmuch as there exists variability in the mechanisms by which these factors stimulate angiogenesis, there is also a "redundancy" of these factors such that no single angiogenic factor alone need be relied on for angiogenesis to occur.

Despite the existence of such a large number of diverse angiogenesis stimulators, it is striking that angiogenesis is a very tightly controlled process that rarely occurs under normal conditions, except for instances of wound healing, embryonic development, and the normal development of the corpus luteum. Normally, vascular turnover is very low. It has been demonstrated that the potential doubling time of capillary endothelium from normal tissues is in the range of 47 to 20,000 d, as opposed to 2.14 to 13 d for tumor capillary endothelium.[9] In fact, capillary endothelial cells of most normal tissue are considered to be "quiescent".

What is/are the mechanism(s) by which angiogenesis is controlled? There is an accumulating body of literature which suggests that, in addition to growth factors, inhibitors of angiogenesis and the extracellular matrix are also key regulators of vascular growth.

The next section of this chapter will focus on inhibitors of angiogenesis, many of which inhibit neovascularization by interfering with one or more of the steps of angiogenesis. Despite the extensive information acquired about angiogenesis stimulators, relatively little is known about angiogenesis inhibitors. To the extent that solid tumor growth is dependent on neovascularization, the potential therapeutic value that an angiogenesis inhibitor could have in controlling solid tumor growth and metastases has prompted a long term search for inhibitors of angiogenesis. This search has been stymied by difficulties in obtaining large enough amounts of purified inhibitors, problems with cytotoxicity of some of the anti-angiogenic agents and a lack of suitable bioassays. Herewith is a brief review of what is currently considered to be the family of angiogenesis inhibitors. A summary of these angiogenesis inhibitors is presented in Table 2.

V. INHIBITORS OF ANGIOGENESIS

A. TISSUE-DERIVED INHIBITORS

1. Cartilage-Derived Inhibitor

The choice of cartilage as a potential source of an angiogenesis inhibitor is a direct function of cartilage's avascularity. Cartilage is a relatively tumor-resistant tissue, and even the tumor associated with cartilage, chondrosarcoma, is the least vascularized of all solid tumors. A number of different groups have shown that cartilage[102] and extracts of cartilage[103-105] inhibit angiogenesis *in vivo* and endothelial cell proliferation *in vitro*.[104,106] Partially purified extracts of cartilage also have been shown to inhibit tumor-induced neovascularization when delivered locally (via controlled release polymer) and when delivered systemically (via infusion).[104,105] However, all of these studies utilized crude or partially purified extracts of cartilage and until recently, no single cartilage-derived macromolecule capable of inhibiting angiogenesis had been purified. The critical role that proteolytic enzymes appear to play in the process of neovascularization suggested that protease inhibitors might be the anti-angiogenic agents.[103,107,108]

Recently, an angiogenesis inhibitor from bovine scapular cartilage has been purified and characterized, and its amino terminal sequence data has been obtained.[109] This acid and heat

TABLE 2
Angiogenesis Inhibitors

Factor	EC Proliferation	EC Migration	Angiogenesis
Cartilage-derived inhibitor	−	−	−
Angiostatic steroids	−	ND	−
Protamine	−	ND	−
Platelet Factor-4	−	ND	−
TGF-β	−	−	+
Thrombospondin	ND	−	−
TNF-α	−	+	+
α-interferon	−	−	−

Note: + = stimulates; − = inhibits; ND = no determination.

stable protein is a collagenase inhibitor (molecular weight 27,650) that also inhibits capillary EC proliferation and migration. It is a potent inhibitor of angiogenesis when tested in the CAM assay (Figure 2). This collagenase inhibitor differs from a tissue inhibitor of metalloproteinase (TIMP) isolated from human amniotic fluid in only two amino acids of the first 28 amino terminal residues.[109]

The fact that this cartilage-derived anti-angiogenic factor is a collagenase inhibitor is consistent with earlier work demonstrating the importance of collagenase in the process of angiogenesis.[108] Proteases, including collagenase, have been shown to be required in several steps of the angiogenic process: the degradation of the parent venule's basement membrane to allow EC "escape" during the process of capillary sprouting, as well as during the process of capillary migration during which endothelial cells must degrade basement membrane to migrate towards a chemotactic stimulus. Additionally, collagenase has been shown to be required for tumor cells to breach the boundaries of the vascular tree during metastases.[111] Metalloproteinases such as collagenase have been strongly implicated in the process of malignant conversion, that point in cancer progression when tumor cells gain the capacity to invade and metastasize. A correlation has been demonstrated between the acquisition of the malignant phenotype and an increase in the expression of metalloproteinases (Type IV collagenase and transin). Additionally, a key metalloproteinase inhibitor, TIMP, is now considered to be a tumor-suppressor gene product.[111,112] The activity of such endogenous protease inhibitors may ultimately serve as a mechanism by which neovascularization and ultimately tumor growth and metastases are regulated.

2. Vitreous-Derived Inhibitor

Another avascular tissue, vitreous, also has been the object of significant efforts to purify an angiogenesis inhibitor. Vitreous extracts have been shown to inhibit neovascularization *in vivo*[113] and endothelial cell proliferation *in vitro.*[114] The identification of the angiogenesis inhibitor(s) in vitreous remains to be determined, however, it appears that vitreous contains two inhibitory species, one 10 kDa and the other 50 kDa.[114]

3. Lens-Derived Inhibitor

Extracts of human and murine lens (also an avascular tissue) have been shown to inhibit endothelial cell proliferation in cell-specific and reversible manner.[115] Purification and identification of this factor remain to be achieved.

4. Cornea-Derived Inhibitor

Bovine corneal extracts recently have been shown to contain an inhibitor of angiogenesis *in vivo* and a stimulator of capillary EC rounding *in vitro.* This negative modulator of

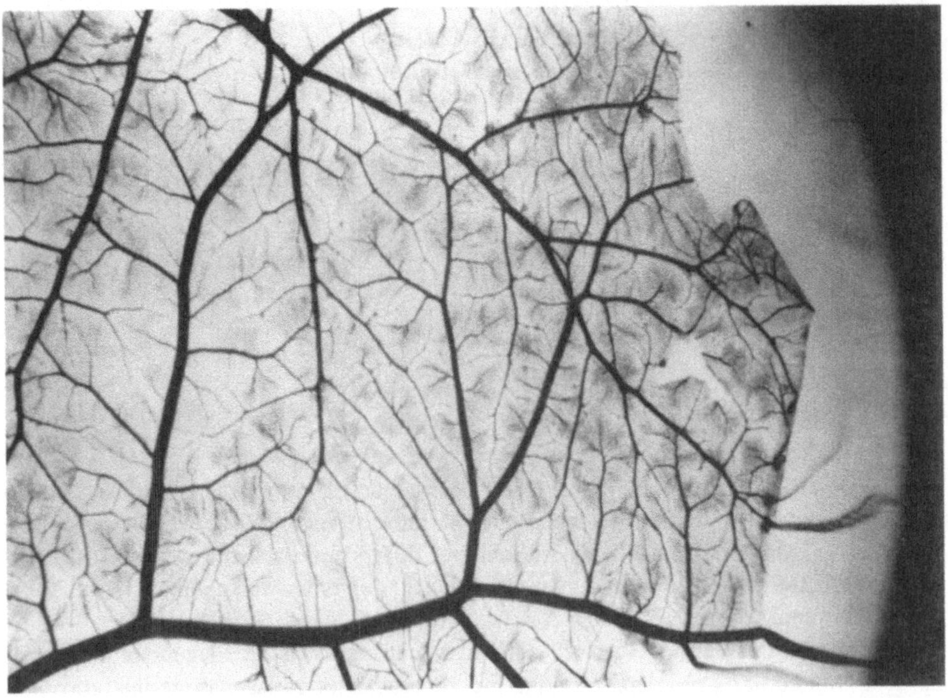

A

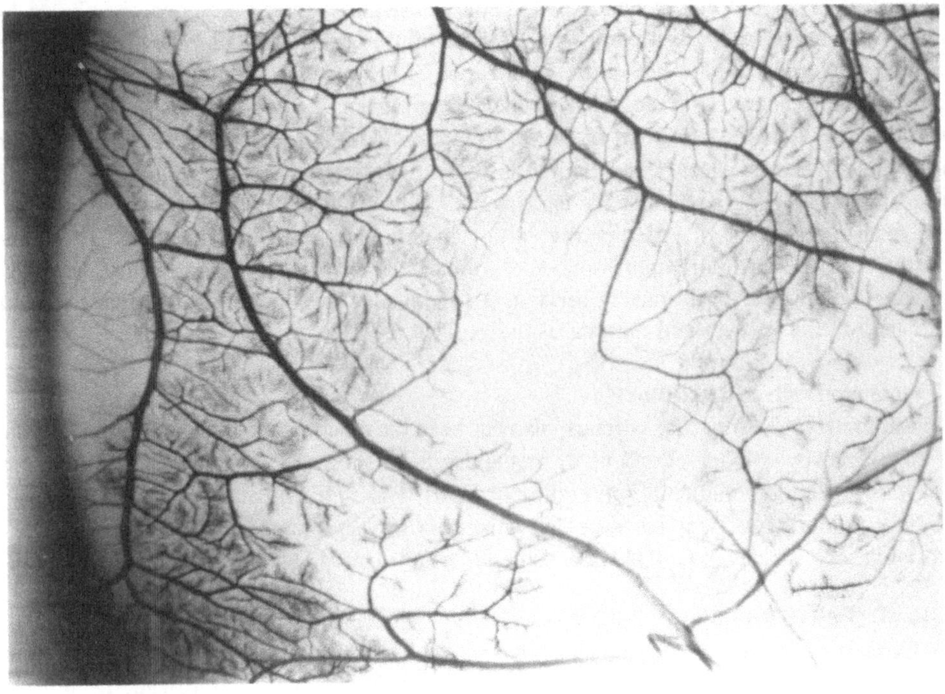

B

FIGURE 2. Inhibition of angiogenesis in the chorioallantoic membrane caused by the cartilage-derived angiogenesis inhibitor. Normal (A) and inhibited (B) showing avascular zone. CAMs were injected intravascularly with India ink. (From Moses, M. A., Sudhalter, J., and Langer, R., *Science*, 248, 1408, 1990. Copyright 1990 by the AAAS. With permission.)

angiogenesis appears to be a low (10 kDa) molecular weight nonpeptide inhibitor whose identity has not yet been determined.[116]

B. ANGIOSTATIC STEROIDS

These steroids are a unique group of molecules whose sole demonstrated biological activity is the inhibition of angiogenesis. Early work on the effects of steroids on angiogenesis demonstrated that heparin or heparin fragments, with no anticoagulant activity, could inhibit angiogenesis *in vivo,* cause tumor regression, and significantly inhibit metastases in the presence of cortisone.[117] These results were striking in their support of the hypothesis that an anti-angiogenic therapy could ultimately influence tumor growth. Subsequent structure-activity studies with steroid analogs demonstrated that the anti-angiogenic activity of the heparin-hydrocortisone combination was not a function of the mineralocorticoid, glucocorticoid, or other known bioactivities of hydrocortisone and resulted in the term "angiostatic steroid".[118] Recently, the use of a synthetic heparin substitute, B-cyclodextrin tetradeca-sulfate, administered with angiostatic steroids, has been shown to inhibit angiogenesis at 100 to 1,000 times the potency of heparin in the standard CAM assay. This drug pair also has been shown to inhibit endotoxin-induced angiogenesis in the rabbit corneal pocket assay when delivered both locally and topically.[119]

A number of mechanisms have been posed to explain the anti-angiogenic effects of these steroids in the presence of heparin. One potential mechanism suggests that these steroids act by causing fragmentation and dissolution of basement membrane components.[120] This matrix disruption is suggested to result in a loss of capillary viability since normal capillary development requires an intact basement membrane. This loss of viability would, in turn, result in the inhibition of angiogenesis and capillary involution.[20] Subsequent studies have shown that the inhibition of collagen deposition can cause capillary regression when tested on the CAM.[121]

An alternative explanation for the anti-angiogenic effect of the steroids focuses on data which demonstrate that the heparin/cortisone combination inhibits capillary endothelial cell proliferation *in vitro.*[122] Additionally, it has been shown that tumor extracts from animals treated with the heparin/cortisone pair inhibited endothelial cell migration to a much greater degree relative to control tumor extracts.[123] These two sets of studies suggested that heparin/cortisone exert their anti-angiogenic effects by directly modulating two key parameters of angiogenesis: endothelial cell proliferation and migration.

C. PROTAMINE

Protamine, a sperm-derived, molecular weight 4.3 kDa, cationic protein has been shown to be a specific inhibitor of angiogenesis. When administered systemically, it inhibited tumor growth and metastases in a number of animal models.[124,125] Due to its strong affinity for heparin and in light of the fact that potent stimuli of angiogenesis (heparin-binding growth factors) also express a strong affinity for this glycosaminoglycan, it has been hypothesized that the anti-angiogenic effect of protamine is a function of its interference with these growth factors. In support of this hypothesis, it has been shown that the mitogenic activity of soluble and matrix-bound FGF is inhibited by protamine.[126]

D. PLATELET FACTOR-4

Platelet factor-4 (PF-4) is a tetrameric polypeptide with a molecular weight of approximately 30,000. It is released from platelets during aggregation as a complex with chondroitin sulfate. This protein was originally tested for its anti-angiogenic potential due to its high affinity for heparin and was shown to be a potent inhibitor of neovascularization *in vivo.*[124] Recent studies using recombinant PF-4 have further shown that it is an inhibitor of endothelial cell proliferation. The angiostatic activity of recombinant PF-4 has been demonstrated to be associated with its heparin-binding region.[127] More recently, PF-4 has been shown to inhibit the growth of murine melanoma and human colon carcinoma.[128]

Other suggestions as to the mechanism by which PF-4 exerts its anti-angiogenic effect include not only its heparin-binding capacity but also its ability to antagonize a recently reported platelet-derived angiogenic factor.[127] Another interesting hypothesis focuses on the anticollagenase activity of this protein and suggests that PF-4's ability to inhibit collagenase may play a role in its anti-angiogenic ability.[109]

E. TRANSFORMING GROWTH FACTOR BETA (TGF-β)

Despite its inclusion in the previous section on angiogenesis factors, TGF-β is a multifunctional modulator of neovascularization.[129] In addition to its ability to stimulate the proliferation of some nonendothelial cell types and its potent stimulatory effect on angiogenesis *in vivo,* TGF-β is also a potent inhibitor of aortic and capillary endothelial cell proliferation and migration as well as being an "inducer" of cellular differentiation.[130,131]

Somewhat surprisingly, it was found that TGF-β was a potent inducer of capillary tube formation *in vitro*.[132] To the extent that angiogenesis can be thought of as a two-stage process, one being proliferative and the other being based on differentiation, it has been hypothesized that TGF-β might shift the balance towards the differentiation of capillary ECs into capillaries by inhibiting their proliferation and their migration.[29] As mentioned earlier, this protein's angiogenic effects also might be indirect ones via TGF-β's ability to attract nonendothelial cell types to a particular site where they can release their angiogenic factors. A particularly interesting role for TFG-β has evolved from a study of the relationship between the pericyte or smooth muscle cell, mural cells intimately associated with endothelial cells, and the endothelial cells themselves. It has been demonstrated, via a coculture system of the two cell types, that contact between them results in the inhibition of endothelial cell proliferation[133] and that this inhibition is mediated by the activation of latent TGF-β. These results have suggested that this protein, by virtue of its ability to inhibit capillary EC proliferation, inhibits angiogenesis, and thereby, maintains the quiescent nature of the normal microvascular system.[134]

F. THROMBOSPONDIN

Recently, a 140 kDa protein (Gp140) homologous in sequence and function to the C-terminus of human thrombospondin (160 kDa) has been shown to inhibit angiogenesis *in vivo* and capillary endothelial cell migration *in vitro*.[135] Most interestingly, this inhibitory factor was purified from the conditioned media of hamster and human hybrid lines when they were expressing an active cancer suppressor gene.[136] Since the onset of angiogenesis and tumorigenesis was concomitant with the loss of GP140 activity, the production of such an angiogenic inhibitor may be a means by which tumor growth is controlled.[135]

G. TUMOR NECROSIS FACTOR ALPHA (TNF-α)

As mentioned earlier, interest in this molecule as an anti-angiogenic factor stemmed from earlier observations that it caused hemorrhagic necrosis in solid tumors and was cytotoxic for some tumor cells.[90] Since then, TNF-α has been shown to inhibit capillary and aortic cell proliferation as well as smooth muscle cell growth.[137] Somewhat paradoxically, TNF-α stimulates angiogenesis *in vivo*. As in the case of TGF-β, this factor may indirectly stimulate angiogenesis by attracting macrophages and mast cells to a particular site where they, in turn, release their stimulants.[29]

H. ALPHA AND GAMMA INTERFERON

Alpha interferon has been shown to inhibit endothelial cell proliferation and capillary tube formation *in vitro* and has been a positive therapy when tested in patients with hemangioendotheliomas.[138] Gamma interferon, a 50 kDa glycoprotein, is also an inhibitor of growth factor-stimulated endothelial cell proliferation as well as a number of transformed cells.[139]

VI. OTHER REGULATORS OF ANGIOGENESIS

A. EXTRACELLULAR MATRIX

Local perturbations in the extracellular matrix via a number of different mechanisms, both direct and indirect, have been shown to play a role in the control of neovascularization. In studies analyzing the mechanism by which angiostatic steroids have their anti-angiogenic effect, evidence was presented to demonstrate that these factors might act to inhibit neovascularization via their dissolution and fragmentation of the basement membrane.[120] *In vitro* studies also support a role for matrix in the control of neovascularization. The growth and differentiation of endothelial cells has been shown to be strongly influenced by the extracellular matrix molecules upon which these cultures are established and maintained.[140] Furthermore, the speed of EC migration is strongly influenced by various extracellular matrix components.[141]

In light of these observations, certain angiogenic factors have been shown to indirectly influence the process of neovascularization by affecting the matrix. Basic FGF has been shown to stimulate capillary EC to secrete collagenase, which causes degradation of the extracellular matrix,[142] an important prerequisite for EC migration; a stimulator of angiogenesis, TGF-β increases the production of Type IV collagen and fibronectin and causes an increase in protease inhibitor production,[143] thereby, perhaps preserving the intact basement membrane required for neovascularization. The fact that a collagenase inhibitor is a potent inhibitor of endothelial cell proliferation and migration as well as being an inhibitor of angiogenesis *in vivo,*[109] suggests that changes in the integrity and/or quantity of intact basement membrane components, in this case collagen, may have significant ramifications on the process of neovascularization. Finally, the extracellular matrix may indirectly influence angiogenesis by functioning as a storage depot for bFGF, which has been demonstrated to be bound to heparin-like sites in the extracellular matrix and may be released by a number of mechanisms.[53,54]

B. COPPER

Much attention has recently been focused on the role of copper in neovascularization. It has been demonstrated that both acidic and basic FGF bind to copper,[144] and when they are complexed to copper, copper-chelating agents have been shown to be angiogenic.[145] Additionally, in work studying the effect of prostaglandin E_1 (PGE_1) on angiogenesis, it was shown that an increase in copper levels preceded the angiogenic response. Rabbits on a copper-deficient diet appear to be unable to respond to angiogenic stimuli.[145] Copper ions have been shown to stimulate endothelial cell migration.[146] To date, despite the lack of a unifying hypothesis, it would appear that copper "modulates the intensity" of the angiogenic response to various stimuli.[31] Further study should elucidate the role of this potentially important angiogenic modifier.

C. HEPARIN

This glycosaminoglycan also appears to play a role in neovascularization by modifying various responses to known angiogenic factors. Heparin enhances the angiogenic effect of angiogenesis factors *in vivo*[124] and can potentiate growth factor-stimulated endothelial cell proliferation and migration *in vitro.*[147,148] It modulates the inhibition of angiogenesis by enhancing the effect of the angiostatic steroids.[118] Whole heparin and nitrous acid-depolymerized heparin have been demonstrated to inhibit capillary EC proliferation in the absence of exogenous growth factors.[149] The exact mechanism(s) by which heparin has these and other modulating effects on the process of neovascularization remains to be elucidated.

VII. SUMMARY

In recent years, much progress has been made in elucidating the role of angiogenesis in the process of tumor metastases. It is now well established that successful solid tumor growth, both primary and secondary, is an angiogenesis-dependent process. Successful propagation of the metastatic cascade also depends on the vascularization of tumors, i.e., blood vessels are required for the growth and metastases of the primary tumor cells to secondary organs; tumor cells in the secondary site also require vascularization to grow, to be shed into the bloodstream, and to colonize other metastatic sites.[20]

Until recently, little was known, either mechanistically or temporally, about the transition to an angiogenic state during early tumor development. Folkman and co-workers have used a transgenic mice model in which the mice express an oncogene (RIP-Tag) in the beta cells of the pancreatic islets. Consequently, they consistently and predictably experience a progression from normality to hyperplasia to neoplasia.[150] In a striking series of experiments, these investigators showed that the induction of angiogenic activity and the resulting neovascularization both preceded tumor formation and correlated with the transition from hyperplasia to neoplasia. Future research efforts will undoubtedly focus on the molecular genetic events that control angiogenesis induction and tumor growth and metastasis.[150]

Angiogenesis is a complex process dependent on a delicate equilibrium between stimulators and inhibitors. It is a phenomenon characterized by key cellular and biochemical events, many of which lend themselves to inhibitory intervention. Therapeutic strategies that accomplish this goal may ultimately lead to the control of those pathological states, including cancer, in which deregulated angiogenesis plays a critical role.

ACKNOWLEDGMENTS

The author gratefully acknowledges Dr. Patricia A. D'Amore for the many helpful discussions and for her critical review of this chapter and Melissa Vultaggio and Judith Sudhalter for their generous help in the preparation of this manuscript.

REFERENCES

1. **Folkman, J. F.,** Angiogenesis: initiation and control, *Ann. N.Y. Acad. Sci.*, 401, 212, 1982.
2. **Algire, G. H., Chalkley, H. W., Legallais, F. Y., and Park, H. D.,** Vascular reactions of normal and malignant tissues *in vitro*. I. Vascular reactions of mice to wounds and to normal and neoplastic implants, *J. Natl. Cancer Inst.*, 6, 73, 1945.
3. **Gimbrone, M. A., Jr., Aster, R. H., Cotran, R. S., Corkery, J., Jandl, J. H., and Folkman, J.,** Preservation of vascular integrity in organs perfused *in vitro* with a platelet-rich medium, *Nature*, 221, 33, 1969.
4. **Gimbrone, M. A., Leapman, S. B., Cotran, R. S., and Folkman, J.,** Tumor dormancy *in vivo* by prevention of neovascularization, *J. Exp. Med.*, 136, 261, 1972.
5. **Folkman, J.,** Anti-angiogenesis: new concept for therapy of solid tumor, *Ann. Surg.*, 1975, 409, 1973.
6. **D'Amore, P. A.,** Antiangiogenesis as a strategy for antimetastasis, *Semin. Thromb. Hemost.*, 14, 73, 1988.
7. **Folkman, J. and Hochberg, M.,** Self-regulation of growth in three dimensions, *J. Exp. Med.*, 138, 745, 1973.
8. **Tannock, I. F.,** The relation between cell proliferation and the vascular system in a transplanted mouse mammary tumor, *Br. J. Cancer*, 22, 258, 1968.

9. **Tannock, I. F.,** Population kinetics of carcinoma cells, capillary endothelial cells, and fibroblasts in a transplanted mouse mammary tumor, *Cancer Res.,* 30, 2470, 1970.
10. **Ausprunk, D. H., Falterman, K., and Folkman, J.,** The sequence of events in the regression of corneal capillaries, *Lab. Invest.,* 38, 284, 1978.
11. **Greenblatt, M. and Shubik, P.,** Tumor angiogenesis: transfilter diffusion studies in the hamster by transparent chamber technique, *J. Natl. Cancer Inst.,* 41, 111, 1968.
12. **Folkman, J., Merler, E., Abernathy, C., and Williams, G.,** Isolation of a tumor factor responsible for angiogenesis, *J. Exp. Med.,* 133, 275, 1971.
13. **Klagsbrun, M., Knighton, D., and Folkman, J.,** Tumor angiogenesis activity in cells grown in tissue culture, *Cancer Res.,* 36, 110, 1976.
14. **Fenseleau, A. and Mello, R. J.,** Growth stimulation of cultured endothelial cells by tumor cell homogenates, *Cancer Res.,* 36, 3269, 1976.
15. **Atherton, A.,** Growth stimulation of endothelial cells by simultaneous culture with Sarcoma 180 cells in diffusion chambers, *Cancer Res.,* 37, 3619, 1977.
16. **McAuslan, B. R. and Hoffman, H.,** Endothelium stimulating factor from Walker carcinoma cells, *Exp. Cell Res.,* 119, 181, 1979.
17. **Weiss, J. B., Brown, R. A., Kumar, S., and Phillips, P.,** An angiogenesis factor isolated from tumours: a potent low-molecular weight compound., *Br. J. Cancer,* 40, 493, 1979.
18. **Fenseleau, A., Watt, S., and Mello, R. J.,** Tumor angiogenic factor. Purification from Walker 256 rat tumor, *J. Biol. Chem.,* 256, 9605, 1981.
19. **Rifkin, D. B., Gross, J. L., Moscatelli, D., and Jaffe, E.,** Proteases and angiogenesis: production of plasminogen activator and collagenase by endothelial cells, in *Pathobiology of the Endothelial Cells,* Nossel, H. L. and Vogel, H. J., Eds., Academic Press, New York, 1982, 191.
20. **Blood, C. H. and Zetter, B. R.,** Tumor interactions with the vasculature: angiogenesis and tumor metastasis, *Biochim. Biophys. Acta,* 1032, 89, 1990.
21. **Folkman, J., Haudenschild, C., and Zetter, B. R.,** Long-term culture of capillary endothelial cells, *Proc. Natl. Acad. Sci., U.S.A.,* 76, 5217, 1979.
22. **Ausprunk, D. H. and Folkman, J.,** Migration and proliferation of endothelial cells in preformed and newly formed vessels during tumor angiogenesis, *Microvasc. Res.,* 14, 53, 1977.
23. **Crocker, D. J., Murand, T. M., and Greer, J. C.,** Role of the pericyte in wound healing. An ultrastructural study, *Exp. Mol. Pathol.,* 13, 51, 1970.
24. **Gross, J. L., Moscatelli, D., and Rifkin, D. B.,** Increased capillary endothelial cell protease activity in response to angiogenic stimuli *in vitro, Proc. Natl. Acad. Sci. U.S.A.,* 80, 2623, 1983.
25. **Glaser, B. M., D'Amore, P. A., Seppa, H., Seppa, S., and Schiffmann, E.,** Adult tissues contain chemoattractants for vascular endothelial cells, *Nature,* 288, 483, 1980.
26. **Gimbrone, M. A., Jr., Cotran, R. S., and Folkman, J.,** Endothelial regeneration and turn-over. Studies with human endothelial cell cultures, *Ser. Haematol.,* 6, 453, 1973.
27. **Gospodarowicz, D.,** Expression and control of vascular endothelial cells: proliferation and differentiation by fibroblast growth factor, *J. Invest. Dermatol.,* 93, 395, 1989.
28. **Montesano, R. and Orci, L.,** Tumor-promoting phorbol esters induce angiogenesis *in vitro, Cell,* 42, 469, 1985.
29. **Klagsbrun, M. and D'Amore, P. A.,** Regulators of angiogenesis, *Ann. Rev. Physiol.,* 53, 217, 1991.
30. **D'Amore, P. A. and Klagsbrun, M.,** Angiogenesis: factors and mechanisms, in *The Pathology of Neoplasia,* Sirica, A. E., Ed., Plenum Press, New York, 1989, 513.
31. **Folkman, J. and Klagsbrun, M.,** Angiogenic factors, *Science,* 235, 442, 1987.
32. **Shing, Y., Folkman, J., Sullivan, R., Butterfield, C., Murray, J., and Klagsbrun, M.,** Heparin affinity: purification of a tumor-derived capillary endothelial cell growth factor, *Science,* 223, 1296, 1984.
33. **D'Amore, P. A. and Klagsbrun, M.,** Endothelial cell mitogen derived from retina and hypothalamus: biochemical and biological similarities, *J. Cell Biol.,* 99, 1545, 1984.
34. **Maciag, T., Mehlman, T., Friesel, R., and Schreiber, A.,** Heparin binds endothelial cell growth factor, the principle mitogen in the bovine brain, *Science,* 225, 932, 1984.
35. **Gospodarowicz, D., Cheng, J., Lui, G. M., Baird, A., and Bohlen, P.,** Isolation of brain fibroblast growth factor by heparin-Sepharose affinity chromatography: identity with pituitary fibroblast growth factor, *Proc. Natl. Acad. Sci., U.S.A.,* 81, 6963, 1984.
36. **Shing, Y., Folkman, J., Haudenschild, C., Lund, D., Crum, R., and Klagsbrun, M.,** Angiogenesis is stimulated by a tumor-derived endothelial cell growth factor, *J. Cell Biochem.,* 29, 275, 1985.
37. **Klagsbrun, M. and Shing, Y.,** Heparin affinity of anionic and cationic capillary endothelial growth factors: analysis of hypothalamus-derived growth factors and fibroblast growth factors, *Proc. Natl. Acad. Sci., U.S.A.,* 83, 805, 1985.
38. **Lobb, R. R. and Fett, J. W.,** Purification of two distinct growth factors from bovine neural tissue by heparin affinity chromatography, *Biochemistry,* 23, 6295, 1984.

39. **Ueno, N., Baird, A., Esch, F., Ling, N., and Guillemin, R.,** Isolation of an amino terminal-extended form of basic fibroblast growth factor, *Biochim. Biophys. Res. Commun.*, 138, 580, 1986.
40. **Moscatelli, D., Joseph, S. J., Presta, M., and Rifkin, D. B.,** Multiple forms of an angiogenesis factor: basic fibroblast growth factor, *Biochimie*, 70, 83, 1988.
41. **Iberg, N., Rogelj, S., Fanning, P., and Klagsbrun, M.,** Purification of 18- and 22-kDa forms of basic fibroblast growth factor from rat cells transformed by the *ras* oncogene, *J. Biol. Chem.*, 264, 19951, 1989.
42. **Florkiewicz, R. Z. and Sommer, A.,** Human basic fibroblast growth factor gene encodes four polypeptides: three initiate translation from non-AUG codons, *Proc. Natl. Acad. Sci. U.S.A.*, 86, 3978, 1989.
43. **Togari, A., Dickens, G., Kuzuya, H., and Guroff, G.,** The effect of fibroblast growth factor on PC12 cells, *J. Neurosci.*, 5, 307, 1985.
44. **Wagner, J. and D'Amore, P. A.,** Neurite outgrowth induced by an endothelial cell mitogen isolated from retina, *J. Cell Biol.*, 103, 1363, 1986.
45. **Walicke, P. A.,** Basic and acidic fibroblast growth factors have trophic effects on neurons from multiple CNS regions, *J. Neurosci.*, 8, 2618, 1988.
46. **Mignatti, P., Tsuboi, R., Robbins, E., and Rifkin, D. B.,** *In vitro* angiogenesis on the human amniotic membrane: requirement for basic fibroblast growth factor-induced proteinases, *J. Cell Biol.*, 108, 671, 1989.
47. **Sato, Y. and Rifkin, D. B.,** Autocrine activities of basic fibroblast growth factor: regulation of endothelial cell movement, plasminogen activator synthesis, and DNA synthesis, *J. Cell Biol.*, 107, 1119, 1988.
48. **Montesano, R., Pepper, M. S., Belin, D., Vassalli, J. D., and Orci, L.,** Induction of angiogenesis *in vitro* by vanadate, an inhibitor of phosphotyrosine phosphatases, *J. Cell Physiol.*, 134, 460, 1988.
49. **Friesel, R., Burgess, W. H., Mehlman, T., and Maciag, T.,** The characterization of the receptor for endothelial cell growth factor by covalent ligand attachment, *J. Biol. Chem.*, 261, 7581, 1986.
50. **Moscatelli, D.,** High and low affinity binding sites for basic fibroblast growth factor on cultured cells: absence of a role for low affinity binding in the stimulation of plasminogen activator production by bovine capillary endothelial cells, *J. Cell. Physiol.*, 131, 123, 1987.
51. **Bikfalvi, A., Dupuy, E., Inyang, A. L., Fayein, N., Leseche, G., Courtois, Y., and Tobelem, G.,** Binding, internalization, and degradation of basic fibroblast growth factor in human microvascular endothelial cells, *Exp. Cell Res.*, 181, 75, 1989.
52. **Bouche, G., Gas, N., Prats, H., Baldin, V., Tauber, J. P., Teissie, J., and Amalric, F.,** Basic fibroblast growth factor enters the nucleolus and stimulates the transcription of ribosomal genes in ABAE cells undergoing G0—G1 transition, *Proc. Natl. Acad. Sci. U.S.A.*, 84, 6770, 1987.
53. **Vlodavsky, I., Folkman, J., Sullivan, R., Fridman, R., Ishai-Michaeli, R., Sasse, J., and Klagsbrun, M.,** Endothelial cell-derived basic fibroblast growth factor: synthesis and deposition into subendothelial extracellular matrix, *Proc. Natl. Acad. Sci., U.S.A.*, 84, 2292, 1987.
54. **Baird, A. and Ling, N.,** Fibroblast growth factors are present in the extracellular matrix produced by endothelial cells *in vitro:* implications for a role of heparinase-like enzymes in the neovascular response, *Biochem. Biophys. Res. Commun.*, 142, 428, 1987.
55. **Bashkin, P., Doctrow, S., Klagsbrun, M., Svahn, C. N. M., Folkman, J., and Vlodavsky, I.,** Basic fibroblast growth factor binds to subendothelial extracellular matrix and is released by heparitinase and heparin-like molecules, *Biochemistry*, 28, 1737, 1989.
56. **D'Amore, P. A. and Thomson, R. W.,** Mechanisms of angiogenesis, *Ann. Rev. Physiol.*, 49, 453, 1987.
57. **Dickson, C., Smith, R., Brookes, S., and Peters, G.,** Proviral insertions within the int-2 gene can generate multiple anomalous transcripts but leave the protein-coding domain intact, *J. Virol.*, 64, 784, 1990.
58. **Tahara, E.,** Oncogenes in human gastric carcinoma, *Gan To Kagaku Ryoho*, 16, 2149, 1989.
59. **Yoshida, T., Muramatsu, H., Muramatsu, T., Sakamoto, H., Katoh, O., Sugimura, T., and Terada, M.,** Differential expression of two homologous and clustered oncogenes, Hst1 and Int-2, during differentiation of F9 cells, *Biochem. Biophys. Res. Commun.*, 157, 618, 1988.
60. **Delli-Bovi, P., Curatola, A. M., Kern, F. G., Greco, A., Ittmann, M., and Basilico, C.,** An oncogene isolated by transfection of Kaposi's sarcoma DNA encodes a growth factor that is a member of the FGF family, *Cell*, 50, 729, 1987.
61. **Zhan, X., Bates, B., Hu, X. G., and Goldfarb, M.,** The human FGF-5 oncogene encodes a novel protein related to fibroblast growth factors, *Mol. Cell. Biol.*, 8, 3487, 1988.
62. **Smith, R., Peters, G., and Dickson, C.,** Multiple RNAs expressed from the int-2 gene in mouse embryonal carcinoma cell lines encode a protein with homology to fibroblast growth factors, *Embo. J.*, 7, 1013, 1988.
63. **Zhou, D. J., Casey, G., and Cline, M.,** Amplification of human int-2 in breast cancers and squamous carcinomas, *Oncogene*, 2, 279, 1988.
64. **Bicknell, R. and Vallee, B. L.,** Angiogenin activates endothelial cell phospholipase C, *Proc. Natl. Acad. Sci. U.S.A.*, 85, 5961, 1988.
65. **Rybak, S. M., Fett, J. W., Yao, Q. Z., and Vallee, B. L.,** Angiogenin mRNA in human and normal cells, *Biochem. Biophys. Res. Commun.*, 146, 1240, 1987.

66. **Shapiro, R., Strydom, D. J., Olson, K. A., and Vallee, B. L.,** Isolation of angiogenin from normal human plasma, *Biochemistry,* 26, 5141, 1987.
67. **Shapiro, R., Riordan, J. F., and Vallee, B. L.,** Characteristic ribonucleolytic activity of human angiogenin, *Biochemistry,* 25, 3537, 1986.
68. **Fox, E. A. and Riordan, J. F.,** The molecular biology of angiogenin, in *The Molecular Biology of the Cardiovascular System,* Chien, S., Ed., Lea and Fabiger, Philadelphia, 1990, 139.
69. **Weiner, H. L., Weiner, L. H., and Swain, J.,** The tissue distribution and developmental expression of the messenger RNA encoding angiogenin, *J. Cell Physiol.,* 102, 267, 1987.
70. **Ferrara, N. and Henzel, W. J.,** Pituitary follicular cells secrete a novel heparin-binding growth factor specific for vascular endothelial cells, *Biochim. Biophys. Res. Commun.,* 161, 851, 1989.
71. **Rosenthal, R. A., Megyesi, J. F., Henzel, W. J., Ferrara, N., and Folkman, J.,** Conditioned medium from mouse sarcoma 180 cells contain vascular endothelial growth factor, *Growth Factors,* 1991, in press.
72. **Conn, G., Soderman, D. D., Schaeffer, M. T., Wile, M., Hatcher, V. B., and Thomas, K. A.,** Purification of a glycoprotein vascular endothelial cell mitogen from a rat glioma-derived cell line, *Proc. Natl. Acad. Sci. U.S.A.,* 87, 1323, 1990.
73. **Connolly, D. T., Heuvelman, D. M., Nelson, R., Olander, J. V., Eppely, B. L., Delfino, J. J., Siegel, N. R., Leimgruber, R. M., and Feder, J.,** Tumor vascular permeability factor stimulates endothelial cell growth and angiogenesis, *J. Clin. Invest.,* 84, 1478, 1989.
74. **Keck, P. J., Hauser, S. D., Krivi, G., Sanzo, K., Warren, T., Feder, J., and Connolly, D. T.,** Vascular permeability factor, an endothelial cell mitogen related to PDGF, *Science,* 246, 1309, 1989.
75. **Levy, A. P., Tamargo, R., Brem, H., and Nathans, D.,** An endothelial cell growth factor from the mouse neuroblastoma cell line NB41, *Growth Factors,* 2, 9, 1989.
76. **Usuki, K., Heldin, N. E., Miyazono, K., Ishikawa, F., Takaku, F., Westermark, B., and Heldin, C. H.,** Production of platelet-derived endothelial cell growth factor by normal and transformed human cells in culture, *Proc. Natl. Acad. Sci. U.S.A.,* 86, 7427, 1989.
77. **Ishikawa, F., Miyazono, K., Hellman, U., Wernstedt, C., Hagiwara, K., Usuki, K., Takuku, F., and Heldin, C. H.,** cDNA cloning and expression of a novel angiogenic factor — platelet-derived endothelial cell growth factor, *Nature,* 338, 557, 1989.
78. **Assoian, R. K., Komoriya, A., Meyers, C. A., Miller, D. M., and Sporn, M. B.,** Transforming growth factor-beta in human platelets. Identification of a major storage site, purification, and characterization, *J. Biol. Chem.,* 258, 7155, 1983.
79. **Roberts, A. B. and Sporn, M. B.,** Transforming growth factor beta, *Adv. Cancer Rev.,* 51, 107, 1988.
80. **Sporn, M. B., Roberts, A. B., Wakefield, L. M., and De Crombrughe, B.,** Some recent advances in the chemistry and biology of transforming growth factor-beta, *J. Cell Biol.,* 105, 1039, 1987.
81. **Lawrence, D. A., Pircher, R., and Julien, P.,** Conversion of a high molecular weight latent TGF-beta from chicken embryo fibroblasts into a low molecular weight active TGF-beta under acidic conditions, *Biochem. Biophys. Res. Commun.,* 133, 1026, 1985.
82. **Frater-Schroder, M., Muller, G., Birchmeier, W., and Bohlen, P.,** Transforming growth factor-beta inhibits endothelial cell proliferation, *Biochem. Biophys. Res. Commun.,* 137, 295, 1986.
83. **Wahl, S. M., Hunt, D. A., Wakefield, L. M., McCartney-Francis, N., Wahl, L. M., Roberts, A. B., and Sporn, M. B.,** Transforming growth factor-beta induces monocyte chemotaxis and growth factor production, *Proc. Natl. Acad. Sci. U.S.A.,* 84, 5788, 1987.
84. **Todaro, G. J., Fryling, C., and DeLarco, J. E.,** Transforming growth factors produced by certain human tumor cells: polypeptides that interact with epidermal growth factor receptors, *Proc. Natl. Acad. Sci. U.S.A.,* 77, 5258, 1980.
85. **Madtes, D. K., Raines, E. W., Sakariassen, K. S., Assoian, R. K., Sporn, M. B., Bell, G. I., and Ross, R.,** Induction of transforming growth factor-alpha in activated human alveolar macrophages, *Cell,* 53, 285, 1988.
86. **Marquadt, H., Hunkapiller, M. W., Hood, L. E., and Todaro, G. J.,** Rat transforming growth factor type I: structure and relationship to epidermal growth factor, *Science,* 233, 1079, 1984.
87. **Derynck, R., Roberts, A. B., Winckler, M. E., Chen, E. Y., and Goeddel, D. V.,** Human transforming growth factor-alpha: precursor structure and expression in *E. coli, Cell,* 38, 287, 1984.
88. **Schreiber, A. B., Winckler, M. E., and Dernyck, R.,** Transforming growth factor-alpha: a more potent angiogenic mediator than epidermal growth factor, *Science,* 232, 1250, 1986.
89. **Hockel, M., Jung, W., Vaupel, P., Rabes, H., Khaledpour, C., and Wisler, J. H.,** Purified monocyte-derived angiogenic substance (angiotropin) induces controlled angiogenesis associated with regulated tissue proliferation in rabbit skin, *J. Clin. Invest.,* 82, 1075, 1988.
90. **Carswell, E. A., Old, L. J., Kassel, R. L., Green, S., Fiore, N., Williamson, B.,** An endotoxin-induced serum that causes tumor necrosis, *Proc. Natl. Acad. Sci. U.S.A.,* 72, 3666, 1975.
91. **Gray, P. W., Aggarwal, B. B., Benten, C. V., Bringman, T. S., Henzel, W. J., Jarrett, J. A., Leung, D. W., Moffat, B., Ng, P., Sverdersky, L. P., Palladino, M. A., and Newdin, G. E.,** Cloning and expression of cDNA for human lymphotoxin, a lymphokine with tumor necrosis activity, *Nature,* 320, 584, 1984.

92. **Leibovich, S. J., Polverini, P. J., Shepard, H. M., Wiseman, D. M., Shively, V., Nuseir, N.,** Macrophage-induced angiogenesis is mediated by tumor necrosis factor-alpha, *Nature,* 329, 630, 1987.
93. **Pober, J. S., Gimbrone, M. A., Jr., LaPierre, L. A., Fiers, W., Rothlein, R., and Springer, T. A.,** Overlapping patterns of activation of human endothelial cells by interleukin-1, tumor necrosis factor, and immune interferon, *J. Immunol.,* 137, 1893, 1986.
94. **Bevilacqua, M. P., Pober, J. S., Wheeler, M. E., Cotran, R. S., and Gimbrone, M. A., Jr.,** Interleukin-1 acts on cultured human vascular endothelium to increase the adhesion of polymorphonuclear leucocytes, monocytes, and related leucocyte cell lines, *J. Clin. Invest.,* 76, 2003, 1985.
95. **Ziche, M., Jones, J., and Gullino, P.,** Role of prostaglandin E1 and copper in angiogenesis, *J. Natl. Cancer Inst.,* 69, 475, 1982.
96. **Form, D. M. and Auerbach, R.,** PGE2 and angiogenesis, *Proc. Soc. Exp. Biol. Med.,* 172, 214, 1983.
97. **Dobson, D. E., Kambe, A., Block, E., Dion, T., Lu, H., Castellot, J. J., Jr., and Speigelman, B. M.,** 1-Butyryl-glycerol: a novel angiogenesis factor secreted by differentiation adipocytes, *Cell,* 61, 223, 1990.
98. **Kull, J. C., Jr., Brent, D. A., Parikh, I., and Cuatrecasas, P.,** Chemical identification of a tumor-derived angiogenic factor, *Science,* 236, 843, 1987.
99. **Dusseau, J. W., Hutchins, P. M., and Malbasa, D. S.,** Stimulation of angiogenesis by adenosine on the chick chorioallantoic membrane, *Circ. Res.,* 59, 163, 1986.
100. **Fraser, R. A., Ellis, M., and Stalker, A. L.,** Experimental angiogenesis in the chorioallantoic membrane, in *Current Advances in the Basic Clinical Microcirculatory Research,* Lewis, S., Ed., S. Karger, Basel, 1979, 25.
101. **Hobson, B. and Denekamp, J.,** Endothelial proliferation in tumors and normal tissues: continuous labelling studies, *Br. J. Cancer,* 49, 405, 1984.
102. **Brem, H. and Folkman, J.,** Inhibition of tumor angiogenesis mediated by cartilage, *J. Exp. Med.,* 141, 427, 1975.
103. **Pauli, B., Memoli, V., and Kuettner, K.,** Regulation of tumor invasion by cartilage-derived anti-invasion factor *in vitro, J. Natl. Cancer Inst.,* 67, 65, 1981.
104. **Langer, R., Brem, H., Falterman, K., Klein, M., and Folkman, J.,** Isolation of a cartilage factor that inhibits tumor neovascularization, *Science,* 193, 70, 1976.
105. **Langer, R., Conn, H., Vacanti, J., Haudenschild, C., and Folkman, J.,** Control of tumor growth in animals by infusion of an angiogenesis inhibitor, *Proc. Natl. Acad. Sci. U.S.A.,* 77, 4331, 1980.
106. **Sorgente, N. and Dorey, C. K.,** Inhibition of endothelial cell growth by a factor isolated from cartilage, *Exp. Cell Res.,* 128, 63, 1980.
107. **Eisenstein, R., Kuettner, K. E., Neopolitan, C., Soble, L. W., and Sorgente, N.,** The resistance of certain tissue to invasion. III. Cartilage extracts inhibit the growth of fibroblasts and endothelial cells in culture, *Am. J. Pathol.,* 81, 337, 1975.
108. **Rifkin, D. B, Gross, S. L., Moscatelli, D., and Jaffe, E.,** Proteases and angiogenesis: production of plasminogen activator and collagenase by endothelial cells, in *Pathobiology of the Endothelial Cell,* Nossel, M. L. and Vogel, H. J., Eds., Academic Press., New York, 1982, 191.
109. **Moses, M. A., Sudhalter, J., and Langer, R.,** Identification of an inhibitor of neovascularization from cartilage, *Science,* 248, 1408, 1990.
110. **Liotta, L. A., Abe, S., Robey, P. G., and Martin, G. R.,** Preferential digestion of basement membrane collagen by an enzyme from a metastatic murine tumor, *Proc. Natl. Acad. Sci. U.S.A.,* 76, 2268, 1979.
111. **Liotta, L. A. and Stetler-Stevenson, W.,** Metalloproteinases and malignant conversion: does correlation imply causality?, *J. Natl. Cancer Inst.,* 81, 556, 1989.
112. **Khokha, R., Waterhouse, P., Yagel, S., Lala, P. K., Overall, G. M., Norton, G., and Denhardt, D. T.,** Antisense RNA-induced reduction in murine TIMP levels confers oncogenicity in Swiss 3T3 cells, *Science,* 243, 947, 1989.
113. **Preis, I., Langer, R., Brem, H., and Folkman, J.,** Inhibition of neovascularization by an extract derived from vitreous, *Am. J. Opthalmol.,* 84, 323, 1977.
114. **Lutty, G. A., Thompson, D. C., Gallup, J. Y., Mello, R. J., Patz, A., and Fenselau, A.,** Vitreous: an inhibitor of retinal extract-induced neovascularization, *Invest. Ophthalmol. Vis. Sci.,* 24, 52, 1983.
115. **Williams, G. A., Eisenstein, R., Schumacher, B., Hsiao, K. C., and Grant, D.,** Inhibitor of vascular endothelial cell growth in the lens, *Am. J. Ophthalmol.,* 97, 366, 1984.
116. **Mun, E. C., Doctrow, S. R., Carter, R., Ingber, D. E., and Folkman, J.,** An angiogenesis inhibitor from the cornea, *Invest. Ophthalmol. Vis. Sci.,* 30, (Suppl.), 151, 1989.
117. **Folkman, J., Langer, R., Linhardt, R. J., Haudenschild, C., and Taylor, S.,** Angiogenesis inhibition and tumor regression caused by heparin or a heparin fragment in the presence of cortisone, *Science,* 221, 719, 1983.
118. **Crum, R., Szabo, S., and Folkman, J.,** A new class of steroids inhibits angiogenesis in the presence of heparin or a heparin fragment, *Science,* 230, 1378, 1985.

119. **Folkman, J., Weisz, P. B., Joullie, M. M., Li, W. W., and Ewing, W. R.**, Control of angiogenesis with synthetic heparin substitutes, *Science*, 243, 1490, 1989.
120. **Ingber, D. E., Madri, J. A., and Folkman, J.**, A possible mechanism for inhibition of angiogenesis by angiostatic steroids: induction of capillary basement membrane dissolution, *Endocrinology*, 119, 1768, 1986.
121. **Ingber, D. E. and Folkman, J.**, Inhibition of angiogenesis through modulation of collagen metabolism, *Lab. Invest.*, 59, 44, 1988.
122. **Sakamoto, N., Tanaka, N. G., Tohgo, A., and Ogawa, H.**, Heparin plus cortisone acetate inhibit tumor growth by blocking endothelial cell proliferation, *Cancer J.*, 1, 55, 1986.
123. **Rong, G. H., Alessandri, G., and Sindelar, W. F.**, Inhibition of tumor angiogenesis by hexuronyl hexosaminoglycan sulfate, *Cancer*, 57, 586, 1986.
124. **Taylor, S. and Folkman, J.**, Protamine is an inhibitor of angiogenesis, *Nature*, 297, 307, 1982.
125. **Majewski, S., Kaminski, M., Szmuro, A., Kaminska, G., and Malejczyk, J.**, Inhibition of tumor-induced angiogenesis by systematically administered protamine sulphate, *Int. J. Cancer*, 33, 831, 1984.
126. **Neufeld, G. and Gospodarowicz, D.**, Protamine sulfate inhibits mitogenic activities of the extracellular matrix and fibroblast growth factor, but potentiates that of epidermal growth factor, *J. Cell Physiol.*, 132, 287, 1987.
127. **Maione, T. E., Gray, G. S., Petro, J., Hunt, A. J., Donner, A. L., Bauer, S. I., Carson, H. F., and Sharpe, R. J.**, Inhibition of angiogenesis by recombinant human platelet factor-4 and related peptides, *Science*, 247, 77, 1990.
128. **Sharpe, R. J., Byers, H. R., Scott, C. F., Bauer, S. I., and Maione, T. E.**, Growth inhibition of murine melanoma and human colon carcinoma by recombinant human platelet factor-4, *J. Natl. Cancer Inst.*, 82, 848, 1990.
129. **Sporn, M. B. and Roberts, A. B.**, Peptide growth factors are multifunctional, *Nature*, 332, 217, 1988.
130. **Muller, G., Behrens, J., Nussbaumer, U., Bohlen, P., and Birchmeier, W.**, Inhibitory action of transforming growth factor beta on endothelial cells, *Proc. Natl. Acad. Sci. U.S.A.*, 84, 5600, 1987.
131. **Muthukkarauppan, V. R. and Auerbach, R.**, Angiogenesis in the mouse cornea, *Science*, 205, 1416, 1979.
132. **Madri, J. A., Pratt, B. M., and Tucker, A. M.**, Phenotypic modulation of endothelial cells by transforming growth factor-beta depends upon the composition and organization of the extracellular matrix, *J. Cell Biol.*, 106, 1375, 1988.
133. **Orlidge, A. and D'Amore, P. A.**, Inhibition of capillary endothelial cell growth by pericytes and smooth muscle cells, *J. Cell Biol.*, 105, 1455, 1987.
134. **Antonelli-Orlidge, A., Saunders, K. B., Smith, S. R., and D'Amore, P. A.**, An activated form of TGF-beta is produced by co-cultures of endothelial cells and pericytes, *Proc. Natl. Acad. Sci. U.S.A.*, 86, 4544, 1989.
135. **Good, D. J., Polverini, P. J., Rastinejad, F., Le Beau, M. M., Lemons, R. S., Frazier, W. A., and Bouck, N. P.**, A tumor suppressor dependent inhibitor of angiogenesis is a fragment of thrombospondin, *Proc. Natl. Acad. Sci. U.S.A.*, 87, 6624, 1990.
136. **Rastinejad, F., Polverini, P. J., and Bouck, N. P.**, Regulation of the activity of a new inhibitor of angiogenesis by a cancer suppressor gene, *Cell*, 56, 345, 1989.
137. **Frater-Schroder, M., Risau, W., Hallman, R., Gautschi, R., and Bohlen, P.**, Tumor necrosis factor type-a, a potent inhibitor of endothelial cell growth *in vitro*, is angiogenic *in vivo*, *Proc. Natl. Acad. Sci. U.S.A.*, 84, 5277, 1987.
138. **Orchard, P. J., Smith, C. M., II, Woods, W. G., Day, D. L., Dehner, L. P., and Shapiro, R.**, Treatment of haemangioendotheliomas with alpha interferon, *Lancet*, 2, 565, 1989.
139. **Friesel, R., Komoriya, A., and Maciag, T.**, Inhibition of endothelial cell proliferation by gamma-interferon, *J. Cell Biol.*, 104, 689, 1987.
140. **Ingber, D. E., Madri, J., and Folkman, J.**, Endothelial growth factors and extracellular matrix regulate DNA synthesis through modulation of cell and nuclear expansion, *In Vitro Cell Dev. Biol.*, 23, 387, 1987.
141. **Young, W. C. and Herman, I. M.**, Extracellular matrix modulation of endothelial cell shape and motility following injury *in vitro*, *J. Cell Sci.*, 73, 191, 985.
142. **Presta, M., Moscatelli, D., Joseph-Silverstein, J., and Rifkin, D. B.**, Purification from a human hepatoma line of a basic fibroblast growth factor-like molecule that stimulates capillary endothelial cell plasminogen activator production, DNA synthesis and migration, *Mol. Cell Biol.*, 6, 4060, 1986.
143. **Roberts, A., Sporn, M. B., Assoian, R. K., Smith, J. M., Roche, N. S., Wakefield, L. M., Liotta, L. A., Falanga, V., Kehrl, J. H., and Fauci, A. S.**, Transforming growth factor beta: rapid induction of fibrosis and angiogenesis *in vivo* and stimulation of collagen formation *in vitro*, *Proc. Natl. Acad. Sci. U.S.A.*, 83, 4167, 1986.
144. **Shing, Y.**, Heparin-copper biaffinity chromatography of fibroblast growth factors, *J. Biol. Chem.*, 263, 9059, 1988.

145. **Raju, K. S., Asessandri, G, and Gullino, P. M.,** Characterization of a chemoattractant for endothelium induced by angiogenesis effectors, *Cancer Res.*, 44, 1579, 1984.
146. **McAuslan, B. R. and Reilly, W.,** Endothelial cell phagokinesis in response to specific metal ions, *Exp. Cell Res.*, 130, 147, 1980.
147. **Gospodarowicz, D. and Cheng, J.,** Heparin protects basic and acidic FGF from inactivation, *J. Cell Physiol.*, 128, 475, 1986.
148. **Azizkhan, R. G., Azizkhan, J. C., Zetter, B. R., and Folkman, J.,** Mast cell heparin stimulates migration of capillary endothelial cells *in vitro, J. Exp. Med.*, 152, 931, 1980.
149. **Sudhalter, J., Folkman, J., Svahn, C. M., Bergendal, K., and D'Amore, P. A.,** Importance of size, sulfation, and anticoagulant activity in the potentiation of acidic fibroblast growth factor by heparin, *J. Biol. Chem.*, 264, 6892, 1989.
150. **Folkman, J., Watson, K., Ingber, D., and Hanahan, D.,** Induction of angiogenesis during the transition from hyperplasia to neoplasia, *Nature,* 339, 59, 1989.

Chapter 17

THE MICROCIRCULATION OF TUMORS

Hans-Inge Peterson

TABLE OF CONTENTS

I. INTRODUCTION

Tumor vascularization and blood supply are of great importance for tumor growth and spread. Tumor vascular morphology has been extensively studied, and some early observations are still of interest. Later contributions have given a fairly good understanding of tumor vascular supply, which is based on two types of vessels, incorporated normal vessels from the tumor host tissue, and newly formed tumor vessels stimulated by one or several tumor angiogenesis factors.

Tumor blood flow also has been extensively studied, mostly in experimental tumors by various techniques. A great heterogeneity in intratumor blood flow distribution has been a main obstacle in finding reproducible techniques for tumor blood flow recording. Thus, after 30 years of intense studies, it still seems that there are many reasons for concentrating again on methodological studies. One reason for this is the heterogeneity in vascular and blood supply to tumors. Another reason is the great differences between the poorly differentiated vessels or vascular channels in rapidly growing transplantable experimental tumors and the often normal blood vessels incorporated in human malignant tumors.

In this chapter, an attempt is made to create a basis for the understanding of the correlations between tumor microcirculation and metastasis by presenting a concentrated review on tumor vascular morphology and on physiological problems in tumor blood supply. This chapter surveys aspects of tumor blood flow, tumor oxygenation, and tumor vascular reactivity to vasoactive drugs and to hyperthermia.

II. TUMOR VASCULAR MORPHOLOGY

Observations on tumor vascular morphology are of great importance for the understanding of tumor vascular physiology. The vascular morphology of experimental and of human malignant tumors was studied early, and some of these observations are still of current interest.

In 1863, on the basis of morphological studies, Virchow[1] reported that solid tumors have their own specific vascular system, which was much more developed than that in healthy tissue. In accordance with this, Ribbert[2] postulated in 1904 that tumors have a vascular supply superior to that of normal tissues. In 1907, Goldmann[3] described the growth of human malignant and some experimental tumors with special reference to the vascular system. He concluded that there was a disturbance of the regular distribution of blood vessels by the invading growth, a formation of new blood vessels most apparent in the zone of proliferation and, as tumor growth increased, development of central tumor necrosis with newly formed blood vessels in the capsule area of the tumor.

In 1945, Lindgren[4] extensively described tumor vascular supply with special reference to the capillary architecture. He found that most malignant tumors were vascularized by poorly differentiated, newly formed vessels that pierce the tumor from various directions. The expanding tumors were found to destroy many preformed vessels in the normal surrounding tissue area, but some coarser vessels could at least temporarily be taken over by the growing tumor.

Malignant tumors growing in the liver were found to have an exclusive arterial blood supply.[5] This had already been reported in 1923[6] and was later verified among others by Nilsson and Zettergren,[7] who investigated primary induced rat hepatic carcinomas and also found vessels filled with contrast material injected into the portal vein around the periphery of the tumors.

In a review of vascular relationships of tumor and host,[8] it was suggested that the discrepancies in the literature on formation, morphology, and physiology of the vascular systems of tumors could be resolved by considering two types of tumor blood supply: one

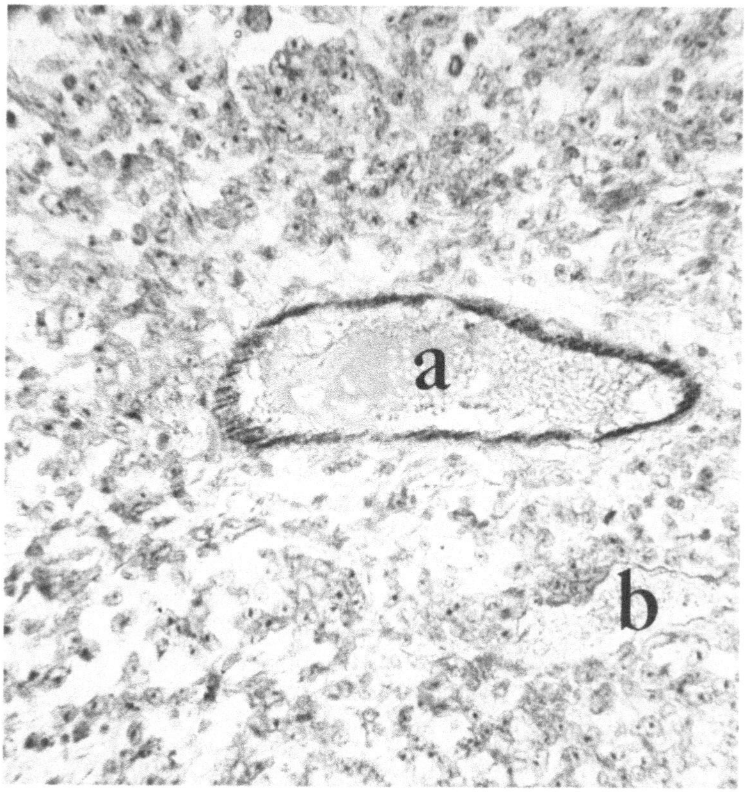

FIGURE 1. Section from a rat fibrosarcoma studied by immunohistochemical technique including factor VIII-related antigen as an endothelial cell marker. Note an endothelial lined vessel (a) but also a vascular channel without any endothelial cell lining (b).

appropriated from existing normal tissue and the other newly generated through a fibrovascular stromal reaction. This latter reaction was earlier compared by Algire et al.[9] to that in wound healing. They found a rapid capillary proliferation in transplantable mouse tumors. Although many vessels became large, no differentiation into arterioles and venules was evident (Figure 1).

In 1979, in an extensive review of tumor vascular morphology, Warren[10] summarized a morphological classification of vessels found within tumor as nine different varieties of vessels: (1) arteries and arterioles, (2) capillaries with basement membrane, (3) capillary sprouts, (4) sinusoidal vessels–interrupted endothelial lining, (5) blood channels without endothelial lining, (6) giant capillaries, (7) capillaries with fenestrated endothelium, (8) venules and veins, and (9) arterio-venous anastomoses. Warren concluded that the arterial system of the host tissue (in contrast to what was suggested by Lindgren) persists in almost all tumors. The main change of the vasculature of small tumors is seen in the transformation of capillaries and veins, which became dilated and tortuous. "The vascular morphology for a specific tumor is characteristic for that tumor, but may not be unique to that tumor." Characteristic vascular patterns for different tumors also have been described in other studies.[11,12]

The presence of intercellular fenestrations in tumor capillaries has been observed in several studies.[13-15] This has provided one explanation for the increased vascular permeability in tumors for large molecules, such as albumin and fibrinogen.[16-20]

Arteriovenous shunting of contrast medium was observed in renal carcinoma.[21-23] In an angiographic-histopathologic correlation of tumor vessels in human renal carcinomas and malignant gliomas, as well as in some experimental tumors,[22] it was concluded that tumor vessels are newly formed, lack contractile tissue in the vessel wall, and are unable to react to vasoactive stimuli. Pancreatic carcinomas were found to be "avascular" when examined angiographically, but microscopically a small number of wide capillary vessels could be demonstrated. Arterial encasement, probably due to pronounced fibrosis within the tumors with compression of vessels, was also observed in all pancreatic carcinomas studied.

A wide heterogeneity in intratumor distribution of vascular and extravascular spaces were found in studies on a transplantable rat tumor.[24] In a recent review,[25] it was also concluded that tumor vasculature is highly heterogenous and does not conform to the normal vascular organization. Quantitative morphometric studies in two-dimensional tumors show that vascular volume, length, and surface area increase during early tumor growth and later decrease with the development of tumor necroses. Great problems are met in identifying specific tumors on the basis of their vascularity due to the considerable intratumor heterogeneities of both vascular structure and function of the vascular bed.[26] The same holds true for an individual tumor at different sizes. Experiments on different human tumor xenografts in nude mice have shown that a similar tumor histology is not necessarily related to a comparable vascular pattern.[27,28] There are still no quantitative data on the vascular morphology of human tumors, which could be obtained by perfusing human tumors *in vivo*.[29]

In conclusion, tumor vascular morphology is characterized by:

1. Two types of tumor blood vessels — newly formed and poorly differentiated vessels on a capillary basis and normal host tissue vessels incorporated in the growing tumor mass, among which arteries and arterioles show a marked resistance against tumor cell invasion.
2. The development of central necroses during progressive tumor growth is related to a decreased vascular supply.
3. A characteristic vascular morphology for a specific type of tumor, but not necessarily unique to that tumor.
4. A wide heterogeneity in intratumor distribution of vascular space and function.

III. VASCULAR AND EXTRAVASCULAR SPACES IN TUMORS

In 1954, Algire[30] found in rapidly growing mouse tumors observed through a transparent chamber that blood vessels reached a volume of 40 to 50% of total space within 5 to 8 d. The tumors elicited a production of new capillary endothelium from the host. This phenomenon of tumor angiogenesis is described in detail in Chapter 16 of this book.

Gullino and Grantham[31] studied the vascular spaces in several different transplantable rat tumors during tumor growth. They used Dextran 500 as a marker substance. The tumors were transplanted either subcutaneously or in the ovary as "tissue-isolated" preparations. The Dextran content in the blood, in the collected interstitial fluid of tumors, and in the homogenized tumor tissue was determined after killing the animals 1 to 5 h after the injection of Dextran 500. The vascular space in the tumor homogenate could only be calculated when the Dextran concentration in blood was constant, and the interstitial fluid was free of Dextran. An early transfer of Dextran was observed, but no reasonable explanation for this was found. The recorded tumor vascular space was found to represent from 1.0 to 12.4% of the tumor mass. The vascular volume varied from one tumor type to another, but was constant within the same tumor group. In small tumors of the same type, a low spread of volume values was found, while in larger tumors, the vascular volume varied from 5 to 25%. There was no remarkable leakage of Dextran into necrotic tumor areas. One potential source of error in this study is the interference of anaphylactoid reactions against Dextran in rats, which are not Dextran-resistant.[32]

In studies of a mouse mammary carcinoma by microangiography and morphometric analyses,[33] the vascular volume, as a percentage of total *viable* tumor volume, was found to remain stable at 17% during tumor growth. Necrotic tumor volume increased progressively during tumor growth and the average vessel diameter increased, while the average vessel length and surface area per mm^3 of viable tumor tissue decreased during tumor growth. In another study,[34] capillary morphometric studies showed a decreased vascular space in growing DS-rat carcinosarcomas, especially distinct during the first period of tumor growth.

In a recent review, typical values of vascular spaces, in different experimental tumors determined by different techniques, were found to vary between 0.8 to 27.5%.[25]

The intratumor distribution of vascular and extravascular spaces were studied in transplantable rat tumors by isotope techniques.[24] In these studies, the residual blood and plasma volume was determined in multiple tumor specimens. Red blood cell volume was calculated after labelling of red blood cells with ^{59}Fe, as milliliters red blood cells/gram tissue. Plasma volume was based on early plasma tissue ratios of ^{125}I and extracellular volume as plasma/tissue ratios of ^{51}Cr-EDTA. Animals were killed by bleeding under ether anesthesia.

In these studies, a wide intratumor distribution of all recorded values were found. The intratumor distribution of red blood cell and plasma volume values was significantly changed towards lower values in older tumors. The intratumor distribution of extracellular space remained unchanged. The unchanged extracellular volume with decreasing erythrocyte and plasma volumes during tumor growth indicates that tumor cell mass increases more rapidly than its vascular supply and at least partially accounts for the development of tumor necroses[35] (Figure 2).

The intratumor distributions of vascular and extravascular spaces were identical in central and peripheral tumor specimens. No significant correlation was found in tumor specimens between plasma volume and blood flow recorded by ^{86}Rubidium chloride, but the reduced plasma volume during tumor growth was accompanied by a continuous reduction of tumor blood flow.

Intravenous administration of norepinephrine changed the distribution of both plasma volume and blood flow to produce low values in a transplantable rat sarcoma.[36]

In humans, vascularization has been found to be most extensive in brain tumors, slightly less in carcinomas, and least in sarcomas.[37] Human renal carcinomas that showed angiographic evidence of hypovascularization were also found to have more frequent and large necrotic areas when examined histopathologically.[22] In a recent study on the correlation of Doppler ultrasound tumor signals with the neovascular morphology, primary human malignant tumors of the liver, kidney, adrenal gland, and pancreas were examined, and some tumors showed prominent vascular spaces.[38]

In an early study by Gullino and Grantham,[39] the interstitial water space was found to be large, accounting for between 30 and 60% of the tumor water. Large extracellular spaces (38%) were found in DS carcinosarcomas of the rat,[40] and similar observations were made in two rat sarcomas[41] where extracellular volumes of approximately 40% were found, compared with 13% in skeletal muscle.

Direct measurements by electron microscopy of human gliomas and meningiomas showed large extracellular spaces in gliomas (20 to 40%) and in meningiomas (13 to 15%) compared with values of 6 to 7% in normal brain.[42] The extracellular volume in human lung-tumor xenografts did not vary with tumor size.[43]

The interstitial fluid pressure in some tumors was found to be higher than that in corresponding normal tissues[44] and to increase during tumor growth, probably due to proliferation of tumor cells compounded by increased vascular permeability[45,46] and ischemic cell swelling.[45] At the same time, a low intravascular pressure has been found in most tumor studies.[47]

In conclusion, although it appears to remain stable in some tumors during growth, the

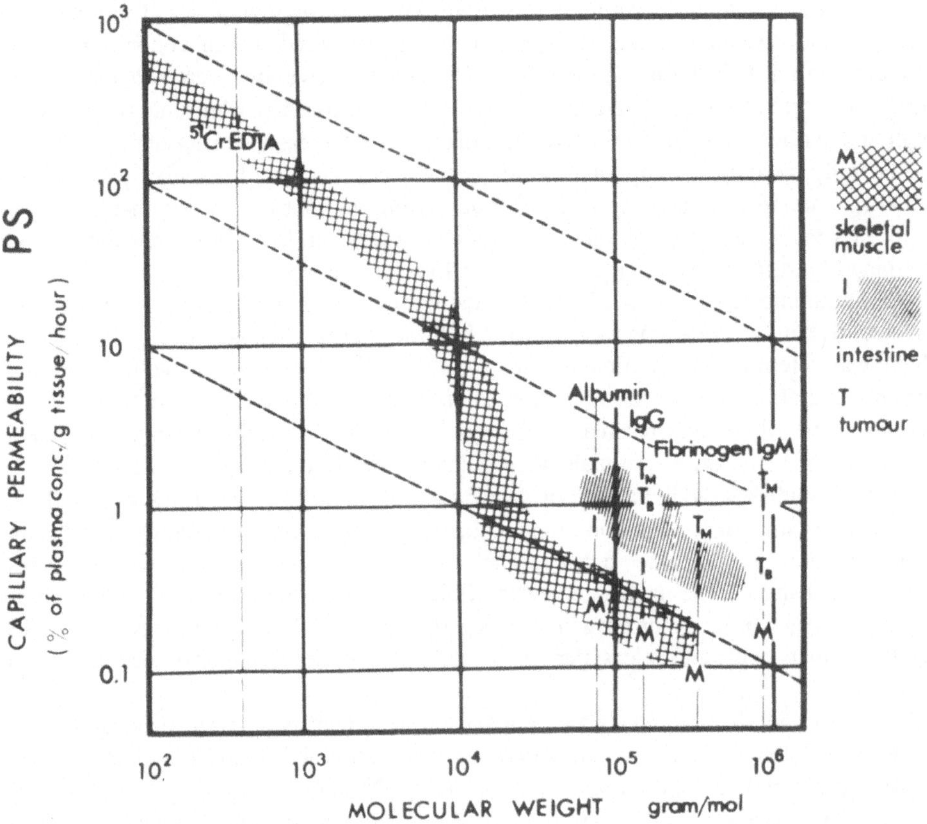

FIGURE 2. Capillary permeability-surface area product (PS: % of plasma concentration/ml/g tissue/h) at different molecular weights. Earlier observations: crosshatched area = skeletal muscle; gray area = gastrointestinal tract. Values of PS are given for two transplantable rat tumors: benzpyrene-induced sarcoma and 20-methylcholanthrene-induced sarcoma (T_B and T_M), small intestine (I), and skeletal muscle (M). The diagonal broken lines indicate the expected reduction of free diffusion with increasing molecular weight. Note the high PS values for tumor. (From Peterson, H.-I., Appelgren, L., Lundborg, G., and Rosengren, B., *Bibl. Anat.*, 12, 511, 1973. With permission.)

vascular volume decreases in most tumors. A large interstitial space has been observed in both experimental and human cancers, and a high interstitial fluid pressure and a low microvascular pressure have been found in experimental tumors. Quantitative morphological studies on human tumors remain to be performed.

IV. TUMOR VASCULAR PERMEABILITY

Morphological alterations of tumor blood vessels, including fenestration, widened intercellular junctions, increase in pinocytotic vessels, and blood channels without endothelial lining may be connected with a high vascular permeability of tumor vessels.

An increased vascular permeability was found in a rat fibrosarcoma after histamine challenge, accompanied by the formation of endothelial gaps in the irregular vascular channels.[48] An extravasation of albumin was found in a mouse lymphosarcoma and was increased by local irradiation of tumors. Irradiated normal muscle also showed increased permeability for albumin. Thus, after extravascular equilibration in irradiated tumors, the albumin space was increased by 200% and in irradiated muscle by 80%.[19] Vascular permeability to Evans blue was studied in Walker carcinosarcoma transplants to the rat liver and in host liver tissue; tumor permeability was significantly higher than liver permeability, and a peak occurred between 6 and 18 h with a T/L ratio of 1.87 at 6 h.[49]

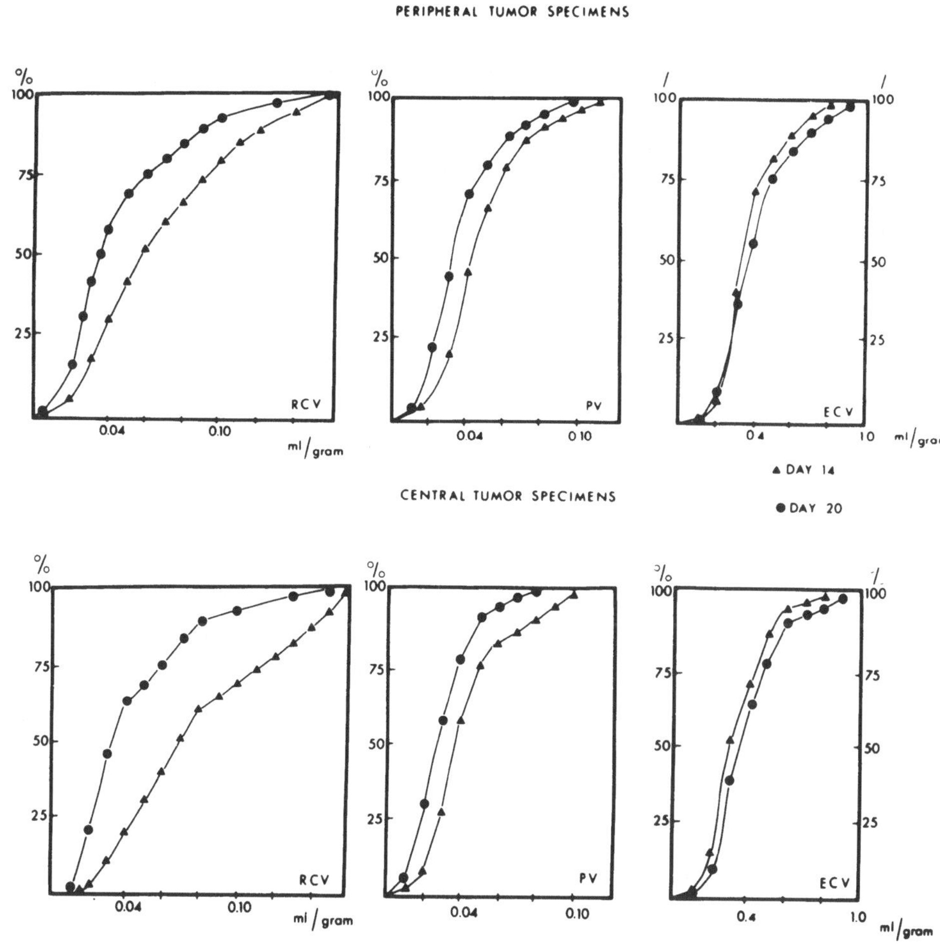

FIGURE 3. Cumulative frequency distribution diagrams based on recorded values of red cell volume (RCV), plasma volume (PV), and extracellular volume (ECV) recorded by isotope technique in a rat fibrosarcoma 14 and 20 d after tumor transplantation. Note an unchanged ECV with decreasing RCV and PV during tumor growth. Similar observations were made in both central and peripheral tumor specimens. (From Karlsson, L., Alpsten, M., Appelgren, K. L., and Peterson, H.-I., *Microvasc. Res.*, 12. 71, 1980. With permission.)

In a series of studies on two rat sarcomas, the capillary permeability of labelled proteins of different molecular weight was examined; a high tumor capillary permeability was observed for large protein molecules such as albumin, immunoglobulin G, and fibrinogen, as compared to various normal tissues.[16-18] Similar observations of a high tumor vascular permeability have since been reported by others[50,51] (Figure 3).

Regional blood-to-tissue transport was measured in experimental brain tumors using alpha-aminoisobutyric acid labelled with carbon 14 and quantitative autoradiography. Estimates of the average fractional extractions by intracranial gliomas and malignant Schwannomas were 0.01 and 0.02, respectively; average fractional extraction for normal brain tissue was approximately 0.003.[52]

Tumor capillary permeability, as measured by the Evans blue extraction technique, markedly increased in transplanted rat liver tumors after a freezing and thawing procedure.[53] However, the same experimental techniques revealed no change in tumor vascular permeability following exposure to histamine, bradykinin, or serotonin, although an increase in tumor vascular permeability was found 5 min after the establishment of reactive hyperemia.[54] Similar observations were made in a transplantable rat sarcoma.[55]

A permeability-enhancing factor in tumor tissue of a rat prostatic carcinoma was reported by Stein-Werblowsky,[56] and Senger et al. have recently attributed the increased vascular permeability of tumor to the activity of a specific 34 to 42 kDa protein—vascular permeability factor (VPF).[57,58]

In studies on a VX2 carcinoma grown in a rabbit ear chamber, moderate hyperthermia (43°C for 1 h) did not induce a statistically significant effect on vascular permeability in either the normal or the tumor tissue, while severe hyperthermia (50°C for 1 h) increased the normal tissue permeability about sixfold and the tumor permeability about twofold. It was concluded that the transport pathways are probably maximally open under control conditions.[59] In a recent review, Jain[47] has summarized observations in semi-quantitative studies of tumor vascular permeability.

Microvascular pressure observations in tumors have been recently reviewed by Jain.[25] The first direct measurements of microvascular pressure were made in a DMBA-induced mammary carcinoma.[60] On the arterial side, there were similar observations for tumor and normal subcutaneous tissue, while venous pressures in the tumor were significantly lower than the corresponding values in subcutaneous tissue. Wiig[61] studied a similar tumor and found a pressure drop during passage of blood into the deeper areas of tumor, which made it difficult to record microvascular pressure in deeper tumor vessels. Endrich and Hammersen[62] studied an amelanotic melanoma growing in a dorsal skin chamber of the hamster at different temperatures and found significantly higher microvascular pressures than that found in a previous study.[60] As temperature was increased, precapillary pressures decreased while venular pressure increased.

The interstitial fluid pressure in tumors has been found to be higher than in normal host tissues[44] and has been explained by the absence of a defined lymphatic system in tumors coupled with increased tumor vascular permeability. An increased interstitial fluid pressure also has been found in central parts of tumor compared to peripheral parts.[47] This, together with the earlier reported hypothesis that tumors grow beyond their own vascular supply has been given as an explanation for the development of central necrosis in growing tumors.

In conclusion, a high tumor vascular permeability has been found in a series of studies, which has been difficult to increase by pharmacologic agents or other procedures.

A low intravascular venous pressure and a high interstitial fluid pressure are also characteristic for tumors; the high interstitial pressure is explained by the lack of an intratumoral lymphatic system coupled with high vascular permeability. An increased interstitial pressure in deeper parts of tumor may be one explanation for the development of tumor necrosis.

V. TUMOR BLOOD FLOW

Studies on tumor blood flow have been limited to the last 30 years due to methodological difficulties. When, in 1961, Gullino and Grantham[63] presented their ingenious techniques for recording the venous outflow from "tissue-isolated" transplanted tumors, they summarized the situation: "to our knowledge the evaluation of the blood supply to a tumor is an unsolved problem." Much of this problem still remains due to the difficulties in finding reproducible techniques, especially in recording the blood flow in human cancers.

The results of different studies on the blood flow of experimental and human tumors have been summarized by Peterson[64] and later by Jain and Ward-Hartley.[65]

In comparing tumor blood flow with normal tissue blood flow,[64] three subdivisions were made based on the different techniques used in the various studies:

1. Total tumor blood flow — techniques used in experimental situations that seldom could be adapted for clinical use.
2. Local tumor blood flow — techniques based on local isotope or heat clearance in addition to direct observations; more recently, the ultrasonic technique has been tested.

These techniques have been used in both experimental and clinical tumor blood flow recording.

3. Intratumor blood flow distribution — techniques mainly based on intratumoral distribution of intravascularly injected isotopes. These techniques mainly have been used in experimental studies.

A. TOTAL TUMOR BLOOD FLOW

Gullino and Grantham[63] introduced the technique of transplanting tumors in isolated kidneys and ovaries in rats and mice; the normal organ was displaced into the subcutis, leaving its vascular pedicle intact. The normal organ was subsequently enveloped in a paraffin sack and resulted in an isolated tumor-system supplied by *one* artery and drained by *one* vein. The venous outflow, which will reflect total tumor blood flow, was measured at a constant blood pressure.

The technique is dependent upon the fact that the isolated growing tumor destroys all or most normal tissues. In ovarian implants larger than 4.0 g, no residues of normal tissue could be found, while in large renal tumors, small residues of normal kidney were still present. The average value of total tumor blood flow in a hepatoma transplanted to isolated kidney was 0.14 ml/min/g calculated to be 20 times less than the blood supply to normal liver. Tumor blood flow decreased with increasing tumor growth and, in tumors with a weight of 12 g, was between 0.09 and 0.12 ml/min/g. These observations were compared in tumors and normal tissues by ^{42}K and ^{85}Rb uptake, which gave tumor flow values in isolated ovarian implants of about 0.15 ml/min/g. The comparatively low tumor blood flow values found in these studies may be explained by the advanced "age" of the tumors because at the time when most normal tissue have been destroyed, the tumor was in a late phase with a reduced blood flow and large necrotic area. In a study on a D5-ascites-carcinoma[66] transplanted and grown in isolated rat kidney, a linear dependence of total tumor blood flow on mean arterial blood pressure was found. With a mean arterial blood pressure of 120 mm Hg, the recorded blood flow in a tumor weighing 2.5 g was 0.32 ml/min/g; in a tumor weighing 8.2 g, the flow was 0.065 ml/min/g.

In a more recent study on blood flow, oxygen consumption, and tissue oxygenation in human breast cancer xenografts in nude mice, an epigastric pouch technique was used to obtain a tissue-isolated tumor preparation.[67] The average total tumor blood flow through medullary carcinomas was significantly higher (0.17 ml/g/min) than in squamous cell carcinomas (0.10 ml/g/min). In both types of cancer, blood flow varied considerably from tumor to tumor, and the total blood flow also decreased with increasing tumor weight. In this study, tumors were also transplanted subcutaneously, and local tumor blood flow was evaluated using a thermoclearance technique. The temperature of the tumor tissue was elevated to 38°C for 60 sec, using localized ultrasonic heating, and the subsequent decline of the tissue temperature was recorded, both in the live and killed animal, to allow separation of convective and conductive heat transfer. The mean local tumor blood flow was calculated in medullary carcinomas at 0.14 ml/g/min with an average wet weight of 3.21 g, and at 0.20 ml/g/min mean in squamous cell carcinomas with a weight of 3.1 g. The differences between the estimates of tumor blood flow using the two different techniques were accounted for by the different transplantation sites.[68]

Blood flow in hamster and mouse tumors was also studied by measuring the uptake in large biopsy specimens or whole tumors of ^{131}I-antipyrine, radioactive microspheres, and lissamine green.[69] The mean blood flow of a hamster melanoma with a weight of 0.5 g remained approximately 0.6 ml/min/g regardless of the site of implantation. In most tumors, the recorded blood flow decreased markedly with increasing tumor growth. The mean tissue blood flow was 2 to 12 times higher in the tumor peripheries than in the central, more necrotic regions.

The total and regional tumor blood flow was also measured using $^{99}Tc^{M}$ labelled microspheres.[70] Mean tumor blood flows in a hepatoma, a methylnitrosoguanidine-induced adenocarcinoma, and a benzpyrene-induced sarcoma were 0.35, 0.38, and 0.92 ml/min/g, respectively, with tumors transplanted into the rat liver. The corresponding flow values in subcutaneously transplanted tumors were 0.47, 0.50, and 2.17 ml/min/g. Tumor blood flow decreased with increasing tumor growth. The high flow observations in the benzpyrene-induced sarcomas were explained by the smaller size of these tumors at the time of tumor blood flow recording. The tumor blood flow results were similar in both transplantation sites. It was concluded that *the discrepancy in tumor blood flow as reported in different studies may be explained not only by different methods for measuring blood flow, but also by varying tumor types and sizes.* One important observation was that the amount of shunted microspheres did not exceed 1%/g of cardiac output. The tumors transplanted to the liver appeared to have the same flow as normal liver parenchyma, while the flow of subcutaneous tumors invariably exceeded that of the skin and muscle.

In apparent contrast to most observations, a study on Guérin carcinoma in rats by ^{86}Rb uptake revealed no significant differences in tumor blood flow between small and large tumors;[71] tumors with a mean weight of 1.21 g showed a mean flow of 20.8 ml/min/100 g, and tumors with a mean weight of 56.6 g showed a mean flow of 19.6 ml/min/100 g. It is difficult to explain these observations.

Various ethylnitrosurea-induced nerve and brain tumors in rats were studied by ^{14}C-antipyrine uptake.[72] In these studies, the mean cerebral cortex blood flow was 1.14 ml/min/g, while the blood flow in tumors varied from 0.44 or 0.79 ml/min/g. Small tumors showed greater flow than large tumors or central tumor growth zones. Well-differentiated tumors also had a considerably larger flow rate than anaplastic tumors.

A plethysmographic technique was elaborated in our laboratory for studies of the total tumor blood flow in rat sarcomas transplanted into the hindpaw of animals.[73] The temperature in the plethysmograph chamber was kept at 31.5°C to minimize the skin flow, and the animal body temperature was kept at 37.5°C. The resting and postischemic flows in tumor-bearing and contralateral normal hindpaws were recorded separately under other anesthesia. The mean resting flow rate for the tumor-bearing paw minus that for the nontumor-bearing paw 21 d after tumor implantation was 58 ml/min/100 g and 22 ml/min/100 g 4 d later. The corresponding blood flow values after 10 min of ischemia were 74 and 30. The decrease of tumor blood flow with tumor growth is in accordance with most other studies, however, the comparatively high recorded tumor blood flow was difficult to explain. Although the technique was used for some time, it has since been abandoned due to considerable methodological and technical difficulties.

B. LOCAL TUMOR BLOOD FLOW

The main technique used in both experimental and clinical studies has been the local isotope clearance of ^{133}xenon, in which tumor blood flow is studied in small tumor regions that may affect the apparent reproducibility of the technique. However, in studies on a rat sarcoma,[74] a good reproducibility was obtained in repeated measurements from the same small tumor area.

The local xenon clearance technique was used in early clinical studies on the effect of hepatic artery ligature on liver-tumor blood flow.[75] A normal liver parenchymal blood flow of 29 ml/min/100 g tissue was found as compared with a mean blood flow in carcinomatous nodules in the liver of 12 ml/min/100 g.[76]

^{133}Xe was injected into central parts of superficial human tumors, and different blood flow values were found in different types of cancer.[77] The mean blood flow in lymphomas was 38 ml/min/100 g, in anaplastic carcinomas 11 ml/min/100 g, and in other different malignant tumors 14 ml/min/100 g. There was a good reproducibility in repeated injections into the same tumor area. In this study, it was stressed that the coefficient of ^{133}Xe-partition between tumor nodule and blood depends strongly upon the fat content of the tissue.

In a later study on human tumors,[78] the same group made more extensive studies on the relative partition coefficient of $^{85}Kr^{M}$, which was found to be slightly smaller than the partition coefficient of ^{133}Xe and was explained by the smaller molecular weight of krypton. The mean value of perfusion rates in tumors calculated from the xenon results was 13 ml/min/100 g as compared with 19 ml/min/100 g from the krypton results. With tumor blood flows >10 ml/min/100 g, a decrease of partition coefficient values was found. It was concluded that the observations were in accordance with relative partition coefficients of krypton and xenon in experimental and in *in vitro* studies, varying between 0.7 and 1.4. Blood perfusion in 19 superficial human tumor metastasis were also studied by injecting three tracers, ^{41}Ar, $^{85}Kr^{M}$, and ^{133}Xe (or ^{135}Xe) simultaneously.[79] The mean blood flow in the tumors studied was 18 ml/min/100 g. The mean values for the ratios of the partition coefficients of the nuclides used were found to be between 0.82 and 1.07.

In experimental studies on methylcholanthrene-induced C3H mouse sarcoma, the tumor blood flow was compared to the blood flow of normal mouse muscle and skin.[80] The mean blood flow in muscle was 0.11 ml/min/g, in skin 0.08 ml/min/g, in small tumors 0.03 to 0.22 ml/min/g, and in larger tumors 0.01 to 0.08 ml/min/g.

In studies on a KHT sarcoma in syngeneic mice,[81] the partition coefficient for ^{133}Xe was found to be 0.891, which was comparatively high when compared to the coefficient of 0.72 observed in some other experimental studies. In unanesthetized mice, a mean tumor blood flow of 21.1 ml/min/100 g was found. Intraperitoneal administration of sodium pentobarbital reduced the mean tumor blood flow to 13.8 ml/min/100 g. There was also a marked decrease of flow with increasing tumor growth.

Local tissue clearance using ^{133}Xe and ^{24}Na ions simultaneously was applied to the study of blood flow in two transplantable mouse tumors.[82] The results showed a wide spread of flow values between tumors as estimated by ^{133}Xe clearance, but a relatively uniform diffusional transport as expressed by the ^{24}Na clearance. The heterogeneity in intratumor blood flow distribution has been verified in a series of studies.[83,84,85]

Regional blood flow was measured in experimental brain tumors using ^{14}C-iodoantipyrine, the Kety tissue-exchange equations, and quantitative autoradiographic techniques.[52] Blood flow was variable within tumor tissue, and the range of blood flow, which was 6 to 138 ml/min/100 g, increased with increasing tumor size.

A direct, noninvasive method based on photon activation–$^{15}0$ decay was used in measurement of tumor blood flow in rat rhabdomyosarcomas and was found to be well suited to studies designed to determine the effect of various agents, such as heat, radiation, and drugs on tumor blood flow. The volume-averaged tumor blood flow varied in different tumors from 9.2 to 35.8 ml/min/100 g.[86]

Blood flow velocity in human tumors has been elevated by color Doppler echography in some studies on human malignant tumors.[87,88] This technique is still in a very early stage, and its future in tumor blood flow recording is not clear.

C. INTRATUMOR BLOOD FLOW DISTRIBUTION

In *in vivo* studies by serial tumor microangiograms, a heterogenous blood flow distribution was observed.[83] Similar observations were reported at the same time from our own laboratory as a wide distribution of local tumor blood flow recordings, using the ^{133}Xe clearance technique.[84,85] The intratumor distribution of ^{86}Rubidium and ^{125}I-antipyrine in transplantable rat tumors was further investigated at our laboratory.[73] A wide distribution of isotope uptake in tumor and in normal muscle was found. With increasing age, a decrease of the fast flow population and an increase of the slow flow population were found, indicating a decreased tumor blood flow with increasing tumor age. A rather wide distribution of isotope uptake also was found in normal muscle, but this remained unchanged during the experimental period and was regarded as a control of the experimental model.

In a later study on a rat sarcoma, the intratumor distribution of blood flow was studied by ^{86}Rb uptake and correlated with the intratumor distribution of vascular volume, which was studied as residual plasma volume with ^{125}I-labelled albumin. A significant change towards lower tumor blood flow was found during tumor growth, accompanied by a reduced plasma volume. The distributions of plasma volume and blood flow were similar in a peripheral and in central parts of tumors. No significant correlation was found in separate tumor specimens between plasma volume and blood flow.[24]

In conclusion, a series of experimental and clinical tumor blood flow studies with different experimental techniques have been reviewed. Some characteristics may be concluded from these studies:

1. In most studies, the blood flow rate in tumors was found to be lower than in normal tissues. However, some remarkable contradictions to this have been reported.
2. In most studies, tumor blood flow rate has been reported to decrease with increasing tumor growth and with the development of central tumor necroses.
3. Regional tumor blood flow could be recorded by isotope techniques in the clinical situation, but the results are dependent upon simultaneous partition coefficient analyses for the isotope studied in the actual tumor.
4. All tumor studies are complicated by the wide heterogeneity in intratumor blood flow distribution.

VI. INFLUENCE OF VASOACTIVE DRUGS ON TUMOR BLOOD FLOW

Malignant tumors derive their vascular bed from newly formed vessels and by incorporation of normal vessels in the host tissue. Willis[89] concluded from a review of the literature and from his own experience that the walls of arteries have a striking immunity against neoplastic invasion. This was supported by Intaglietta et al.,[90] who, by the Algire chamber technique, found that arterioles were incorporated in a growing tumor mass without apparent structural changes. Arterioles with a diameter of 20 to 40 μm showed a strong vasomotor activity, which modulated the blood flow to the tumors. Contrary to this, Lindgren[4] could only find remaining parts of the preformed vessels in the periphery of growing tumors.

Three transplantable rat tumors were studied by the Falk-Hillarp histochemical technique without any findings of adrenergic innervation related to tumor vessels.[91,92] In a human renal adenocarcinoma, no adrenergic innervation was found in the main parts of the tumor, but a scarce adrenergic innervation was localized to arteries included in the tumor mass.[93] The absence of adrenergic innervation of tumor vessels does not exclude the possibility of alpha receptors, and the vessels may still be influenced by vasoactive drugs.

Systemically administered drugs can modify the tumor blood flow by affecting the systemic blood pressure.[30,66] Gullino and Grantham[63] found a marked fall in total tumor blood flow recorded by venous outflow in tissue isolated tumors after intravenous administration of epinephrine. Intravenous injection of epinephrine and norepinephrine induced a rapid but temporary fall in tumor blood flow or rat hepatomas.[94] The same authors also found that 5-hydroxytryptamine, in a dose which had little effect on muscle blood flow, arrested temporarily the tumor blood flow. From this they concluded that tumor vessels may be extremely sensitive to circulating amines. In another study, norepinephrine increased the resistance of the tumor vascular bed approximately 13 times.[95] However, a progressive loss of the ability of tumor vessels to respond to vasoactive drugs also has been observed.[96] Hafström et al.[92] studied the effect of epinephrine and norepinephrine in tumors transplanted into the rat liver. Epinephrine had no effect on tumor/liver flow ratios while norepinephrine infusion was followed by increasing tumor/liver blood flow ratios. The authors explained these observations saying that it was a failing reaction of tumor vessels to vasoconstriction as compared with normal liver vessels.

Studies at our laboratory on the influence of intravenous administration of norepinephrine on the intratumor blood flow distribution of two transplantable rat tumors showed that norepinephrine changed the distribution of tumor blood flow values towards low values; a similar observation was made in normal muscle.[97] In a later investigation,[74] the influence of norepinephrine on local tumor blood flow in a rat sarcoma was studied by local ^{133}Xe clearance. This study was made in an attempt to differentiate between a direct effect of tumor vessels or an indirect effect on normal afferent vessels supplying the transplantation area. Norepinephrine reduced significantly the blood flow in both tumor and in normal tissues. Since norepinephrine was added to the injected ^{133}Xe, it was suggested that the tumor vascular bed could be influenced by vasoactive drugs. In a similar study[98] on tumors transplanted subcutaneously into the rat hindpaw, a dose-response experiment showed that the tumor and subcutaneous vascular beds were equally sensitive to norepinephrine. Local administration of isoprenaline did not influence the blood flow in either subcutaneous tissue or tumor, while local administration of papaverine increased subcutaneous tissue blood flow significantly without influencing tumor blood flow. From this we suggested that *the tumor vascular bed is normally in a state close to maximal dilatation* (Figures 4 and 5).

Blood flow during "resting conditions" and during norepinephrine infusion was studied by microsphere technique in a DMBA-induced mammary tumor and in some normal tissues of the rat.[99] The mean blood flow to tumors (49 ml/min/100 g) was markedly decreased by norepinephrine to 5 ml/min/100 g, producing a pressure elevation of 35 mm Hq. The vascular resistance in tumor increased dramatically, while it was unchanged in normal muscle. Shunted systemic blood flow to the lungs decreased, indicating reactivity of large arteriovenous passages in the tumors. In a later study, the same authors found a striking similarity in blood flow and reactivity to norepinephrine of nontransplanted and autotransplanted DMBA tumors with insignificant reactions in normal muscle. This favored the idea that tumors regulate their blood supply irrespective of host tissue.[100]

Tumor vessel reactivity to a vasoactive substance may change markedly during various phases of tumor growth and may differ in various experimental models. Thus, in studies of some mouse tumors, the cardiac output distribution to tumors was only influenced at either an early or a late phase of tumor growth.[101]

In a recent study, the capillary blood flow was investigated with a laser Doppler probe in normal liver and in a Walker carcinosarcoma transplanted into the liver of rats.[102] Epinephrine injected into the portal system induced a short but significant increase in capillary blood flow within central parts of the tumors and apparently in the "avascular" regions.

In a study on two transplantable rat tumors, both prolonged administration of a prostaglandin synthesis inhibitor and induced thrombocytopenia significantly increased tumor blood flow.[103] The tumor capillary surface area product was increased by administration of a prostaglandin synthesis inhibitor, but not by thrombocytopenia. We concluded from this study that a release of prostaglandins and serotonins may be included in the regulation of both tumor blood flow and tumor vascular permeability.

Calcium channel blockers produced a marked increase in tumor blood flow, which was observed by the microsphere technique.[104,105] A calcium antagonist (Nisoldipine) and 5-hydroxytryptamine (5HT) were both found to significantly decrease the blood flow of some rat tumors as studied by the ^{133}xenon wash-out technique and the ^{11}C-butanol fractional distribution technique.[106] We found conflicting results in recording an increased tumor blood flow by microsphere technique after administration of a calcium channel blocker, while no effect was observed in a similar experimental situation using local ^{133}Xe clearance technique for recording tumor blood flow.[107]

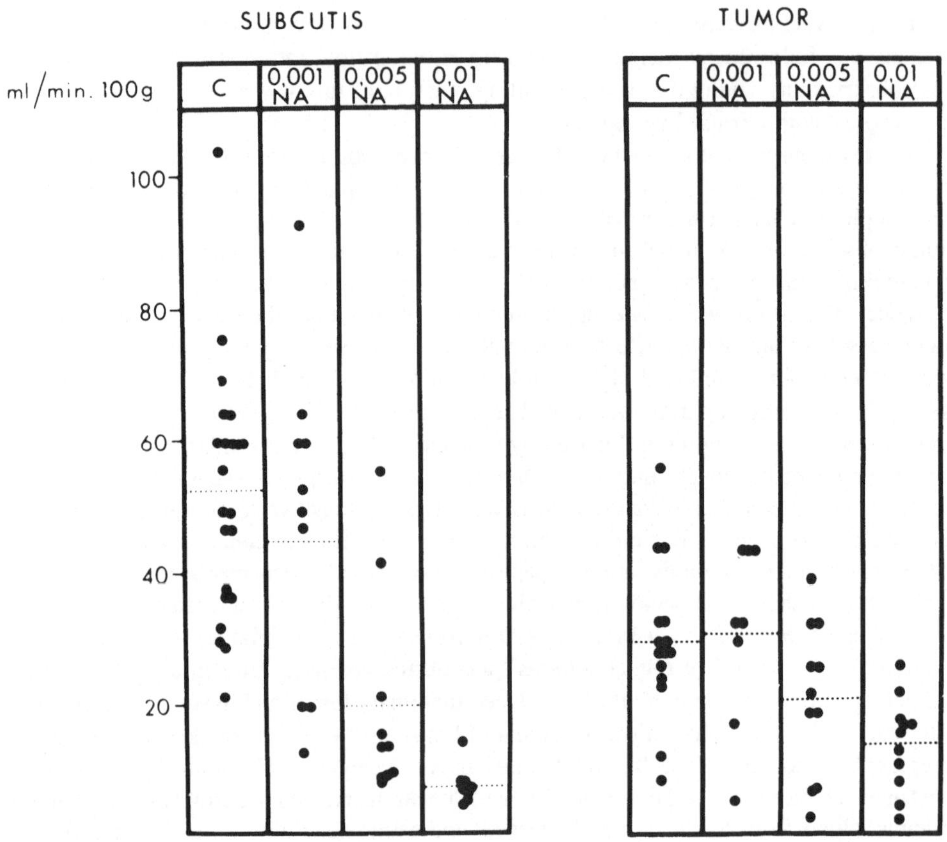

FIGURE 4. Local tumor and subcutaneous tissue blood flow in a rat fibrosarcoma transplanted into one hindpaw and recorded by local xenon clearance technique. Noradrenaline was added to the xenon solution in concentrations of 0.001, 0.005 and 0.01 mg/ml (NA) with corresponding control recordings (C). A significant reduction of local blood flow ($P < 0.01$) was observed in both tumor and subcutaneous tissue from a noradrenaline concentration of 0.005 mg/ml. (From Mattson, J., Lilja, J., and Peterson, H.-I., *Eur. J. Cancer Clin. Oncol.*, 18, 677, 1982. With permission.)

Regional blood flow, measured by microsphere technique in transplantable rat tumors, was not influenced by the vasodilator hydralazine, but some tumors reacted with decreased blood flow after administration of a vasoconstrictor, phenylephrine. Histological studies of tumor vessel walls revealed an absence of smooth muscle capable of responding to vasoactive drugs. It was concluded that by their selective action on normal vessels, vasoactive drugs can change the ratio of tumor:normal tissue perfusion.[108] These observations may also support our previous hypothesis of the tumor vascular bed normally in a state close to maximal dilatation.

It has also been shown that infusion of angiotensin II may significantly increase tumor blood flow and tumor oxygen tension by elevation of blood pressure. The hydrostatic pressure difference between the tumor vessel and the extravascular tissue was also markedly increased.[109]

In conclusion, adrenergic innervation has been found in normal vessels that were probably incorporated into human tumors, but was not found in newly formed vessels in rapidly growing experimental tumors.

In different studies, the sensitivity of tumor vessels to vasoactive drugs has been found to be lower, similar, or higher than that of vessels in the corresponding normal tissue.

In most studies, tumor blood flow was decreased by vasoconstricting drugs. However,

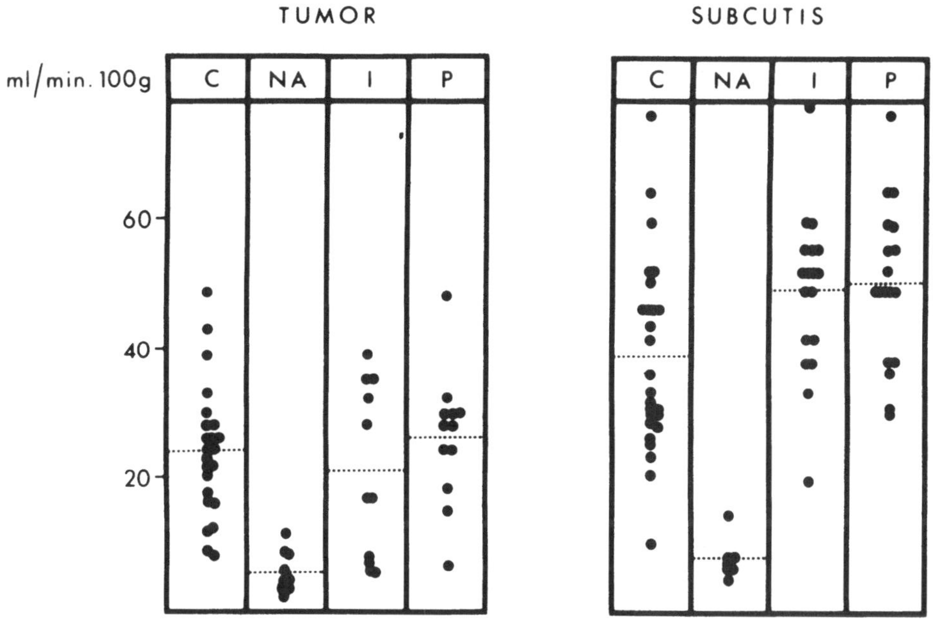

FIGURE 5. Local blood flow recordings in a rat fibrosarcoma and in subcutaneous tissue similar to the experimental model used in Figure 4. Noradrenaline (NA) in a concentration of 0.01 mg/ml reduced the tumor and subcutaneous blood flow significantly. Isoprenaline (I) had no significant influence on the blood flow recordings, while papaverine (P) increased the subcutaneous tissue blood flow significantly. (From Mattson, J., Lilja, J., and Peterson, H.-I., *Eur. J. Cancer Clin. Oncol.*, 18, 677, 1982. With permission.)

in attempts to increase pharmacologically tumor blood flow, conflicting results have been observed in which differences were obtained with the same tumor and drug, but with different techniques for measuring tumor blood flow. There is considerable support for the hypothesis that the tumor vascular bed is normally in a state close to maximal dilatation.

VII. TUMOR TISSUE OXYGENATION

The oxygen supply to tumor tissue is strictly correlated to tumor vascular and blood supply. A series of important contributions on this subject have been published by Vaupel and his group.[110] In an early study on rat D5 carcinosarcoma, they found, by capillary morphometry, that the mean volume of vascular space was reduced during tumor growth and that the intercapillary distances and length of capillaries were enlarged. At the same time, the total tumor blood flow and the regional microcirculation diminished, and the mean tissue oxygen pressure values decreased with a decrease in O_2-tension and glucose uptake;[34] a regional inadequacy in glucose and O_2, therefore, occurs during tumor proliferation.[111] Inadequate tumor neovascularization, increased resistance to vascular flow, broadening of vessel diameter, widening of intercapillary distances, and a heterogenous intratumor blood flow distribution are all factors that diminish the O_2-transport capacity and uptake in tumor tissue.[112] Vaupel concluded that hypoxia/anoxia in addition to glucose depletion in neoplastic tissue must be held responsible for cytolysis/necrosis during progressive tumor growth.

In polarographic measurements of the local tissue oxygen tension by gold microelectrodes, very low PO_2 values were observed in C3H mouse mammary carcinoma.[113] Low pH values were found in tumor tissues due to an elevated rate of lactic acid production and its subsequent inadequate removal.

The oxygenation of human tumors was studied primarily in solid cancer tissue of the oral cavity by a cryophotometric micromethod.[114] The intracapillary oxyhemoglobin saturation curves showed significantly lower values than normal mucosa. The extent of the oxyhemoglobin saturation could be related to the degree of tumor vasculature reduction.

In a study on tissue-isolated human breast cancer xenografts,[67] using the epigastric pouching technique, the tumor blood flow and oxygen supply were investigated. At comparable tumor sizes, the average tumor blood flow was higher in medullary than in squamous cell carcinomas. The mean oxygen consumption rates were 10.4 μl O_2 g/min in medullary and 7.7 μl O_2 g/min in squamous cell carcinomas. A decreased O_2 consumption rate following a decline of tumor blood flow was observed during tumor growth. The authors concluded that the O_2 utilization of human breast cancer xenografts is high due to a restricted blood supply. Thus, tissue hypoxia and anoxia were found in early tumor growth stages. Heterogeneities in tumor tissue oxygenation are characteristic features of human breast cancer xenografts.

As stressed by Denekamp,[115] physiological hypoxia is important in cancer therapy. "It is a two-edged sword that can confer resistance to therapy or can be itself cytotoxic." This has been obvious, not only in tumor radiation therapy but also in tumor chemotherapy and tumor hyperthermia.

In conclusion, studies on tumor oxygenation in experimental tumors and in human cancer xenografts have revealed a pronounced hypoxia, local acidosis, and glucose depletion. A high O_2 utilization has been explained by a restricted blood supply. The heterogeneity in tumor blood supply is reflected in a heterogenous O_2 distribution in tumor tissue.

VIII. INFLUENCE OF HYPERTHERMIA ON TUMOR BLOOD FLOW

The effect of hyperthermia on vascular volume and vascular permeability of a subcutaneously transplanted Walker rat carcinoma and of normal skin and muscle in the rat was studied by isotope techniques.[116] Tumor and normal tissues were heated to 43°C for 60 min. A marked increase in vascular volume and vascular permeability were found in normal tissues, while the increase in tumor vascular volume and in vascular permeability during hyperthermia was insignificant. These results indicated that the increased vascular volume in normal tissues was associated with increased circulation, which may enhance the dissipation of heat and result in a differential effect of hyperthermia on normal tissues and tumor tissue. However, the Walker carcinosarcoma seems to be more resistant to hyperthermia than other experimental tumors, in which a decreased blood flow is observed at a temperature of 43°C.

Thermal clearance and temperature profiles were measured in canine mast cell sarcomas and compared to surrounding normal muscle tissue.[117] Tumors and normal tissues were heated to a temperature of 44°C for 40 min, and all animals were treated four times during a 9-d period. Normal tissue blood flow was increased during the 40 min hyperthermia, and a maximal increase was found during the fourth treatment; tumor blood flow was unchanged during the first hyperthermia treatment, but was increased during later treatment. This was interpreted as "compensatory changes", and it was concluded that the response of a tumor to hyperthermia may depend upon the delivery of adequate thermal doses during the initial treatments.

There seems to be a wide variation in the response of blood flow to heat among different tumor models investigated.[118] After less than 60 min of heating at 42 to 44°C, the blood flow in most tumors decreases markedly, and vascular stasis is often observed. Normal blood vessels are reported to tolerate temperatures up to 45°C for 1 h without obvious injuries.[118,119]

Human tumor blood flow was studied under whole-body hyperthermia to 41.5°C for 2 h, and in some tumors, a decreased blood circulation was observed.[120] In another clinical investigation,[121] tumor blood flow was studied in patients with well-defined superficial lesions, undergoing local hyperthermia induced by 915 MH_2 microwaves, and was determined from thermal clearance measurements by use of the bio-heat transfer equation.[122] Local hyperthermia was induced for 1 h. Tumor blood flow increased initially during treatment, and reached a maximum after 30 to 50 min of heating at approximately 44°C. The magnitude of increase in blood flow ranged from 15 to 250%. No sharp reductions of tumor blood flow or vascular stasis were observed as in experimental tumors, and this difference may be explained by differences in the vascular structure between rapidly growing transplantable tumors and human spontaneous malignant tumors.

Intratumor pH decreases during experimental tumor heating to a minimum temperature of 42°C.[123] The development of edema in the tumor interstitium also has been reported by the same author.[124] In studies of an amelanotic hamster melanoma by chamber technique, Endrich observed a decrease of the arterio-venous pressure gradient over the tumor during hyperthermia as well as during arteriolar vasoconstriction.[125] Fibrin accumulation in tumors observed during hyperthermia may contribute to the development of vascular stasis.[126] In a study on the microcirculatory response to hyperthermia of five different rat tumors, the various tumors required significantly different exposure times to induce a 50% stoppage of the tumor microcirculation. From this it was concluded that the differences in the characteristics of the tumor cells are more important for a tumor microcirculatory stoppage than the sensitivity of tumor blood vessels.[127] However, the mechanisms underlying circulatory disturbances in tumors subjected to hyperthermia can only be explained on a multifactorial basis.[128]

In conclusion, a decreased tumor blood flow and vascular stasis have been observed after hyperthermia. Differences in reactions to hyperthermia between experimental and human malignant tumors may be explained by differences in vascularization. However, differences in sensitivity to hyperthermia may also be explained by differences in sensitivity of tumor cells to hyperthermia. The mechanisms behind circulatory disturbances in tumors subjected to hyperthermia are probably explained on a multifactorial basis.

REFERENCES

1. **Virchow, R.,** *Die Krankhaften Geschwulste,* August Hirschwald, Berlin, 1863.
2. **Ribbert, H.,** Über das Gefäss-system und die Heilbarkeit der Geschwulste, *Dtsch. Med. Wochenschr.,* 30, 801, 1904.
3. **Goldmann, E.,** Growth of malignant disease in man and the lower animals with special reference to vascular system, *Proc. R. Soc. Med.,* 1, 1, 1907.
4. **Lindgren, A. G. H.,** The vascular supply of tumors with special references to the capillary angioarchitecture, *Acta Pathol. Microbiol. Scand.,* 22, 493, 1945.
5. **Breedis, C. and Young, G.,** The blood supply to neoplasms in the liver, *Am. J. Pathol.,* 30, 969, 1954.
6. **Segall, H. N.,** An experimental anatomical investigation of the blood and bile channels of the liver, *Surg. Gynecol. Obstet.,* 37, 152, 1923.
7. **Nilsson, L. A. V. and Zettergren, L.,** Blood supply and vascular pattern of induced primary hepatic carcinoma in rats, *Acta Pathol. Microbiol. Scand.,* 71, 179, 1967.
8. **Day, E. D.,** Vascular relationships of tumor and host, *Prog. Exp. Tumor Res.,* 4, 57, 1964.
9. **Algire, G. H., Chalkley, H. W., Legallais, F. Y., and Park, H. D.,** Vascular reactions of normal and malignant tissues *in vivo.* I. Vascular reactions of mice to wounds and to normal and neoplastic transplants, *J. Natl. Cancer Inst.,* 6, 73, 1945.
10. **Warren, B. A.,** The vascular morphology of tumors, in *Tumor Blood Circulation: Angiogenesis, Vascular Morphology and Blood Flow of Experimental and Human Tumors,* Peterson, H.-I., Ed., CRC Press, Boca Raton, FL, 1979, 1.

11. **Goodall, C. M., Feldman, R., Sanders, A. G., and Shubik, P.,** Vascular patterns of four transplantable tumors in the hamster, *Angiology,* 16, 622, 1965.
12. **Hammersen, F. U., Osterkamp-Baust, U., and Endrich, B.,** Ein Beitrag zum Feinbau terminaler Strombahnen und ihrer Entstehung in bösartigen Tumoren, *Mikrozirk. Forsch. Klin.,* 2, 15, 1983.
13. **Warren, B. A.,** The ultrastructure of the microcirculation of the advancing edge of Walker 256 carcinoma, *Microvasc. Res.,* 2, 443, 1970.
14. **Hirano, A. and Matsui, T.,** Vascular structures in brain tumors, *Hum. Pathol.,* 6, 611, 1975.
15. **Waggener, J. D. and Beggs, J. L.,** Vasculature of neural neoplasms, *Adv. Neurol.,* 15, 27, 1976.
16. **Peterson, H.-I., Appelgren, K. L., and Rosengren, B. H. O.,** Experimental studies on the mechanisms of fibrinogen uptake in a rat tumor, *Eur. J. Cancer,* 8, 677, 1972.
17. **Peterson, H.-I., Appelgren, L., Lundborg, G., and Rosengren, B.,** Capillary permeability of two transplantable rat tumours as compared with various normal organs of the rat, *Bibl. Anat.,* 12, 511, 1973.
18. **Peterson, H.-I., Appelgren, L., Javelin, L., and Rosengren, B.,** Influence of intravenously injected ^{131}I-labeled albumin on the growth rate of sarcoma transplanted into the rat stomach, *Eur. J. Cancer,* 13, 1357, 1977.
19. **Potchen, E. J., Kinzie, J., Curtis, C., Siegel, B., and Studer, R. K.,** Effect of irradiation on tumor microvascular permeability to macromolecules, *Cancer (Philadelphia),* 30, 693, 1972.
20. **Ackerman, N. B.,** Differences in vascular permeability between normal and tumor vessels produced by vasoactive agents, *Surg. Forum,* 24, 105, 1973.
21. **Folin, J.,** Angiography in renal tumor. Its value in diagnosis and differential diagnosis as a complement to conventional methods, *Acta Radial.,* Suppl., 267, 1967.
22. **Ekelund, L., Jonsson, N., and Lunderquist, A.,** Tumor vessels. Angiographic-histopathologic correlation, *Radiologe,* 17, 95, 1977.
23. **Göthlin, J.,** Arteriovenous shunting in carcinomas evaluated by a dye dilution technique, *Scand. J. Urol. Nephrol.,* 11, 159, 1977.
24. **Karlsson, L., Alpsten, M., Appelgren, K. L., and Peterson, H.-I.,** Intratumor distribution of vascular and extravascular spaces, *Microvasc. Res.,* 19, 71, 1980.
25. **Jain, R. K.,** Determinants of tumor blood flow: a review. *Cancer Res.,* 48, 2641, 1988.
26. **Vaupel, P. and Gabbert, H.,** Evidence for and against a tumor type-specific vascularity, *Strahlenther. u. Onkol.,* 162, 633, 1986.
27. **Solesvik, O. V., Rofstad, E. K., and Brustad, T.,** Vascular structure of five human malignant melanomas grown in athymic nude mice, *Br. J. Cancer,* 46, 557, 1982.
28. **Kraus, W., Fiebig, H. H., Schuchhardt, C., Koch, H., and Strecker, E. P.,** Mikroangiographische Untersuchungen vershciedener menschlicher Tumoren nach Transplantation auf thymusaplastische Nacktmause, *Res. Exp. Med.,* 182, 63, 1983.
29. **Tveit, E., Weiss, L., Lundstam, S., and Hultborn, R.,** Perfusion characteristics and norepinephrine reactivity of human renal carcinoma, *Cancer Res.,* 47, 4709, 1987.
30. **Algire, G. H.,** Vascular reactions of normal and malignant tissues *in vivo.* VII. Observations of vascular reactions in destructions of tumor homografts, *J. Natl. Cancer Inst.,* 15, 483, 1954.
31. **Gullino, P. M. and Grantham, F. H.,** The vascular space of growing tumors, *Cancer Res.,* 24, 1727, 1964.
32. **Ivarsson, L., Appelgren, L., and Rudenstam, C.-M.,** Plasma volume after dextran infusion in rats sensitive and non-sensitive to dextran, *Eur. Surg. Res.,* 7, 315, 1975.
33. **Hilmas, D. E. and Gillette, E. L.,** Tumor microvasculature following fractional X-irradiation, *Radiology,* 116, 165, 1975.
34. **Vaupel, P., Braunbeck, W., Schultz, V., Günther, H., and Thews, G.,** Critical O^2 and glucose supply and microcirculation in tumor tissue, *Bibl. Anat.,* 12, 527, 1972.
35. **Tannock, I. F.,** Population kinetics of carcinoma cells, capillary endothelial cells, and fibroblasts in a transplanted mouse mammary tumor, *Cancer Res.,* 30, 2470, 1970.
36. **Karlsson, L., Alpsten, M., Mattsson, J., and Peterson, H.-I.,** Influence of vasoactive drugs on the intratumor distribution of blood flow and vascular volume in a transplantable rat fibrosarcoma, *J. Cancer Res. Clin. Oncol.,* 105, 212, 1983.
37. **Brem, S., Cotran, R. S., and Folkman, J.,** Tumor angiogenesis: a quantitative method for histologic grading. *J. Natl. Cancer Inst.,* 48, 347, 1972,
38. **Taylor, K. J. W., Ramos, I., Carter, D., Morse, S. D., Snower, D., and Fortune, K.,** Correlation of Doppler US tumor signals with neovascular morphologic features, *Radiology,* 166, 57, 1988.
39. **Gullino, P. M., Grantham, F. H., and Smith, S. H.,** The interstitial water space of tumor, *Cancer Res.,* 25, 727, 1965.
40. **Rauen, H. M., Norpoth, K., and van Husen, N.,** Extracellulären Raum und Blutraum von DS-Carcinosarkom auf der Chorioallantois Membran des Hühnerembryos, *Naturwissenschaften,* 54, 540, 1967.
41. **Appelgren, L., Peterson, H.-I., and Rosengren, B.,** Vascular and extravascular spaces in two transplantable tumors of the rat, *Bibl. Anat.,* 12, 504, 1973.

42. **Bakay, L.**, The extracellular space in brain tumors. I. Morphological considerations, *Brain*, 93, 693, 1970.
43. **Wist, E., Millar, J. L., and Shorthouse, A. J.**, Melphalan cellular space of human long-tumour xenografts, *Br. J. Cancer*, 43, 458, 1981.
44. **Young, J. S., Lumsden, C. E., and Stalker, A. L.**, The significance of the "tissue pressure" of normal testicular and of neoplastic (Brown-Pearce carcinoma) tissue in the rabbit, *J. Path. Bact.*, 62, 313, 1950.
45. **Wiig, H., Tveit, E., Hultborn, R., Reed, R. K., and Weiss, L.**, Interstitial fluid pressure in DMBA-induced rat mammary tumors, *Scand. J. Clin. lab. Invest.*, 42, 159, 1982.
46. **Hori, K., Suzuki, M., Abe, I., and Saito, S.**, Increased tumor pressure in association with the growth of rat tumors, *Jpn. J. Cancer Res. (Gann)*, 77, 65, 1986.
47. **Jain, R. K.**, Transport of molecules across tumor vasculature, *Cancer Metast. Rev.*, 6, 559, 1987.
48. **Papadimitriou, J. M. and Woods, A. E.**, Structural and functional characteristics of the microcirculation in neoplasms, *J. Pathol.*, 116, 65, 1975.
49. **Ackermann, N. B. and Hechmer, P. A.**, Studies on the capillary permeability of experimental liver metastases, *Surg. Gynecol. Obstet.*, 146, 884, 1978.
50. **Song, C. W., Kang, M. S., Rhee, J. G., and Levitt, S. H.**, Effect of hyperthermia on vascular function in normal and neoplastic tissues, *Ann. N.Y. Acad. Sci.*, 335, 35, 1980.
51. **Sands, H., Shan, S. H., and Gallagher, B. M.**, Vascular volume and permeability of human and murine tumors grown in athymic mice, *Cancer Lett.*, 27, 15, 1985.
52. **Blasberg, R. G., Kolayashi, T., Horowitz, M., Rice, J. M., Groothuis, D., Molnar, P., and Fester-macher, J. D.**, Regional blood-to-tissue transport in ethylnitrosurea-induced brain tumors, *Ann. Neurol.*, 14, 202, 1983.
53. **Ackerman, N. B. and Makohon, S.**, The effects of cooling, freezing, and thawing on vascular permeability and perfusion in experimental liver metastases, *Surg. Gynecol. Obstet.*, 152, 262, 1981.
54. **Ackerman, N. B., Hechmer, P. A., and Makohon, S.**, Failure of histamine type mediators to enhance vascular permeability in experimental liver metastases, *Surg. Gynecol. Obstet.*, 151, 647, 1980.
55. **Underwood, J. C. E. and Carr, I.**, The ultrastructure and permeability characteristics of the blood vessels of a transplantable rat sarcoma, *J. Pathol.*, 107, 157, 1972.
56. **Stein-Werblowsky, R.**, A permeability-enhancing factor produced by tumor, *J. Cancer Res. Clin. Oncol.*, 97, 315, 1980.
57. **Senger, D. R., Galli, S. J., Dvorak, A. M., Peruzzi, C. A., Harvey, V. S., and Dvorak, H. F.**, Tumor cells secrete a vascular permeability factor that promotes accumulation of ascites fluid, *Science*, 219, 983, 1983.
58. **Senger, D. R., Peruzzi, C. A., Feder, J., and Dvorak, H. F.**, A highly conserved vascular permeability factor secreted by a variety of human and rodent tumor cell lines, *Cancer Res.*, 46, 5629, 1986.
59. **Gerlowski, L. E. and Jain, R. K.**, Effect of hyperthermia on microvascular permeability of normal and neoplastic tissues, *Int. J. Microcirc. Clin. Exp.*, 4, 336, 1985.
60. **Peters, W., Texeira, M., Intaglietta, M., and Gross, J. F.**, Microcirculatory studies in a rat mammary carcinoma. I. Transparent chamber method, development of microvasculature and pressures in tumor vessels, *J. Natl. Cancer Inst.*, 65, 631, 1980.
61. **Wiig, H.**, Microvascular pressures in DMBA-induced mammary tumors, *Scand. J. Clinc. Lab. Invest.*, 42, 165, 1982.
62. **Endrich, B. and Hammersen, F.**, Morphologic and hemodynamic alterations in capillaries during hyperthermia, in *Hyperthermia in Cancer Treatment*, Anghileri, L. J. and Roberts, J., Eds., CRC Press, Boca Raton, FL, 1986.
63. **Gullino, P. M. and Grantham, F. H.**, Studies on the exchange of fluids between host and tumor. II. The blood flow of hepatomas and other tumors in rats and mice, *J. Natl. Cancer Inst.*, 27, 1465, 1961.
64. **Peterson, H.-I.**, Tumor blood flow compared with normal tissue blood flow, *Tumor Blood Circulation: Angiogenesis, Vascular Morphology and Blood Flow of Experimental and Human Tumors*, Peterson, H.-I., Ed., CRC Press, Boca Raton, FL, 1979, 103.
65. **Jain, R. K. and Ward-Hartley, K.**, Tumor blood flow characterization, modifications and role in hyperthermia, *IEEE SU 31*, 504, 1984.
66. **Vaupel, P.**, Interrelationship between mean arterial blood pressure, blood flow and vascular resistance in solid tumor tissue of D5-carcino-sarcoma, *Experientia*, 31, 587, 1975.
67. **Vaupel, P., Fortmeyer, H. P., Runkel, S., and Kallinowski, F.**, Blood flow, oxygen consumption, and tissue oxygenation of human breast cancer xenografts in nude rats, *Cancer Res.*, 47, 3496, 1987.
68. **Vaupel, P. and Mueller-Klieser, W.**, Cell line and growth site as relevant parameters governing tumor tissue oxygenation, *Adv. Exp. Med. Biol.*, 200, 633, 1986.
69. **Rogers, W.**, Tissue blood flow in transplantable tumors of the mouse and hamster, *Diss. Abstr. Int. B.*, 28, 5185, 1968.
70. **Sundqvist, K., Hafström, L., and Persson, B.**, Measurements of total and regional tumor blood flow and organ blood flow using $99Tc^{M}$ labelled microspheres, *Eur. Surg. Res.*, 10, 433, 1978.

71. **Takács, L., Debreczeni, L. A., and Farsang, C. S.**, Circulation in rats with Guérin carcinoma, *Appl. Physiol.*, 38, 696, 1975.
72. **Allen, N., Goldman, H., Gordon, W. A., and Clendenon, N. R.**, Topographic blood flow in experimental nervous system tumors and surrounding tissues, *Trans. Am. Neurol. Assoc.*, 100, 157, 1975.
73. **Kjartansson, I., Applegren, L., and Peterson, H.-I.**, Tumor Circulation. An experimental study in the rat with a comparison of different methods for estimation of tumor blood flow, *Acta Chir. Scand.*, Suppl., 471, 1976.
74. **Mattsson, J., Alpsten, M., Appelgren, L., and Peterson, H.-I.**, Influence of noradrenaline on local tumour blood flow, *Eur. J. Cancer*, 16, 99, 1980.
75. **Gelin, L.-E., Lewis, D. H., and Nilsson, L.**, Liver blood flow in man during abdominal surgery, *Acta Hepato-Splenol.*, 15, 13, 1968.
76. **Plengvanit, U., Suwanik, R., Chearanai, O., Instrasupt, S., Satayvanich, S., Kalayasiri, C., and Viranuvatti, V.**, Regional hepatic blood flow studied by intrahepatic injection of ^{133}Xenon in normals and in patients with primary carcinoma of the liver with particular reference to the effect of hepatic artery ligation, *Aust. N.Z.J. Med.*, 1, 44, 1972.
77. **Mäntylä, M. Kuikka, J., and Rekonen, A.**, Regional blood flow in human tumors with special reference to the effect of radiotherapy, *Br. J. Radiol.*, 49, 335, 1976.
78. **Heikkonen, J., Mäntylä, M., and Perkkiö, J.**, Partition coefficient ratios and tumor perfusion studied with ^{85}Kr^{M} and ^{133}Xe, *Nucl. Med.*, 26, 253, 1987.
79. **Mäntylä, M., Heikkonen, J., and Perkkiö, J.**, Regional blood flow in human tumors measured with argon, krypton and xenon, *Br. J. Radiol.*, 61, 379, 1988.
80. **Robert, J., Martin, J., and Burg, C.**, Evolution de la vascularisation d'une tumeur isologue solide de la souris au cours de sa croissance, *Strahlenterapie*, 133, 621, 1967.
81. **Kallman, R. F., de Nardo, G. L., and Stasch, M. J.**, Blood flow in irradiated mouse sarcoma as determined by the clearance of Xenon^{133}, *Cancer Res.*, 32, 483, 1972.
82. **Peterson, H.-I., Appelgren, K. L., Rudenstam, C.-M., and Lewis, D. H.**, Studies on the circulation of experimental tumours. I. Effect of induced fibrinolysis and antifibrinolysis on capillary blood flow and the capillary transport function of two experimental tumors in the mouse, *Eur. J. Cancer*, 5, 91, 1969.
83. **Reinhold, H. S.**, Improved microcirculation in irradiated tumors, *Eur. J. Cancer*, 7, 273, 1971.
84. **Kjartansson, I. E., Lewis, D. H., Peterson, H.-I., Rosengren, B., and Rudenstam, C.-M.**, Effect of X-irradiation on blood circulation in two experimental tumours, *Microvasc. Res.*, 3, 438, 1971.
85. **Kjartansson, I., Appelgren, L., Peterson, H.-I., Rosengren, B., Rudenstam, C.-M., and Lewis, D. H.**, Capillary blood flow, transport and flow distribution in two transplantable rat tumors, *Bibl. Anat.*, 12, 519, 1973.
86. **Ten Haken, R. K., Nussbaum, G. H., Emami, B., and Hughes, W. L.**, Photon activation — ^{15}O decay studies of tumor blood flow, *Med. Phys.*, 8, 324, 1981.
87. **Itoh, K., Suzuki, O., Yasuda, Y., and Aihara, T.**, Evaluation of blood flow in tumor masses by using 2D-Doppler flow mapping — case reports, *Angiology*, 38, 705, 1987.
88. **Shimamoto, K., Sakuma, S., Ishigaki, T., and Makino, N.**, Intratumoral blood flow: evaluation with color Doppler echography, *Radiology*, 165, 683, 1987.
89. **Willis, R. A.**, The spread of tumours in the human body, *Butterworths*, London, 1973.
90. **Intaglietta, M., Myers, R. R., Gross, J. F., and Reinhold, H. S.**, Dynamics of microvascular flow in implanted mouse mammary tumors, *Bibl. Anat.*, 15, 273, 1977.
91. **Mattsson, J., Appelgren, L., Hamberger, B., and Peterson, H.-I.**, Adrenergic innervation of tumour blood vessels, *Cancer Lett.*, 3, 347, 1977.
92. **Hafström, L., Nobin, A., Persson, B., and Sundqvist, K.**, Effects of catecholamines on cardiovascular response and blood flow distribution to normal tissue and liver tumors in the rat, *Cancer Res.*, 40, 481, 1980.
93. **Mattsson, J., Appelgren, L., Hamberger, B., and Peterson, H.-I.**, Tumor vessel innervation and influence of vasoactive drugs on tumor blood flow, in *Tumor Blood Circulation: Angiogenesis, Vascular Morphology and Blood Flow of Experimental and Human Tumors*, Peterson, H.-I., Ed., CRC Press, Boca Raton, FL, 1979, 29.
94. **Cater, D. B., Grigson, D. M. B., and Watkinsson, D. A.**, Changes of oxygen tension in tumors induced by vasoconstrictor and vasodilator drugs, *Acta Radiol.*, 58, 401, 1962.
95. **Rankin, J. H. G. and Phernetton, T.**, Effects of prostaglandin E2 on blood flow to the V2 carcinoma, *Fed. Proc. Am. Soc. Exp. Biol.*, 35, 297, 1976.
96. **Wickersham, J. K., Barret, W. P., Furukawa, S. B., Puffer, W. H., and Warner, N. E**, An evaluation of the response of the microvasculature in tumors in C3H mice to vasoactive drugs, *Bibl. Anat.*, 15, 291, 1977.
97. **Mattsson, J., Appelgren, L., Karlsson, L., and Peterson, H.-I.**, Influence of vasoactive drugs and ischaemia on intra-tumor blood flow distribution, *Eur. J. Cancer*, 14, 761, 1978.

98. **Mattsson, J., Lilja, J., and Peterson, H.-I.**, Influence of vasoactive drugs on local tumor blood flow, *Eur. J. Cancer,* 18, 677, 1982.
99. **Hultborn, R., Tveit, E., and Weiss, L.**, Vascular reactivity and perfusion characteristics in 7,12-Dimethylbenz(a)anthracene-induced rat mammary neoplasia, *Cancer Res.*, 43, 363, 1983.
100. **Tveit, E., Weiss, L., and Hultborn, R.**, Blood flow and reactivity to noradrenaline in induced and autotransplanted DMBA rat mammary neoplasia and autotransplanted DMBA mammary neoplasia, *Eur. J. Cancer Clin. Oncol.*, 20, 707, 1984.
101. **Quintana, A., Raczka, E., Latallao, Z. S., and Donati, M. D.**, Cardiac output redistribution induced by noradrenaline in two murine tumor models, *Eur. J. Cancer Clin. Oncol.*, 19, 1031, 1983.
102. **Ackerman, N. B. and Jacobs, R.**, The blood supply of experimental liver metastases. VIII. Increased capillary blood flow within liver tumors with administration of epinephrine, *Microcirc. Endothel. Lymphat.*, 2, 457, 1985.
103. **Peterson, H.-I., Alpsten, M., Skolnik, G., and Karlsson, L.**, Influence of a prostaglandin synthesis inhibitor and of thrombocytopenia on tumor blood flow and tumor vascular permeability. Experimental studies in the rat, *Anticancer Res.*, 5, 253, 1985.
104. **Kaelin, W. G., Shrivastav, S., Shand, D. G., and Jirtle, R. L.**, Effect of verapamil on malignant tissue blood flow in SMT-2A tumor-bearing rats, *Cancer Res.*, 42, 3944, 1982.
105. **Kaelin, W. G., Shrivastav, S., and Jirtle, R. L.**, Blood flow to primary tumor and lymph node metastases in SMT-2A tumor-bearing rats following intravenous flunarizine, *Anticancer Res.*, 44, 896, 1984.
106. **Knapp, W. H., Debatin, J., Lager, K., Helus, F., Altmann, A., Sinn, H. J., and Ostertag, H.**, Selective drug-induced reduction of blood flow in tumor transplants, *Int. J. Radiat. Oncol. Biol. Phys.*, 11, 1357, 1985.
107. **Mattsson, J., Hafström, L., Naredi, P., and Peterson, H.-I.**, Techniques for measuring regional blood flow, *Int. J. Radiat. Oncol. Biol. Phys.*, 13, 945, 1987.
108. **Chan, R. C., Babbs, C. F., Vetter, R. J., and Lamar, C. H.**, Abnormal response of tumor vasculature to vasoactive drugs, *J. Natl. Cancer Inst.*, 72, 145, 1984.
109. **Suzuki, M., Hori, K., Abe, I., Saito, S., and Sato, H.**, Functional characterization of the microcirculation in tumors, *Cancer Metast. Rev.*, 3, 115, 1984.
110. **Vaupel, P.**, Oxygen supply to malignant tumors, in *Tumor Blood Circulation: Angiogenesis, Vascular Morphology and Blood Flow of Experimental and Human Tumors,* Peterson, H.-I., Ed., CRC Press, Boca Raton, FL, 1979, 143.
111. **Vaupel, P. and Thews, G.**, PO^2 distribution in tumor tissue of DS-carcinosarcoma, *Oncology,* 30, 475, 1974.
112. **Vaupel, P.**, Hypoxia in neoplastic tissue, *Microvasc. Res.*, 13, 399, 1977.
113. **Vaupel, P. W., Frinak, S., and Bicher, H.-I.**, Heterogenous oxygen partial pressure and pH distribution in C3H mouse mammary adenocarcinoma, *Cancer Res.*, 41, 2008, 1981.
114. **Mueller-Klieser, W., Vaupel, P., Mauz, R., and Schmidseder, R.**, Intracapillary oxyhemoglobin saturation of malignant tumors in humans, *Int. J. Radiat. Oncol. Biol. Phys.*, 7, 1397, 1981.
115. **Denekamp, J.**, Does physiological hypoxia matter in cancer therapy, in *The Biological Basis of Radiotherapy,* Steel, G. G., Adams, G. E., and Peckham, S., Eds., Elsevier, Amsterdam, 1983.
116. **Song, C. W.**, Effect of hyperthermia on vascular functions of normal tissues and experimental tumors-brief communication, *J. Natl. Cancer Inst.*, 60, 711, 1978.
117. **Milligan, A. J. and Panjehpour, M.**, Canine normal and tumor tissue estimated blood flow during fractionated hyperthermia, *Int. J. Radiat. Oncol. Biol. Phys.*, 11, 1679, 1985.
118. **Song, C. W.**, Effect of local hyperthermia in blood flow and microenvironment: a review, *Cancer Res.*, 44 (Suppl.), 4721, 1984.
119. **Dudar, T. E. and Jain, R. K.**, Differential response of normal and tumor microcirculation to hyperthermia, *Cancer Res.*, 44, 605, 1984.
120. **Karino, M., Koga, S., Maeta, M., Hamazoe, R., Kumane, T., and Oda, M.**, Experimental and clinical studies on effect of hyperthermia on tumor blood flow, in *Hyperthermic Oncology,* Vol. 1, Overgaard, J., Ed., Taylor and Francis, London, 1984, 79.
121. **Waterman, F. M., Nerlinger, R. E., Moylan, D. J., III, and Leeper, D. B.**, Response of human tumor blood flow to local hyperthermia, *Int. J. Radiat. Oncol. Biol. Phys.*, 13, 75, 1987.
122. **Milligan, A. J., Conran, P. B., Ropar, M. A., McCulloch, H. A., Ahuja, R. K., and Dobelbower, R. R.**, Predictions of blood flow from thermal clearance during regional hyperthermia, *Int. J. Radiat. Oncol. Biol. Phys.*, 9, 1335, 1983.
123. **Vaupel, P.**, Einfluss einer lokalisierten Mikrowellen-Hyperthermie auf die pH-Verteilung in bösartigen Tumoren, *Strahlentherapie,* 158, 168, 1982.
124. **Vaupel, P., Müller-Klieser, W., Otte, J., Manz, R., and Kallinowski, F.**, Blood flow, tissue oxygenation, and pH distribution in malignant tumors upon localized hyperthermia. Basic pathophysiological aspects and the role of various thermal doses, *Strahlentherapie,* 159, 73, 1983.
125. **Endrich, B.**, Mikrozirkulation maligner Tumoren, Ph.D. Thesis, University of Heidelberg, 1984.

126. **Lee, S. Y., Song, C. W., and Levitt, S. H.,** Change in fibrinogen uptake in tumors by hyperthermia, *Eur. J. Cancer Clin. Oncol.*, 21, 1507, 1985.
127. **Reinhold, H. S. and Van den Berg-Blok, A. E.,** Differences in the response of the microcirculation to hyperthermia in five different tumours, *Eur. J. Cancer Clin. Oncol.*, 25, 611, 1989.
128. **Vaupel, P.,** Lokale Hyperthermie-Behandlung, *Fortschr. Med.*, 104, 263, 1986.

INDEX

A

D

E

F

G

H

I

K

L

M

N

O

P

R

S

W

X

Z